ESSENTIAL EYE CARE

THE JOHNS HOPKINS WILMER HANDBOOK

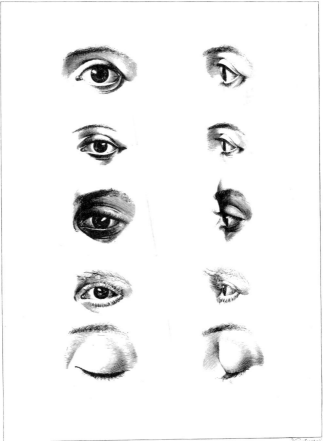

S. TH. SOEMMERRING ICONES OCULI HUMANI

Prostat apud Varrentrapp & Wenner

ESSENTIALS OF EYE CARE

THE JOHNS HOPKINS WILMER HANDBOOK

Edited by
Rohit Varma, M.D.

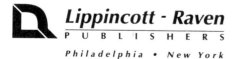

Lippincott - Raven
PUBLISHERS

Philadelphia • New York

Manufacturing Manager: Dennis Teston
Associate Managing Editor: Kathleen Bubbeo
Production Service: Hockett Editorial Service
Cover Designer: Tom Jackson
Indexer: Corinne Ferrara
Compositor: Compset
Printer: R.R. Donnelley—Crawfordsville

Printed in the United States of America

9 8 7 6 5 4 3 2 1

Library of Congress Cataloging-in-Publication Data
Essentials of eye care : the Johns Hopkins Wilmer handbook / edited by
 Rohit Varma.
     p.   cm.
  Includes index.
  ISBN 0-397-51317-8
  1. Ophthalmology—Handbooks, manuals, etc.   I. Varma, Rohit.
  [DNLM: 1. Eye Diseases—therapy.   WW 166 E78 1996]
RE48.9.E87   1996
617.7—DC20
DNLM/DLC
for Library of Congress   96-17976
                                                                         CIP

Frontispiece: Courtesy of the Museum of Ophthalmology of the American Academy
of Ophthalmology.

Care has been taken to confirm the accuracy of the information presented and to describe generally accepted practices. However, the authors, editors, and publisher are
not responsible for errors or omissions or for any consequences from application of
the information in this book and make no warranty, express or implied, with respect
to the contents of the publication.

The authors, editors, and publisher have exerted every effort to ensure that drug
selection and dosage set forth in this text are in accordance with current recommendations and practice at the time of publication. However, in view of ongoing research, changes in government regulations, and the constant flow of information re-
lating to drug therapy and drug reactions, the reader is urged to check the package
insert for each drug for any change in indications and dosage and for added warnings
and precautions. This is particularly important when the recommended agent is a
new or infrequently employed drug.

Some drugs and medical devices presented in this publication have Food and Drug
Administration (FDA) clearance for limited use in restricted research settings. It is
the responsibility of the health care provider to ascertain the FDA status of each drug
or device planned for use in their clinical practice.

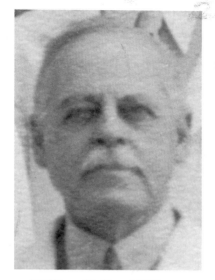

William Holland Wilmer

Wilmer Ophthalmological Institute—Directors

William Holland Wilmer, MD—1925–1934
Alan Churchill Woods, MD—1934–1955
Alfred Edward Maumenee, MD—1955–1979
Arnall Patz, MD—1979–1989
Morton Falk Goldberg, MD—1989–

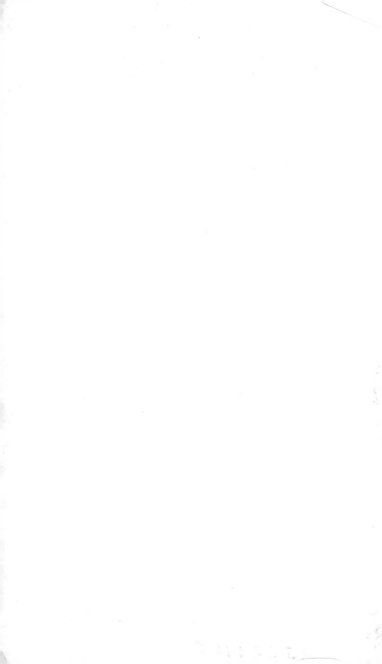

REVIEWERS

Eugene de Juan, Jr., M.D.

James P. Dunn, M.D.

Morton F. Goldberg, M.D.

W. Richard Green, M.D.

David L. Guyton, M.D.

Julia A. Haller, M.D.

Nicholas T. Iliff, M.D.

Henry D. Jampel, M.D.

Neil R. Miller, M.D.

Harry A. Quigley, M.D.

Michael X. Repka, M.D.

Andrew P. Schachat, M.D.

Elias I. Traboulsi, M.D.

Walter J. Stark, M.D.

Daniel Finkelstein, M.D.

To my friend and partner, *Carol,*
and the joy of our lives, our son, *Kesar*

CONTENTS

CONTRIBUTORS

Lisa S. Abrams, M.D.

Lloyd P. Aiello, M.D.

Robert L. Avery, M.D.

Thomas B. Connor, Jr., M.D.

Martin G. Edwards, M.D.

Dean Eliott, M.D.

Sharon Fekrat, M.D.

Tamara R. Fountain

Subba R. Gollamudi, M.D.

Katrinka L. Heher, M.D.

Deborah G. Keenum, M.D.

Thomas Leitman, M.D.

Mathew W. MacCumber, M.D.

Albert M. Maguire, M.D.

John J. Michon, M.D.

Fernando Murillo-Lopez, M.D.

Terrence P. O'Brien, M.D.

Dante Pieramici, M.D.

Timothy Schneider, M.D.

Rohit Varma, M.D.

FOREWORD

This useful handbook on ophthalmology has been written "by residents for residents" and for other predoctoral and postdoctoral students of clinical ophthalmology. In training programs such as that of the Wilmer Ophthalmological Institute, residents have traditionally represented the heart and soul of the institution. Their presence lends vitality and excitement. In the American system of graduate medical education, residents are entrusted with major responsibilities that reflect the dual role of graduate student and young physician. These two ostensibly separate roles almost always harmonize with each other; indeed, they often create a synergy.

The learning process in the academic medical center should be a combination of formal instruction and properly supervised clinical experience, and, ideally, the clinical challenges encountered daily by residents will provide meaningful stimuli for a vigorous commitment to continual self-education. Both components of the resident's life—education and clinical care—are time consuming and demanding. Efforts to assist the resident in acquiring the salient features of a clinical education are, therefore, highly desirable. This handbook is a valuable contribution by a talented group of residents and faculty preceptors; it makes important clinical components of the ophthalmology education both accessible and up to date. This handbook also highlights many of the clinical principles and procedures favored by our current group of residents. We believe that it will help others to acquire and implement key components of the clinical ophthalmic education. This concise compilation will assist current and future generations of residents in the valuable combination of active self-education and exemplary medical care that our patients have learned to expect and to trust.

Morton F. Goldberg, M.D.
Director, the Wilmer Ophthalmological Institute
Johns Hopkins Hospital
Baltimore, Maryland

PREFACE

In 1970, "Survey of Ophthalmology—Manual for Medical Students" edited by Stephen J. Ryan, M.D., under the guidance of Dr. A. Edward Maumenee, was published by the Johns Hopkins Medical Institutions. It is interesting to note the authors of specific chapters in that manual: Cornea (D. A. Schlernitzauer), Lens and Vitreous (R. E. Smith), Uvea (M. A. Naidoff), Retina (C. P. Wilkinson), Intraocular Tumors (W. J. Stark), Glaucoma (P. E. Michelson), Conjunctiva (R. N. Frank), Lids (A. D. Jensen), Lacrimal Apparatus (R. G. Michels, Late), Orbit (S. J. Ryan), Optics and Refraction (A. L. Norton), Strabismus (D. D. Pfaffenbach), Neuro-ophthalmology (M. H. Barlow, Late), Genetics (H. E. Cross), Trauma (H. Holcomb), and Ocular Therapeutics (J. M. Emery). While all of these individuals went on to excel, for many it was in areas quite different from the chapters they wrote.

Twenty-six years later we now have what might be considered a second edition. *The Essentials of Eye Care: The Johns Hopkins Wilmer Manual* has been written by a group of Wilmer residents dedicated to educating medical students, residents, and eye care/providers. This handbook provides an understanding of the various disease entities in addition to the essentials of diagnosis and treatment. The chapters are succinct and concise to allow the reader to obtain accurate, "cutting-edge" information on ocular disease in a time-efficient manner. The format for most conditions covered is standardized to facilitate consistent and cohesive exposition of each ocular disease. In addition, we have included a section on common surgical procedures, an introduction to optics, and a drug formulary. (While every attempt has been made to verify drug dosage and frequency of usage, we recommend that all practitioners check with the drug insert/their pharmacist/the drug manufacturer prior to administering any drug.)

I would like to thank Dr. Morton F. Goldberg, Ophthalmologist-in-Chief, Wilmer Ophthalmological Institute, Johns Hopkins

Hospital, for supporting and indeed encouraging this endeavor. The Wilmer faculty served as peer-reviewers/advisors and their contributions have been invaluable. I would also like to thank Albert Maguire, M.D. for going the extra mile, Dean Eliott, M.D. for helping with the conception, and Ranjit Dhaliwal, M.D. for reviewing the initial chapters. I am indebted to Susan Clarke for her diligent copyediting. And finally I thank Stuart Freeman for sticking with me through thick and thin and helping bring this project to completion.

In reading this handbook we hope that you the reader will gain a sound understanding of ocular disease. Our endeavor will have been successful if this handbook is able to help educate eye care providers so that their patients may achieve a better quality of life.

Rohit Varma, M.D.

Essentials of Eye Care, edited by Rohit Varma.
Lippincott–Raven Publishers,
Philadelphia © 1997.

1

Anatomy, Embryology, and Physiology of the Eye

I. DEVELOPMENT OF THE EYE

Derivatives of embryonic tissues (by tissue type)

A. Neuroectoderm
   1. Iris
      a. sphincter and dilator muscles of iris
      b. pigmented iris epithelium
   2. Ciliary body
      a. pigmented/nonpigmented ciliary epithelium
   3. Vitreous
   4. Neurosensory retina
   5. Retinal pigment epithelium (RPE)
   6. Optic nerve
      a. axons and glia

B. Surface Ectoderm (anterior to posterior)
   1. Lids and caruncle
      a. epithelium, glands, and cilia
   2. Lacrimal gland and drainage system
   3. Conjunctiva
      a. epithelium
   4. Cornea
      a. epithelium
   5. Lens
   6. Vitreous

C. Cranial Neural Crest Cells
   1. Cornea
      a. stroma and endothelium
   2. Trabecular meshwork
   3. Iris
      a. connective tissue
   4. Ciliary body
      a. ciliary muscles
   5. Choroid
      a. stroma
   6. Sclera (except portion of sclera temporally)

      7. Extraocular muscles
         a. sheaths and tendons
      8. Optic nerve
         a. meningeal sheaths
      9. Melanocytes ciliary nerve
         a. Schwann cells
     10. Ciliary ganglion
     11. Orbit
         a. bones
         b. connective tissue
     12. Vasculature
         a. all muscular layer and connective tissue sheaths of all ocular and orbital vessels

D. Mesoderm
    1. Vitreous
    2. Sclera
       a. portion of sclera temporally
    3. Extraocular muscles
       a. fibers
    4. Vasculature
       a. endothelial lining of all vessels

Derivatives of Embryonic Tissues (By Anatomical Location)

Conjunctiva

epithelium	surface ectoderm

Cornea

epithelium	surface ectoderm
stroma and endothelium	neural crest

Trabecular Meshwork	neural crest

Iris

sphincter and dilator muscles of iris	neuroectoderm
pigmented iris epithelium	neuroectoderm
connective tissue	neural crest

Ciliary Body

pigmented/nonpigmented ciliary epithelium	neuroectoderm
ciliary muscles	neural crest

Lens	surface ectoderm

Vitreous

	neuroectoderm surface ectoderm mesoderm
Neurosensory Retina	neuroectoderm
RPE	neuroectoderm
Choroid	
stroma	neural crest
Sclera	neural crest
temporal portion	mesoderm
Optic Nerve	
axons and glia meningeal sheaths	neuroectoderm neural crest
Lids and Caruncle	
epithelium, glands, and cilia	surface ectoderm
Lacrimal Gland and Drainage System	surface ectoderm
Extraocular Muscles	
sheaths and tendons fibers	neural crest mesoderm
Melanocytes	neural crest
Ciliary Nerve	
Schwann cells	neural crest
Ciliary Ganglion	neural crest
Orbit	
bones connective tissue	neural crest neural crest
Vasculature	
all muscular layer and connective tissue sheaths of all vessels endothelial lining of all vessels	neural crest mesoderm

Derivatives of Embryonic Tissues (By Anatomical Location) (*continued*)

Chronological Development of the Eye

morula → blastula → gastrula embryonic plate primitive streak → formation of three cell types (ectoderm, mesoderm, endoderm) → ectoderm forms the neural plate → neural folds form → neural folds close, forming a neural tube, and ectoderm differentiates into three subtypes (neuroectoderm lines inner folds, surface ectoderm covers outer folds, neural crest cells at summit of folds)

Neuroectoderm

optic pit (22 days) → optic vesicle (25 days) → induces surface ectoderm to form lens placode (28 days) → during 2nd month, optic cup and lens vesicle formed (by invagination of optic vesicle); outer layer becomes RPE and inner layer becomes neurosensory retina with potential space—subretinal space—between the two layers; optic cup closes when two lips of the embryonic fissure meet and fuse (closure near equator first)

By Structure, By Month

Mo.	Cornea	Angle	Lens
2	neural crest cells of endothelium, then stroma migrate centrally		cavity of lens vesicle obliterated
3		ciliary body develops	
4	Descemet's membrane	ciliary process Schlemm's canal	
5		iris stroma vascularized	
6		dilator muscle of iris	
7		circular muscle of ciliary body	
8		iris sphincter angle complete	
9		pupillary membrane disappears	

	Vitreous	Retina/RPE	Nerve
2	hyaloid artery fills embryonic fissure	pigment granules in RPE retinal differentiation begins (nuclear/ marginal) Bruch's membrane	axons from ganglion cells migrate to optic nerve optic nerve lamina cribrosa (glial portion)

	Vitreous	Retina/RPE	Nerve
3		precursor rods/ cones	
		vortex veins	
4	regression of hyaloid	retinal vessels grow into nerve fiber layer (NFL) near disc	
5		photoreceptors develop inner segments	
6		ganglion cells thicken in macula	
7		outer segments differentiate	lamina cribrosa (fibrous portion)
		central fovea thins	
8	disappearance of hyaloid	retinal vessels reach periphery	myelination complete to lamina cribrosa

	Choroid	Lids/Adnexae	Muscles
2	vasculature develops	lid folds appear	primordia of lateral rectus and superior oblique grow
3		lid folds meet and fuse	
5	vessels from layers	lids begin to separate	
6	recurrent arterial branches join choroidal vessels		
7	melanocytes produce pigment		

II. ORBIT AND CRANIAL NERVES

 A. Bony Orbit (Seven Bones)
    frontal
    zygoma
    maxilla

ethmoid
sphenoid
lesser wing
greater wing
lacrimal
palatine

1. Roof (2)
   a. frontal and lesser wing of sphenoid
   b. location of fossa for lacrimal gland and trochlea
2. Medial wall (4)
   a. maxilla, lacrimal, ethmoid, frontal lacrimal fossa formed by maxilla and lacrimal
   b. lacrimal sac fossa continuous with nasolacrimal canal which connects to inferior meatus of the nose
   c. medial wall is thin lamina papyracea
3. Orbital floor (3)
   a. maxilla, palatine, zygoma
   b. inferior orbital fissure located on floor
   c. inferior oblique (IO) muscle originates from floor just lateral to opening of nasolacrimal canal
4. Lateral wall (2)
   a. zygoma, greater wing of sphenoid
   b. lateral orbital Whitnall's tubercle (on orbit margin, 11 mm below frontal-zygomatic suture)
   c. site of attachment for
      1) check ligament of lateral rectus
      2) suspensory ligament of eyeball (Lockwood's ligament)
      3) lateral canthal ligament
      4) aponeurosis of levator muscle
      5) not Whitnall's ligament, which inserts 10 mm above Whitnall's tubercle
5. Superior orbital fissure
   a. located between greater (lateral wall) and lesser (roof) wings of the sphenoid bone
   b. lateral to optic foramen
   c. superior part (outside muscle cone)
      1) lacrimal nerve, frontal nerve, trochlear nerve (cranial nerve [CN] IV)
   d. inferior part (inside lateral rectus muscle)
      1) oculomotor nerve (III) (superior and inferior divisions), nasociliary nerve
      2) abducens nerve (VI), sympathetic nerve plexus,
      3) superior ophthalmic vein
6. Inferior orbital fissure
   a. located between lateral wall and floor of orbit

        b. trigeminal nerve (maxillary division) pterygoid nerve, nerve from pterygopalatine ganglion

        c. inferior ophthalmic vein

    7. Foramina

        a. optic foramen

           1) optic nerve, ophthalmic artery, sympathetic fibers from carotid plexus

        b. supraorbital foramen (notch)

           1) supraorbital nerve (V1 branch)

        c. infraorbital foramen

           1) infraorbital nerve (V2 branch)

B. Cranial Nerves

    1. Optic nerve (discussed later)

    2. Oculomotor nerve (CN III)

        a. superior branch—superior rectus and levator

        b. inferior branch—medial rectus, inferior rectus, inferior oblique, motor root of ciliary ganglion (pupillary constriction)

        c. loss of CN III function (complete):

           1) ptosis, dilated pupil, inability to move eye up, down, or in

    3. Trochlear nerve (CN IV)

        a. longest intracranial course (75 mm)

        b. nucleus supplies contralateral superior oblique muscle

        c. through superior orbital fissure (outside annulus of Zinn) to enter superior oblique

        d. loss of CN IV function: elevation and extorsion of involved eye

    4. Trigeminal nerve (CN V)

        a. motor—mastication

        b. sensory

           1) ophthalmic (V1): lacrimal, frontal, nasociliary branches

           2) maxillary (V2)

           3) mandibular (V3)

    5. Abducens nerve (CN VI)

        a. innervates only lateral rectus muscle

        b. relatively long course: vulnerable to trauma

    6. Facial nerve (CN VII)

        a. orbicularis oculi and muscles of facial expression

        b. secretory branches to lacrimal gland

        c. Nadbath facial block (stylomastoid foramen)

           1) hemifacial paralysis (main trunk of facial nerve exits)

        d. O'Brien and Van Lint—more distal blocks of CN VII

C. Ciliary Ganglion

     1. located between optic nerve and lateral rectus muscle

     2. Receives three roots:

        a. long (sensory) root from nasociliary nerve (V1 branch); sensory fibers from cornea, iris, and ciliary body (synapse in trigeminal ganglion)

        b. short (motor) root from lower division of CN III

           1) Fibers *synapse* in ganglion and carry parasympathetic axons to supply iris sphincter muscle.

     3. Sympathetic root from plexus around internal carotid artery (ICA) fibers pass through ganglion and innervate vessels, carry sensation from eye (synapse in superior cervical ganglion)

     4. Short ciliary nerves formed by nonsynapsing sympathetic and sensory fibers and postganglionic parasympathetic fibers (1, 2, 3 above); 6–10 short ciliary nerves pierce sclera (with long ciliary nerves) around optic nerve; pass between choroid and sclera to ciliary muscle

     5. There is dual sympathetic innervation to the eye; all the third-order sympathetic neurons to eye begin in superior cervical ganglion, travel along ICA to cavernous sinus

        a. pupillomotor fibers of sympathetic neurons join V1, the nasociliary nerve (branch of V1), pass through the ciliary ganglion (without anastomosing) and then the long ciliary nerve to dilate pupil (via superior orbital fissure)

        b. sympathetic nerves to lacrimal gland, Müller's muscle, orbital, and uveal vasomotor nerves enter orbit with ophthalmic artery (via optic foramen), form sympathetic root of ciliary ganglion, and are distributed with the short ciliary nerves

III. OCULAR APPENDAGES

    A. Extraocular Muscles

      1. Annulus of Zinn: lateral, inferior, medial, superior rectus originate from annulus

      2. Spiral of Tillaux: four rectus muscles insert on anterior portion of globe in the following distances from limbus: medial, 5.5; inferior, 6.5; lateral, 6.9; superior, 7.7 mm

      3. Blood supply to extraocular muscles

        a. each rectus muscle receives two anterior ciliary arteries derived from inferior and superior branches of ophthalmic artery, the lacrimal artery, and the infraorbital artery (except lateral rectus supplied by one anterior ciliary artery derived from lacrimal artery)

B. Eyelids

Seven layers from dermal surface inward

Skin
Subcutaneous connective tissue
Orbicularis oculi muscle
Orbital septum
Levator muscle
Tarsus
Conjunctiva

1. Skin
  a. gray line—no histologic counterpart
  b. along lid margin, eyelashes anterior to line
  c. meibomian glands posterior to line
  d. mucocutaneous junction posterior to gray line, at level of meibomian glands
  e. 30 to 40 meibomian gland orifices above, 20 to 30 below

2. Subcutaneous connective tissue
  a. contains no fat

3. Orbicularis oculi
  a. orbital part inserts into medial canthal tendon
  b. voluntary muscle
  c. palpebral part both voluntary and involuntary (blinking)
  d. preseptal and pretarsal portions meet along superior palpebral furrow

4. Orbital septum
  a. extension on periosteum of roof and floor of orbit
  b. attaches to anterior surface of levator muscle
  c. posterior to orbital septum is fat barrier to spread of infection

5. Levator muscle
  a. body of muscle overlies superior rectus horizontally
  b. near Whitnall's ligament, it changes from horizontal to vertical and divides into aponeurosis and Müller's muscle (superior tarsal muscle)
  c. aponeurosis inserts into medial and canthal tendons
  d. levator muscle and tendon 50 mm long

6. Tarsus/Müller's muscle
  a. dense connective tissue (*not* cartilage)
  b. contains the meibomian glands (modified holocrine sweat glands)

      c. trichiasis—misdirection in orientation of eye-lashes
      d. distichiasis—aberrant growth through meibomian glands
      e. Müller's muscle—attaches to upper border of upper tarsus and lower border of lower tarsus; sympathetically innervated muscle—Horner's syndrome ptosis, dysthyroid ophthalmopathy lid retraction

  7. Conjunctiva
      a. nonkeratinized epithelium (contains goblet cells which produce mucin)

  8. Vascular supply of eyelids
      a. facial system, from external carotid artery (ECA)
      b. orbital system, from internal carotid artery (ICA) via ophthalmic artery
      c. marginal arterial arcade—3 mm from lid margin, between tarsal plate and orbicularis muscle
      d. peripheral arcade—along upper margin of tarsal plate within Müller's muscle
      e. venous drainage
         1) pretarsal drains to internal/external jugular veins;
         2) post-tarsal drains to cavernous sinus

  9. Lymphatics of eyelids
      a. medial group to submandibular lymph nodes
      b. lateral group to preauricular lymph nodes

 10. Plica semilunaris
      a. fold of conjunctiva just lateral to caruncle

 11. Caruncle
      a. modified skin, contains nonkeratinized, stratified, squamous epithelium, with hairs, sebaceous glands

C. Lacrimal Glands
  1. Divided in two parts by lateral expansion of levator aponeurosis
  2. Smaller palpebral lobe, larger orbital lobe
  3. Lacrimal gland ducts empty into superior conjunctival fornix
  4. Lacrimal glands are exocrine (also known as eccrine)
  5. Glands of Krause and Wolfring (eccrine), under sympathetic control, furnish basal tear secretion

D. Lacrimal Drainage System
  1. Lacrimal puncta, upper and lower canaliculi, lacrimal sac, nasolacrimal duct
  2. Puncta, on margin, between cilia and meibomian gland openings, 0.3 mm diameter

    3. Inferior punctum 6.5 mm from medial canthus
    4. Superior punctum 6.0 mm from medial canthus
    5. 90% of people, common canaliculus present
    6. 30% of neonates, outlet (Hasner's valve) closed at birth
    7. 90% open spontaneously by 6 months
    8. Remainder need probing at a minimum

IV. CONJUNCTIVA, TENON'S CAPSULE, AND LIMBUS

  A. Conjunctiva
    1. Palpebral, forniceal, bulbar
    2. Nonkeratinized squamous epithelium and goblet cells, covering substantia propria containing blood and lympatic vessels
  B. Tenon's Capsule
    1. Collagen fibers and fibroblasts
    2. Perforated by optic nerve sheath, posterior ciliary vessels and nerves, vortex veins
  C. Limbus
    1. Structure
      a. conjunctiva
      b. Tenon's capsule
      c. episclera
      d. corneoscleral stroma
      e. aqueous outflow apparatus
    2. Clinical significance—relationship to chamber angle and use as a surgical landmark
    3. Definition
      a. Pathologists termination of Bowman's layer to iris root (about 1.5 mm)
      b. Surgeons two equal zones (2 mm total)
        1) anterior bluish gray zone over clear cornea from Bowman's layer to Schwalbe's line (termination of Descemet's membrane) (about 1 mm)
        2) posterior white zone over trabecular meshwork from Schwalbe's line to iris root (about 1 mm)

V. SCLERA

  A. Structural Features:
    1. Posterior 4/5 of surface of globe
    2. Opening at cornea and optic nerve

   3. Rectus muscle tendons insert into superficial collagen
   4. Tenon's capsule and bulbar conjunctiva cover sclera (firmly attached at limbus)
   5. Thinnest (0.3 mm) at insertion of rectus muscles
   6. Thickest (1.0 mm) at posterior pole
   7. 0.4 to 0.5 mm at equator
   8. 0.6 mm anterior to muscle insertions
   9. Collagen bundles vary in size and shape resulting in opaque appearance
   10. Clinical significance: most common site scleral rupture following blunt trauma; superonasal quadrant near limbus
B. Blood Supply
   1. Essentially avascular except for superficial vessels of episclera and intrascleral vascular plexus posterior to limbus
   2. Emissary (channels) through sclera for passage of vessels

VI. CORNEA AND TEAR FILM

A. Precorneal Tear Film
   1. Composed of:
      a. outer oily layer; meibomian glands, glands of Zeis (holocrine) and Moll (apocrine)
      b. middle watery layer; lacrimal glands
      c. inner mucous layer; goblet cells (holocrine) of conjunctival epithelium
   2. Function:
      a. lubrication, smooth optical surface, oxygen and other nutrients, lysozymes and immunoglobulins
B. Cornea
   Composed of:
   1. Epithelium and basal lamina
      features:
      a. nonkeratinized, stratified squamous epithelium
      b. basal columnar cell layer attached to basal lamina by hemidesmosomes
      c. clinical significance: recurrent corneal erosions
      d. middle wing cell layer (2 to 3 cells thick)
      e. superficial cells, apical surfaces contain microvilli
      f. nonepithelial cells; histiocytes, macrophages, lymphocytes
   2. Bowman's layer (also known as Bowman's membrane)
      features:

      a. not a true membrane, not replaced following injury

      b. randomly dispersed collagen fibrils 8 to 14 microns thick

  3. Stroma

    features:

      a. ninety percent of total corneal thickness (500 microns)

      b. collagen producing fibroblasts (keratocytes)

      c. ground substance; mucoprotein and glycoprotein

      d. collagen lamellae; obliquely oriented lamellae anterior 1/3, parallel lamellae posterior 2/3

  4. Descemet's membrane

    features:

      a. basement membrane of the corneal epithelium

      b. PAS-positive

      c. anterior banded zone (in utero); 3 to 4 microns

      d. posterior nonbanded zone (during life); 7 to 9 microns

      e. clinical significance—peripheral Hassal-Henle warts, and central corneal guttata

  5. Endothelium

    structural features:

      a. not true endothelium (*not* mesodermal origin)

      b. neuroectodermal (neural crest) origin

      c. hexagonal shape

      d. interlock with tight junctions, not desmosomes

      e. function: active transport; maintenance of deturgescence of stroma

      f. clinical significance—if endothelial cells injured (surgery, increased intraocular pressure), don't regenerate, leads to corneal edema

VII. ANTERIOR CHAMBER: CHEMISTRY OF AQUEOUS HUMOR, TRABECULAR MESHWORK (TM), GONIOSCOPIC VIEW

A. Chemistry of Aqueous Humor

    aqueous humor, optically clear, yet acts as substitute blood supply to lens, cornea, TM

  1. Inorganic ions concentration compared to plasma

      a. Na, K, Mg, Fe, Cu, Zn   same

      b. Ca, phosphate   less

      c. Cl, bicarbonate   variable

  2. Organic anions concentration compared to plasma

      a. lactate   more

      b. ascorbic acid   more (by 10- to 50-fold)

  3. Carbohydrates concentration compared to plasma

      a. glucose   less (80%)

facilitated diffusion,
not active transport

  4. Proteins
  - **a.** almost complete absence of protein, normally 0.02 gm/100 ml vs 7 gm/100 ml in plasma
  - **b.** protein content increases after breakdown of blood-aqueous barrier (seen as aqueous flare)
  5. Oxygen and carbon dioxide
  - **a.** oxygen present at partial pressure of 55 mm Hg
  - **b.** corneal endothelium dependent on aqueous oxygen supply
  - **c.** (no net flux of oxygen from atmosphere across cornea)
  - **d.** Carbon dioxide of aqueous at partial pressure of 40 to 60 mm Hg
  - **e.** CO_2 and HCO_3—determine pH of aqueous; usually 7.5 to 7.6

B. Trabecular Meshwork
  1. Meshwork
  - **a.** series of thin, perforated connective tissue sheets arranged in laminar pattern
  - **b.** sheets composed of collagen and elastic fibrils surrounded by basal lamina and endothelial cells with multiple pinocytotic vesicles
  - **c.** endothelial cells contain pigment granules; the melanin granules located in the trabecular meshwork are structurally identical to those found in the posterior pigmented layer of the iris
  2. Schlemm's canal
  - **a.** large venous channel, formed by nonfenestrated endothelium and a thin connective tissue wall
  3. Collector channels
  - **a.** arise from Schlemm's canal and drain into intrascleral venous plexus, the deep scleral plexus, and then into the aqueous veins, which are visible in the conjunctiva by biomicroscopy

C. Gonioscopy
  1. Clinical Anatomy
  - **a.** pupillary margin; look for pseudoexfoliation, posterior synechiae
  - **b.** iris; look at contour of iris plane, width of angle, look for neovascularization (normal radial vessels may be observed within iris stroma)
  - **c.** ciliary body; above iris root
  - **d.** scleral spur; white line of varying width, composed of band of collagen fibers which marks the attachment of the ciliary body
  - **e.** trabecular meshwork and Schlemm's canal; Schlemm's canal appears as faint gray line, or if

blood refluxed from episcleral veins, red line between middle and posterior third of TM
  f. Schwalbe's line; TM terminates at Schwalbe's, slit beam converges to point at Schwalbe's
2. Depth of angle
  a. deeper in aphakia and myopia
  b. shallower in hyperopia
  c. 3 mm deep at center is average

VIII. LENS

A. Structure—biconvex, located in posterior chamber; four to 5 mm in anterior-posterior diameter until age 40, increased width with age; nine to 10 mm in equatorial diameter
B. Features—lacks innervation; depends totally on aqueous and vitreous for nourishment (after regression of hyaloid vascular system during fetal life); entirely enclosed by a basement membrane
  1. Capsule
    a. periodic acid Schiff-positive basement membrane, produced by lens epithelium
    b. anterior twice as thick as posterior and increases in thickness throughout life
  2. Epithelium
    a. beneath anterior and equator capsule only, not beneath posterior capsule
    b. bases face capsule, apices face lens interior, lateral borders of cells interdigitated
    c. at equator "nuclear bow," mitotic division
    d. divided cells elongate, transformed from tall cuboidal cells to fibers
  3. Fibers
    a. "lens sutures" formed by arrangement of interdigitations of apical cell processes (anterior sutures) and basal cell processes (posterior sutures), Y-sutures within nucleus of lens
  4. Zonules
    a. originate from basement membrane of non-pigmented epithelium of pars plana and pars plicata of ciliary body
    b. attach to lens capsule anterior and posterior to equator
    c. zonular fiber made of multiple filaments of collagen
C. Lens Function, Metabolism and Biochemistry
  1. Function

a. forms the second refracting unit of eye, adding 20 diopters to approximately 43 diopters of corneal accommodation
2. Metabolism and biochemistry
   a. specific internal ionic-osmotic balance important for normal lens metabolism
   b. by active transport, sodium is 20 mM and potassium 120 mM inside lens, vs 150 mM and 5 mM respectively in aqueous
   c. primary site for active transport in lens is in epithelium

IX. UVEAL TRACT

The vascular compartment of the eye; comprises three parts: iris, ciliary body, choroid; attached firmly to sclera only at three sites:
1. scleral spur
2. exit point of vortex veins
3. the optic nerve

clinical significance—these attachments account for the characteristic ophthalmoscopic findings in bullous choroidal detachments

A. Iris
  1. Stroma
     a. composed of pigmented (melanocytes) and nonpigmented cells, collagen fibrils, and a matrix of hyaluronidase-sensitive mucopolysaccharide
     b. anterior surface not covered by continuous layer of cells
     c. aqueous humor flows freely through loose iris stroma
  2. Vessels
     a. blood vessels from bulk of iris stroma, majority radial course from pupil
     b. in the region of the collarette (thickest portion of the iris), anastomoses occur between the arterial and venous arcade; however, no true minor iris circle exists. (The major arterial circle is located in the ciliary body)
     c. anterior border layer is avascular
     d. clinical significance—the normally avascular anterior border layer of the iris is the site of rubeosis iridis
  3. Posterior pigmented layer
     a. densely pigmented; continuous with the non-pigmented epithelium of the ciliary body and neurosensory retina

      b. polarity of cells is maintained from embryogenesis; basal surface borders posterior chamber, apical surface faces stroma

      c. curves around pupillary margin and extends for short distance on anterior border layer of iris stroma (physiologic ectropion)

      d. clinical significance—in rubeosis iridis, the pigmented layer extends further onto the anterior surface of the iris (pathologic ectropion)

    4. Dilator muscle

      a. neuroectoderm

      b. parallel and anterior to the posterior pigmented epithelium

      c. innervation:

        1) morphologically, dual sympathetic and parasympathetic innervation;

        2) functionally, sympathetic only

      d. first order neuron:

        1) ipsilateral posterolateral hypothalamus to syn-apse in intermediolateral gray matter of spinal cord, C8 and T2

      e. second order neuron:

        1) exits spinal cord, passes over pulmonary apex, through stellate ganglion without synapsing, to synapse in the superior cervical ganglion

      f. third order:

        1) postganglionic neuron joins the internal carotid plexus, enters the cavernous sinus, travels with ophthalmic division of trigeminal nerve (VI) to orbit, and then to dilator muscle

    5. Sphincter muscle

      a. neuroectoderm

      b. circular band of smooth muscle fibers

      c. near pupillary margin in deep stroma

      d. innervation

        1) from Edinger–Westphal nucleus, following inferior division CN III after it bifurcates in cavernous sinus; fibers continue with branch supplying inferior oblique muscle; exits branch to synapse with postganglionic fibers in the ciliary ganglion

        2) postganglionic fibers travel with short ciliary nerves to the iris sphincter

B. Ciliary Body

    1. Function

      a. aqueous humor formation

      b. accommodation

       c. uveoscleral outflow of aqueous humor
2. Ciliary epithelium and stroma
   a. pars plana
      1) 3 to 4 mm from the corneal limbus, 4 mm in width, extends from the pars plicata to the ora serrata
      2) clinical significance—safest posterior approach to the vitreous cavity is via the pars plana
   b. pars plicata
      1) seventy radial folds or ciliary processes, highly vascularized
      2) zonular fibers attach primarily in the valleys of the ciliary process, but also along pars plana
   c. epithelium
      1) double layer of epithelial cells: inner, nonpigmented epithelium; outer, pigmented epithelium
      2) apices of nonpigmented and pigmented cell layers are fused by a complex system of tight junctions and cellular interdigitations
      3) along lateral surfaces of nonpigmented epithelium are zonulae occludentes, maintaining blood-aqueous barrier
      4) basal surface of nonpigmented epithelium, which borders posterior chamber, covered by basement membrane
      5) basal surface of pigmented epithelium also covered by basement membrane
      6) pigmented epithelium: cuboidal shape throughout ciliary body; multiple basal infoldings, large nucleus, abundant melanosomes, mitochondria, endoplasmic reticulum
      7) nonpigmented epithelium: cuboidal in pars plana and columnar in pars plicata; multiple basal infoldings, large nucleus, rare melanosomes, endoplasmic reticulum and Golgi's complex present in these cells play an important role in aqueous humor formation
   d. stroma
      1) composed of large fenestrated capillaries, collagen fibrils, and fibroblasts
      2) main arterial supply, long posterior and the anterior ciliary arteries, which form the major arterial circle of the iris located in ciliary body

      3) venous system: drain posteriorly through vortex system

  3. Ciliary muscle

      outer longitudinal (attach to scleral spur)

      middle radial

      inner circular

    a. clinical significance—presbyopia related to aging changes of lens rather than ciliary muscles

    b. innervation—parasympathetic fibers of CN III

    c. clinical significance—pilocarpine lowers IOP by contraction of the longitudinal fibers of the ciliary muscle, producing tension on the scleral spur and on the trabecular meshwork lamellae. This results in an increase in outflow facility (also causes miosis)

C. Neurotransmitters and Receptors in the Iris-Ciliary Body

  1. Sphincter muscle and ciliary muscles innervated by CN III (parasympathetic)

  2. Cholinergic impulses transmitted by acetylcholine

  3. Dilator muscle fibers innervated by sympathetic nerves from superior cervical ganglion

  4. Adrenergic nerve impulses transmitted by norepinephrine (NE)

  5. Cholinergic receptors divided into muscarinic and nicotinic

  6. Iris sphincter and ciliary muscles are of cholinergic muscarinic type

  7. Adrenergic receptors divided into α- and β-adrenergic type

      dilator muscle is of α-adrenergic receptor type

  8. Miotics act by

    a. stimulating the sphincter directly (e.g., pilocarpine) or indirectly by inhibiting acetylcholine esterase (e.g., phospholine iodide)

    b. blocking the dilator by inhibiting release of NE or by blocking the a-adrenergic receptors

  9. Mydriatics act by

    a. stimulating the dilator by

      1) increasing NE release (hydroxyamphetamine)

      2) interfering with NE reuptake (cocaine)

      3) directly stimulating the a-receptors (phenylephrine)

    b. blocking the sphincter

      1) anticholinergic (atropine, cyclopentolate, tropicamide)

D. Choroid

    .25 mm thick

arterial flow from anterior ciliary arteries (ACA), long posterior ciliary arteries (LPCA), and short posterior ciliary arteries (SPCA)

1. Bruch's membrane
   a. not a true membrane
   b. five layers:
      1) basal lamina of the RPE
      2) inner collagenous zone
      3) elastic fibers
      4) outer collagenous zone
      5) basal lamina of inner layer of choriocapillaris
   c. permeable to small molecules like fluorescein
2. Choriocapillaris
   a. lobular pattern of large fenestrated capillaries; acts like an end-arteriole system
3. Middle and outer choroidal layers
   a. vessels not fenestrated, fluorescein molecules do not diffuse
   b. degree of pigmentation of fundus dependent on number of pigmented melanocytes in choroid, not RPE

X. RETINA AND RPE

A. Retina
   1. Structure
      a. rods and cones (120 million and 6 million)
      b. rod discs are not attached to the cell membrane; cone discs are attached to the cell membrane
      c. bipolar cells: dendrites synapse with rod's spherule and cone's pedicle and axons syn-apse with ganglion cells
      d. horizontal cells provide horizontal connections in the outer plexiform layer (OPL)
      e. amacrine cells provide horizontal connections in the inner plexiform layer (IPL)
      f. ganglion cell axons form nerve fiber layer (NFL)
      g. glial cells: Müller cells (nucleus located in inner nuclear layer [INL]) and astrocytes provide structural support
      h. vascular elements
      i. cilioretinal artery contributes to macular circulation in about 15% of individuals
      j. site of inner blood-retinal barrier is endothelial cell with tight junctions
      k. retinal blood vessels lack an internal elastic lamina unlike blood vessels of middle and outer layers of choroid

    l. retinal blood vessels extend as deep as inner portion of inner nuclear layer
    m. layers of the retina
      1) external limiting membrane (ELM); deepest location of Müller's cells, where they attach to photoreceptors; not a true membrane
      2) OPL also known as fiber layer of Henle; accumulation of lipid/blood within this layer accounts for star pattern seen in some cases of systemic hypertension
      3) INL: contains nuclei of bipolar, Müller, horizontal and amacrine cells
      4) middle limiting membrane (MLM) not a true membrane; region of synaptic bodies of the photoreceptor cells
      5) IPL axons of bipolar and amacrine; dendrites of ganglion cells
      6) ganglion cell layer (GCL)
      7) NFL axons of ganglion cells
      8) internal limiting membrane (ILM) not a true membrane formed by footplates of the Müller cells and attachments to the basal lamina

Macula

Anatomist	Clinician		
"fovea"	foveola	350 microns	cones only
	FAZ	250–600 u	(often quoted at 500 u)
"macula"	fovea	1500 microns	(optic disc size)
"posterior pole"	macula	area within temporal arcades	

    n. ora serrata
      1) distance from limbus (Schwalbe's line) to ora serrata: 5.75 mm nasally and 6.50 mm temporally
      2) diameter is 20 mm vs. 24 mm at equator
      3) ora smooth temporally and serrated nasally
2. Retinal function
    a. biochemical reactions of the light cycle: the light-evoked reactions in photoreceptor cells are associated with three reactions

    b. chemical changes in visual pigments following photon absorption:

        1) rhodopsin to bathorhodopsin to lumirhodopsin to metarhodopsin I to metarhodopsin II to all-trans-retinaldehyde and opsin

        2) the conversion from metarhodopsin I to metarhodopsin II is the step that initiates visual excitation

        3) rhodopsin regenerated by condensation of 11-*cis*-retinaldehyde with opsin

    c. the vitamin A cycle

        1) vitamin A stored in liver as retinyl ester hydrolyzed to retinol, which combines with serum RBP in 1:1 ratio complex bound to prealbumin

        2) all-trans-retinol delivered to RPE

        3) net movement of vitamin A derivatives from the outer segments of retina to the RPE during light adaptation and the reversal of this flow in the dark during light exposure

        4) 11-*cis*-retinaldehyde required for formation of pigment (rhodopsin = opsin + 11-*cis*-retinaldehyde) capable of absorption of photons and initiation of visual excitation

        5) action of light is to isomerize 11-*cis*-retinaldehyde to all-trans-retinaldehyde in visual pigment

        6) all-*trans*-retinaldehyde reduced to all-*trans*-retinol in outer segments

        7) all-*trans*-retinol transported to RPE

        8) all-*trans*-retinol to 11-*cis*-retinol in RPE

        9) 11-*cis*-retinol transported to outer segment where oxidized back to 11-*cis*-retinaldehyde

            Key: RPE is site of isomerization from all-*trans*-retinol to 11-*cis*-retinol

            Key: outer segment is site of isomerization from 11-*cis*-retinaldehyde to all-*trans*-retinaldehyde

            Key: outer segment is site of conversion from alcohol to aldehyde and aldehyde to alcohol

    d. cyclic nucleotide metabolism

        1) levels of cyclic guanosine monophosphate (cGMP) in rod outer segments are controlled by changes in levels of illuminance

        2) effect of light on plasma membrane activities in rod photoreceptor cells

        3) in the dark (dark current), high levels of cGMP in outer segments keep sodium channels open, allowing for passive entry of sodium (Na+) into the outer segment; Na+ diffuses through the connecting cilium into the inner segment

4) Na+ actively transported to the extracellular space by sodium potassium adenosinetriphosphatase (ATPase)

5) in this depolarized state, neurotransmitter is released from the synaptic terminal

6) in the light, decreased levels of cGMP lead to closure of Na+ channels and hyperpolarization of the rod cell

7) results in decrease in neurotransmitter release at the synaptic terminal

 e. turnover of photoreceptors

1) new membrane material added at the inner–outer segment junction

2) old membranes are shed from the apical tips of both rods and cones

3) phagocytized by RPE

4) renewal rate of mammalian rods is 9 to 13 days

5) rods shed disks at dawn, cones shed at dusk (when functionally less active)

B. RPE

 1. Five major functions

  a) vitamin A metabolism

  b) blood-retinal barrier maintenance

  c) phagocytosis of the photoreceptor outer segments

  d) formation of the basal lamina

  e) active transport of metabolites to and from retina

 2. polarized with basal side facing Bruch's membrane and apical side facing neurosensory retina

 3. junctional complexes provide outer blood-retinal barrier

 4. cells in foveal area are taller, narrower, and contain more melanosomes (pigment granules), accounting for darker appearance in fluoresceins

 5. melanosomes develop in situ in RPE cells, in contrast to pigment granules in melanocytes in uveal tract, which are derived from the neural crest and migrate into uvea later

XI. VITREOUS

A. Structure

 1. 4/5 of volume of globe

 2. 4 gm and 4 ml

   3. 99% water
   4. 2 times as viscous as water, due to hyaluronic acid
   5. Anterior vitreous base extends 2 mm anterior to the ora serrata
   6. Posterior vitreous base extends 4 mm posterior
   7. Fetal vasculature remnants include Mittendorf's dot, vascular loops, and Bergmeister's papilla
   8. Ultrastructurally, vitreous composed of hyalocytes and fine collagen fibrils

XII. OPTIC NERVE

A. Prelaminar
   1. Ganglion cell axons divided into fascicles by neuroglial cells (astrocytes)
   2. Müller cells of retina replaced by astrocytes of optic nerve
B. Laminar
   1. Lamina cribrosa composed of collagenous connective tissue and elastic fibers which act as a scaffold for optic nerve axons
C. Retrolaminar
   1. From lamina cribrosa to apex of orbit
   2. Posterior to lamina cribrosa, ganglion cells are myelinated
   3. Diameter increases from 1.5 mm to 3.0 mm
D. Meningeal Sheaths—Pia, Arachnoid, Dura
   1. Pial septae originate in posterior lamina cribrosa; enclose the neurofascicles
   2. Arachnoid mater is continuous with subarachnoid space of brain
   3. Dura mater fuses with outer layer of sclera
E. Central Retinal Artery and Vein
   1. Artery:
      a. nonfenestrated endothelial cells, fenestrated internal elastic lamina, outer layer of smooth muscle cells
   2. Vein:
      a. endothelial cells, thin basal lamina, thick collagenous adventitia
F. Intracranial Portion
   1. Optic nerves pass posteriorly to join in optic chiasm
G. Chiasm
   1. 12 mm wide by 8 mm long by 4 mm thick (lima bean)
   2. Wilbrand's knee—contralateral inferonasal fibers
   3. Macular projections constitute 80 to 90% of volume
   4. Nasal macular fibers cross in posterior part
   5. Temporal macular fibers uncrossed

      6. 53% crossed, 47% uncrossed; unlike albinism where more fibers uncrossed

H. Optic Tract
    1. Fibers from superior retina travel medially
    2. Fibers from inferior retina travel laterally
    3. Fibers from macula travel dorsolateral

 I. Lateral Geniculate Nucleus
    1. Layers 1, 4, 6 contain contralateral axons
    2. Layers 2, 3, 5 contain ipsilateral axons

 J. Optic Radiation
    1. Superior fibers leaving lateral geniculate body (LGB) proceed directly to occipital cortex
    2. Inferior fibers leaving LGB loop around temporal horn of lateral ventricle (Meyer's loop)

K. Visual Cortex
    1. Also called striate cortex or area 17
    2. Located along superior and inferior lips of calcarine fissure
    3. Macular vision projects to occipital tip
    4. Peripheral vision projects to anterior visual cortex
    5. Most anterior portion of calcarine fissure is occupied by contralateral nasal retinal fibers only (temporal crescent syndrome)
    6. Posterior cerebral artery, branch of basilar artery supplies visual cortex

Essentials of Eye Care, edited by Rohit Varma.
Lippincott–Raven Publishers,
Philadelphia © 1997.

2

Ocular Examination

The basic ocular exam should assess function and note anatomic appearance within the context of the patient's presenting problem and ability to cooperate. Special adjuncts to the exam may be added, depending on the patient's problem.

I. VISUAL ACUITY

A. Use—single most important test in visual assessment. Reflects refractive errors, media abnormalities, and abnormal retinal, optic nerve, or cortical function.

B. Instruments—ability to cover/occlude one eye at a time. Optotype eye chart, reading card.

C. How to Perform—depends on age and ability to cooperate. Essential to test each eye independently. Subject should be wearing existing spectacle correction.

1. Infants—Objection to occlusion? Response to light? Response to threat? Response to objects by fixing and following?

2. Small children—pick up small objects (coins, paper clips), identify familiar pictures. Illiterate E or Landolt C—child indicates direction that E or C is open. Matches displayed letters to those on a card. Allen picture card. All scored as to farthest distance at which subject performs task reproducibly. Children often need one eye occluded with an adhesive patch to avoid intentional or unintentional cheating.

3. Literate subject—Snellen letters/optotypes on stationary or projected chart. While wearing appropriate near correction, smallest line read correctly at whatever distance with near card.

4. Illiterate subject—E game, Landolt C as above, picture identification, numerical chart.

5. Poor vision—finger counting (CF) or hand motions (HM) at best distance. Light projection (directional perception of light), light perception (LP)

   D. Findings—recorded as sc (without correction) or cc (with correction). For literate subjects, could appear as 20/20—1 (missed one letter on 20/20 line) down to 6/200 (20/200 E seen at 6 feet), CF 8 ft., HM 2 ft., LP with projection 4 quadrants, LP, no light perception (NLP).

   E. Special/Additional Features—Color vision may be assessed in each eye independently with color plates or more formally with anomoloscope 100-hue test. Color vision may be crudely assessed in children by identification of simple colors in objects (i.e., crayons).

      1. Low vision charts (Early Treatment of Diabetic Retinopathy Study [ETDRS], Sloane charts) can better define acuities between 20/80 and 20/200.

      2. Contrast sensitivity charts also define another aspect of visual acuity and may be useful in confirming subtle visual difficulties not detected with Snellen letters.

      3. Entoptic phenomenon (moving bright light over closed lids, revealing shadowed retinal vessel image) may be used in the case of hazy media. It is commented on as present or absent.

II. REFRACTIVE ERROR NEUTRALIZATION

   A. Use—to estimate or neutralize refractive error, completely or partially, to improve vision.

   B. Instruments—pinhole (PH), stenopeic slit, phoropter, trial lenses, retinoscope, equipment from visual acuity assessment.

   C. How to Perform

      1. Pinhole, slit: subject holds pinhole before eye that is tested.

      2. Retinoscopy: neutralizing lenses, from phoropter or trial lenses, are placed before examined eye while light reflex pattern is observed via retino-scope until neutralization is achieved. Estimating techniques may be used with the retinoscope alone to approximate refractive error. Either method may be used in state of cycloplegia, especially in hyperopia.

      3. Subjective refraction: subject is asked to view optotypes and indicate what corrective lenses, presented via phoropter or trial lenses, make image sharp and clear.

      4. Use patient's own correction: spectacles or contact lenses.

    D. Findings—recorded as sc or cc followed by PH and resulting Snellen acuity with pinhole. No improvement may be recorded as NI.

        1. RNS represents retinoscopy with prefix A (atropine), M (mydriacyl), C (cyclopentolate), or S (scopolamine) referring to cycloplegic used followed by spherocylindrical notation of refraction = resulting acuity.

        2. M represents manifest subjective refraction followed by spherocylindrical notation of refraction = resulting acuity.

        3. W represents present correction worn in spherocylindrical notation.

    E. Special/Additional Features—Potential Acuity Meter (PAM) is a type of projected pinhole which can neutralize refractive error in some cases of opaque media, especially cataract, by revealing potential vision improvement if opacity was removed. Automated refractors are available for cycloplegic estimation as well as manifest refraction.

III. PUPIL EXAMINATION

    A. Requires—darkened room, hand-held bright light source (indirect ophthalmoscope, Finoff transilluminator, pen light).

    B. Tests—sympathetic, parasympathetic, and afferent visual system portion of CN III.

    C. To Perform—first look at each eye individually.

        1. Round or irregular? Irregular pupils suggest trauma, inflammation, neurologic abnormality, or prior surgery.

        2. Reactive or nonreactive? Have patient look into distance and apply light source briefly to each eye individually and characterize briskness of response and range of pupil size. If light reaction is abnormal, test for accommodative response. In moderately lighted room, have patient look in distance and then at an accommodative target at near and observe pupil reaction. If normal response to near and abnormal response to light, light-near dissociation present is suggestive of pretectal or anterior afferent visual system lesion, lues, or diabetes. If light and near reactions are abnormal, consider mechanical damage to iris (trauma to sphincter or dilator or synechiae from old inflammation), autonomic nerve abnormality, or pharmacologic blockade.

        3. Compare both eyes; are pupils equal in size/reactivity? Inequality could mean previous surgery, trauma, inflammation, or pharmacologic agent (mydriatic such as atropine or miotic such as pilocarpine) or neurologic abnormality (CN III abnormality, Horner's syndrome, Adie's syndrome).

4. Swing flashlight from one eye to the other and look for Marcus Gunn pupil and consensual response. Marcus Gunn pupil demonstrates relative afferent pupillary defect; suggests abnormality in ipsilateral retina, ipsilateral prechiasmatic optic nerve, or contralateral optic tract lesion.

D. Special/Additional Features
   1. Pharmacologic testing (see neuro-ophthalmology section)

IV. VISUAL FIELDS—CONFRONTATIONAL

A. Requires—ability to cover one of patient's eyes at a time to allow independent testing of each eye. Red test object (pen, bottle cap, etc.).

B. To Perform
   1. Examiner faces subject and positions self about 4 feet from subject with examiner's face at same level as subject's face. Cover subject's left eye (use subject's hand, patch, or occluder). Examiner closes right eye and has subject fixate on examiner's open left eye. Examiner then holds up one or both hands equidistant from subject and examiner to test upper, middle, or lower visual fields. One, two, five, or no fingers are held up on either or both of the examiner's hands, and the subject is asked for the total number of fingers seen. Fixation is monitored by the examiner's open left eye. Examiner uses his/her own visual field to map extent of subject's visual field. Any areas of difficulty are examined again to confirm the deficit. Examiner's fingers are kept still, as immobile targets are more difficult to see than moving ones.

   2. If subject fails to correctly identify still finger counting in an area of normal visual field, subject has at least a relative scotoma in that area. Retesting the area for the ability to see moving fingers, hand, or objects in that same area will confirm the presence of a relative scotoma or an absolute scotoma (inability to see anything in that area).

   3. Examination is then repeated for the other eye.

   4. Additional techniques may be used for children or uncooperative patients, such as monitoring responses to movement or threat in each of four quadrants of each eye's visual field.

C. Findings—Visual field abnormalities may come from any part of the afferent visual system—from abnormalities of spectacle edges, ptotic lids, media abnormalities of cornea, lens, or vitreous, but most often represent abnormalities of the retina, retinal ganglion cells, optic nerve tract radiation, or visual cortex. The type, pattern, laterality, or congruity of the defect are all helpful in localizing the source of the visual field defect.

D. Special/Additional Features—Using a red test object in each quadrant of the visual field may help elicit subtle/early signs of an optic neuropathy. The subject's eye is presented with one or more red test objects and asked if the color or richness of red is maintained or absent/washed out/dull in any of the quadrants.

   1. An Amsler grid is a square pattern containing an homogenous grid—initially white on black background or red, most often reproduced as black on white background—that may be used as a subjective measure of central vision. It initially consisted of a series of different grid patterns, but now one simple pattern is commonly used. The subject wears appropriate near correction and has one eye occluded. Subject is asked to look at the center of the grid pattern, so marked by a black dot. While fixating there, any abnormalities, distortions, duplications, or absences of the pattern are noted and drawn onto the grid by the subject. This test may be especially useful in following changes in macular disease (see retina section).

   2. A tangent screen, a 2×2 meter square of dark cloth, may be used to plot a patient's central 20 degrees of field with the use of targets moved by the examiner. Large Goldmann bowl perimeters may give a quantified representation of the entire visual field and may be used to further define defects uncovered in confrontational testing. Static automated perimetry is now available to further rigorously analyze the visual field, and with the help of databases, provide useful insights into early detection and progression of optic nerve disease, particularly glaucoma (see glaucoma section).

V. MOTILITY

A. Use—assesses extraocular muscle movements, cranial nerves III, IV, and VI, and other central nervous system (CNS) higher motor centers.

B. Instruments—small penlight, occluder, distance target, near target.

C. How to Perform—Observe both eyes in primary position. Are they aligned, steady (i.e., any nystagmus)? Any head tilt?

1. Light reflexes—Handlight is held about 2 feet from subject, who is looking straight ahead and not at the light. Reflexes should be symmetrically placed, slightly nasal to center. Any deviation is either a manifest tropia or an angle kappa. If centered, phoria may be present.

2. Cover test—requires useful vision in both eyes. Subject looks at distance target with both eyes in primary position. One eye is covered, and the uncovered eye is observed for realignment movement, demonstrating tropia in that eye. Finds may be more easily observed with simultaneous light reflex examination. Any deviation detected in primary position should be examined in the six cardinal positions of gaze (up and right, far right, down and right, down and left, far left, up and left) as well as up gaze and down gaze to determine if the deviation is comitant or incomitant. Prisms may be used to neutralize the deviation to quantify the amount. Exam may be repeated with near target.

3. Uncover test—Subject looks straight ahead in primary gaze at distant target. One eye is occluded and then uncovered. This same eye is observed for any realignment movement following cover removal. This movement demonstrates either a phoria or a tropia. If cover test was negative, it is a phoria. Phorias may be quantified with prisms.

4. Ductions—With the subject facing forward, subject's eyes are directed to extremes of gaze in each of the six cardinal positions of gaze as well as up gaze and down gaze. Patient should be able to move each eye to direction of gaze and bury the sclera.

5. Versions—With both eyes open and facing straight ahead, subject is asked to follow nonaccommodative target through all six cardinal positions of gaze as well as up gaze and down gaze.

6. Pursuit—Subject is asked to follow slow target horizontally in smooth, steady manner.

7. Saccades—Subject is asked to fixate on one point and then rapidly look at another point in subject's visual field without moving subject's head. Saccades should be accurate and rapid without correcting movements.

        8. Near-point convergence—Fixation object is placed at 40 cm in the midplane of the patient's head and moved slowly toward patient until one eye loses fixation and turns out. That point is the near point of convergence, usually 8 to 10 cm.

  D. Findings

      1. Fixation: steady or nystagmus (horizontal, vertical, rotatory, bilateral, unilateral, pendular, jerk, high or low velocity, and high or low amplitude)

      2. Head position: chin up or down, face turn, head tilt

      3. Deviation: tropia or phoria, horizontal, vertical, or both, comitant or incomitant

      4. Ductions/versions: underactive, overactive, paralytic, restricted

  E. Special/Additional Features

      1. Old photographs may note long-standing head position abnormality.

      2. Prisms may be used to quantify deviations in primary and all positions of gaze. Accommodation may be relaxed with +3.00 lenses before the patient while having deviations remeasured.

      3. Maddox rods and other tests of dissimilar images (Worth 4-dot, amblyoscope, etc.) can also quantify deviations as well as detect amblyopia.

      4. Stereo and vectographic tests may demonstrate degree of stereopsis, which is abnormal in amblyopia.

      5. Forced ductions with cotton tip or forceps on the conjunctiva of anesthetized globe can differentiate paralytic from restrictive strabismus.

      6. Optokinetic nystagmus (OKN) drum, oculocephalic maneuvers may be used to detect supranuclear causes of ocular misalignment.

VI. EXTERNAL EXAM

  A. Use—to evaluate the lids, lashes, lacrimal system, orbit, and associated cranial nerves V and VII.

  B. Instruments—inspection with a handlight, use of cotton applicator for corneal and facial sensation.

  C. How to Perform

      1. Inspect the gross position of the eyes and lids—are the upper lids too low (ptosis)? or too high (lid retraction)? Are the lower lids too low (scleral show)? Are the lids symmetric or asymmetric? Are the lid creases in normal position? Are the eyes equally set apart, too wide, too narrow, or asymmetric? Are the eyes too proptotic or sunken in (best viewed while looking up from the subject's chin)? Do the lids follow a smooth contour or do they make an S-turn in the lacrimal region? Do the lashes turn in or out? Are the lashes free of scale, crusting, or foreign matter? Are the puncta everted? Is there a normal height of the lacrimal lake? Are there skin lesions on the lids or areas of erythema?

2. Have subject open and close eyes passively and then actively open against the force of the observer's fingers, observing lid position and orbicularis strength. If ptosis is present, assess levator function by measuring distance upper lid traverses from straight ahead to up while frontalis is neutralized.

3. Palpate the orbital rim and lacrimal areas for irregularities and tenderness. Press on the lacrimal sac and examine for purulent punctal reflux. Assess sensation with a cotton applicator along forehead and malar region. Assess corneal sensation with cotton applicator stroked gently along peripheral cornea, and look for symmetric blink response.

D. Findings—may indicate external eye abnormalities, be part of a panophthalmic condition, or indicative of a neurological or systemic disorder.

E. Special/Additional Features—Schirmer's strips (filter paper strips) may be placed inside the temporal lower lid to assess tear production in basal and stimulated states. Exophthalmometry may be performed with various instruments (i.e., Hertel device) to quantify degrees of exophthalmus or enophthalmus. CT scanning may also be performed to evaluate the orbit or lacrimal region. Jones testing and irrigation of the lacrimal system may be performed in the office to define the location of lacrimal system obstruction (see plastics section). Testing cranial nerve VIII or quantitating corneal sensation with an esthesiometer may be helpful in certain neuro-ophthalmic situations (see neuro-ophthalmology section).

VII. TONOMETRY

A. Use—to measure intraocular pressure (IOP). While statistical guidelines have given a normal range of 8 to 21 mm Hg, visually threatening diseases can occur within this normal range, and eyes can function normally outside this range. IOP measurements are a useful component in assessing the health of the eye in conditions of inflammation, trauma, glaucoma, and following surgery, among others.

B. Instruments—Goldmann-type applanation tonometer along with topical anesthetic and fluorescein; Schiotz tonometer, pneumotonometer, tonopen, each with topical anesthetic; finger tactile tension estimation.

C. How to Perform

  1. A cooperative subject may be assessed with a Goldmann-type tonometer at a slit lamp or with a portable unit. Topical anesthetic and fluorescein solution are applied to the eye to be examined. The conical tonometer tip is placed on the center of the cornea while illuminated obliquely with a cobalt blue light, revealing a prism-split image of half circles. A dial is used to align these properly and yields the IOP. High amounts of astigmatism may necessitate adjustments in tonometer tip orientation.

  2. Tonopen or pneumotonometer measurements are made with an upright or supine subject whose eye has been anesthetized; such techniques may be used in infirmed or uncooperative patients or children. Very crude estimates of IOP may be made by gently palpating the globe through closed lids and comparing the feel to the examiner's own eyes.

  3. It is important to avoid putting undue pressure on the globe in a traumatized or recently postsurgical eye until it has been determined that the eye's integrity has not been violated. Pressure on an open globe can cause prolapse of intraocular contents.

VIII. ANTERIOR SEGMENT

A. Use—to evaluate anterior segment components: conjunctiva, sclera, cornea, aqueous, iris, lens, anterior vitreous. May also be used for magnified look at lids and lashes and tear film.

B. Instruments—may be crudely performed with a handlight or a direct ophthalmoscope with +10 diopters, but is best performed with a slit lamp. Supine or sedated patients may be examined with a portable slit lamp, operating microscope, or a hand lens as situation allows.

C. How to Perform—Slit lamp allows illumination directly, obliquely, with sclerotic scatter, or specular reflection to examine conjunctival and corneal surfaces and stroma. Direct and oblique illumination are useful in examining aqueous, lens, and anterior vitreous. Retroillumination is a useful tool to examine ocular media for subtle opacities of cornea, lens, or anterior vitreous as well as iris defects.

  1. Direct illumination—light beam is on line with axis of observation.

2. Oblique illumination—light beam is adjusted to thin beam and is directed from side while object of regard is viewed straight on. Yields optical section of lens and cornea. By turning beam intensity up and beam height down and quite small and aiming through the pupil, aqueous and anterior vitreous may be examined for cell and flare.

3. Retroillumination—light beam is sized to fit through pupil completely and aligned with axis of observation while cornea is examined straight on. By moving slit lamp toward and away from patient, red reflex will appear on retroillumination.

4. Sclerotic scatter—adjustment knob allowing concentric pivoting of light source is loosened to allow off-axis illumination of limbus/sclera with wide beam. Observer looks straight on at cornea, concentrating on tear film and then epithelium.

5. Specular reflection—thin beam of light is directed at angle greater than 45 degrees while observer looks straight on at corneal level of endothelium. Careful movement toward and away from patient will eventually reveal hexagonal shapes of corneal endothelium.

   Anterior vitreous and lens are best examined in the dilated state.

D. Findings

1. Tear film—height of lacrimal lake, foamy? Debris, decreased tear break-up time (less than 15 seconds, aided by fluorescein strip or solution—time for "holes" to form in corneal fluorescein film in unblinking eye).

2. Conjunctiva—fornices, hyperemia, discharge, follicles, papillae, foreign material, ulceration, pigmentation, concretions. May be aided with strips or solution of fluorescein. Rose bengal may be used to detect devitalized areas.

3. Sclera—vascular engorgement, staphylomata, nodules.

4. Cornea—normal five layers, clarity, opacities, surface defects, edema, ulcerations, pigmentation, precipitates, vessels. May be aided with fluorescein or rose bengal.

5. Aqueous/anterior chamber—cell, flare, hypopyon, hyphema, foreign material, pigment.

6. Iris—transillumination defects, corectopia, nevi, vessels, masses, synechiae, material at pupillary border, sphincter tears.

7. Lens—opacities, dislocation, color, pigment, zonular material.

8. Anterior vitreous—clarity, mobility, cell, flare, blood, debris, cysts, vessels, foreign material, syneresis.
9. Special/Additional Features—Lids may be everted with cotton applicator or retractors to evaluate conjunctival fornices, especially after corneal abrasion, foreign body, or chemical injury.
   a. deep episcleral vessels will often not blanch after topical application of phenylephrine, while superficial vessels will—useful in determining episcleral vs. scleral inflammation. Areas of scleritis are often tender to palpation despite topical anesthetic.
   b. gonioscopy enables examination of the anterior chamber angle by means of a mirrored prism placed on an anesthetized cornea. Useful in IOP abnormalities, uveitis, iris lesions, trauma, glaucoma.
   c. fluorescein strips are soluble in topical anesthetic while rose bengal strips are not; they are soluble in balanced salt solution or tears.

IX. OPHTHALMOSCOPY

A. Use—to examine retina, optic nerve head, and posterior vitreous.
B. Instruments—direct ophthalmoscope and indirect ophthalmoscope with hand-held lens (14, 20, 28, or 30 diopter).
C. How to Perform—Limited information may be obtained with undilated examination using small pupil equipment, small light beam, and 28 to 30 diopter hand lens; best examination is performed with pupillary dilation.
   1. Direct ophthalmoscopy—With subject's eyes dilated, subject's right eye is examined with examiner's right eye as examiner places self on subject's right side and faces subject. Room is darkened, and ophthalmoscope is placed on bright setting with large diameter spot size. While peering through peephole, observer looks at subject's pupil from 2 to 3 feet, observing red reflex. Diopter wheel is dialed until retinal/vascular detail is appreciated, and examiner moves up to subject's eye. Diopter wheel is dialed as needed for best view. Disc is observed, and each of the four vascular arcades are followed from the disc out to near the equator; macula is then observed. Subject's unobserved eye should be open and looking straight ahead. Posi-

tions are changed for examiner to examine subject's left eye with examiner's left eye. Direct ophthalmoscopy yields a real, noninverted, nonreversed image.

2. Indirect ophthalmoscopy—Subject may be viewed sitting upright in situations of examining a retinal detachment or in the face of a settling vitreous hemorrhage, but examinations are usually best performed with patient supine in darkened room. Indirect ophthalmoscope is placed on examiner's head and adjusted for comfort. Light beam is then aimed by adjusting mirror and any aperture adjustments so that it might fall on the subject's pupil at 3/4 of examiner's arm's length. A hand lens, usually a 20 diopter lens, is placed with marked side to patient, about 2 inches in front of the subject's eye. The lens is slowly moved back until a panoramic fundus image pops into view; lens is carefully and slowly pulled back to examiner until the fundus view fills the lens. The goal of indirect ophthalmoscopy is to align subject's pupil, lens, light, and examiner's eyes. This alignment is crucial for success, and light should be adjusted to fit within the dilated pupil, as any extra light is wasted and can cause distracting glare and reflections. By maintaining this alignment, a sweeping view of the fundus may be obtained, beginning in the posterior pole and sweeping anteriorly along each quadrant. Viewing peripheral retina may be aided by having the subject look in the direction of the area to be observed. Scleral depression through the lids or on the anesthetized globe provides a view of far peripheral and anterior structures via gentle indentation of the sclera in the region to be examined. Additionally, this indentation adds a dynamic feature to the exam quite useful in the detection of retinal breaks and detachment. Indirect ophthalmoscopy gives an inverted, reversed image.

D. Findings
   1. Vitreous—clarity (sharpness of view of retina), condensations, opacities, blood.
   2. Optic nerve head—color/pallor, shape, orientation of nerve head, cup size, swelling, hemorrhage, pulsations, exudate.
   3. Retina, overall—hemorrhage, pallor, lipid, masses, attachment, extraretinal vessels, nevi/pigmentation.
   4. Vessels—arterial/venous size ratio, tortuosity, vascular sheathing, sclerotic vessels, exudate, hemorrhage, emboli/occlusion.

    5. Macula: normal foveal reflex, epiretinal abnormalities, holes, perfusion, hemorrhage, exudate, drusen, attachment.

    6. Periphery: breaks, detachment, hemorrhage, oral abnormalities, dialyses, extraretinal vessels/abnormalities, ciliary nerves, vortex veins.

    7. Fundus findings are best recorded with colored pencils according to standard color schemes.

       a. red—arteries, intra-, sub-retinal hemorrhage, attached retina

       b. yellow—chorioretinal or intraretinal exudate

       c. blue—retinal veins, detached retina

       d. green—media opacity, vitreous hemorrhage

E. Special/Additional Features—Dilation may be performed with 0.5 to 1.0% tropicamide and 2.5 to 10% phenylephrine. 10% phenylephrine may cause blood pressure elevation in some patients and should be used with caution. 0.5 to 2.0% cyclopentolate may be used. Higher concentrations may have mild psychotropic effects in some children, and may cause ileus in neonates. Cyclomydril (R) is used for neonates and infants.

    1. Slit lamp biomicroscopy, with Hruby lens, indirect lens (60, 78, or 90 diopter), or fundus contact lens may be used for detailed view of posterior vitreous, nerve head and retina. Mirrored fundus contact lenses can provide detailed views of equatorial and peripheral retina and pars plana.

    2. Opaque media and mass lesions require echographic evaluation.

    3. Photographs may be useful to document fundus abnormalities.

Essentials of Eye Care, edited by Rohit Varma.
Lippincott–Raven Publishers,
Philadelphia © 1997.

3

Eyelid, Lacrimal System, and Orbit

I. EYELID ANATOMY

A. Eyebrow Muscles
   1. Frontalis
   2. Procerus—creates horizontal glabellar furrows
   3. Corrugator superciliaris—creates vertical glabellar wrinkles
   4. Orbicularis oculi
B. Eyelid
   1. Layers
      a. skin
      b. orbicularis oculi
      c. tarsus
      d. conjunctiva
   2. Orbicularis oculi muscle divided into three portions:
      a. orbital
      b. pretarsal
      c. preseptal
   3. Orbital septum
      a. continuation of periosteum that confines orbital fat
      b. inserts into levator aponeurosis 8 to 10 mm above superior tarsal border (lower in Asians)
      c. inserts in lower lid into capsulopalpebral fascia
   4. Upper lid has two orbital fat pads, lower lid has three
   5. Meibomian glands
      a. 25 to 30 in the upper lid
      b. 15 to 20 in the lower lid
      c. drain into a single row of orifices posterior to the mucocutaneous junction

6. Glands of Zeis are associated with lash follicles
7. Approximately 100 lashes in the upper lid, 50 in lower
8. Whitnall's ligament
   a. condensation of levator aponeurosis
   b. found 14 to 20 mm above tarsus
   c. acts as a fulcrum directing horizontal pull of levator vertically over lid
9. Müller's muscle
   a. sympathetic smooth muscle
   b. arises from terminal fibers of levator
   c. lies posterior to aponeurosis
   d. firmly adherent to conjunctiva
   e. attaches to superior tarsus
10. Inferior lid
    a. capsulopalpebral fascia formed from portion of inferior rectus muscle and is analogous to the levator muscle
    b. Lockwood's ligament is analogous to Whitnall's ligament

II. LACRIMAL ANATOMY

A. Secretory System
   1. Lacrimal gland divided by levator aponeurosis into a larger orbital and smaller palpebral lobe
   2. 12 ducts drain lacrimal gland into superior cul-de-sac
   3. Lacrimal (eccrine) gland primarily responsible for reflex secretion
   4. Accessory (eccrine) glands of Wolfring, located at superior tarsal border, and Krause, located in conjunctival fornix, are responsible for basal secretion
   5. Three layers of tear film:
      a. inner mucin layer secreted by goblet cells (holocrine)
      b. middle aqueous layer secreted by lacrimal glands (eccrine)
      c. superficial lipid layer secreted by meibomian glands (holocrine)
B. Excretory System
   1. Superior punctum lies 5 mm from medial commissure
   2. Inferior punctum is slightly lateral to superior punctum

3. Each canaliculus begins as a 2 mm vertical segment, then turns horizontally for another 8 mm
4. In 90% of people, both canaliculi form one common canaliculus which empties through the valve of Rosenmüller into lacrimal sac
5. Lacrimal sac is 14 mm, 4 mm of which is superior to entrance of common canaliculus
6. Lacrimal duct is 12 mm long and empties through valve of Hasner into inferior nasal meatus
7. Distance from valve of Hasner to external nares is 40 mm in adults
8. Distance from punctum to valve of Hasner is 20 to 25 mm in infants, 30 to 35 mm in adults

III. ORBITAL ANATOMY

A. Bones
  1. Orbit formed from seven bones:
     a. ethmoid
     b. palatine
     c. lacrimal
     d. zygomatic
     e. frontal
     f. maxillary
     g. sphenoid
  2. Medial wall: ethmoid, lacrimal, maxillary, sphenoid
  3. Inferior wall: maxillary, palatine, zygomatic
  4. Lateral wall: greater wing of sphenoid, zygomatic, frontal
  5. Roof: frontal, lesser wing of sphenoid
  6. Volume is 30 cc
  7. Entrance is 40 mm high by 35 mm wide
  8. The two medial walls are 45 mm long and parallel to each other
  9. The two lateral walls are 47 mm long and form a 90 degree angle with each other
B. Foramina
  1. Superior orbital fissure
     a. divides greater from lesser wing of sphenoid
     b. transmits cranial nerves III, IV, VI, V (ophthalmic division), sympathetics, and the superior orbital vein
  2. Inferior orbital fissure
     a. passes between sphenoid, maxillary, and palatine bones

        b. transmits cranial nerve V (maxillary division), zygomatic nerve, and inferior orbital vein

  3. Optic canal
      a. lies within lesser wing of sphenoid
      b. transmits ophthalmic artery, optic nerve, and sympathetic nerves

  4. Anterior and posterior ethmoid foramina
      a. lie in medial wall along frontoethmoid suture

  5. Zygomaticotemporal and zygomaticofacial foramina
      a. located in lateral wall
      b. transmits zygomatic nerve

  6. Frontosphenoidal foramen
      a. passes through frontosphenoidal suture
      b. transmits lacrimal and middle meningeal arteries

C. Sinuses
  1. Frontal—fully developed by age six
  2. Maxillary—largest sinus, fully developed as secondary teeth erupt
  3. Ethmoid—grows into puberty, outpouchings are called air cells
  4. Sphenoid—fully developed by adulthood

D. Annulus of Zinn
  1. Fibrous ring continuous with periorbita
  2. Gives rise to four rectus muscles
  3. Encircles optic canal and portion of superior orbital fissure

E. Vascular Supply
  1. Arterial
      a. internal carotid artery branches
          1) ophthalmic
          2) central retinal
          3) dorsal nasal
          4) supratrochlear
          5) palpebral
          6) 6 to 8 short posterior ciliary
          7) posterior/anterior ethmoid
          8) muscular (two to each rectus muscle except lateral rectus which receives one)
      b. external carotid artery branches
          1) maxillary
          2) infraorbital
          3) superficial temporal
          4) transverse facial
          5) zygomaticofacial
          6) frontal
  2. Venous

      a. superior orbital vein drains the following veins to cavernous sinus
- **1)** angular
- **2)** supraorbital
- **3)** supratrochlear
- **4)** veins of globe

      b. infraorbital vein drains floor of inferomedial orbit to pterygoid plexus

  3. Lymphatics—none in orbit

F. Nerves

  1. Optic nerve
- **a.** approximately 50 mm long
- **b.** four divisions
  - **1)** intraocular—0.7 to 1.0
  - **2)** intraorbital—30 to 33 mm
  - **3)** intracanalicular—7 mm
  - **4)** intracranial—10 to 12 mm
- **c.** 1.5 mm diameter at disc
- **d.** 4 mm diameter posterior to Tenon's capsule due to myelin sheathing
- **e.** covered by pia, arachnoid and dura which fuses with sclera anteriorly and with periosteum posteriorly at optic canal

  2. Oculomotor nerve
- **a.** both divisions exit superior orbital fissure
- **b.** superior division supplies superior rectus and levator palpebrae muscles
- **c.** inferior division supplies medial rectus, inferior rectus, inferior oblique, and pupillary parasympathetics

  3. Trochlear nerve
- **a.** exits superior orbital fissure above annulus of Zinn
- **b.** supplies superior oblique muscle

  4. Trigeminal nerve (ophthalmic division)
- **a.** sensory
- **b.** exits superior orbital fissure
- **c.** three branches:
  - **1)** frontal—supraorbital, supratrochlear
  - **2)** nasociliary—long posterior ciliary, anterior/posterior ethmoids, infratrochlear
  - **3)** lacrimal

  5. Trigeminal nerve (maxillary division)
- **a.** sensory
- **b.** exits inferior orbital fissure
- **c.** two branches
  - **1)** infraorbital—nasal, labial, palpebral
  - **2)** zygomatic—zygomaticofacial, zygomaticotemporal

      6. Abducens nerve
- a. exits superior orbital fissure within annulus of Zinn
- b. supplies lateral rectus muscle

      7. Cranial nerve VII
- a. exits stylomastoid foramen
- b. branches
  - 1) temporal
  - 2) zygomatic
  - 3) buccal
  - 4) mandibular
  - 5) cervical
- c. motor supply to muscles of facial expression

G. Extraocular Rectus Muscles
1. About 40 mm long
2. 9.2 to 10.6 mm wide at tendinous insertions
3. Tendons insert along spiral of Tillaux at level of ora serrata
4. Distance from insertion to limbus
- a. medial—5.5 mm
- b. inferior—6.5 mm
- c. lateral—6.9 mm
- d. superior—7.7 mm

IV. CONGENITAL EYELID DEFORMITIES

A. Epidemiology
1. Coloboma
- a. usually unilateral
- b. may be bilateral and affect all four lids
- c. usually involves medial upper lid and less commonly lower lateral lid
- d. can be isolated or part of a syndrome of oculofacial malformations

2. Epicanthus
- a. bilateral but may be asymmetric
- b. can affect mostly upper or mostly lower lid or both equally

3. Telecanthus
- a. nearly always associated with epicanthus except in congenital ectropion or Waardenburg syndrome

4. Blepharophimosis syndrome
- a. bilateral
- b. autosomal dominant or sporadic

5. Ankyloblepharon
- a. sporadic with some autosomal dominant cases reported

6. Epiblepharon

      a. familial cases reported
- **7.** Euryblepharon
  - **a.** unilateral or bilateral
  - **b.** affects all lids but lower lid involvement more clinically evident
  - **c.** autosomal dominant cases reported

B. Clinical Features
- **1.** Coloboma
  - **a.** ranges from small notch to full thickness loss of lid
  - **b.** most involve no more than 1/3 of eyelid margin
  - **c.** lower lid involvement commonly seen with Treacher Collins syndrome
  - **d.** other associations include microphthalmos, iris coloboma, anterior polar cataract, and nasolacrimal duct obstruction
- **2.** Epicanthus
  - **a.** isolated or associated with blepharophimosis
  - **b.** often resolves as facial bones mature
- **3.** Telecanthus
  - **a.** increased intercanthal width
- **4.** Blepharophimosis syndrome
  - **a.** decreased interpalpebral width
  - **b.** varying degrees of telecanthus, epicanthus and severe ptosis
  - **c.** lids foreshortened horizontally and vertically
  - **d.** associated features: high arching eyebrows, flattened supraorbital ridge, strabismus, and nystagmus
- **5.** Ankyloblepharon
  - **a.** partial or complete fusion of eyelids
  - **b.** usually affects lateral portion of lids
- **6.** Pseudo-exotropia
  - **a.** pseudo-esotropia when medial lids involved
  - **b.** occasional association with anophthalmos, microphthalmos, and congenital phthisis bulbi
- **7.** Epiblepharon
  - **a.** horizontal fold of skin across upper or lower lid
  - **b.** eyelashes rotate against globe without in-turning of lid margin (i.e., entropion)
  - **c.** spontaneous resolution can occur
- **8.** Euryblepharon
  - **a.** inferotemporal displacement of lateral canthus

      b. symmetric enlargement of horizontal palpebral apertures

      c. antimongoloid slant

      d. corneal exposure due to lagophthalmos and poor lid apposition

      e. may be associated with ptosis, telecanthus, and esotropia

C. Pathology

    1. Coloboma

      a. incomplete union of frontonasal or maxillary mesoderm

      b. etiology uncertain

      c. possible causes: pressure necrosis from amniotic bands, localized failure of mesoblastic folds to fuse, intrauterine viral infection, vitamin imbalance, or inadequate placental circulation

    2. Ankyloblepharon

      a. thought to represent arrested embryonic lid development

    3. Epiblepharon

      a. pretarsal muscle and skin ride above lid margin forming a horizontal fold that forces lashes to assume vertical position

    4. Euryblepharon

      a. etiology unknown

      b. possible causes: orbicularis hypoplasia, excess skin tension, shortened lid skin or defective lid separation

D. Diagnosis

    1. all by physical exam

E. Indications

    1. Cosmesis for all disorders

    2. Occasionally keratitis due to coloboma, epiblepharon or euryblepharon

F. Treatment

    1. Coloboma

      a. medical—lubricants, bandage contact lens

      b. surgical—delay until preschool age if possible

        1) if less than 1/3 margin involved, pentagonal resection with direct closure in layer, cantholysis may be necessary

        2) if more than 1/3 but less than 1/2 margin involved, perform lateral cantholysis or canthotomy followed by direct closure

        3) if more than 50% margin involved, utilize full thickness rotational flaps. Lid-sharing

procedures are contraindicated in children because they block the visual axis
2. Epicanthus
   a. treatment not usually necessary
   b. when associated with blepharophimos syndrome, perform Y-to-V plasty. Delay surgery until age 3 to 5 years of age
3. Telecanthus
   a. Y-to-V plasty
4. Blepharophimosis
   a. sequential, staged surgical approach addresses, in order:
      1) epicanthus and telecanthus as described above
      2) ptosis—frontalis sling (severely deficient levator function)
      3) vertical skin shortage—full thickness graft from preauricular or supraclavicular area
5. Ankyloblepharon
   a. clamp lid margin with a hemostat, then divide
   b. reapproximate conjunctiva and skin
6. Epiblepharon
   a. excise skin and muscle away from lid margin and reapproximate skin edges to anterior tarsus
7. Euryblepharon
   a. tarsorraphy for mild cases
   b. for more severe cases, lateral canthoplasty with full thickness resection of excess eyelid skin. If vertical foreshortening is present, utilize a full thickness skin graft to the anterior lamella
G. Complications
   scar contraction causing further lid malposition

V. ENTROPION

A. Epidemiology
   1. Unilateral or bilateral
   2. Involves all lids, though more commonly the lower lid
   3. Classified by four etiologies:
      a. involutional
      b. cicatricial
      c. spastic
      d. congenital

B. Clinical Features
  1. In-turning of eyelid margin
  2. Skin or lashes abrade cornea
  3. Conjunctival hyperemia
  4. Epiphora
  5. Keratitis
  6. Corneal ulceration
C. Pathology
  1. Involutional
      a. lid laxity results from involutional enophthalmos and attenuation of lower lid retractors or canthal tendons
  2. Cicatricial
      a. vertical shortening of tarsus and conjunctiva due to inflammation (Stevens-Johnson syndrome, ocular cicatricial pemphigoid, trachoma) or trauma (burns, post-surgical)
  3. Spastic
      a. ocular irritation or blepharospasm
  4. Congenital
      a. primary—dysgenesis of lower lid retractors
      b. secondary—epiblepharon, epicanthus, microphthalmos
D. Diagnosis
  1. Presence of eyelid margin in-turning with or without lash involvement
  2. If entropion is suspected but not observed, have patient forcefully squeeze eyes shut
  3. Evaluate lid tension by pulling lid margin from globe and observing how quickly it returns to position (snapback test)
E. Indications for Surgery
  1. Severe ocular irritation
  2. Keratitis, corneal ulceration
F. Method/Technique
  1. Treatment choice must be guided by each patient's etiology and severity
  2. Involutional
      a. erythromycin or lubricating ointment in conjunction with lid taping, suture marginal rotation, or vertical and horizontal lid tightening procedures
  3. Cicatricial
      a. marginal rotation
      b. tarsoconjunctival graft in select cases; prognosis guarded in inflammatory or traumatic settings
  4. Spastic and congenital
      a. same as involutional

   G. Complications
      1. Undercorrection
      2. Overcorrection
      3. Exposure
      4. Wound dehiscence

VI. ECTROPION

   A. Epidemiology
      1. Unilateral or bilateral
      2. Involves lower lid more commonly due to gravity
      3. Classified by the following etiologies:
         a. involutional
         b. cicatricial
         c. paralytic
         d. congenital
      4. Congenital cases can be associated with euryblepharon, blepharophimosis, or Treacher Collins syndrome
   B. Clinical Features
      1. Eversion of eyelid margin
      2. Can be asymptomatic
      3. Epiphora due to punctal eversion
      4. Conjunctival hyperemia, edema
      5. Corneal exposure
   C. Pathology
      1. Involutional
         a. medial and lateral canthal tendon laxity
         b. may see lower lid retractor laxity and involutional enophthalmos
      2. Cicatricial
         a. vertical shortening of eyelid skin and sometimes orbicularis
         b. etiologies include chronic inflammation and trauma
      3. Paralytic
         a. facial nerve palsy causes loss of orbicularis muscle tone
      4. Congenital
         a. deficiency of skin and orbicularis muscle
         b. hypoplasia of canthal tendons or maxillary bone
   D. Diagnosis
      1. Look for signs of inflammation or previous trauma
      2. Evaluate lid tension by pulling lid margin away from globe and observing how quickly it returns to position (snapback test)

        3. Punctal displacement indicates medial canthal tendon laxity
        4. Test orbicularis muscle strength by having patient squeeze eyes shut
        5. Manually elevate lower lid to rule out mechanical restriction

E. Indications for Surgery
        1. Corneal or conjunctival exposure
        2. Ocular irritation

F. Method/Technique
        1. As for entropion, surgical approach must be individualized
        2. Involutional
            a. plication of canthal tendons
            b. horizontal lid tightening
        3. Cicatricial
            a. three-step approach:
                1) resection of cicatrix
                2) vertical lengthening of lid with a full thickness skin graft
                3) horizontal lid tightening
        4. paralytic
            a. lubrication, moisture chambers
            b. lateral tarsorrhaphy in chronic cases
            c. lid reanimation by lid load or palpebral spring
        5. Congenital
            a. vertical lengthening with a full thickness skin graft

G. Complications
        1. Overcorrection
        2. Undercorrection

VII. BLEPHAROPTOSIS

A. Epidemiology
        1. 60% congenital, 40% acquired
        2. Acquired cases classified by etiology:
            a. aponeurotic (comprises vast majority)
            b. myogenic
            c. neurogenic
            d. mechanical
            e. traumatic

B. Clinical Features
        1. Lower than normal position of upper eyelid due to inadequate retraction
        2. In congenital ptosis, lid is higher in downgaze than contralateral upper lid because the poorly

contracting levator muscle also doesn't relax well

   3. In acquired ptosis, lid remains lower than the contralateral lid in all positions of gaze
   4. Variability suggests myasthenia gravis

C. Pathology

   1. Congenital
      a. localized dystrophy of striated muscle fibers, unilateral in 75%
   2. Aponeurotic
      a. attenuation or dehiscence of levator aponeurosis
      b. a superiorly displaced lid crease results from upward dragging of the levator attachment to skin and orbicularis muscle
   3. Myogenic
      a. myasthenia gravis
      b. chronic progressive external ophthalmoplegia
      c. myotonic dystrophy
   4. Neurogenic
      a. inadequate innervation to levator (third nerve palsy) or Müller's muscle (Horner's syndrome)
   5. Mechanical
      a. lid tumors
      b. forniceal conjunctival scarring
      c. blepharochalasis
      d. lid edema
   6. Traumatic
      a. surgical or nonsurgical injury to levator, aponeurosis or third nerve

D. Diagnosis

   1. History
      a. onset at birth, antecedent trauma, variability, associated neuromuscular symptoms
   2. Physical exam
      a. assess levator function by measuring excursion in extreme upgaze and downgaze (normal, 12 to 17 mm). Fix brow to nullify any contribution from frontalis muscle.
      b. measure palpebral fissure width, upper lid margin to pupillary reflex distance, and superior lid crease to lid margin distance
      c. note any abnormal head or chin position
      d. observe position of ptotic lid in downgaze relative to contralateral lid
      e. note any synkinetic facial or ocular movements

       f. rule out pseudoptosis caused by dermatocha-
          lasis, contralateral lid retraction, or ipsilat-
          eral hypotropia
       g. tensilon or ice test if indicated

E. Indications for Surgery
    1. Abnormal head or chin position
    2. Amblyopia
    3. Ocular fatigue
    4. Cosmesis
    5. Vision complaints

F. Method/Technique
    1. Dependent on underlying cause and amount of levator function
    2. Congenital
       a. levator resection if adequate levator function present
       b. frontalis sling for poor/absent levator function
    3. Aponeurotic
       a. if tendon dehisced, reattach to tarsus
       b. if tendon attenuated, a tuck or resection is performed
    4. Myogenic
       a. myasthenia gravis patients require only anti-cholinesterase therapy
       b. conservative approach to CPEO and myotonic dystrophy; Bell's reflex is often poor—lubrication may be helpful
    5. Neurogenic
       a. observation may be indicated if correction of ptosis will cause exposure
       b. amount of levator function will dictate surgical choice
       c. in third nerve paresis, address ophthalmoplegia with strabismus surgery and/or prisms
    6. Mechanical
       a. address underlying problem; perform blepharoplasty, excise any tumor or conjunctival scar. Any residual ptosis is addressed as in aponeurotic cases.
    7. Trauma
       a. reapproximate any lacerated structures.
       b. delay further ptosis surgery for 6 months since levator function often improves as it heals
       c. post-operative ptosis is managed as in aponeurotic cases

G. Complications
    1. Lagophthalmos

2. Corneal exposure
3. Overcorrection
4. Undercorrection (more likely)
5. Lid asymmetry
6. Adverse reaction to stored fascia used in frontalis sling procedure

VIII. TRICHIASIS

A. Epidemiology
  1. May be isolated or associated with entropion, lid trauma, ocular cicatricial pemphigoid, Stevens-Johnson syndrome, or chronic blepharoconjunctivitis
B. Clinical Features
  1. Posterior misdirection of lashes
  2. Eyelashes are of normal texture
  3. Involvement may be segmental or generalized
  4. Foreign body sensation and epiphora
  5. Corneal ulceration and vascularization
C. Pathology
  1. Idiopathic
  2. Conjunctival scarring
  3. Lid malposition (entropion, mechanical insults, post-trauma or postoperative)
D. Diagnosis
    physical exam
E. Indications for Surgery
    ocular irritation
    corneal ulceration
F. Method/Technique
  1. Mechanical epilation is quick, easy, and temporary; cilia will return in 2 to 6 weeks
  2. Electrolysis, while more permanent, has only a 30 to 50% success rate
  3. Surgical wedge resection useful for localized involvement
  4. Entropion repair if this underlying condition is present
  5. Cryotherapy
    a. double freeze thaw technique
    b. cool to −20 degrees Celsius with thermocouple monitoring
    c. antibiotic ointment for several days
    d. epilate lashes 10 days after treatment (no resistance should be encountered)
    e. 90% success rate, any recurrences can be retreated

    G. Complications
        1. Lid scarring and malposition from electrolysis
        2. Post-surgical infection
        3. Cryotherapy can cause edema, skin depigmentation, loss of normal, adjacent lashes, and epithelial sloughing
        4. Secondary scarring, entropion, lid deformity

IX. DISTICHIASIS

    A. Epidemiology
        1. Rare
        2. Usually congenital
    B. Clinical Features
        1. Extra row of abnormal eyelashes growing from meibomian gland orifices
        2. Generalized lid involvement
        3. Lashes are finer and softer than normal lashes
        4. Generally less ocular irritation than in trichiasis
        5. May be associated with ocular cicatricial pemphigoid, Stevens-Johnson syndrome, or chemical burns
    C. Pathology
        1. Congenital
            a. improper differentiation of meibomian pilosebaceous units
        2. Acquired
            a. severe conjunctival injury causes meibomian gland metaplasia and generation of a second line of abnormal cilia at gland orifices
    D. Diagnosis
        1. Physical exam
    E. Indications for Surgery
        1. Ocular irritation
        2. Corneal ulceration
    F. Method/Technique
        1. See *Trichiasis*
        2. Also, aberrant hair bulbs can be excised via lid-splitting or conjunctival surgery
    G. Complications
        1. See *Trichiasis*

X. ESSENTIAL BLEPHAROSPASM

    A. Epidemiology
        1. Onset usually after age 50

       2. Females predominate

B. Clinical Features

    1. Bilateral

    2. Begins as frequent blinking

    3. Progresses to spasms of involuntary forceful closure of eyelids

    4. Patient rendered functionally blind during these episodes

    5. Worsened by fatigue, ocular irritation, noise, reading, or eye or head movement

    6. Improved by rest, mental concentration, and facial maneuvers like chewing, yawning, or whistling

C. Pathology

    1. Thought to be of central origin, perhaps from abnormality of basal ganglia, rostral brain stem, or bulbar reticular formation

D. Diagnosis

    1. Detailed neurologic and ophthalmologic exam

    2. Rule out reflex blepharospasm caused by dry eye, entropion, ectropion, trichiasis, or blepharitis. If topical anesthesia alleviates spasm, corneal irritation is the cause.

    3. Lower facial musculature involvement suggests Meige's syndrome

    4. Antihistamines and sympathomimetics may cause blepharospasm

    5. Rule out Huntington's chorea, Parkinson's disease, and tardive dyskinesia

    6. Hemifacial spasm is unilateral and does not disappear during sleep

E. Indications

    1. Functional blindness

    2. Patient discomfort

F. Method/Technique

    1. Botulinum toxin

        a. multiple subcutaneous injections around brow and upper and lateral lid

        b. 2.5 to 5.0 units at each site

        c. relief begins in 2 to 3 days and lasts 2 to 3 months

        d. repeat injections required

    2. Orbicularis myectomy

        a. with or without blepharoplasty

        b. 80 to 90% success rate at 2 years

G. Complications

    1. Botulinum can lead to exposure keratopathy, ptosis, and diplopia

   2. Surgery may cause supraorbital nerve damage, transient lagophthalmos, and exposure

XI. BASAL CELL CARCINOMA

A. Epidemiology
   1. Most common eyelid malignancy (90% of all eyelid tumors)
   2. Older patients (average age 60)
   3. Males predominate 2:1
   4. 67% lower lid, 20% upper lid, 10% medial canthus, and 3% lateral canthus
   5. Risk factors include sun exposure and fair skin
B. Clinical Features
   1. Locally invasive but rarely metastasizes
   2. Canthal tumors are more infiltrative and more commonly invade orbit or recur
   3. Orbital invasion and death more likely with canthal tumors and previously irradiated or clinically neglected tumors
   4. Two clinical types:
      a. nodular
         1) most common
         2) small, painless, umbilicated nodule with sharp pearly borders and superficial telangiectasias; rarely pigmented
         3) further divided into:
            a) ulcerative—crusting within central umbilication (known as rodent ulcer)
            b) multicentric—multiple tumor lobules
      b. morpheaform (sclerosing or fibrosing)
         1) appears as flat, indurated plaque
         2) lacks clinically distinct margins
         3) predilection for medial canthus
         4) often ulcerated
C. Diagnosis Is Based on Clinical Features and Pathologic Features Following an Excisional or Incisional Biopsy
D. Pathology
   1. Cell of origin is basal epithelial cell
   2. Cells appear basophilic on H&E stain due to high nuclear/cytoplasmic ratio
   3. Nodular
      a. dermis is infiltrated by large nests of cells with peripheral palisading. Upward migration causes central necrosis and ulceration. Cystic variant results from mucin accumulation within nests. Adenoid variety demonstrates pseudoglandular units in cellular nests.

Occasional melanocyte proliferation accounts for the rare pigmented tumor.

    4. Morpheaform
        a. same bluish cells but instead of nests with peripheral palisading, cells are tightly packed in fingerlike cords that invade dermis

E. Treatment
    1. Surgical excision with frozen section control is favored for most primary lesions and all canthal or recurrent tumors
    2. Mohs surgery also has high cure rate but it is expensive and limited by inability to monitor tumor margin within orbital fat
    3. Radiation and cryotherapy, due to high recurrence rates and inability to monitor margins, is used only for palliation or when surgery is not possible
    4. Lid reconstruction should proceed after intraoperative frozen section report confirms margins are clear

F. Complications
    1. Recurrence if margins not monitored

XII. SQUAMOUS CELL CARCINOMA

A. Epidemiology
    1. Second most common eyelid malignancy
    2. Affects upper and lower lids equally
    3. Still much rarer than basal cell carcinoma by 10 to 40 fold
    4. Like basal cell, risk factors include fair skin and sun exposure
    5. Male preponderance may reflect greater occupational and recreational sun exposure
    6. May arise de novo or from actinic keratosis (better prognosis)
    7. Squamous cell tumors on lids have better prognosis than on other parts of face

B. Clinical Features
    1. Indurated, flat, or elevated plaque often with ulcerated crater
    2. Low metastatic rate but locally destructive
    3. Faster growth than basal cell carcinoma
    4. Predilection for lid margin and canthus

C. Pathology
    1. Cell of origin is more differentiated and superficial than in basal cell carcinoma
    2. Eosinophilic on H&E stain due to abundant cytoplasm

3. Intraepithelial dysplasia seen in actinic keratosis but orderly progression of cellular maturation from basal to superficial layers is preserved
4. In-situ carcinoma shows anaplasia. Unlike actinic keratosis, the orderly maturation of cells is disrupted. The basement membrane is intact though underlying dermis may demonstrate reactive inflammation.
5. With advanced disease, differentiated cells invade dermis
6. Bowen's disease felt by some to be in-situ tumor. Others believe it represents a pre-malignant dermatosis characterized by a scaling patch and radial intraepithelial growth. There is a 50% association with other skin tumors and an 80% association with internal malignancies.

D. Diagnosis
   1. Biopsy
   2. In the past, commonly misdiagnosed as basal cell carcinoma, keratoacanthoma, inverted follicular keratosis, or pseudoepitheliomatous hyperplasia

E. Treatment
   1. Same as in basal cell except with wider (2 to 5 mm) margins
   2. Lymph node dissection when indicated

XIII. SEBACEOUS CELL CARCINOMA

A. Epidemiology
   1. Rare
   2. No gender or racial predilection
   3. Elderly (average age 61)
   4. Upper lid more commonly affected (may reflect the greater concentration of meibomian glands)
   5. Arises most commonly from meibomian glands and less commonly from glands of Zeis or sebaceous glands, of eyelid or brow skin
   6. Not related to sun exposure
   7. Rarely occurs outside of eye area
   8. Prognosis worsened when associated with:
      a. multicentric origin
      b. tumor diameter greater than 10 mm
      c. duration of symptoms greater than 6 months
      d. intraepithelial pagetoid invasion
      e. lymphatic, vascular, or orbital invasion
      f. poor cellular differentiation

       9. Mortality 23 to 41% overall, up to 83% when both lids involved

B. Clinical Features
    1. Painless, insidious onset
    2. Ulcerated, erythematous nodule with associated lid swelling
    3. Destruction of meibomian gland orifices and loss of lashes
    4. Simulates unilateral blepharitis, blepharoconjunctivitis, or chalazion
    5. Metastasizes via parotid, cervical, or submaxillary lymph nodes to lung, brain, and liver

C. Pathology
    1. Lobules of large eosinophilic sebaceous cells
    2. Foamy, vacuolated cytoplasm
    3. Dermis invaded by cords of tumor cells that may be multicentric and show skip areas
    4. Invasion of overlying epidermis demonstrates intraepithelial pagetoid spread like squamous cell carcinoma but with more anaplasia
    5. Mitoses, multinucleated cells, disorganized ductules, and acini are also seen

D. Diagnosis
    1. Full thickness biopsy since tumor arises deep in tarsal plate
    2. Alert pathologist since lesion often misdiagnosed
    3. Oil-red-O stain will identify intracytoplasmic lipid droplets

E. Treatment
    1. Total excision with wide margins (at least 5 mm) under frozen section control
    2. Some advocate exenteration for evidence of pagetoid spread, or tumors larger than 20 mm
    3. Because tumor may show skip areas, Mohs surgery not beneficial
    4. Radiotherapy is contraindicated due to frequent recurrence

XIV. MALIGNANT MELANOMA

A. Epidemiology
    1. Rare (less than 1% of all eyelid lesions)
    2. Middle to late age
    3. Arises from either skin or conjunctival melanocytes

      4. Conjunctival lesion arises de novo, from pre-existing nevus or primary acquired melanosis

      5. Prognosis related to histology, depth of invasion, and tumor thickness

      6. Three histologic types:

        a. lentigo maligna—most common eyelid melanoma. Older patients, sun exposure a risk factor. Best prognosis.

        b. superficial spreading—most common melanoma elsewhere in body. Can appear on non-sun-exposed skin.

        c. nodular—very rare on eyelid; worst prognosis

B. Clinical Features

    1. Lentigo maligna melanoma

      a. begins as flat, tan to brown lesion with spreading, irregular borders

      b. enlarges radially and acquires dark brown and black flecks of pigment

      c. appearance of elevated, palpable nodule heralds vertical growth and dermal invasion

      d. focal loss of visible pigment reflects areas of immune-mediated tumor regression

    2. Superficial spreading melanoma

      a. begins as flat, variegated tumor with multi-colored hues

      b. tends to invade dermis and become palpable sooner than lentigo maligna melanoma nodular

      c. palpable, uniformly brown or black nodule appears over several months

      d. occasionally amelanotic

C. Pathology

    1. All types arise from atypical epidermal melanocytes

    2. Lentigo maligna and superficial spreading melanomas have biphasic growth pattern. Intraepithelial radial phase lasts months to years. Only when dermis is invaded are metastases possible.

    3. Lentigo maligna melanoma—in radial phase, atypical melanocytes appear at dermo-epidermal junction singly or in nests. This pre-invasive lesion is called Hutchinson's freckle, or simply lentigo maligna. Skin markings are preserved and there is a tendency to invade adnexal structures.

    4. Superficial spreading melanoma—unlike lentigo maligna melanoma, atypical melanocytes

are not confined to basal layer but invade upwards. Skin markings are obliterated. Tumor does not invade adnexal structures.
5. Nodular—no radial phase. Epithelioid-type melanocytes invade dermis.
- **D.** Diagnosis
    1. Incisional or excisional biopsy. Unlike uveal melanomas, one may incise cutaneous melanomas without fear of tumor seeding
    2. Frozen sectioning is contraindicated because it destroys fine detail necessary to distinguish tumor from other pigmented lesions
    3. Evert lid to rule out conjunctival involvement
    4. Refer patient for thorough dermatologic evaluation
- **E.** Treatment
    1. Surgical excision with wide margins
    2. For lentigo maligna and superficial spreading melanoma in the radial growth phase, this should approximate a 100% cure rate
    3. Exenteration for more advanced tumors—controversial
    4. Palliative role for cryotherapy or radiation

XV. CANALICULITIS

- **A.** Epidemiology
    1. Unilateral
    2. Typically one but sometimes both canaliculi involved
- **B.** Clinical Features
    1. Punctal edema and erythema
    2. Canalicular swelling and tenderness
    3. Epiphora
    4. Chronic unilateral follicular conjunctivitis
- **C.** Pathology
    1. Actinomycoses and proprionobacterium proprionicus are most common pathogens
    2. Other microbes include Nocardia, Aspergillus, and Candida
- **D.** Diagnosis
    1. Rule out uncomplicated nasolacrimal duct obstruction (no erythema, normal punctum)
    2. Rule out dacryocystitis (tenderness over sac not canaliculitis, swelling over sac)
    3. Manually express any concretions and submit for Gram and Giemsa stains, potassium hydrox-

ide prep, and inoculation of Sabouraud's medium and thioglycolate broth
        4. Dacryocystography may show a dilated canalicular diverticulum
    E. Indications for Surgery
        1. Chronic conjunctivitis
        2. Epiphora
        3. Pain
    F. Treatment
        1. Debride retained concretions by incising canaliculus horizontally through the conjunctiva. Start inferomedial to the punctum and carry incision medially a few millimeters and express and curette concretions. No suture closure necessary
        2. In upright position, irrigate incised punctum with penicillin G (PCN G) (100–160,000 U/ml)
        3. Topical PCN G (60,000 U/ml) and warm compresses TID for 5 days
    G. Complications
        1. Canalicular or punctal trauma
        2. Epiphora
        3. Recurrence

XVI. DACRYOCYSTITIS

    A. Epidemiology
        1. Bimodal incidence: under age two or over age 40
        2. Females and whites predominate due to narrower, more tortuous nasolacrimal channels
    B. Clinical Features
        1. Inflammation of lacrimal sac
        2. Acute infection
            a. erythema, edema, and pain over sac
            b. fistulous tract formation to anterior ethmoid sinus or overlying skin may lead to preseptal or orbital cellulitis
            c. swelling of sac
        3. Chronic infection
            a. chronic ipsilateral conjunctivitis, eyelash matting, and mucopurulent discharge may arise spontaneously or evolve from acute infection
            b. swelling of sac
    C. Pathology
        1. Nasolacrimal duct obstruction results in tear stasis, inflammation, mucocele formation, and ultimately infection

      2. Predisposing factors: dacryolith formation, sinusitis, and systemic infections

      3. Acute infection can produce persistent sac dilatation which promotes chronic infection

      4. In acute infections, responsible microbes include *Staph aureus, staph epi,* and beta *streptococcus. Pneumococcus* and *Haemophilus influenzae* predominate in chronic infections.

  D. Diagnosis

      1. Note any epiphora, cellulitis, pain or tenderness in the area of the sac

      2. Rule out orbital cellulitis by noting any decreased vision, pupillary abnormality, proptosis, or restriction of extraocular movements

      3. Apply pressure over sac. Document and culture any expressed material.

      4. Note any swelling or palpable mass

  E. Treatment

      1. Acute

         a. warm compresses for comfort and to promote antibiotic penetration

         b. analgesics (narcotics may be necessary)

         c. oral antibiotics based on culture and sensitivity results

         d. empiric dicloxacillin or Keflex 500 mg/q6 hours for 14 days

         e. topical sulfa or penicillin 10,000 to 50,000 U/ml

         f. surgical aspiration and antibiotic irrigation with topical penicillin for pointing, fluctuant abscess

      2. Chronic

         a. dacryocystorhinostomy with or without bicanalicular intubation

  F. Complications

      1. Fistulization from surgical drainage

      2. Postoperative hemorrhage and infection

      3. Epiphora

      4. Recurrence

XVII. CONGENITAL NASOLACRIMAL DUCT OBSTRUCTION

  A. Epidemiology

      1. Clinically significant in 1 to 6% of infants

      2. Majority will spontaneously open by 6 to 12 months of age

  B. Clinical Features

      1. Epiphora

      2. Mucopurulent discharge

       3. Matting of eyelashes

       4. May produce dilatation of lacrimal sac (mucocele) or acute dacryocystitis

C. Pathology

       1. Most common etiology is failure of duct to canalize at its opening beneath inferior turbinate (valve of Hasner)

       2. Other causes include punctal atresia, canalicular stenosis, and nasolacrimal duct atresia

D. Diagnosis

       1. Rule out other causes of neonatal epiphora such as conjunctivitis, glaucoma, and corneal irritation

E. Indications for Probing

       1. Chronic discharge beyond 12 months of age

       2. Acute dacryocystitis

       3. Severe inflammation

F. Treatment

       1. Topical sulfacetamide drops TID

       2. Massage over sac, stroking downward toward nose to promote perforation of mucous membrane

       3. Therapeutic probing

          a. timing is controversial

          b. early probing (up to 6 months) may be more successful and may obviate need for general anesthesia

          c. late (less than 13 months) probing favored by some because children will spontaneously canalize by then and the number of unnecessary probings is then minimized

G. Technique

       1. Cannulate superior punctum for the passage is more directly aligned with the nasolacrimal duct

       2. Probe should enter the space beneath the inferior turbinate after passing about 20 mm

       3. Check success of probing by irrigating Neosporin-Bacitracin-Polymyxin solution stained with 2% fluorescein and try to recover in nose

       4. While primary probings may be attempted in the office setting, all subsequent probings should be performed under general anesthesia in the operating room

       5. If multiple probings fail, silastic intubation for 4 to 6 months is indicated

          a. Dacryocystorhinostomy (DCR) is needed in some cases

H. Complications

       1. Creation of blind passage during probing

      2. Failure to obtain drainage
      3. Bleeding
      4. Infection

XVIII. ACUTE INFECTIOUS DACRYOADENITIS

A. Epidemiology
   1. Primary infections usually unilateral
   2. Secondary infections usually bilateral
   3. Most often seen in children and young adults

B. Clinical Features
   1. Painful swelling of superolateral orbit due to bacterial or viral infection of lacrimal gland
   2. S-shaped lid contour
   3. Superotemporal forniceal conjunctivitis
   4. May see fever, leukocytosis, and preauricular adenopathy
   5. Generally benign course with resolution over 10 to 14 days

C. Pathology
   1. Lacrimal gland predisposed to infection due to its communication with the external environment and its rich blood and lympatic supply
   2. Secondary infections caused by gonorrhea, mumps, mononucleosis, herpes zoster, or histoplasmosis are generalized
   3. Secondary infections caused by conjunctivitis, hordeola, cellulitis, or facial trauma tend to be localized

D. Diagnosis
   1. Based on clinical findings
   2. Culture any discharge and if patient febrile, obtain complete blood count (CBC) and blood cultures
   3. Consider orbital cellulitis in setting of proptosis and restricted ocular motility

E. Indications for Therapy
   1. Fever
   2. Pain
   3. Discharge

F. Treatment
   1. Choice of antibiotic guided by exam and culture results
   2. Bacterial—suggested regimen
      a. outpatient adult—amoxicillin/clavulanate 500 mg po q8 or cephalexin 500 mg po q6
      b. outpatient child—amoxicillin/clavulanate 20 to 40 mg/kg po divided q8 or cephalexin 25 to 50 mg/kg po divided q6

> **c.** inpatient adult—ticarcillin/clavulanate 3.2 gram IV q6 or cefazolin 1.0 gram IV q8
>
> **d.** inpatient child—ticarcillin/clavulanate 200 mg/kg IV divided q6 or cefazolin 50 to 100 mg/kg IV divided q8
>
> **3.** Viral
>
> > **a.** cool compresses QID
> >
> > **b.** acetaminophen 650 mg po q4h

G. Complications

> **1.** Antibiotic sensitivity
>
> **2.** Progression to orbital cellulitis

XIX. CHRONIC DACRYOADENITIS

A. Epidemiology

> **1.** Usually bilateral
>
> **2.** Inflammatory etiologies far outnumber infectious though the two are clinically indistinguishable
>
> **3.** Causative inflammatory syndromes include idiopathic pseudotumor, Mikulicz's syndrome, Graves' disease, sarcoidosis, and Sjögren's syndrome
>
> **4.** Infectious agents include syphilis, tuberculosis, mumps, leprosy, and trachoma

B. Clinical Features

> **1.** Variable lacrimal gland enlargement (except in Mikulicz's or Sjögren's syndromes)
>
> **2.** Lid edema and S-shaped lid curve
>
> **3.** Pain is a variable feature and when present, should raise the suspicion of malignancy
>
> **4.** Inferomedial globe displacement

C. Pathology

> **1.** Localized inflammations
>
> > **a.** pseudotumor—polyclonal surface immunoglobulins, mostly T-cells
> >
> > **b.** benign lymphoepithelial lesion (Mikulicz's syndrome)—lymphocytes
>
> **2.** Systemic inflammations
>
> > **a.** Graves' disease—lymphocytic infiltrate with connective tissue edema
> >
> > **b.** sarcoidosis—noncaseating epithelioid cell granulomas
> >
> > **c.** Sjögren's syndrome—lymphocytic and plasma cell infiltration

D. Diagnosis

> **1.** Incisional biopsy for definitive diagnosis is advised since the differential diagnosis includes life-threatening malignancies

      2. Excisional biopsy if a benign, mixed-cell, or dermoid tumor is suspected

      3. On neuroimaging, infectious and inflammatory processes respect the contours of surrounding structures and generally do not cause bony destruction

      4. PPD, FTA-ABS, angiotensin converting enzyme and chest x-ray as indicated

E. Treatment

      1. Infections require appropriate antimicrobials

      2. Inflammations

          a. Graves' disease—steroids (see dysthyroid orbitopathy)

          b. sarcoidosis—prednisone 60 to 100 mg po qd

          c. Sjögren's/Mikulicz's syndromes—ocular lubrication, supportive therapy

          d. pseudotumor—prednisone 80 to 120 mg/d $\times$ 4 days with rapid taper to 20 mg/d then taper gradually over 5 to 6 weeks

F. Complications

      1. Antibiotic sensitivity

      2. Steroid side effects

      3. Recurrence

XX. LACRIMAL GLAND TUMORS

A. Epidemiology

      1. Benign mixed cell tumor (pleomorphic adenoma)

          a. wide age range but more common in fourth and fifth decade

          b. most common epithelial tumor of lacrimal gland

      2. Adenoid cystic carcinoma (cylindroma)

          a. younger adults

          b. most common epithelial malignancy

      3. Malignant mixed cell tumor (pleomorphic adenocarcinoma)

          a. older patients

B. Clinical Features

      1. Benign mixed cell tumor

          a. slow growing, long duration of symptoms

          b. good prognosis with low rate of recurrence or malignant transformation when properly excised

          c. in setting of incomplete excision or recurrence, 20% rate of malignant transformation over 3 years

    2. Adenoid cystic carcinoma
      a. painful
      b. aggressive, fast-growing tumor with short duration of symptoms
      c. poor prognosis
    3. Malignant mixed cell tumor
      a. rapid growth, short duration of symptoms
      b. painful
      c. usually arises from malignant change in an incompletely excised or recurrent benign mixed cell tumor
      d. can arise de novo

C. Pathology
    1. Benign mixed cell tumor
      a. mixtures of duct, tubule, and acini-type structures with epithelial and mesenchymal elements
      b. variable histologic appearance between individuals and within the same tumor
      c. pseudocapsule forms from pressure exerted by enlarging gland
    2. Adenoid cystic carcinoma
      a. sheets of epithelial cells mimic glandular structures and contain mucin-filled cystic spaces (Swiss cheese appearance)
      b. lack of capsule promotes perineural infiltration and posterior orbital invasion
    3. Malignant mixed cell tumor
      a. similar in histology to benign mixed cell tumor except mitoses and anaplastic elements are present

D. Diagnosis
    1. CT findings help differentiate inflammatory from neoplastic processes
      a. inflammatory lesions cause enlargement of lacrimal gland that molds to contours of adjacent structures. There is no bony destruction.
      b. neoplastic lesions cause globular lacrimal gland enlargement
      c. benign mixed cell tumors cause lacrimal fossa enlargement but, like inflammatory lesions, no bony destruction
      d. malignant tumors cause bony destruction and create irregular contours of surrounding bony cavities
    2. Definitive diagnosis requires biopsy; note—perform a wide excisional biopsy if benign mixed cell tumors suspected because incision may promote recurrence and malignant transformation

E. Treatment
  1. Benign mixed cell tumor
     a. complete excision via lateral orbitotomy
  2. Adenoid cystic carcinoma/malignant mixed cell tumor
     a. orbital exenteration can be considered if no metastases present but questionable. This improves prognosis for adenoid cystic carcinoma. Include eyelid skin and any involved bone
     b. radiation therapy indicated as (1) adjuvant to exenteration, (2) alternative when exenteration not possible, or (3) palliation for locally advanced or metastatic disease
F. Complications
  1. Malignant recurrence
  2. Malignant transformation due to incomplete removal of benign lesion
  3. Bleeding

XXI. DYSTHYROID ORBITOPATHY

A. Epidemiology
  1. Most common cause of unilateral or bilateral adult proptosis
  2. Women predominate by as much as 8:1
  3. Onset in third or fourth decade
  4. Bilateral involvement the rule though marked asymmetry common
  5. Orbitopathy may precede or follow diagnosis of hyperthyroidism
  6. Severity of orbitopathy does not correlate with degree of hyperthyroidism
  7. Orbitopathy may progress even in clinically euthyroid Graves' patients
  8. Active stage of inflammation resolves spontaneously over months to years
  9. Secondary fibrotic changes do not resolve
  10. Extraocular myopathy affects all rectus muscles but most commonly inferior and medial recti
B. Clinical Features
  1. Upper and lower eyelid retraction
  2. Lid lag on downgaze (von Graefe's sign)
  3. Exophthalmos
  4. Restrictive ophthalmoplegia
  5. Diplopia
  6. Eyelid edema
  7. Conjunctival vascular congestion

8. Exposure keratopathy
9. Optic neuropathy leading to decreased central acuity, dyschromatopsia, and visual field defects
10. Lacrimal gland involvement with decreased tear production
11. Resistance to retropulsion of globe

C. Pathology
1. Pathogenesis unclear; believed to be a multifactorial autoimmune phenomenon
2. Initial inflammatory phase marked by lymphocyte, plasma cell and mast cell infiltration of extraocular muscle and orbital fat
3. In contrast to pseudotumor, muscle tendons spared by inflammatory process
4. Fibroblasts proliferate and produce mucopolysaccharides (including hyaluronic acid) which bind water and cause massive interstitial edema
5. Secondary stage marked by disorganization and loss of muscle striations. Fibrosis and contracture seen in late stages.

D. Diagnosis
1. Thorough ophthalmic exam including orthoptics, exophthalmometry, and forced ductions
2. Tonometry in primary gaze and upgaze to detect any intraocular pressure increase attributable to inferior rectus restriction
3. Orbital imaging will demonstrate enlarged muscles
4. Thyroid function tests: T4, T3RU, thyroid stimulating hormone (TSH) for screening. Thyroid releasing hormone (TRH) stimulation test (hyperthyroid patient will suppress pituitary TSH response) useful when Graves' suspected but screening thyroid function tests (TFTs) are normal.
5. In the presence of optic neuropathy, a visual field test may show central or paracentral scotoma
6. Tensilon test to rule out myasthenia gravis

E. Indications
1. Corneal exposure
2. Cosmesis
3. Strabismus
4. Optic neuropathy

F. Treatment
1. Co-management with internist/endocrinologist advised
2. Ideally, radiation or surgical treatment delayed until a hyperthyroid patient is treated and made clinically euthyroid

3. Supportive therapy for corneal exposure—lubrication, moisture chambers, and taping lids closed during sleep
4. Oral steroids indicated in early, soft tissue inflammatory stage—prednisone 60 to 100 mg po divided BID for 3 weeks, tapering by 5 mg/week. In menopausal women at risk for osteoporosis, consider supplementation with vitamin D 50,000 units q week and $CaCO_3$ 0.5 gram po
5. Steroids much less effective for restrictive myopathy, lid retraction, or proptosis
6. radiation therapy for severe inflammation, optic neuropathy and steroid failures—2000 rads divided into multiple sessions over 2 weeks with or without steroids
7. Surgery
   a. for mild corneal exposure—lateral tarsorraphy or canthorraphy
   b. for more severe exposure or cosmesis related to lid retraction, lagophthalmos or proptosis-levator, Müller's and/or inferior retractor recessions with or without scleral spacers
   c. for optic neuropathy and some cases of severe proptosis—medial and inferior and lateral orbital decompression

      two surgical approaches:
      1) transantral (Caldwell-Luc)—allows direct visualization and greater access to posterior orbit
      2) transcutaneous (or transconjunctival)—easier for most ophthalmologists and creates less interference with oral intubation; oral steroids are given preoperatively and tapered thereafter
   d. for strabismus—rectus muscle recessions should be delayed until ocular deviations stable for 6 months and any orbital surgery is completed

G. Complications
   1. Steroid side effects
   2. Radiation side effects
   3. Orbital decompression—cerebrospinal fluid (CSF) leak, oral-antral fistula, diplopia, globe ptosis, or loss of vision
   4. inferior rectus recession—lower lid retraction, limitation of upgaze, globe perforation, and worsened proptosis due to anterior migration of globe

XXII. ORBITAL INFLAMMATORY PSEUDOTUMOR

A. Epidemiology
   1. No sexual or racial predilection
   2. Onset usually in middle age
   3. Typically unilateral, though bilateral involvement seen in up to one third of affected children
   4. Variable course, recurrences common
   5. Tolosa-Hunt variant (painful ophthalmoplegia) is localized to area of superior orbital fissure, optic canal, and anterior cavernous sinus
B. Clinical Features
   1. Myositis, dacryoadenitis, scleritis, or perineuritis
   2. Orbital pain
   3. Restricted eye movement
   4. Proptosis
   5. Decreased vision and diplopia
   6. Eyelid edema
   7. Conjunctival chemosis
   8. Paresthesias along ophthalmic branch of trigeminal nerve
   9. In children: fever, headache, vomiting, papillitis, and iritis
C. Pathology
   1. Histologic composition:
      a. reactive inflammation—lymphocytes, plasma cells, and eosinophils
      b. fibrosis—reticulum cells, macrophages, fibroblasts, capillaries, and collagen
   2. Lymphocytic infiltration is polymorphous, polyclonal, and comprised mostly of T-cells (unlike lymphoma which is monoclonal and mostly B cells)
D. Diagnosis
   1. Rule out history of malignancy
   2. CT—thickened posterior sclera, inflamed orbital fat or lacrimal gland, irregular EOM thickening with tendon involvement
   3. Orbital biopsy indicated in setting of recurrence, suspected malignancy, or steroid failure. Open biopsy better demonstrates gross histologic architecture and is preferred over fine needle.
   4. Erythrocyte sedimentation rate, complete blood count with differential, antinuclear antibody, blood urea nitrogen, serum creatinine, or fasting blood sugar indicated in atypical cases
E. Indications

      1. Pain

      2. Cosmesis

      3. Decreased vision

  F. Treatment

      1. Prednisone 80 to 100 mg po divided BID times 2 weeks. Expect response in 24 to 48 hours. More effective for reactive inflammation than fibrosis.

      2. Radiation 2500 rads divided into 12 sessions over 2 to 3 weeks is indicated when steroids are ineffective or contraindicated

      3. Topical prednisone for iritis

  G. Complications

      1. Steroid or radiation side effects

XXIII. CONGENITAL ORBITAL DEFORMITIES

  A. Epidemiology

      1. Synophthalmia (two incomplete eye structures which fuse posteriorly) and cyclopia (single median eye)

        a. extremely rare

        b. affected infants usually stillborn

        c. females predominate

        d. association with Trisomy 13

      2. Anophthalmia

        a. rare

        b. sporadic and usually bilateral

        c. patients often stillborn

      3. Microphthalmia

        a. small, abnormal eye

        b. unilateral or bilateral

        c. sporadic or inherited

      4. Cryptophthalmia

        a. failure of eyelid formation

        b. sporadic

        c. usually bilateral and symmetric

        d. slight male predominance

      5. Orbital hypertelorism

        a. increased distance between medial orbital walls

      6. Orbital hypotelorism

        a. decreased distance between medial orbital walls

      7. Cranial synostoses (Crouzon's disease or Apert's syndrome)

        a. premature closure of cranial sutures

        b. often autosomal dominant

        8. Mandibular dysostosis (Treacher Collins syndrome)
          a. autosomal dominant with variable penetrance and expressivity

B. Clinical Features

    1. Synophthalmia/cyclopia
      a. hypoplastic mid-face and lids
      b. single midline orbit and optic canal
      c. microcephaly
      d. in synophthalmia, eye structures are dual anteriorly and become less differentiated posteriorly and medially
      e. in cyclopia, eye is well-defined but optic nerve is absent

    2. Anophthalmia
      a. normal-appearing lids
      b. reduced interpalpebral fissure and orbital volume
      c. extraocular muscles are present but insert abnormally into orbital soft tissue
      d. lacrimal gland usually normal

    3. Microphthalmia
      a. coloboma or cyst often seen
      b. narrowed interpalpebral fissure
      c. anterior chamber shallowing
      d. hyperopia

    4. Cryptophthalmia
      a. three clinical variants:
        1) complete
          a) most common
          b) lid is replaced by skin which passes over eye continuously from superior orbital rim to maxilla
          c) skin adheres to underlying, abnormal corneal epithelium
          d) posterior pole disorganized. Vision is usually no light perception.
        2) incomplete
          a) only medial globe affected
        3) congenital symblepharon
          a) upper lid is fused to an abnormal keratinized cornea
      b. associated with mental retardation, deafness, and facial bone deformities

    5. Hypertelorism
      a. associated with dermoids, encephaloceles, and orbito-facial clefts

    6. Hypotelorism

       a. associated with a variety of cranial synostoses, cranial synostosis
       b. cleft lip and palate
       c. maxillary hypoplasia
       d. cranial vault deformities
       e. prominent forehead
       f. exophthalmos due to reduced orbital volume
       g. dental malocclusions
  7. Mandibular dysostosis
       a. zygoma hypoplasia
       b. lower eyelid coloboma
       c. loss of lashes in medial lid
       d. antimongoloid slant
       e. external ear abnormalities

C. Diagnosis
  1. All by physical exam and clinical findings
  2. True anophthalmia can only be differentiated from severe microphthalmia by histologic examination
  3. Neuroimaging may aid in diagnosis of microphthalmia, hypertelorism, and hypotelorism

D. Treatment
  1. Synophthalmia/cyclopia
       a. none available
  2. Microphthalmia
       a. in a growing child, socket expansion with progressively larger conformers
       b. avoid enucleation since even a small eye promotes orbital growth
       c. in adults, orbital enlargement may be attempted surgically by utilizing buccal membrane and split thickness skin grafts
  3. Cryptophthalmia
       a. if there is light perception vision or electrophysiologic evidence of visual function, lids may be surgically separated. However, subsequent conjunctival and corneal scarring limits ultimate visual outcome.
  4. Hypertelorism
       a. medial orbital translocation
  5. Hypotelorism
       a. lateral orbital translocation
  6. Cranial synostosis
       a. craniofacial surgery utilizing advancement osteotomy techniques
  7. Mandibular dysostosis
       a. bone graft augmentation of zygomaticomaxillary area

          b. mandibular advancement osteotomy
          c. rhinoplasty and eyelid surgery

XXIV. ORBITAL RHABDOMYOSARCOMA

  A. Epidemiology
     1. Most common childhood malignant orbital tumor
     2. Males predominate 5:3
     3. Unilateral
     4. No racial predilection or known heritable transmission
     5. Presents in first two decades, usually by age 7
     6. Arises in orbit or paranasal sinuses
     7. Tissue of origin is NOT pre-existing muscle but undifferentiated mesenchyme that differentiates to striated muscle
     8. If diagnosed early and appropriately treated, there is a 3 to 5 yr survival
  B. Clinical Features
     1. Rapidly progressive proptosis over several days
     2. Eyelid edema, discoloration
     3. Headache, epistaxis, and sinusitis indicate sinus extension
     4. A mass may be palpated in the superonasal orbit
     5. Hematogenous dissemination to lung and bone
  C. Pathology
     1. Four histologic types
          a. embryonal—most common (70%) of all types. Syncytium of stellate cells with eosinophilic cytoplasm. Cross striations seen in 50% of cells.
          b. alveolar—(20 to 30%) most malignant. Anaplastic cells line fibrovascular trabeculae and fill center alveolar spaces. Few cross striations seen.
          c. pleomorphic—(less than 10%) most differentiated, best prognosis solid, circumscribed tumor. Patients are generally older. Cross striations readily observed.
          d. botryoid—rare, arises in sinuses or conjunctiva. Bundles of spindle cells with eosinophilic cytoplasm and hyperchromatic nuclei
  D. Diagnosis
     1. Urgent incisional biopsy for light and electron microscopy
     2. CT shows no bony erosion

   3. A-scan ultrasound demonstrates intermediate internal reflectivity
   4. B-scan ultrasound shows good sound transmission
   5. Metastatic workup: chest and abdominal CT, bone marrow aspirate, bone scan, and lumbar puncture
 E. Treatment
   1. Combined radiation and chemotherapy. 5000 to 6000 rads divided 200/day, 5 days/week over 6 weeks. 5000 rads delivered via anterior portal and 1000 rads via lateral portal. Triple chemotherapy with vinscristine, d-actinomycin, and cyclophosphamide in 84-day cycles.
 F. Complications
   1. Radiation keratitis, cataract, and retinopathy
   2. Arrested development of orbital bones due to irradiation

XXV. OPTIC NERVE GLIOMA (JUVENILE PILOCYTIC ASTROCYTOMA)

 A. Epidemiology
   1. 75% are symptomatic in first decade
   2. May occur in teenagers or adults
   3. Slightly more common in females
   4. 10 to 70% incidence of associated neurofibromatosis
   5. Chiasm involved in up to half of cases
   6. Most cases sporadic; heritable cases are associated with neurofibromatosis
 B. Clinical Features
   1. Painless, gradual unilateral proptosis
   2. Insidious loss of vision with afferent pupillary defect
   3. Optic disc edema and pallor
   4. Strabismus
   5. Central retinal vein compression can cause central retinal vein occlusion (CRVO), venous stasis retinopathy, optociliary shunt vessels, rubeosis irides, and neovascular glaucoma
   6. Intracranial extension may cause nystagmus, headache, or vomiting
 C. Pathology
   1. Histologically benign, felt by some to be hamartoma rather than neoplasm
   2. Mature astrocytes predominate. Some contain fusiform, eosinophilic intracytoplasmic struc-

ture (Rosenthal fibers). Glial and multinucleated cells are also seen
3. Surrounding meninges show reactive hyperplasia and examined in isolation, these areas
may lead to an erroneous diagnosis of meningioma
4. Microcystic degeneration, calcification, and pia
septal thickening may occur
5. Rare mitoses
D. Diagnosis
1. Biopsy unnecessary in most cases due to accuracy of neuroimaging
2. CT shows fusiform intradermal nerve enlargement. Buckling and low density areas of intra-
neural cystic infarction may be demonstrated
3. Concentric enlargement of optic canal, when
present, may indicate intracranial extension
E. Indications for Surgery
1. No standard treatment protocol exists because
of the variable clinical course
F. Treatment
1. If vision is good, observation with follow-up
and neuroimaging every 6 to 12 months is ac-
ceptable
2. In the event of tumor growth, symptomatic
proptosis, or visual deterioration, surgical excision via craniotomy or, less commonly, an orbital approach is attempted
3. Radiation therapy indicated when excision not
possible
G. Complications
Attendant risks of intracranial surgery

XXVI. ORBITAL MENINGIOMA

A. Epidemiology
1. Median age at diagnosis is 38
2. Females predominate 2:1
3. Primary site usually cranium; orbit may be involved by secondary invasion
4. Primary orbital tumors outnumber primary intracranial tumors in pediatric age group
5. Primary tumors have a better prognosis
6. Tumors more aggressive in young patients
B. Clinical Features
1. Variable clinical course
2. Slowly progressive proptosis

       3. Subjective loss of vision, contrast sensitivity, and color discrimination

       4. Visual field defects

       5. Transient visual obscurations

       6. Lid edema

C. Pathology

       1. Histologically benign

       2. In optic nerve, arises from arachnoid villi between arachnoid and dural sheaths

       3. Two major cell populations: meningocytes (epithelioid cell) and fibroblasts

       4. Psammoma bodies are meningocytes that form whorls around concretions of hyalinized calcium salts

       5. Three major histologic categories

          a. meningoepitheliomatous

          b. psammomatous (transitional)

          c. mixed

             (a) and (b) comprise 65% of all meningiomas

D. Diagnosis

       1. CT will show one of several patterns of optic nerve enlargement:

          a. diffuse tubular thickening

          b. localized fusiform enlargement

          c. apical globular thickening

       2. CT may show ring-like calcification of outer nerve (railroad track sign) or bony erosion of optic canal

E. Indications

       1. Like gliomas, treatment is controversial and tailored to the individual patient. In general, younger patients are treated more aggressively.

F. Treatment

       1. Observe patients with good vision and full fields with biannual exams, visual fields, and annual CTs

       2. Tumor resection via lateral orbitotomy for deteriorating visual function or evidence of intracranial tumor extension. Apical tumors may not be resectable.

       3. Optic nerve extirpation via craniotomy for total loss of vision or evidence of intracranial extension

       4. Radiation used as adjuvant to surgery or as palliation for nonresectable tumors

G. Complications

       1. Intracranial surgical risks

       2. Radiation side effects

XXVII. CAPILLARY HEMANGIOMA

A. Epidemiology
   1. Very common, benign pediatric tumor
   2. One third present at birth, nearly all present in first few months of life
   3. Predilection for medial eyelid and superonasal orbit
   4. Can be associated with nonocular hemangiomatosis
B. Clinical Features
   1. Superficial orbital lesions impart a bluish hue to normal, overlying skin
   2. Eyelid lesions appear red and dimpled (strawberry nevus)
   3. Blanches with pressure (unlike nevus flameus)
   4. Can cause amblyopia by obstructing visual axis and distorting globe
   5. Enlarges over first year, stabilizes, then regresses. Complete resolution over 1 to 4 years is typical.
C. Pathology
   1. Represents hamartoma rather than true neoplasm
   2. Anastomosing, blood-filled channels lined by plump endothelial cells
   3. Fibrous septa contain large feeding and draining vessels which traverse solid nests of proliferating endothelial cells
   4. Reticulum stain outlines basement membranes
D. Diagnosis
   1. Clinical history, physical exam
   2. CT shows contrast-enhancing lesion that enlarges orbit and may erode surrounding bone
   3. Biopsy rarely needed except in deep orbital tumors
E. Indications for Surgery
   1. Since complete resolution is the rule and there are risks with all treatment, intervention should be avoided except in the event of:
      a. occlusion of visual axis
      b. amblyopia
      c. strabismus
      d. optic nerve compression
      e. question of diagnosis
      f. excessive orbital enlargement or dystopia
F. Treatment
   1. Prednisone 2 mg/kg po qd or 4 mg/kg po qod. Expect response in 1 to 2 weeks, then taper.

  2. Intralesional triamcinolone/betamethasone so-
     dium phosphate mixture, 1 ml with 27-gauge
     needle
  3. Surgical excision difficult due to infiltrative na-
     ture of tumor and lack of encapsulation. Best re-
     served for small, localized tumors and then only
     as a last resort.
G. Complications
  1. Oral prednisone may cause rebound tumor
     growth, adrenal suppression, and iatrogenic
     Cushing's syndrome
  2. Intralesional steroids can lead to cutaneous de-
     pigmentation, soft tissue atrophy, and subcuta-
     neous steroid retention
  3. Surgery may produce scarring

XXVIII. LYMPHANGIOMA

A. Epidemiology
  1. Appears in first decade of life
  2. Grows along with child's body, ceasing at adult-
     hood
  3. Three sites of involvement: subcutaneous, con-
     junctival, and deep orbital
B. Clinical Features
  1. Slowly progressive, sometimes exhibiting inter-
     mittent proptosis
  2. Rapid growth seen in two settings:
     a. upper respiratory infection which causes re-
        active lymphoid hyperplasia
     b. spontaneous or traumatic vessel rupture
        which creates a blood or "chocolate" cyst.
        Massive enlargement can appear over hours.
  3. May spontaneously regress
  4. Can cause severe facial deformities
  5. Sometimes associated with oropharyngeal
     lymphangioma
C. Pathology
  1. Pathogenesis unclear as orbit contains no lym-
     phatic channels
  2. Hamartoma of vascular channels lined by
     monolayer of flattened endothelial cells
  3. Vascular channels contain eosinophilic material
     but no red blood cells
  4. Stroma demonstrates connective tissue, lym-
     phoid follicles and, over time, cholesterol,
     thrombi, and calcium

  5. Unlike capillary and cavernous hemangiomas respectively, endothelium does not contain pericytes or smooth muscle cells
D. Diagnosis
  1. Plain films show diffuse orbital enlargement
  2. Ultrasound and CT demonstrate a nonencapsulated, irregular mass with scattered cystic spaces
  3. MRI useful to differentiate normal from abnormal tissue planes in anticipation of surgery
E. Indications
  1. Deprivational or anisometropic amblyopia
  2. Proptosis
  3. Cosmetic deformity
F. Treatment
  1. Oral steroids can shrink the reactive inflammation caused by upper respiratory infections
  2. Drain blood cysts with large-bore needle
  3. Surgical decompression for fibrovascular proliferation. Excision is technically difficult due to vascular and infiltrative nature of tumor. Cryotherapy and unipolar cautery aid in hemostasis.
  4. Intraoperative steroids can shrink residual tumor, retard recurrence, and minimize postoperative inflammation
  5. Preoperative evaluation should include a blood type and screen
G. Complications
  1. Both needle drainage and surgical excision carry a high risk of trauma to adjacent vessels and subsequent hemorrhage
  2. Intraoperative hemorrhage
  3. Tumor recurrence
  4. Scarring

XXIX. CAVERNOUS HEMANGIOMA

A. Epidemiology
  1. Most common benign orbital tumor in adults
  2. Onset in third to fifth decades
  3. Females predominate
  4. Predilection for retrobulbar space
B. Clinical Features
  1. Slowly progressive proptosis
  2. Posterior pressure on globe may cause hyperopia, optic nerve compression, choroidal folds, ocular hypertension, and strabismus
  3. Recurrence rare if completely excised

        4. Pregnancy can accelerate growth

C. Pathology
    1. Round to oval, purple-red hamartoma
    2. Well-defined fibrous capsule
    3. Fibrous septa divide large vascular channels which are lined by flattened endothelial cells. These channels also contain smooth muscle cells in their walls.
    4. Limited communication with systemic circulation

D. Diagnosis
    1. Ultrasound shows high amplitude internal echoes and good sound transmission
    2. CT shows an isolated, well-defined mass usually within the muscle cone
    3. MRI reveals heterogenous internal signal densities

E. Indications for Surgery
    1. Cosmesis
    2. Proptosis
    3. Corneal exposure
    4. Strabismus
    5. Optic nerve compression
    6. Diagnosis

F. Treatment
    1. Surgical excision via lateral orbitotomy

G. Complications
    1. Optic nerve damage

XXX. HEMANGIOMPERICYTOMA

A. Epidemiology
    1. Rare tumor of middle-aged adults
    2. Predilection for superior orbit
    3. Orbital tumors represent (1) a primary focus, (2) extension from an adjacent sinus, or (3) a metastasis

B. Clinical Features
    1. Slow, painless proptosis
    2. Restricted ocular motility and strabismus
    3. Conjunctival prolapse and chemosis
    4. Recurrences common after incomplete excision and may occur up to ten years later
    5. A recurrent tumor is more aggressive—it invades locally, metastasizes, and can be fatal

C. Pathology
    1. Histology ranges from benign to malignant
    2. Oval, purple-red encapsulated tumor

        3. Aggregates of pericytes surround numerous capillary-like lacunae

        4. More malignant varieties exhibit nuclear atypia, increased mitoses, and prominent vascularity

        5. Silver stain highlights reticulum fibers

    D. Diagnosis

        1. CT shows diffuse orbital enlargement without bony erosion

        2. A-scan ultrasound demonstrates minimal internal reflectivity

    E. Indications

        1. Proptosis

        2. Cosmesis

        3. Strabismus

    F. Treatment

        1. Total excision taking care not to rupture capsule

        2. Irradiation if question about completeness of excision

        3. Regular postop follow-up to detect any recurrences

    G. Complications

        1. Recurrence after incomplete removal

XXXI. DERMOID

    A. Epidemiology

        1. Congenital tumor but may not be manifest at birth

        2. Most common orbital tumor of childhood

        3. 90% present in the first decade and are located anterior to the orbit along the superotemporal orbital rim. They may be fixed to the zygomaticofrontal suture.

        4. Only 3 to 7% are deep-seated lesions. These present in adulthood and are located in the superotemporal orbit.

    B. Clinical Features

        1. Firm, painless, minimally mobile mass over the lateral brow

        2. Downward globe displacement and diplopia

        3. Ptosis

        4. Proptosis

        5. Decreased tear production if lacrimal gland involved

    C. Pathology

        1. Congenital choristoma arises from ectoderm that became isolated along bony sutures during fetal development

2. Epidermal tissue combined with one or more dermal appendages (hair follicles, sebaceous or sweat glands)
3. Cyst wall composed of keratinized, stratified squamous epithelium. Cyst lumen contains keratin debris.
4. Pedicle attachment to periorbita, or in posterior lesions, attachment to dura can be seen

D. Diagnosis
1. CT shows well-defined, thin-walled cyst. Deep orbital dermoids erode and enlarge surrounding bone. Calcium may be seen around or within the cyst. There can be intracranial extensions. Contents are fatty, and nonenhancing ultrasound reveals smooth contours, good sound transmission, and variable internal echo amplitudes.

E. Indications for Surgery
1. Amblyopia
2. Diplopia
3. Cosmesis
4. Diagnosis

F. Treatment
1. Important to preserve capsule because inadvertent rupture incites exuberant postoperative granulomatous inflammation
2. Approach anterior orbital rim lesions transcutaneously. If a pedicle is present, cut and remove it
3. Deep orbital tumors, depending on location, are approached from a superonasal anterior or later orbitotomy. The capsule is difficult to completely excise in posterior lesions.
4. Adjuvant intraoperative chemical and thermal cautery, or CO_2 laser treatment may help destroy any remaining cyst wall

G. Complications—orbital
1. Inflammation from ruptured cyst

XXXII. ORBITAL FIBRO-OSSEOUS TUMORS

A. Epidemiology
1. Osteoma
a. rare
b. most common bony orbital tumor
c. onset can range from teens to late sixties
d. invades orbit from paranasal sinuses, commonly frontal

      e. can be associated with familial polyposis and intestinal adenocarcinoma

  2. Osteosarcoma

      a. second most common primary bone malignancy behind multiple myeloma

      b. most common primary bone malignancy in young patients

      c. 70% diagnosed by age 20

      d. many orbital tumors arise after radiation for retinoblastoma

      e. may arise in areas of chronic osteomyelitis, Paget's disease, and previous fracture in orbit

  3. Chondrosarcoma

      a. rare before age 20

      b. more common in females

      c. presents in medial orbit

      d. often bilateral

      e. tumors in the orbit represent secondary invasion from a primary site in the medial orbital wall, nasopharynx, or nasal septum

  4. Fibrous dysplasia

      a. unknown etiology

      b. histologically benign but locally aggressive

      c. two thirds present by age 10

      d. rapid growth seen during pubertal growth spurts

      e. growth ceases in adulthood

      f. may affect one bone (monostotic) or many (polyostotic)

      g. 85% of patients have pathologic long-bone fractures

  5. Paget's disease (osteitis deformans)

      a. unknown etiology

      b. commonly seen in sixth and seventh decades

      c. affects skull, pelvis, and lumbosacral spine

B. Clinical Features

  1. Osteoma

      a. slow growth

      b. exophthalmos

      c. globe displacement away from tumor

      d. nasolacrimal duct obstruction

      e. epiphora

      f. conjunctival chemosis

      g. headache

      h. decreased vision

      i. optic atrophy

  2. Osteosarcoma

      a. presents as a palpable mass in an anophthalmic socket 5 to 20 years after orbital radiation
- **3.** Chondrosarcoma
  - **a.** proptosis
  - **b.** temporal globe displacement
  - **c.** nasal obstruction
  - **d.** sinus disease
  - **e.** intracranial extension (typically fatal)
- **4.** Fibrous dysplasia
  - **a.** painless, progressive facial deformation
  - **b.** occipital hypertrophy
  - **c.** globe displacement away from involved orbital wall
  - **d.** sinus obstruction
  - **e.** nasolacrimal duct obstruction
  - **f.** mucocele formation
  - **g.** metabolic derangements from sella turcica involvement
- **5.** Paget's disease
  - **a.** facial enlargement
  - **b.** increased head circumference
  - **c.** proptosis
  - **d.** ptosis
  - **e.** diplopia
  - **f.** retinal hemorrhages
  - **g.** choroidal sclerosis
  - **h.** angioid streaks
  - **i.** optic atrophy
- **C.** Pathology
  - **1.** Osteoma
    - **a.** mature bone with fibrous stroma molds to surrounding uninvolved bone
  - **2.** Osteosarcoma
    - **a.** anaplastic sarcoma with prominent vascularity and varying degrees of osteoid and cartilaginous fibrous tissue
  - **3.** Chondrosarcoma
    - **a.** richly cellular and undifferentiated mesenchymal cells and well-differentiated hyaline cartilage. Chondrocytes show atypia, marked cellularity, hyperchromatic nuclei, and calcium deposition.
  - **4.** Fibrous dysplasia
    - **a.** gritty texture on gross exam. Lamellar bone of trabecula is replaced with woven bone, often in a C-shape. Stroma is richly vascular with varying amounts of fibrous and osteoid tissue.
  - **5.** Paget's disease

      a. normal bone replaced by a process of destructive deossification, reactive hyperplasia, and sclerosis

D. Diagnosis is made by clinical exam combined with the following findings on neuroimaging:
  1. Osteoma
    a. well-circumscribed, dense calcific lesion of posterior orbit, frontal or ethmoid sinus
  2. Osteosarcoma
    a. sclerotic, lytic, calcified tumor
  3. Chondrosarcoma
    a. irregular bony erosion and calcification
  4. Fibrous dysplasia
    a. diffuse bony sclerosis with ground glass appearance on plain films. Radiolucent lesions of frontal and parietal bones. Increased density of greater and lesser wings of sphenoid. Thickened occiput.
  5. Paget's disease
    a. mottled, lytic lesion

E. Treatment
  1. Osteoma
    a. observation
    b. complete excision is performed when visual function is threatened, or intracranial extension is documented
  2. Osteosarcoma, chondrosarcoma, fibrous dysplasia, Paget's disease
    a. there is no role for medical therapy. Surgical intervention is technically difficult and at best palliative. Clinical cure is virtually never possible in these diseases.

XXXIII. LYMPHOMA/REACTIVE LYMPHOID HYPERPLASIA

A. Epidemiology
  1. Presents in middle to late age
  2. Most orbital lymphomas are non-Hodgkin's B-cell tumors
  3. Diffuse growth pattern
  4. Benign and malignant lymphoid lesions are clinically indistinguishable

B. Clinical Features
  1. Slow progression
  2. Minimal proptosis

   3. Predilection for superior anterior orbit
   4. Occasionally presents as a salmon-colored conjunctival lesion
   5. Vision loss
   6. Diplopia
C. Pathology
   1. Lymphoma
      a. atypical mature lymphocytes
      b. growth pattern is either a diffuse proliferation or a follicular aggregation
      c. most cells are monoclonal B-cells with some reactive T-cells
   2. Reactive lymphoid hyperplasia
      a. mature lymphocytes
      b. unlike lymphoma, T-cells predominate with only 20 to 40% B-cells which are polyclonal
      c. may see germinal centers
      d. multiple cell types including fibroblasts, capillary endothelial cells, plasma cells, and eosinophils
      e. presence of atypia signifies a borderline lesion that should be followed closely
D. Diagnosis
   1. Orbital biopsy yields definitive diagnosis. Submit for immunohistochemistry, light and electron microscope.
   2. CT reveals irregular mass which molds to surrounding bone with no evidence of bony erosion
   3. Monoclonality is associated with malignant tumors
   4. Systemic workup is advised on all patients with lymphoid tumors since benign lesions can undergo malignant change
E. Treatment
   1. Lymphoma
      a. for isolated orbital disease, radiation with 2400 to 3000 rad divided 200/day, 5 day/week. Follow these patients closely for signs of systemic spread.
      b. for systemic disease, chemotherapy
   2. Reactive lymphoid hyperplasia
      a. radiation with 1000 to 2500 rad divided 200 rad/week, 5 day/week
F. Complications
   1. Radiation keratitis, cataract, and retinitis
   2. Radiation can retard orbital growth in children

XXXIV. METASTATIC ORBITAL TUMORS

A. Epidemiology
  1. Leukemia
     a. usually first decade of life
     b. all forms affect orbit
     c. may be bilateral
  2. Neuroblastoma
     a. most common metastatic orbital lesion in pediatric age group
     b. second most common orbital malignancy in children behind rhabdomyosarcoma
     c. presents in first decade, most often by age 4
     d. adrenals are primary site in 50%
     d. metastasizes to orbit more than globe
     e. predilection for zygoma
     f. poor prognosis with median survival at diagnosis 3.5 months
  3. Breast adenocarcinoma
     a. most common metastatic orbital lesion in adults
     b. may often present years after apparently successful eradication of primary tumor
  4. Lung adenocarcinoma
     a. second most common tumor metastatic to orbit
     b. often presents before diagnosis of primary tumor
  5. Other tumors that metastasize to the orbit are prostatic and colonic adenocarcinoma and melanoma.
B. Clinical Features
  1. Leukemia
     a. rapid onset of painful proptosis
     b. lid edema and chemosis
  2. Neuroblastoma
     a. unilateral or bilateral
     b. abrupt-onset proptosis
     c. eyelid ecchymosis
     d. lateral facial mass
     e. Horner's syndrome and heterochromia in congenital cervical ganglion tumors
     f. patients are extremely ill and debilitated
     g. two clinical presentations:
        1) Pepper variant presents in infancy, metastasizes to liver
        2) Hutchinson variant presents in older children and metastasizes to bone. Poorer prognosis.

      3. Breast adenocarcinoma
        a. proptosis
        b. pain
        c. may see enophthalmos due to fibrotic contracture of malignant orbital soft tissue
        d. choroidal and intracranial metastases
        e. papilledema
      4. Lung adenocarcinoma
        a. painful proptosis
        b. choroidal and intracranial metastases

C. Pathology
    1. Leukemia
      cellular infiltrate of atypical, immature lymphocytes
    2. Neuroblastoma
      undifferentiated embryonic cells of neural crest origin
    3. Breast adenocarcinoma
      adenocarcinoma with possible estrogen and progesterone receptors
    4. Lung adenocarcinoma
      adenocarcinoma cells

D. Diagnosis
    1. Leukemia
      a. CT shows irregular mass without bony erosion
      b. characteristic serum abnormalities
      c. biopsy
    2. Neuroblastoma
      a. CT shows poorly defined mass, and bony erosion, particularly of lateral wall
      b. increased urine levels of vanillymandelic acid (VMA) or homovanillic acid (HVA)
      c. biopsy
    3. Breast adenocarcinoma
      a. increased carcinoembryonic antigen (greater than 5.0 ng/ml)
      b. biopsy
    4. Lung adenocarcinoma
      a. radiographic evidence of pulmonary lesion
      b. biopsy

E. Treatment
    1. Leukemia
      a. systemic chemotherapy
      b. some role of orbital radiation for early, localized disease or optic nerve compromise
    2. Neuroblastoma
      a. orbit biopsy if needed for diagnosis. Chemotherapy is then begun, employing triple

therapy with cyclophosphamide, vincristine, and imidazolecarboxamide.
    b. if multiple metastases are present, local radiation and systemic chemotherapy are indicated
  3. Breast/lung adenocarcinoma
    a. metastatic disease is extremely poor prognostic sign
    b. treatment is palliative and consists of chemotherapy and local radiation
    c. for breast tumors with estrogen or progesterone receptors, hormone therapy may benefit
  F. Complications
    1. Radiation and chemotherapy side effects
    2. Local radiation

XXXV. NONTRAUMATIC ORBITAL EMERGENCIES

  A. Preseptal Cellulitis
    1. Epidemiology
        most common in children; often concurrent upper respiratory infection or may occur after minor skin trauma to periorbital area
    2. Clinical Features
        a. visual acuity, pupillary reactivity, motility are all within normal limits; see generalized lid swelling, erythema, periocular pain in absence of proptosis, conjunctival chemosis
        b. may be afebrile or mildly febrile, with increased WBC count
    3. Pathology
        a. infection of the soft tissue anterior to the orbital septum, often with contiguous ethmoiditis or dacryocystitis
        b. *Staphylococcus* and *Streptococcus* species are common causes; *H. influenzae* infection is commonly seen in children less than 5 years of age; children less than 2, in particular, have a decreased antibody response to the *H. influenzae* capsular antigen; may have associated otitis, sinusitis, pneumonitis, or systemic infection; a well-demarcated purple-red skin discoloration is characteristic for *H. influenzae* infection
        c. anaerobic cellulitis is suggested by a history of trauma, tissue necrosis, crepitus, or a malodorous discharge from the affected area

4. Diagnosis
   a. clinical exam with attention to acuity, pupillary reactivity, motility, and degree of proptosis
   b. may have concurrent upper respiratory, facial, or sinus infection; consider CT scan if facial or sinus infection present or suspected; examine closely for a laceration, puncture wound, or evidence of a retained foreign body

5. Treatment
   a. culture any purulent material; warm compresses tid to qid to the periocular area may increase local blood flow
   b. children should generally be admitted to the hospital for IV antibiotics under comanagement with a pediatrician
   c. incision and drainage of any fluctuant or pointing abscess may be indicated
   d. older children and adults without systemic symptoms may be given oral antibiotics as outpatient (e.g., dicloxacillin); close follow-up, initially with daily examination, is indicated until the infection resolves; adults should receive IV nafcillin or oxacillin 1 to 2 grams q4 to 6 hours in moderate to severe infections; children should receive cefuroxime 100 mg/kg/day IV in three divided doses if *H. influenzae* infection is suspected
   e. if little or no response to systemic antibiotics, then get CT scan and look for evidence of abscess formation or orbital extension of the infectious process

B. Orbital Cellulitis
   1. Epidemiology
      a. may be due to contiguous sinusitis, especially in children; other etiologic factors include penetrating orbital trauma with or without foreign body, midfacial trauma with paranasal sinus fracture, contiguous lid or facial infection, or septic emboli from infected teeth, heart valves, bladder, or other sites, recent orbital surgery (especially with placement of an orbital implant)
      b. there may be a history of sinusitis, dacryocystitis, or trauma
   2. Clinical Features
      a. see proptosis, motility defects and pain on eye movement, decreased visual acuity, af-

ferent pupillary defect, decreased sensation in distribution of first division of trigeminal nerve, retinal vein engorgement, choroidal folds, disc edema

b. often febrile with increased WBC, chills, malaise, rhinorrhea, concurrent URI in children; may have bacteremia or full-blown sepsis, therefore aggressive management is indicated when systemic signs are present

3. Pathology

a. thin or frankly defective ethmoid walls may allow rapid spread of infection from adjacent sinuses due to lack of orbital lymphatics and valveless orbital veins

b. fungal orbital cellulitis is rare except in the immunocompromised

4. Diagnosis

a. clinical exam and CT scan (with contrast); scan may show well-defined intraorbital or subperiosteal abscess or more diffuse inflammatory process; abscess enhances with contrast

b. differential diagnosis of acute inflammatory proptosis includes preseptal cellulitis, inflammatory pseudotumor, rhabdomyosarcoma (in children)

c. often polymicrobial infection, including anaerobes in adults; anaerobes may predominate when chronic sinusitis coexists; in adults may culture *Staphylococcus, Streptococcus, E. coli, Pseudomonas;* in children see *H. influenzae, Staphylococcus, Streptococcus*

5. Treatment

a. hospitalize all pediatric cases for IV antibiotics and close observation for clinical deterioration (as often as q2 to q4 hours initially); monitor acuity, pupillary response, motility, confrontation fields, and degree of proptosis; culture and Gram stain any orbital or sinus discharge; monitor mental status and check for signs of meningeal irritation; the ocular surface should be lubricated if significant proptosis is present

b. a diffuse cellulitis may be treated with intravenous antibiotics and close observation for clinical deterioration; orbital or subperiosteal abscess requires surgical drainage; in mild cases, cefuroxime 1 to 2 grams q6 to 8 hours in adults (in children 100 mg/kg/day in three divided doses) may be used; in severe cases, oxacillin or nafcillin 1 to 2 grams q4 to 6 hours (pediatric dose 100 mg/kg/day divided into four doses), combined with a third generation cephalosporin or chloramphenicol 100 mg/kg/day divided into four doses

c. development of decreased vision or pupillary abnormalities despite appropriate antibiotic therapy are indications for surgical drainage

d. permanent visual deficits are more common in adults; adults more often develop subperiosteal abscess and require open surgical drainage

e. blood cultures and pediatric or medical consultation are indicated if systemic toxicity is present; an ENT or neurology consultation should be obtained as appropriate

f. unchecked infection may lead to cavernous sinus thrombosis; CNS toxicity, headache, nausea/vomiting, cranial nerve palsies, coma, and death

C. Orbital Mucormycosis

uncommon but potentially lethal fungal infection that may have fulminant course

1. Epidemiology
   a. primarily affects diabetics (especially in metabolic acidosis) and immunocompromised patients; only rarely seen in healthy adults
   b. may be increasing in prevalence due to prolonged survival of debilitated patients
   c. often has preceding or concurrent bacterial infection, either locally or systemically
   d. high mortality (70% in one case series) due to aggressive, invasive infection, and underlying condition of affected patients

2. Clinical Features
   a. initially see sinusitis, rhinorrhea, facial or orbital pain; later see proptosis, decreased vision (secondary to central retinal artery occlusion or ischemic optic neuropathy), ophthalmoplegia, chemosis, orbital apex syndrome, cavernous sinus thrombosis
   b. ultimately invades brain and may cause obtundation, convulsions, hemiplegia, coma, and death

      c. black necrotic skin lesions are the classic sign of mucormycosis but are usually seen after the onset of the previous signs and symptoms

  3. Pathology

      a. infection by fungi of the order *Mucorales,* nonseptate fungi found ubiquitously in air, soil, and vegetable matter

      b. spores usually inhaled and colonize naso- and oropharynx and germinate as hyphae; characteristically invades and occludes blood vessels, particularly arteries, causing thrombotic vasculitis and ischemic necrosis; necrotic tissue is then further colonized and the infection spreads rapidly to sinuses, orbit, and CNS

  4. Diagnosis

      a. clinical suspicion and early diagnosis are critical; suspect in any patient with risk factors and progressive orbital pain, swelling and sinusitis

      b. hyphae can usually be demonstrated in biopsy specimens of nasal or paranasal sinus mucosa, palate, or skin

      c. black skin eschar is nearly pathognomonic for mucormycosis

  5. Treatment

      a. stat CT scan, ENT consult are required to perform nasal and sinus endoscopy and obtain material for biopsy and culture

      b. wide surgical debridement, often necessitating orbital exenteration

      c. intravenous amphotericin B and local irrigation (1 mg/ml solution) at the time of surgery

      d. infectious disease consultation, control of ketoacidosis (if present)

      e. parenteral antibiotic therapy for any concurrent bacterial infection

D. Acute Dacryocystitis

  1. Epidemiology

      a. bimodal distribution:

        1) infants with congenitally imperforate nasolacrimal duct (at the valve of Hasner); present in 2 to 5% of all births and is bilateral in up to one third of cases

        2) middle-aged and elderly (with female preponderance) with acquired nasolacrimal duct stenosis; also may be seen after trauma, particularly nasal and medial orbital wall fractures; often there is history of recurrent discharge, epiphora, chronic blepharoconjunctivitis

2. Clinical Features
   a. pain, redness, edema over medial canthal area, distended lacrimal sac, purulent discharge from puncta, epiphora; may be febrile, especially in children
3. Pathology
   a. infection of lacrimal sac associated with obstructed tear outflow and tear stasis; common organisms are *Staphylococcus* and *Streptococcus*
   b. obstruction of the nasolacrimal duct with a dacryolith (calcified epithelial cells and debris) may be associated with infection with the filamentous bacterium *Actinomyces israelii* or chronic use of topical medications such as epinephrine
   c. complications include mucocele or fistula formation, infectious keratitis, or orbital cellulitis
4. Diagnosis
   a. see pain, redness, purulent discharge from puncta upon gentle sac pressure; occasionally fluctuant abscess over medial canthus; history of trauma, previous nasolacrimal surgery
   b. a mass extending above the medial canthal tendon or bloody discharge from the puncta are suspicious for a lacrimal sac tumor (e.g., papilloma, adenoma, or carcinoma)
5. Treatment
   a. definitive therapy is restoration of lacrimal outflow through probing (infants) or silicone intubation or dacryocystorhinostomy (DCR) (infants to adults); infants may be successfully probed until age 12 months; thereafter probing is less effective and silicone intubation should be attempted
   b. acute dacryocystitis in young children due to congenital obstruction should be treated with probing
   c. acute dacryocystitis in adults can be treated acutely with DCR—but if it is severe and fluctuant, it can be drained, treated with antibiotics, and then a DCR can be performed
   d. if acute dacryocystitis in adults is not fluctuant, antibiotics can be used to treat the infection and then a DCR can be performed

E. Acute Proptosis in Children
always a frightening and alarming event; requires immediate, careful, and thorough workup
  1. Differential diagnosis
  a. orbital cellulitis—most common cause of acute proptosis in children; important to suspect contiguous ethmoiditis; often systemically ill and may have meningitis or otitis media; see separate section
  b. inflammatory pseudotumor—may be bilateral in children; usually idiopathic; see separate section
  c. rhabdomyosarcoma—most common malignant primary orbital tumor in children; must be diagnosed and treated promptly to spare vision and life; 70% of cases occur in first decade of life; present with acute proptosis, rapidly enlarging lesion, lid swelling and erythema; often a palpable mass present, especially superonasally; symptoms may be confused with orbital cellulitis or other orbital inflammatory disease; treatment consists of chemotherapy and radiation with 95% five-year survival
  d. orbital leukemia (granulocytic sarcoma)—rapidly developing proptosis (10% of cases bilateral) of first decade of life; occurs as variant of acute myelogenous leukemia; see frequent and early orbital involvement, chronic leukemias involve orbit late in disease and present with slowly progressive proptosis, often with leukemic optic nerve infiltration; treatment includes systemic chemotherapy and local radiotherapy
  e. retrobulbar hemorrhage—most commonly traumatic, occasionally due to spontaneous hemorrhage in vascular tumors such as lymphangioma or orbital varix; see separate section
  f. ruptured dermoid cyst—most common superotemporally; invaginated embryonic ectoderm proliferates and secretes keratin into cystic cavity; may burst spontaneously or with minor trauma with intense inflammatory response; therapy is steroids and surgical evacuation with removal of cyst wall to prevent recurrence
  g. neuroblastoma—most common metastatic orbital tumor in children; see acute unilat-

eral (60%) or bilateral (40%) proptosis, systemic disease (usually abdominal); 8% of cases present with eye disease as initial finding; CT scan shows an irregular, contrast-enhancing soft tissue lesion with adjacent bony destruction

    h. lymphangioma—slowly growing benign hamartomatous proliferation of lymphatic channels, presents acutely when bleeds spontaneously, often after minor trauma; CT or MRI shows low density cyst-like structures organized into lobules in intra- or extraconal locations; should be excised if optic nerve compromised or motility disturbance sufficient to cause strabismic amblyopia exists; may have concurrent conjunctival or skin lesions that suggest diagnosis

F. Acute Proptosis in Adults

  1. Differential diagnosis

    a. orbital cellulitis—see separate section

    b. inflammatory pseudotumor—see separate section

    c. metastatic cancer—most patients have known primary tumor at the time of orbital presentation; may be increasing in prevalence due to prolonged survival of cancer patients; most common primaries are breast (may cause enophthalmos), lung, prostate, GI; CT scan shows ill-defined mass which conforms to orbital structures, often with bony erosion; palpable mass may be present through eyelids

    d. thyroid orbitopathy—rarely causes acute proptosis; usually have preceding or concurrent systemic thyroid disease; may see periocular inflammation, injection over rectus muscle insertions, lid retraction and lid lag on downgaze or diplopia on upgaze; exposure keratitis, or compressive optic neuropathy in severe cases; CT shows fusiform muscle enlargement that spares tendon

    e. carotid-cavernous sinus fistula—high flow communication between carotid and cavernous sinus; seen post-trauma or spontaneously, especially in middle-aged or elderly females; see pulsating proptosis, pain, vascular engorgement, orbital bruit, increased intraocular pressure; differential diagnosis includes inflammatory orbitopathies such as cellulitis and pseudotumor; definitive diagnosis requires carotid angiography

f. orbital leukemia—almost always there is a history of chronic leukemia; may be seen in chronic myeloid leukemia or chronic lymphocytic leukemia with blast crisis

g. retrobulbar hemorrhage—most likely after trauma or surgery; see separate section

G. Chalazia/Hordeola

1. Epidemiology

   a. may be multiple and recurrent; may affect any age group; may be associated with ocular rosacea in older men

2. Clinical features

   a. often history of chronic blepharitis and prior excision of chalazia

   b. lid tenderness, pain, swelling, edema, often associated with blepharitis and acne rosacea; inspissated meibum may be seen along lid margins or occluding meibomian gland orifices

3. Pathology

   a. chalazion is a lipogranulomatous inflammation of meibomian glands within tarsal plate; a stye (external hordeolum) is an inflammation of glands of Zeis or Moll

4. Diagnosis

   a. history and clinical exam, presence of coexisting blepharitis

5. Treatment

   a. warm compresses for 10 to 15 minutes bid or as often as tolerated, with gentle massaging; lid hygiene with gentle debridement of lid margin with cotton tip applicator; antibiotic ointments (e.g., Bacitracin, Erythromycin, Neomycin qid) are helpful with underlying blepharitis

   b. tissue from any recurrent chalazion or atypical in middle-age or older should be sent to pathology lab to rule out sebaceous cell carcinoma; frozen sections stained with oil-red-O stain should be prepared; loss of lashes, involvement of both upper and lower lids, prior history of chalazion excision are all suspicious for sebaceous cell carcinoma

   c. may inject with steroid triamcinolone 40 mg/ml up to 1.0 ml if patient refuses surgery; may cause permanent depigmentation of lid skin

    d. surgical technique—consider surgical therapy if persists for 3 to 4 weeks despite patient compliance with medical regimen

    e. incision and curettage may be performed through transconjunctival or transcutaneous approach; because lesion is usually contained within tarsal plate, the transconjunctival approach is preferred, which also provides a better cosmetic result; the incision must be made vertically in order to spare the meibomian glands:

        1) evert lid, infiltrate anesthesia locally, and apply chalazion clamp

        2) incise at least 2 mm from lid margin directly over lid mass

        3) curette widely, breaking fibrous adhesions and attempting to remove remnants of pseudocapsule; do not remove normal tissue; no sutures are required with a transconjunctival incision

        4) continue compresses and antibiotic ointment postoperatively

    f. a transcutaneous incision directly over the inflammatory mass may be made horizontally, along the lines of relaxed skin tension; curette as above and close skin with interrupted 6-0 or 7-0 nylon sutures

H. Retrobulbar Hemorrhage

  1. Epidemiology

    a. trauma, intraoperative (after retrobulbar injection), postoperative (after blepharoplasty), rarely spontaneous (e.g., lymphangioma, cavernous hemangioma, varices, aneurysm)

    b. risk factors include systemic hypertension, atherosclerosis, and impaired blood clotting (e.g., aspirin consumption, thrombocytopenia, vitamin K deficiency)

  2. Clinical features

    a. acute proptosis, pain, increased intraocular pressure, motility defects, tense periorbital swelling and erythema; severe hemorrhage may cause decreased vision, afferent pupillary defect, visual field deficits; may see pulsating central retinal artery in impending central retinal artery occlusion

  3. Pathology

    a. extravasated orbital blood is confined by bony walls and orbital septum anteriorly; increased intraorbital pressure may cause ischemia of the small nutrient vessels that supply the optic nerve or the central retinal artery itself; uncommonly see nerve sheath hemorrhage

4. Diagnosis
   a. history, clinical exam; occasionally need to get CT to make diagnosis and define location and extent of hemorrhage; MRI is preferred if a preexisting vascular lesion is suspected

5. Treatment
   a. no treatment is needed if visual acuity is unaffected and intraocular pressure remains within normal limits using medical therapy (e.g., topical beta-blockers bid, Diamox 500 mg po bid); if hemorrhage has followed surgery, prompt evacuation of clotted blood and control of bleeding is mandatory if decreased acuity, decreased pupillary response, or increased IOP
   b. the surgical wound should be opened and evacuated, if present; lateral canthotomy followed by cantholysis should be performed next; if this fails, creation of a limited orbital floor fracture with a curved hemostat introduced at the lateral lower lid may allow drainage of blood into the maxillary sinus; if high intraorbital pressure still persists, then proceed to the operating room with surgical removal of the orbital floor or medial wall for direct observation and ligation of bleeding points
   c. there is value in treating patients even with no light perception, for some may have some return of vision if treatment instituted within 4 to 6 hours; attempt anterior chamber paracentesis to reduce IOP only if CRAO impending and lateral canthotomy/cantholysis is ineffective.
   d. consider optic nerve sheath decompression if nerve sheath hemorrhage is documented by CT scan, or ultrasound and decreased vision or APD present; there may also be value to intravenous methylprednisolone loading dose 30 mg/kg and then 250 mg qid for 48 to 72 hours followed by an oral steroid taper

I. Acute Inflammatory Pseudotumor
   1. Epidemiology
      a. equal sex incidence, except lacrimal form has 4:1 female predominance

      b. average age 40 years but may affect children and elderly

      c. a small number of patients may go on to develop Wegener's granulomatosis, lymphoma, or leukemia

  2. Clinical features

      a. most forms present with some degree of eye pain, red eye, and proptosis; may have diplopia due to mass effect of lesion or direct muscular involvement

      b. may classify according to area of involvement: apical—may have subnormal acuity and motility out of proportion to inflammatory signs; neuroimaging may show fluid in the optic nerve sheath

          1) anterior—globe may be prominently involved with secondary uveitis, scleritis, papillitis, exudative retinal detachment and decreased vision; neuroimaging may show thickened sclera adjacent to an irregular, poorly defined density

          2) lacrimal—acuity and motility generally good, may see characteristic S-shaped deformity of lateral upper lid

          3) myositic—pain on eye movement, local injection over muscle insertion, diplopia, ptosis; may simulate thyroid eye disease clinically; CT scan shows diffuse muscle enlargement involving muscle tendon in contrast to thyroid myopathy with fusiform enlargement and tendon sparing; inflammatory changes to adjacent orbital fat may leave an irregular muscle contour

          4) diffuse—multiple orbital structures affected with inflammation; may have any combination of the above signs

  3. Pathology

      a. generally idiopathic; if occurs bilaterally in an adult, should suspect and rule out systemic vasculitis or lymphoma; bilateral involvement in children is not unusual

      b. consists of aggregation of benign mononuclear cells including lymphocytes, plasma cells, and macrophages

  4. Diagnosis

      a. generally afebrile with normal white blood cell count

      b. differential diagnosis includes orbital cellulitis, ruptured dermoid cyst, hemorrhagic vascular lesion, scleritis/uveitis; in children must consider rhabdomyosarcoma, metastatic neuroblastoma, orbital leukemia

c. CT scan should be obtained in nearly all cases

d. may be difficult to distinguish histologically between polyclonal benign lymphoid proliferations and monoclonal malignant proliferations

5. Treatment
   a. rapid response is usually observed to steroids 1 mg/kg/day for 48-hour trial, then gradual taper if response; if no response, biopsy if indicated; biopsy-proven pseudotumor resistant to steroids may benefit from adjunctive radiotherapy
   b. recurrence is fairly common, especially in the diffuse variant

Essentials of Eye Care, edited by Rohit Varma.
Lippincott–Raven Publishers,
Philadelphia © 1997.

4

Strabismus

I. ANATOMY AND PHYSIOLOGY OF THE EXTRAOCULAR MUSCLES

A. Muscle Origins: The rectus muscles, the superior oblique muscle, and the levator muscle originate from the annulus of Zinn. The functional origin of the superior oblique, however, is the trochlea. The inferior oblique, the shortest of the extraocular eye muscles, originates from the maxilla near the nasolacrimal canal.

B. Muscle Insertions: The recti insert onto the globe in the spiral of Tillaux (medial rectus [MR] 5.5 mm, inferior rectus [IR] 6.5 mm, lateral rectus [LR] 6.9 mm, and superior rectus [SR] 7.7 mm, posterior to the limbus, respectively). The superior oblique tendon inserts underneath and about 4 mm posterior to the insertion of the superior rectus, extending to about 14 mm posterior to the limbus. The inferior oblique muscle inserts beneath the lateral rectus into the posterior globe, extending close to the macula.

C. Definitions:

1. **Agonist:** the primary muscle moving the eye in a given direction

2. **Synergist:** a muscle which acts with the agonists to produce a given movement (e.g., for intorsion, the superior oblique and the superior rectus are synergists)

3. **Antagonist:** a muscle which acts in the direction opposite to that of the agonist (e.g., the left MR is the antagonist to the left LR)

4. **Hering's Law of Equal Innervation of Yoke Muscles** states that synergistic muscles are stimulated equally.

5. **Sherrington's Law of Reciprocal Innervation** states that contraction of a muscle is accompanied by decreased (reciprocal) contraction of the antagonist muscle.

6. **Ductions:** eye movements examined monocularly

7. **Versions:** conjugate binocular eye movements (for example, gaze left)
8. **Vergences:** disconjugate binocular eye movements (for example, convergence to a near target)

II. DEVIATIONS

A. Definitions:
   1. **Phoria:** a latent deviation controlled by fusional mechanisms
   2. **Tropia:** a manifest deviation resulting in misalignment of the eyes which exceeds fusional control
   3. **Comitant deviation:** a deviation which is constant across all directions of gaze and with either eye fixating
   4. **Incomitant deviation:** a deviation which varies with position of gaze or with change of fixating eye; usually paralytic or restrictive
   5. **Primary deviation:** deviation measured with non-paretic eye fixating
   6. **Secondary deviation:** deviation measured with paretic eye fixating; is larger than the primary deviation as a consequence of Hering's law

III. BINOCULAR VISION

A. Definitions:
   1. **Corresponding retinal areas:** retinal areas in the two eyes which, when stimulated simultaneously, result in the sensation that the stimulus has come from the same direction in space
   2. **Normal retinal correspondence:** when corresponding retinal areas in the two eyes share identical relationships to the fovea in each eye
   3. **Empirical horopter:** the locus of points in space which stimulate corresponding retinal areas and thus, are seen singly
   4. **Panum's area of single binocular vision:** the area within which objects stimulating disparate retinal areas are still seen singly. Objects outside of Panum's area are seen as coming from different visual directions and elicit diplopia.
   5. **Fusion:** simultaneous stimulation of corresponding retinal areas which results in cortical unification
      a. sensory—corresponding retinal points project to the same locus in the visual cortex
      b. motor—vergence movement which prevents diplopia by causing similar retinal images to fall on corresponding retinal areas

6. **Stereopsis:** relative ordering of visual objects in depth which occurs when retinal disparity is too great to permit fusion of two visual directions, but not great enough to elicit diplopia

IV. EXAMINATION OF THE PEDIATRIC PATIENT

A. Visual Acuity:
  1. Birth—blinks to bright light
  2. 3 months—fixation behavior is central, steady, and maintained (CSM)
     a. central—light reflex is central or paracentral on the pupil
     b. steady—no nystagmoid movements in fixing eye
     c. maintained—maintenance of fixation with an eye when converting from monocular to binocular conditions
  3. Infants—monocular occlusion fixation behavior, Teller cards (forced choice preferential looking)
  4. 2 yrs—picture optotypes (e.g., Allen pictures), matching identification with letter optotypes (e.g., HOTV)
  5. 3 yrs—tumbling E's
  6. 5 yrs—Snellen letters
  7. Ancillary acuity tests
     a. optokinetic nystagmus (OKN) drum
     b. visual evoked potentials (VEP)—only test that does not require an intact efferent system for acuity assessment
B. Binocular Sensory Testing:
  All tests of binocular function should be performed prior to occlusion of either eye.
  1. **Titmus stereo testing:** Different images are presented to the two eyes using polarized targets and spectacles. These images are stereo pairs with varying degrees of disparity. The patient's stereopsis is quantitated by noting the smallest amount of disparity which the patient can detect.
     a. fly: 3000 seconds of arc
     b. animals: (3) 400, 200, and 100 seconds of arc
     c. circles: (9) 800 to 40 seconds of arc
  2. **Randot stereo testing:** also measures stereopsis, without the monocular clues present in the Titmus test. Includes shapes, animals, and circles.
  3. **Worth 4-dot testing:** assesses binocularity and determines suppression involving the peripheral retina (as the targets are relatively large) by dissociating the eyes' images with color filters. The

patient wears a pair of spectacles with a red glass over the right eye and a green glass over the left eye. The patient is then shown a four-dot image—two green, one red, and one white—at distance and near. Possible responses are:

a. four dots (normal)

b. five dots (diplopia)

c. two or three dots (suppression)

4. Bagolini's striated glasses: lenses with no dioptric power in which one lens has many striations oriented at 45° while the other lens has parallel striations at 135° meridian. Used to test for suppression and anomalous retinal correspondence.

5. Afterimage testing: for retinal correspondence is performed by flashing a vertical line with a central target in one eye (the deviating eye) and a horizontal line in the other (fixating) eye. The patient then draws the afterimages which he sees; the positioning of the afterimages indicates the retinal correspondence. In normal retinal correspondence the afterimages will form a cross, even if the patient has strabismus. In anomalous retinal correspondence, the lines do not form a cross—the afterimages appear to be separated.

6. Motor Testing:

ductions and versions

deviation: measured in the primary and secondary positions (25 to 30 degrees from primary gaze) of gaze, measured in degrees or in prism diopters (PD) (*not* in diopters!). A one-prism diopter prism deflects a ray of light one centimeter at a distance of one meter.

> Deviation in prism diopters =
> about 2* deviation in degrees
> (this relationship is accurate
> up to 45 degrees or 90 PD)

A and V patterns (incomitance) should be noted.

7. Hirschberg corneal light reflection test: The patient views an accommodative target approximately one-third meter away, and the examiner estimates the degree of deviation by the position of the corneal light reflex in the deviating eye (about 7 to 20 PD per mm of decentration). A reflex found at the pupillary margin represents a deviation of 15 degrees or about 30 PD; a reflex at the mid-iris stroma represents a deviation of 30 degrees or about 60 PD; and a reflex at the corneal limbus of the deviating eye would represent a deviation of 45 degrees or about 90 PD.

8. **Krimsky test:** Performed as the Hirschberg test; however, the examiner places a prism in front of the *fi* eye which centers the corneal light reflex of the deviating eye. This is more quantitative than the Hirschberg test.

9. **Prism and cover testing:** Type of test selected can detect phoria or tropia, depending on whether or not it dissociates the two eyes. In each case, prisms of increasing power are placed before one or both eyes until there is no movement of the eyes (no shift). The power of the prism equals the size of the deviation. Note that although a horizontal and a vertical prism can be stacked, two horizontal or two vertical prisms should not be stacked because the effects are not linearly additive. One prism may be placed over each eye instead.

   If the patient's spectacle lenses are greater than 5 diopters in power, the measured deviation cannot be considered the same as the actual deviation. The measured deviation measures larger than the actual deviation with myopic correction and smaller than the actual deviation with a hyperopic correction.

   a. **cover/uncover test:** Detects tropias or phorias; should be performed at distance and near for each eye. The patient fixates a target as a cover is placed over one eye while observing the opposite eye for movement. If the opposite eye moves to take up fixation, a tropia has been detected. If no tropia is seen, the cover is removed, and the covered eye is observed for a fixation movement, thus detecting a phoria.

   b. **simultaneous prism and cover test:** Measures tropia; the patient fixates on a target and the fixating eye is covered; at the same time an increasing prism is placed in front of the deviating eye until it stops moving.

   c. **alternate cover test:** Measures combined latent and manifest deviation (tropia plus phoria); should be performed at distance and at near, both with and without correction. The cover is placed in front of one eye and then alternated from one eye to the other. Prisms are placed in front of one eye until no movement occurs as the cover is moved.

10. **Parks-Bielschowky three-step test:**
    a. step 1: determine which eye is hypertropic in primary gaze
    b. step 2: determine whether the vertical deviation is greater in right or left gaze
    c. step 3: (Bielschowsky test) determine whether the vertical deviation is greater in right or left head tilt (45 degrees)
    d. IVth nerve palsy will classically show a hypertropia, worse with gaze to the opposite side and worse on head tilt to the same side.

11. **Lancaster red-green test:** A subjective test for deviations, including cyclodeviations. Useful in incomitant deviations. Eyes are dissociated with red-green glasses. The patient and the examiner face a screen with the examiner behind the patient. The examiner projects a red streak onto the screen. The patient aligns a green streak with the red streak so that the two streaks appear to be superimposed. The actual positions of the two lights on the screen are recorded in the diagnostic positions of gaze. The higher (or more intorted, etc.) streak represents the higher (or more intorted, etc.) eye.

12. **Maddox rod testing** can dissociate the eyes by color filter and isolate horizontal and vertical deviations by cylindrical lenses. The rod consists of a series of parallel cylinders such that a streak of light appears 90° to the orientation of the cylinders. The rod is placed in front of the right eye and the cylinders are oriented horizontally. The patient fixates on a white light. If the patient is orthophoric, the light will be seen intersecting the line created by the rod. If the image of the light and the line are crossed (i.e., the line is seen to the left of the white light), an exodeviation is present. If the images are separated but uncrossed, an esodeviation is present. The rod is then oriented vertically to identify a vertical deviation.

13. **Double Maddox rod** (one red and one white before the two eyes) testing in a trial frame can be used to measure subjective torsion (cyclodeviations) while gazing at a light.

14. **Indirect ophthalmoscopy** can be used to measure objective torsion. Normally the vertical position of the fovea is level with the lower third of the optic disc (or the upper third of the disc in the inverted image of the indirect ophthalmo-

scope). A higher fovea (lower in the indirect ophthalmoscopic view) represents intorsion and a
lower fovea (higher in the indirect ophthalmoscopic view) represents extorsion.
15. **Near point of convergence:** the patient fixates on
an object which is moved toward the patient until one eye loses fixation (normal less than 8 to
10 cm)
16. **AC/A ratio** (accommodative convergence/accom-
modation ratio). High AC/A ratio implies an esodeviation greater at near than at distance, or an
exodeviation greater at distance than at near.
Two methods for measuring the AC/A ratio are
available. The ratio determined by the heterophoria method tends to be larger than the gradient method. Normal ratios range from three to
six (prism diopters/diopter).
   a. **heterophoria method:** The deviation in prism
   diopters is measured with full distance correction at distance and at near. The inter-pupil-
   lary distance in centimeters (IPD) is measured
   or approximated. The diopters of accommodation necessary for the near distance is determined (D). Esodeviations are defined as positive and exodeviations as negative.

AC/A = IPD + (near deviation − distance deviation)/D

   b. **gradient method:** The deviation in prism
   diopters is determined at distance (Δ_1). A minus lens of power D (usually −2.00 sphere) is
   then placed in the spectacle plane and the deviation is redetermined (Δ_2).

$$AC/A = (\Delta_2 - \Delta_1)/D$$

V. ESODEVIATIONS

A. The eye is rotated such that the cornea is deviated
nasally and the fovea is rotated temporally. The
types of esodeviations are essential infantile esotropia, accommodative esotropia, and miscellaneous
esodeviations.
B. Differential Diagnosis: Sixth nerve palsy (unilateral
or bilateral), nystagmus blockage syndrome, sensory
esotropia, cyclic esotropia, Duane's syndrome type I,
spasm of the near reflex, thyroid myopathy, myasthenia gravis, medial orbital wall fracture, pseudostrabismus, Möbius' syndrome, consecutive ET.
C. Essential Infantile Esotropia
1. Esotropia developing by 6 months of age

2. Epidemiology:
   a. More common than exodeviations by 3:1, present in up to 30% of children with cerebral palsy and hydrocephalus; family history common
3. Clinical Features:
   a. commonly equal visual acuities with cross-fixation and alternating fixation; amblyopia may be present if no cross-fixation
   b. usually greater than 30 PD, equal near and distance deviations (normal convergence)
   c. normal refractive error for age (low hyperopia)
   d. associated features
      1) Dissociated vertical deviation (DVD)—75%, usually occurs after 1 year of age
      2) latent nystagmus—30%
      3) 1 to 2 diopters of hyperopia
      4) overaction of inferior obliques—75%, usually occurs by age 2 to 3 years
      5) accommodative esotropia—will develop in 25% of congenital esotropia patients by age 3 to 4 years
      6) abnormal monocular smooth pursuit
4. Treatment:
   a. prescribe full cycloplegic refraction, begin treatment of amblyopia if present
   b. if there is a residual deviation with spectacle correction, then consider bilateral medial rectus recessions
   c. goals of surgery: early restoration of binocular vision, expansion of visual field, restoration of normal eye contact with others
D. Accommodative Esotropia
   1. Clinical Features:
      a. onset at 2.5 years on average (range, 6 months to 7 years), initially intermittent
      b. amblyopia common, if not detected or treated early
      c. associated with significant hyperopia
      d. positive family history not uncommon
      e. three types:
         1) refractive—high hyperopia (+3.00 to +10.00 diopters, average +4.00 diopters) with normal AC/A ratio; moderate esotropia (20 to 30 prism diopters); distance and near deviations within 10 prism diopters of each other
         2) nonrefractive—esodeviation greater at near than at distance (high AC/A ratio); refractive error normal for age (average +2.25

diopters); near deviation 20 to 30 prism diopters with little deviation at distance; near deviation reduced by +3.00 spectacles

    3) combined—high hyperopia with moderate deviation at distance, greater deviation at near

2. Treatment:

    a. spectacle correction based on cycloplegic refraction; atropine 1% solution may be rarely used (for about one week) to help patient accept spectacles. If spectacles correct nearly all of the deviation and the patient has some degree of fusion, corrective lenses may be slowly reduced, as long as no tropia is induced.

    b. if near deviation exceeds distance deviation by greater than 10 prism diopters and patient fuses at distance, then prescribe bifocals (+2.50 to +3.00 add). If the deviation remains greater than 10 prism diopters at near, surgery should be considered to restore binocular function.

    c. long-acting cholinesterase inhibitors (echothiophate 0.125% solution for example) potentiate accommodation and thus lessen accommodative convergence; dose should be titrated to the minimum effective dose (begin with 0.06%). Complications include development of iris cysts and increased susceptibility to depolarizing agents which must be communicated to the anesthesiologist if the patient is to undergo surgery.

    d. treatment of amblyopia

        1) surgery: indicated for deviations greater than 12 PD

        2) bilateral medial rectus recessions; recession of medial rectus with resection of ipsilateral lateral rectus if significant amblyopia present

        3) prism adaptation (more commonly used for acquired, nonaccommodative esotropia): the patient wears the full hyperopic correction with Fresnel prisms to correct residual deviation for one to two weeks and then is reexamined; if the esodeviation increases, the prisms are increased until there is no further change. Surgery is planned to correct the full prism-adapted deviation.

        4) goals of surgery: restoration of binocular function, eliminate need for bifocals

        5) complications: approximately 20% of patients undercorrected, 10% overcorrected

E. Miscellaneous Esodeviations

1. Acquired, Nonaccommodative Esotropia
   a. cyclic esotropia
      1) rare; intermittent esotropia which occurs with a 48-hour cycle, often with a V pattern; may become constant with time
      2) amblyopia uncommon
      3) patients usually have normal binocular vision and good stereoacuity when the esotropia is not present
   b. treatment:
      1) prescribe full hyperopic correction if greater than +1.50 diopters
      2) surgery: for maximum deviation
2. Stress Induced Acquired Esotropia
   a. esotropia which results from breakdown of fusional divergence secondary to stress such as illness, emotional or physical trauma, or aging
   b. treatment:
      surgery usually required
3. Nystagmus blockage syndrome
   a. congenital nystagmus which is dampened by accommodation, resulting in convergence and variable esotropia based on presence or absence of fixation
4. Manifest latent nystagmus with infantile esotropia
   a. nystagmus which becomes manifest intermittently
   b. patients may adopt a head turn to place the fixating eye in adduction which is the null point of the nystagmus
5. Spasm of the near response
   a. intermittent episodes of accommodative spasm and miosis accompanying sustained convergence
   b. diagnosis made by horizontal versions—the patient displays convergent movement rather than a gaze movement while monocular duction is normal
6. Monofixation Syndrome
   a. small angle esodeviation (<10 prism diopters), suppression scotoma in the fixating eye with peripheral fusion, and amblyopia
   b. diagnosis: 4 PD base out test—a 4 PD prism is placed base out over each eye; as the prism is introduced, the nonamblyopic eye will make a small refixation movement toward the prism apex; on the opposite (amblyopic) eye, no movement, or only a slow sustained movement, will be seen
7. Consecutive esodeviation

      a. esotropia occurring after surgery for exodeviation

      b. often improves spontaneously if surgery is recent

      c. differential diagnosis:
          1) rule out slipped or lost muscle

      d. treatment:
          1) base out prism
          2) hyperopic correction
          3) miotics
          4) alternating occlusion (temporizing measure in acquired esotropia to prevent suppression)
          5) surgery—wait for 6 months after previous surgery before considering re-operation.

VI. SIXTH NERVE PARESIS

  A. Clinical Features:
      1. Incomitant esodeviation with increasing esotropia with gaze toward the paretic side
      2. Limited abduction of the affected side in paresis, absence of abduction past the midline in paralysis
      3. Usually associated with a head turn
      4. Amblyopia uncommon
      5. May be present at birth secondary to increased intracranial pressure during labor and delivery—often resolves spontaneously
  B. Differential Diagnosis:
      1. May occur spontaneously (children), secondary to inflammation or infection, after trauma, secondary to compressive lesions, or due to ischemia (adults)
  C. Evaluation:
      1. History looking for other neurologic and/or systemic symptoms
      2. Neuroimaging if neurologic symptoms or signs are present
  D. Treatment:
      1. Patching to prevent amblyopia in the deviated eye
      2. Fresnel prisms
      3. Botulinum toxin injection to the ipsilateral medial rectus—may prevent contracture of the MR and promote earlier rehabilitation
      4. Surgery—if no resolution after 12 months (except in patients with intracranial lesions); large recess/resect on the affected eye, or vertical muscle transposition if total paralysis present

VII. EXODEVIATIONS

A. Epidemiology:
  1. Less common than esotropias (about 1:3), onset from infancy to 4 years, often initially intermittent; congenital exotropia may be associated with neurological impairment; possible female preponderance, incidence is probably unrelated to refractive error.
B. Clinical Features:
  1. **Exophoria**—usually asymptomatic; asthenopia may occur with prolonged visual work; may be associated with A or V pattern or vertical deviation; amblyopia uncommon
  2. **Intermittent exotropia**—most common type of exodeviation; onset 6 months to 4 years; exodeviation intermittently controlled by fusional mechanisms; worse when sick, tired, or stressed, often without diplopia; hemiretinal suppression and anomalous retinal correspondence may occur; amblyopia uncommon; one-third are stable, one-third improve, one-third worsen with time
  3. **Basic exotropia**—distance and near deviations are equal; onset in infancy to 4 years of age, often older patients with a decompensated intermittent exotropia or sensory deprivation; often associated with oblique muscle overaction especially if angle of the deviation is large
  4. **Divergence excess**—deviation with distance fixation is larger than with near fixation; true divergence excess differentiated from simulated divergence excess when the near deviation is not increased by monocular occlusion for 30 to 40 minutes (to disrupt binocular fusion)
  5. **Convergence insufficiency**—deviation with near fixation is larger than with distance fixation; asthenopia; blurred vision at near; remote near point of convergence, may be secondary to accommodative insufficiency (Adies' syndrome, post head trauma, systemic illness such as multiple sclerosis)
C. Differential Diagnosis:
  1. Pseudostrabismus, intermittent exotropia (XT), basic XT, divergence excess, convergence insufficiency, sensory deprivation, consecutive XT, Duane's syndrome type II, third nerve palsy, orbital tumor or pseudo tumor, trauma, thyroid myopathy, myasthenia gravis, chronic progressive external ophthalmoplegia (CPEO), and internuclear ophthalmoplegia (INO). May be idiopathic, after neuro-

logical disease, fragile X syndrome, mental retardation, adrenoleukodystrophy, pseudoexotropia (positive angle kappa, wide interpalpebral distance).
D. Treatment:
1. Exophoria—no treatment
2. Intermittent and basic exotropia—treat amblyopia; minus lenses to stimulate accommodative convergence may be considered but also may induce myopia; base-in prisms to compensate for the deviation may be considered; alternate day patching to prevent suppression and create diplopia forcing convergence may be effective in some patients; orthoptic exercises to stimulate fusional convergence and diplopia awareness
3. Convergence insufficiency: orthoptic exercises (convergence training, e.g., base-out prisms to stimulate fusional convergence); base-in prism reading spectacles or bifocals with prisms; reading glasses without prisms for patients with primary accommodative insufficiency; if patient orthophoric at distance and prisms ineffective, perform bilateral medial rectus resections—operate for the near deviation
4. Indications for surgery: consider for intermittent exotropia if deviation progressing to increased frequency or increased magnitude (preferably not before age 3) or if the patient demonstrates a decline in binocularity; for manifest exotropia of >15 PD
5. Surgery: bilateral lateral rectus recessions (especially with divergence excess) or unilateral recess/resection; operate for the deviation at distance and aim for initial overcorrection

VIII. VERTICAL DEVIATIONS

A. More common in adults; nearly always incomitant.
B. Differential Diagnosis:
1. Dissociated vertical deviation (DVD), inferior oblique (IO) overaction, superior oblique (SO) overaction, SO palsy, IO palsy, double elevator palsy, Brown's syndrome, orbital floor fracture, inferior rectus (IR) paresis, thyroid myopathy, myasthenia gravis, chronic progressive external ophthalmoplegia (CPEO).

IX. DISSOCIATED VERTICAL DEVIATION

A. Elevation of either eye during periods of inattention or under occlusion; when the deviated eye returns to

primary position, there is no corresponding downward movement of the fellow eye (i.e., DVD does not
obey Herring's law). The etiology is unknown.

B. Clinical Features:

    1. Elevation, with abduction and extorsion of non-fix-
ating eye; constant horizontally, no A or V pattern

    2. Usually bilateral, often asymmetric

    3. Often associated with congenital esotropia

    4. May be associated with latent nystagmus

    5. May be measured with base down prisms in front
of the deviating eye, or graded as a slight to large
deviation (+1 to +4)

C. Treatment:

    1. Treatment of amblyopia—may improve the DVD

    2. Surgical treatment indicated if the deviation oc-
curs spontaneously, is frequent, and is cosmetically significant:

        a. superior rectus recessions, 6 to 10 mm, bilat-
eral surgery if patient fixates with either eye;
lid retraction may occur as a complication

X. INFERIOR OBLIQUE OVERACTION

A. May be primary or secondary to a superior oblique
palsy.

B. Clinical Features:

    1. Elevation of the adducting eye, incomitant across
horizontal (i.e., hyper on adduction greater than
on abduction); cross cover testing with the ad-
ducting eye fixating will reveal hypotropia of the
abducting eye (i.e., obeys Hering's law—helps to
differentiate from DVD)

        a. fundus extorsion

        b. V pattern

        c. often concurrent with DVD

C. Treatment:

    1. Surgical: inferior oblique recession or myectomy;
inferior oblique recession with anterior transposition if associated with DVD

XI. SUPERIOR OBLIQUE OVERACTION

A. Clinical Features:

    1. Hypotropia of the ipsilateral eye on adduction

    2. Fundus intorsion

    3. A pattern

    4. May be associated with horizontal deviations, of-
ten exotropia

B. Treatment:

1. Indicated for significant ocular deviation or A pattern (>10 prism diopters)
2. Surgical: superior oblique tenotomy or lengthening of the muscle by a nonabsorbable spacer or simple "chicken" suture
3. Complications include superior oblique palsy; patients with binocular fusion may develop torsional diplopia from SO tenotomy

XII. DOUBLE ELEVATOR PALSY

A. Etiology unknown, may result from a supranuclear defect
B. Clinical Features:
   1. Monocular elevation weakness on versions and ductions, both in adduction and abduction, with hypotropia of involved eye that increases in upgaze
   2. Chin up head position
   3. Amblyopia in hypotropic eye
   4. May have ptosis or pseudoptosis
   5. May be unilateral or bilateral
   6. Inferior rectus muscle restriction with poor Bell's phenomenon
   7. Three types
      a. IR restriction—positive forced ductions, no muscle paralysis (by forced generations testing), normal SR saccade
      b. elevator weakness—negative forced ductions, elevator muscle paralysis, reduced upward saccadic velocities
      c. combination—positive forced ductions, muscle paralysis, and abnormal saccades
C. Treatment:
   1. Surgical: indicated if large vertical deviation or ptosis in primary position or unacceptable head position. If IR restriction present, then IR recession performed; otherwise, transposition of MR and LR towards SR insertion (Knapp procedure) performed.

XIII. BROWN'S SYNDROME

A. Etiology unknown, but may be due to a primary anomaly or due to mechanical restriction secondary to inflammation or scarring of the superior oblique tendon.
   1. May be congenital or acquired, occasionally familial. Bilateral in 10%.
B. Differential Diagnosis:

1. Paralysis of the inferior oblique, orbital floor fracture
   C. Clinical Features:
      1. Limited elevation in adduction, with better elevation in abduction
      2. Restriction of passive elevation on forced duction
      3. Exotropia in upgaze (V pattern)
      4. Hypotropia in primary position and/or abnormal head posture
      5. Acquired cases may improve spontaneously
   D. Treatment:
      1. Surgical: indicated for large hypotropia in primary gaze or unacceptable head posture—superior oblique tenotomy, or superior oblique weakening with spacer or "chicken" suture
      2. Complication: superior oblique palsy

XIV. SUPERIOR OBLIQUE PALSY

   A. Most common form of paralytic strabismus; decompensated congenital IVth nerve palsy occurs most often, followed by post-traumatic, idiopathic, and rarely neurologic.
   B. Differential Diagnosis:
      1. Must rule out bilateral superior oblique palsy—usually associated with V-pattern esotropia, greater than 15° extorsion, positive Bielschowsky head tilt test to both sides, and limited ductions of both superior oblique muscles
   C. Clinical Features:
      1. If patient fixating the nonparetic eye, a hypertropia of the involved eye will be present; if patient fixates with the paretic eye, a hypotropia of the opposite eye will be present
      2. Head tilt toward side opposite paretic muscle
      3. Fundus extorsion
      4. Often IO overaction
   D. Evaluation:
      1. Bielschowsky head tilt test, double Maddox rod test (<10 degrees in downgaze implies unilateral, >15 degrees implies bilateral), examination of old photos for head tilt to determine duration; vertical fusional amplitudes (often large with congenital palsies), Lancaster red-green testing
   E. Treatment:
      1. Prisms or patching to avoid diplopia (prisms effective for small, comitant deviations with minimal torsional component)

2. Surgical: indicated for cosmetically unacceptable head position, large vertical deviation, diplopia not alleviated by prisms

Surgical Approach to Superior Oblique Palsy

Ipsilateral IO Overaction	Deviation in Primary Position	Surgical Procedure
present	<15 PD	weaken ipsilateral IO
present	>15 PD	weaken ipsilateral IO weaken contralateral IR
absent		weaken contralateral IR if ipsilateral depression limited weaken ipsilateral SR
present	>35 PD	weaken ipsilateral IO +/− tuck SO vertical rectus surgery

a. SO tuck best for bilateral SO paresis, or when deviation is greatest in downgaze to opposite side
b. If the deviation is primarily torsional, a Harada-Ito procedure is recommended—anterotemporal displacement of the anterior one-third of the SO tendon (does not correct vertical deviation in primary position)

XV. A AND V PATTERNS

A. Common (15 to 25%) in strabismic patients. Early onset small V pattern is often asymptomatic and may be a normal variant. A patterns are seen in SO overaction; V patterns are seen in IO overaction, Brown's syndrome, SO palsy, associated with Apert syndrome and Crouzon's disease.
B. Clinical Features:
1. Incomitant horizontal deviation which changes in amount from gaze 25 degrees above to 25 degrees below primary position; considered clinically significant if greater than 15 prism diopters for V pattern and greater than 10 prism diopters for A pattern
C. Treatment:
1. Surgical: indicated for clinically significant patterns to gain or improve single binocular vision or to correct an unacceptable head position; primary and reading positions are most important. Horizontal deviations in primary position should be addressed separately.

2. Options:
   a. IO myectomy or SO tuck (may correct 15 to 25 prism diopters of V pattern)
   b. SO tenotomy (bilateral surgery may correct 35 to 45 prism diopters of an A pattern)
   c. horizontal muscle transposition if no oblique dysfunction—MR towards direction of vertical gaze with greater esotropia (apex), LR towards direction of greater exotropia (empty space) [Mnemonic = MALE]

Surgical Approach to A and V Patterns

(In all cases bilateral rectus muscle recession with vertical displacement may be replaced by recess/resect with displacement of MR to apex and LR to base, but astigmatism may be induced)

Deviation	Overaction/Underaction	Surgical Procedure
V esotropia	IO overaction	Weaken bilateral IO and weaken bilateral MR
	No IO overaction	Weaken bilateral MR with downward transposition
V exotropia	IO overaction	Weaken bilateral IO and weaken bilateral LR
	No IO overaction	Weaken bilateral LR with upward transposition
A esotropia	SO overaction	Bilateral SO tenotomies and weaken bilateral MR
	No SO overaction	Weaken bilateral MR with upward transposition
A exotropia	SO overaction	Bilateral SO tenotomies and weaken bilateral LR
	No SO overaction	Weaken bilateral LR with downward transposition

XVI. MISCELLANEOUS SYNDROMES

A. Duane's Syndrome: Congenital syndrome characterized electrophysiologically by decreased firing of the LR on abduction and paradoxical innervation of the LR on adduction. Proposed etiologies include hypoplasia of the abducens nuclei and nerve, midbrain pathology, and fibrosis of LR; the LR may be innervated by a branch of CN III. Usually sporadic, but autosomal dominant inheritance occurs in 5 to 10%. Occurs more often in the left eye (75%) and in females; usually unilateral (80%). May be associated with hearing deficits, other ear malformations, spinal anomalies, and Goldenhar syndrome.

1. Clinical Features:
   a. type 1: (most common) marked limitation of abduction, slight or no limitation of adduction, narrowing of palpebral fissure secondary to globe retraction on adduction, and widening of palpebral fissure on abduction; vertical upshoot or downshoot of the eye with adduction; occasionally esotropia. Unilateral cases associated with head turn.
   b. type 2: marked limitation of adduction, less limitation of abduction, narrowing of palpebral fissure secondary to globe retraction on adduction, and exotropia in primary position
   c. type 3: marked limitation of adduction and abduction, with globe retraction on adduction; sometimes orthophoric in primary position
2. Treatment:
   a. correction of refractive errors and treatment of amblyopia
   b. surgical: indicated if there is a large deviation in primary position, or if there is an intolerable head turn.
      1) MR recession +/− LR recession to decrease globe retraction
      2) posterior fixation sutures may decrease upshoot and downshoot

B. Möbius' Syndrome: Gaze palsies suggestive of a lesion in the parapontine reticular formation (PPRF); agenesis of the VI and VII nerve nuclei have been seen.
   1. Clinical features:
      a. VI and VII nerve palsies, may be incomplete
      b. limited abduction and adduction, worse with versions than convergence
      c. orthophoric or esotropic in primary position
      d. poor eyelid closure
      e. mask-like facies
      f. associated with skeletal and orofacial malformations
   2. Treatment:
      a. treat amblyopia if present
      b. surgical: if deviation cosmetically significant—MR recession, unless adduction significantly limited

XVII. AMBLYOPIA

A. Unilateral or bilateral decrease in visual acuity not attributable to a structural abnormality of the eye or visual pathways. Incidence is 2 to 4% of population. May be associated with strabismus, anisometropia, isoametropia (in which case amblyopia may be bilateral), or image degradation (example, cataract).

B. Clinical Features:
   1. Decreased visual acuity
   2. Fixation preference
   3. Vision not as affected by neutral density filters as retinal diseases
   4. Crowding phenomenon—Snellen acuity worse if measured with a full line or chart of letters than when measured with single letters; may be due to increased receptive field of neurons in amblyopic eyes
   5. Color vision often normal
   6. No, or very minimal, afferent pupillary defect
   7. Often have deficient accommodation

C. Types:
   1. **Strabismic**—most common, amblyopia occurs in the deviating eye; acuity tested by grating detection better than that detected by Snellen chart
   2. **Anisometropic**—occurs when there is unequal refractive error resulting in a chronically defocused retinal image in one eye; hyperopic differences more amblyogenic than myopic differences; often detected at later age unless strabismus also present
   3. **Isoametropic**—bilateral decreased visual acuity due to large, symmetric, uncorrected refractive errors, usually greater than +5.00 or −10.00 diopters
   4. **Deprivation**—least common form of amblyopia; due to congenital or early onset media opacities, may also occur after excessive therapeutic patching in occluded eye

D. Histopathology:
   1. Reduced number and size of cells in layers of lateral geniculate nucleus and striate cortex corresponding to amblyopic eye. Animal models of amblyopia demonstrate that cells of the visual cortex lose their ability to respond to stimulation of the eye and/or the eye shows fixational deficiencies.

E. Treatment:
   1. Correct refractive error—usually full cycloplegic refraction
   2. Remove media opacity
   3. Limit use of the better eye to force use of poorer eye:

    a. full-time occlusion—patch one week per year of age of patient initially and reevaluate for occlusion amblyopia; reserved for patients where a constant strabismus eliminates chance of developing binocular vision

    b. part-time occlusion—patching time proportional to degree of amblyopia, with at least 1 to 2 waking hours per day of binocular vision

    c. penalization—degradation of optical image of dominant eye such that use of the amblyopic eye is favored while binocularity is maintained

        1) optical penalization—plus lenses which reduce the visual acuity in the better eye till the amblyopic eye is preferred for distance vision

        2) pharmacologic—atropine 0.5 to 1.0% solution, one drop each morning (or every other morning in blue-eyed children) in conjunction with the full cycloplegic refraction (ultraviolet light protection recommended). For milder cases, intermittent atropine penalization with drop in good eye one to two consecutive mornings each week.

4. Complications: occlusion amblyopia of sound eye due to patching; atropine may cause fever, flushing, nausea, allergy

5. Follow-up:

    a. evaluate at the end of each patching session for improvement of acuity of amblyopic eye, decrease in acuity of occluded/penalized eye. Goal is to achieve Snellen acuity that differs less than 1 line between the two eyes or spontaneous alternation of fixation. Once this is achieved, therapy may be titrated to patching 1 to 3 hours per day or that which preserves acuity; or mild penalization; continue maintenance therapy till age 8 to 10 years.

    b. once acuity stable, follow every 6 months

    c. if no progress after 3 to 6 months with good compliance, recheck cycloplegic retinoscopy (CRNS) and dilated fundus exam. If no significant changes, therapy may be discontinued.

XVIII. EXTRAOCULAR MUSCLE SURGERY

A. General Considerations:

1. When medial rectus surgery is performed, the amount of correction is planned based on the deviation measured at near, whereas the deviation measured at distance is used for lateral rectus surgery. Each millimeter of vertical rectus muscle recession yields about 3 prism diopters of vertical correction.

2. Anesthesia—general versus local, consider age (>15 years for local)
   local—4% lidocaine sub-Tenon's injection; avoid bupivacaine if adjustable sutures are to be used
3. Unilateral vs. bilateral—unilateral if densely amblyopic or poorly seeing eye
4. Adjustable suture—consider age, cooperation, reoperation (less predictable without adjustable)
5. Postoperative care: antibiotic-steroid drops or ointment are given for 1 week. Patients are generally evaluated for effect 6 weeks after surgery, at which time the alignment should be fairly stable
6. Forced ductions are performed at the beginning of every procedure

B. Recession of a Rectus Muscle:
1. Conjunctival incision is made in the fornix (e.g., inferotemporal to isolate the LR), approximately 8 mm from the limbus, a second incision through Tenon's capsule is dissected to bare sclera. A small muscle hook followed by a larger muscle hook is used to isolate the muscle. The muscle is freed from its attachments to Tenon's capsule and conjunctiva by sharp and blunt dissection. It is imperative to be sure that all insertional fibers are included on the muscle hook. Using a double armed 6-0 polyglactin suture, a central bite of muscle is taken 3 to 4 mm posterior to its insertion and the suture is tied. One arm of the suture is then used to take a partial thickness bite at the insertional corner; a full thickness bite follows from beneath the muscle, and this arm of the suture is tied, locking it at the muscle corner. The other arm of the suture is tied similarly at the other corner. The muscle is then disinserted from the globe. The muscle is refixated to the globe by passing each suture arm through the original insertion site, but the muscle is not pulled up to the insertion site; rather, the sutures are tied such that the muscle "hangs back" from the original insertion site by the desired amount. Alternatively, the sutures may be placed directly into the sclera at the site of the recession. The conjunctiva is smoothed over the area with a large muscle hook, excising protruding tags of Tenon's tissue.

C. Resection of a Rectus Muscle:

1. The muscle is isolated as for a recession (see above). Once the muscle is freed from its local soft-tissue attachments, it is isolated on two Jamison muscle hooks and the amount of resection is marked posterior to the insertion with the cautery. The double armed 6-0 polyglactin suture is then placed in the muscle as described above, approximately 2 mm posterior to the cautery mark, slanting the suture bites at the corner such that the suture exits in line with the cautery mark. The muscle is clamped along the cautery line with a small straight clamp for several seconds and then cut with the Wescott scissors. The anterior muscle remnant is then excised from the globe. Each arm of the suture is then placed through the sclera at the original muscle insertion site and the sutures are pulled up and tied to each other. The conjunctiva is smoothed over the area with a large muscle hook, excising protruding tags of Tenon's tissue.

D. Inferior Oblique Weakening:

1. The conjunctiva is incised in the inferotemporal quadrant and dissection is carried down to bare sclera. The lateral rectus muscle is isolated on a large muscle hook and retracted superonasally. The inferior oblique is isolated on a small muscle hook, while the assistant uses a small Desmarre's lid retractor to provide exposure. The fascial attachments are incised temporally and reflected over the muscle hook, and the muscle is freed from its soft-tissue attachment by sharp dissection, avoiding penetration of fat pockets. A small clamp is placed on the IO, 1 to 2 mm away from its insertion, and the muscle is then disinserted from the globe with Wescott scissors; the end of the muscle is cauterized. (For IO disinsertion, the procedure is completed here and the conjunctiva is smoothed over the incision.) The muscle is held with a small clamp more posteriorly while a double-armed polyglactin suture is placed through the end as described above. The muscle is sutured to the globe 2 mm temporal and 3 mm posterior to the temporal edge of the IR insertion (8 mm IO recession), or straddling the vortex vein (14 mm IO recession). The conjunctiva is smoothed over the area with a large muscle hook, excising protruding tags of Tenon's tissue.

E. Superior Oblique Tenotomy:

1. The SO is approached through a superonasal fornix incision. The superior rectus is engaged on a

large muscle hook and the globe is rotated
laterotemporally. The SO tendon is engaged on a
small muscle hook; the encapsulating membrane is
incised, and the tendon is transected. The conjunctiva is smoothed over the area with a large muscle
hook, excising protruding tags of Tenon's tissue.

F. Superior Oblique Strengthening:

1. A superotemporal fornix incision is made and the
superior rectus is engaged on a large muscle hook.
The SO is isolated on a small muscle hook and elevated. Using a small straight clamp, the muscle
is folded upon itself for the desired amount (usually till moderate resistance is felt) and secured
with two interrupted mattress sutures. An additional suture is placed at the apex of the tuck and
secured to the sclera along the line of action of the
muscle. The conjunctiva is smoothed over the
area with a large muscle hook, excising protruding tags of Tenon's tissue.

G. Complications:

1. Anterior segment ischemia (1:6000 cases, usually
after operating on three or more rectus muscles),
retrobulbar hemorrhage, endophthalmitis (rare),
orbital cellulitis, slipped muscle (decreased action), lost muscle (no action), scleral perforation
(less common with current spatula needles),
dellen, antibiotic toxicity, suture reaction, astigmatism (with a resection), diplopia, visual confusion, pain, nausea, vomiting, allergic reaction to
suture material.

Horizontal Rectus Muscle Surgery (Hang-Back Recession Technique)

Devia-tion (PD)	Esotropia			Exotropia		
	Bilateral MR Recession	*MR Recession*	*LR Resection*	*Bilateral LR Recession*	*LR Recession*	*MR Resec-tion*
15	3	3	4	4	4	3
20	3.5	3.5	5	5	5	3.5
25	4	4	6	6	6	4
30	4.5	4.5	7	7	7	5
35	5	5	8	7.5	7.5	5.5
40	5.5	5.5	8.5	8	8	6
50	6	6	9	9	9	7
60	6.5	6.5	9.5	10	10	8

Essentials of Eye Care, edited by Rohit Varma.
Lippincott–Raven Publishers,
Philadelphia © 1997.

5

Pediatric Ophthalmology

I. **NEONATAL CONJUNCTIVITIS (OPHTHALMIA NEONATORUM)**
   A. Purulent conjunctivitis occurring during the first month of life
   B. Epidemiology:
      1. Affects 1.6% of U.S. newborns and 7 to 12% worldwide
      2. Most common cause is Chlamydia trachomatis (Trachoma inclusion conjunctivitis—TRIC). Other causes are viral, bacterial, especially gonorrhea, and chemical.
   C. Clinical Features:
      1. Purulent discharge
      2. Lid edema
      3. Conjunctival hyperemia
      4. Occasionally preauricular adenopathy
   D. Differential Diagnosis:
      1. Chemical, chlamydial, viral and bacterial agents may cause ophthalmia neonatorum
      2. The period of time from birth until onset of symptoms may be helpful in diagnosing the causative agent:
         a. chemical (e.g., silver nitrate) occurs first 24 hours after drops and lasts 24 to 36 hours; usually mild with a watery discharge
         b. gonococcal occurs in 2 to 4 days with hyperacute onset and purulent discharge; Neisseria gonorrhoeae can rapidly penetrate intact epithelial cells and cause corneal ulceration; thus diagnosis should not be delayed
         c. staphylococcal or haemophilus occurs in 4 to 5 days
         d. herpes simplex occurs in 5 to 7 days
         e. chlamydia occurs in 5 to 14 days
   E. Pathogenesis:

1. N. gonorrhoeae and chlamydia contracted from maternal genital tract
2. Evaluation:
   a. smears and cultures should be taken from the palpebral conjunctiva and therapy begun immediately
   b. N. gonorrhoeae—gram-negative intracellular diplococci seen on Gram stain
   c. C. trachomatis—basophilic intracytoplasmic inclusion bodies in conjunctival epithelial cells, polys, or lymphocytes with Giemsa stain or fluorescent antibody staining
   d. bacteria seen with routine Gram stain
   e. herpes simplex virus—multinucleated giant cells on Giemsa stain
3. Treatment:
   a. based on clinical findings, and modified pending culture results:
      1) C. trachomatis—with systemic erythromycin 40 mg/kg/day in divided doses p.o. for 2 to 3 weeks; topical 10% sulfacetamide or tetracycline ointment 4 times a day for 3 weeks; must treat mother and her sexual partners
      2) N. gonorrhoeae—admit patient and treat with systemic penicillin G 50,000 units/kg IM or IV every 12 hours for 7 days and periodically irrigate eyes with saline; topical bacitracin ointment QID. Mother and her sexual partners must be treated.
   b. Current prophylaxis includes tetracycline and erythromycin ointment and povidone-iodine solution at birth
4. Complications:
   a. N. gonorrhoeae—corneal ulceration, perforation, rarely endophthalmitis. Occasionally associated with pulmonary infiltrates, meningitis, sepsis.
   b. C. trachomatis—conjunctival scarring, micropannus; rhinitis, nasopharyngitis, tracheitis; chlamydial pneumonia may develop at 3 to 13 weeks
   c. herpes simplex virus—chorioretinitis, encephalitis

II. THE BLIND INFANT

A. Evaluation of visual function in pediatric patient:
   1. Newborn: pupillary response to light; at several days, the infant should exhibit a blink reflex; skew deviation and tonic downward deviation may occur transiently

    2. 4–6 weeks, infancy: follow light of large objects; hold eye contact

    3. 3 months: fix and follow

    4. Childhood: visual acuity should be 20/40 or better by age 3 years

    5. Signs of poor visual development: constant deviation of one eye; nystagmus (onset at 2–3 months if secondary to decreased sensory input); wandering eye movements, lack of response to familiar faces, staring at bright lights, forceful rubbing of eyes (oculodigital sign).

B. Evaluation:

    1. History: birth trauma or history of prematurity, maternal drug use, infection, trauma or radiation exposure, family history of eye disease, exposure to oxygen

    2. Exam:

        a. ability to fix and follow with each eye individually

        b. pupillary exam

        c. ocular alignment and motility, nystagmus

        d. iris transillumination defects or anterior segment abnormalities

        e. detailed retinal exam

        f. cycloplegic refraction

        g. ERG, VEP, CT or MRI of brain, if etiology unclear

        h. If the exam appears normal, two diagnoses should come to mind: Leber's congenital amaurosis and achromatopsia. Both diagnosed with ERG.

C. Differential Diagnosis:

    1. Conditions often associated with nystagmus and decreased visual function:

        a. macular scars (e.g., toxoplasmosis)

        b. macular hypoplasia (e.g., albinism, aniridia)

        c. achromatopsia

        d. retinal degeneration, e.g., Leber's congenital amaurosis

        e. optic nerve hypoplasia

        f. congenital optic atrophy

        g. infantile nystagmus

    2. If strabismus present: must rule out organic lesion in the deviating eye (e.g., retinoblastoma)

    3. Other causes of impaired vision in infants and young children:

        a. microphthalmia

        b. anterior segment anomalies (Peter's anomaly)

        c. glaucoma

        d. cataracts

        e. toxoplasmosis, rubella, cytomegalovirus, herpes simplex, syphilis/congenital infection

   f. coloboma
   g. retinopathy of prematurity (ROP)
   h. X-linked retinoschisis
   i. delay in visual maturation—delayed visual development secondary to neurologic dysfunction
   j. cortical blindness—may have some visual function
   k. albinism
D. Treatment:
   1. Parental counseling with caution in giving hopeless prognosis
   2. Genetic counseling
   3. Information regarding educational services for the visually handicapped

III. LEBER'S CONGENITAL AMAUROSIS

A. A congenital rod-cone dystrophy that presents at birth or in the first few months and accounts for 10% of congenital blindness
   1. Infants are blind or nearly blind at birth
B. Clinical Features:
   1. Poor pupillary reaction to light
   2. Visual acuity ranges from 20/200 to bare LP
   3. Nystagmus presenting at 2 to 3 months
   4. Oculodigital sign common, possibly an effort to induce entopic stimulation of the retina
   5. Autosomal recessive
   6. Fundus exam may be normal, abnormalities include: a diffuse pigmentary change with tiny clumps of delicate bone spicules similar to those in RP; may be progressive
   7. Optic nerve pallor
   8. Attenuation of the vessels
   9. Cataracts
   10. Commonly hyperopic
   11. Macular coloboma
   12. Glaucoma
   13. Keratoconus
   14. Keratoglobus
       a. associations:
          1) cerebral anomalies with abnormal EEG, mental retardation
          2) microcephaly
          3) hydrocephaly
          4) seizures
          5) skeletal changes: acrocephaly, hemifacial hypoplasia, polydactyly, kyphoscoliosis, arachnodactyly, and osteoporosis
          6) deafness

7) renal anomalies

C. Evaluation:
1. ERG: nonrecordable or severely subnormal photopic and scotopic; must test both scotopic and photopic to distinguish from congenital stationary night blindness (CSNB) or achromatopsia
2. EOG: reduced

D. Histopathology:
1. Disorganized or absent rods and cones

E. Treatment
1. No treatment exists. Counseling of the parents in taking care of blind children. Referral to institutions that provide special education for blind children.

IV. ACHROMATOPSIA (ROD MONOCHROMATISM)

A. Stationary retinal dystrophy in which there is an absence of functioning cones in the retina

B. Clinical Features:
1. Autosomal recessive
2. Total color blindness
3. Reduced vision, 20/200 range
4. Nystagmus—may be less at near than distance
5. Marked photophobia in an attempt to keep rods dark-adapted
6. Vision better in dimly illuminated environments
7. Fundus exam is normal but an abnormal foveal reflex may develop with age
8. Small central scotoma can often be detected, peripheral field is normal

C. Evaluation:
1. ERG: normal scotopic response, abnormal photopic response to white light, red light, and flicker
2. EOG: normal

D. Histopathology:
1. Absence of cones; abnormally structured cones and rarely normal appearing cones; rods are normal

E. Treatment:
1. Correction of refractive error
2. Extra-dark sunglasses with side shields
3. Low-vision aids

V. CONGENITAL NYSTAGMUS

A. Nystagmus of all forms present at birth or within the first 4 months of life; congenital idiopathic nystagmus implies lifelong nystagmus of unknown etiology
1. Motor defect nystagmus—defect in efferent control; occurs shortly after birth. Not associated with ocular anomalies. Usually horizontal. No oscillopsia.

2. Latent nystagmus—nystagmus which occurs during monocular fixation; usually horizontal and conjugate, direction changes with change in fixating eye; associated with strabismus; etiology unknown

3. Secondary nystagmus—nystagmus secondary to afferent defect; loss of neural control of ocular function; associated with any cause of severely impaired vision at birth. Onset 8 to 12 weeks of age, severity proportional to severity of visual loss. Usually horizontal.

B. Epidemiology
   1. Usually sporadic, may be X-linked recessive, or autosomal dominant

C. Clinical Features
   1. Typically pendular, may be jerk; horizontal, vertical, circular, or elliptical
   2. Binocular
   3. Similar amplitude in both eyes
   4. No oscillopsia (illusion of environmental movement)
   5. Abolished in sleep (key feature of history)
   6. May have associated head oscillation
   7. Dampened on convergence
   8. Increased by fixation effort
   9. May have superimposed latent nystagmus (nystagmus seen only when one eye covered)
   10. Inversion of the optokinetic reflex, i.e., induced nystagmus in the opposite direction to that expected
   11. Increased velocity exponential of the slow phase on eye movement recording
   12. Uniplanar (usually horizontal) remains unchanged in all positions of gaze including vertical gaze
   13. Mild to moderately reduced visual acuity
   14. Null zone where nystagmus is reduced in amplitude and visual acuity best, often with a head turn
   15. Occasionally with high astigmatism
   16. May be associated with strabismus

D. Differential Diagnosis:
   1. Opsoclonus—irregular, repetitive, multidirectional eye movements, chaotic, stop during sleep, saccadomania
   2. Nystagmus associated with brain stem or cerebellar disease
   3. Post-viral encephalitis—nystagmus self-limited and benign
   4. Neuroblastoma—dancing eyes and feet
   5. Remote effect of visceral carcinoma in adults
   6. Spasmus nutans—triad of head turn (torticollis), head nodding, and nystagmus; begins first 12

months of life, usually resolves clinically by 2 years of age but is evident on eye movement recordings years later. Horizontal or vertical, pendular, low-amplitude, high-frequency nystagmus. May be unilateral or asymmetrical. Diagnosis of exclusion; obtain neuroimaging to rule out intracranial tumors. Etiology unknown.

   7. Central nervous system tumors
   8. Monocular blindness
 E. Treatment:
   1. Directed toward moving the null point toward the primary position of gaze
   2. Correct refractive error; contact lenses may minimize the effect of eye wiggling behind glasses
   3. Prisms oriented with base opposite to the direction of the null zone, or base out to induce convergence to maximize its nystagmus dampening effect
   4. Amblyopia therapy—usually pharmacologic penalization
   5. Surgery—indicated for head turn which is cosmetically or functionally unacceptable
   6. Kestenbaum procedure—eyes rotated in direction of head turn (away from the null zone) by bilateral, equal recession/resection to shift the null point to primary position; surgery modified if strabismus present

VI. PERSISTENT HYPERPLASTIC PRIMARY VITREOUS (PHPV)

 A. Congenital, nonhereditary, unilateral malformation of the eye caused by failure of the primary vitreous to regress
 B. Clinical Features:
   1. Unilateral leukocoria recognized soon after birth
   2. Microphthalmus, shallow anterior chamber with dilated radial iris vessels
   3. Vascularized retrolental membrane—may contain cartilage
   4. Intralenticular vessels
   5. Posterior cortical cataract often develops
   6. Nystagmus and strabismus common
   7. Dilated iris vessels
   8. Prominent, elongated ciliary processes
   9. Other complications: vitreous hemorrhage, retinal detachment, angle-closure glaucoma and phthisis bulbi
   10. Range of severity:
      a. mild—prominent hyaloid remnants, Mittendorf's dot, Bergmeister's papillae

  b. severe—progressive anterior chamber shallowing and angle closure glaucoma due to fibrovascular invasion of the posterior lens capsule and retinal detachment
 C. Differential Diagnosis:
  1. All causes of leukocoria
 D. Evaluation:
  1. History—rule out prematurity
  2. Ultrasound or CT to rule out retinoblastoma—retinoblastomas are almost never found in microphthalmic eyes
 E. Treatment:
  1. Goals: avoid glaucoma and phthisis bulbi
  2. Early enucleation causes failure of normal orbital development
  3. Eyes can be saved with early cataract surgery combined with membrane excision—limbal or pars plana/plicata; aggressive amblyopia therapy should be attempted
  4. Visual prognosis is poor but depends on severity of posterior involvement

VII. INTRAUTERINE AND PERINATAL INFECTIONS (TORCHS)

The TORCHS infections (i.e., TO—toxoplasmosis, R—rubella, C—cytomegalovirus [CMV], H—herpes simplex, and S—syphilis), as well as HIV and varicella may damage the developing fetus, and affect the eyes. Visual acuity may be decreased secondary to ocular involvement, encephalitis, meningitis, arachnoiditis, optic neuritis, and/ or chorioretinitis.

Infection may occur by hematogenous spread, ascending infection at the time of passage through the birth canal. Diagnosis is facilitated by the neonate's IgM antibody titers (elevated titer suggests an intrauterine neonatal infection as maternal IgM is too large to cross the placenta-blood barrier).

VIII. TOXOPLASMOSIS

 A. A protozoan, obligate intracellular parasite
  1. three forms: oocyst, tissue cyst, active or proliferative form
  2. affinity for the CNS, including the eye
  3. cats shed oocysts in their feces—humans ingest oocysts in raw meat
 B. Epidemiology:
  1. Common with (+) serology increasing with age—70% of obstetric population serologically (–), therefore at risk

2. 1/1000 newborns affected, 65% symptomatic, 15% have serious disease
3. The earlier in gestation the disease is contracted the more serious the outcome

C. Clinical Features:
  1. Nonocular findings:
     a. intracranial calcifications
     b. seizures
     c. hydrocephalus or microcephalus
     d. abnormal CSF
     e. anemia
     f. mental retardation
     g. jaundice, hepatosplenomegaly
     h. fever
     i. diarrhea/vomiting
  2. Ocular findings:
     a. necrotizing chorioretinitis, may be granulomatous
     b. bilateral
     c. frequently involves the macula
     d. inactive lesion is a flat scar
     e. active lesions develop near the scar, are white, elevated, and exude cells, protein in the vitreous
     f. microphthalmos and cataracts are rare

D. Evaluation:
  1. Antibodies—IgM in newborn diagnostic
  2. Indirect hemagglutination test and the indirect fluorescent antibody test
  3. RPR
  4. CxR
  5. PPD

E. Differential Diagnosis:
  1. Tuberculosis, syphilis, Coat's disease, retinoblastoma, presumed ocular histoplasmosis syndrome (POHS), congenital hypertrophy of the retinal pigment epithelium (CHRPE), traumatic scar, toxocariasis, Aicardi syndrome, Best's disease, fungal infection, cytomegalovirus retinitis

F. Treatment:
  1. Pyrimethamine—4 mg/kg loading dose, then 1 mg/kg bid for 2 to 4 days, then 0.5 mg/kg/day for 6 weeks
  2. Sulfadiazine—100 mg/kg/day in four doses for 6 weeks (daily dose not to exceed 4000 mg)
  3. Prednisone—1–2 mg/kg/day for 6 weeks (prednisone is only used if macula or optic nerve is threatened)
  4. folinic acid—3–9 mg IM q day for 3 days or 5 mg p.o. qd
  5. Clindamycin—3 to 4 week course
  6. Reactivation of treated disease always possible

IX. RUBELLA (GERMAN MEASLES)

A. Epidemiology:
   1. 10 to 15% of women of childbearing age are susceptible to rubella
   2. 50% of mothers with clinical evidence of rubella infection during the first 8 weeks of gestation will bear offspring with congenital malformations; lower incidence of congenital anomalies if infection occurs later in gestation, unusual if infection occurs after 20 weeks gestation
   3. Congenitally infected infants shed virus for several months or years after birth and may infect others

B. Clinical Features:
   1. Ocular findings:
      a. nuclear cataract in newborn period which is most dense centrally
      b. microphthalmos, uni- or bilateral
      c. chronic nongranulomatous iridocyclitis with focal necrosis of the pigment epithelium of the ciliary body
      d. congenital or infantile glaucoma (rarely occurs in eye with congenital cataract)
      e. transient opacification of the cornea independent of elevated IOP
      f. speckled appearance of the RPE—salt and pepper retinopathy—does not affect vision early in life
      g. iris hypoplasia, often slow to dilate
   2. Nonocular findings:
      a. congenital heart disease
      b. neurosensory deafness, which may be acquired and not congenital, most common defect
      c. encephalitis
      d. hepatosplenomegaly
      e. microcephaly and mental retardation in severe cases

C. Evaluation:
   1. Diagnosis based on clinical and laboratory findings
   2. Serologic diagnosis based on specific IgM and IgG antibodies
   3. IgM antibodies in the cord sera establishes diagnosis of fetal infection as it does not cross the placenta
   4. Pharyngeal swabs or lens aspirates for live virus (virus has been isolated in the lens material as late as 3 years of age)

D. Differential Diagnosis:
   1. Pigmentary retinopathy: syphilis; Leber's congenital amaurosis; radiation retinopathy; other viral diseases—measles, varicella, and influenza

E. Treatment:
  1. Cataract surgery at an early age especially if bilateral with special attention to possibility of severe post-op inflammation
  2. Careful monitoring of glaucoma
  3. Vaccination for future generations

X. CYTOMEGALOVIRUS (CMV)

A. Virus of the herpes family; infection of the fetus occurs from maternal viremia or contact with the cervix at birth
B. Epidemiology:
  1. 60–90% of women of childbearing age seropositive
  2. the most common intrauterine infection—0.5 to 2.5% of all newborns infected, but only 10 to 20% develop congenital abnormalities
  3. ocular manifestations uncommon
C. Clinical Features:
  1. Ocular findings:
    a. chorioretinitis—15 to 29% of severely affected infants; usually multiple and bilateral foci
    b. microphthalmos/anophthalmos
    c. cataracts
    d. keratitis
    e. optic atrophy/disc anomalies
    f. uveitis
    g. Peters' anomaly
    h. nystagmus
    i. strabismus
  2. Systemic findings:
    a. fever
    b. anemia, thrombocytopenia
    c. jaundice/hepatosplenomegaly
    d. microcephaly
    e. psychomotor retardation
    f. periventricular calcifications
    g. sensorineural deafness
    h. petechial rash
    i. encephalitis
    j. pneumonitis
D. Histopathology:
  1. Infected retinal cells are large (cytomegalic) with intranuclear and cytoplasmic inclusions
  2. Retinal necrosis
  3. Secondary granulomatous choroiditis
E. Evaluation:
  1. Virus recovery from body fluids—maternal cervical secretions; aqueous humor
  2. Neonatal IgM
  3. CT—periventricular calcifications

F. Differential Diagnosis:
   1. Tuberculosis, syphilis, Coat's disease, retinoblastoma, presumed ocular histoplasmosis syndrome (POHS), congenital hypertrophy of the RPE (CHRPE), traumatic scar, toxocariasis, Aicardi syndrome, Best's disease, fungal infection, toxoplasmosis

G. Treatment:
   1. Ganciclovir
   2. Foscarnet

XI. HERPES SIMPLEX VIRUS (HSV)

A. Epidemiology:
   1. In the presence of active genital lesions the risk of congenital infection approaches 50% following vaginal birth
   2. Most neonatal infections are HSV-2 (genital)
   3. 13% of infants with neonatal herpes will have eye involvement
   4. Clinical signs may develop during the first month of life
   5. Overall mortality 60%—two thirds of those infected will have disseminated disease with 75 to 80% mortality; CNS involvement carries a 50% mortality

B. Clinical Features:
   1. Ocular findings:
      a. keratitis with epithelial dendrites, progression to stromal involvement if left untreated
      b. chorioretinitis (massive yellow-white exudates) with accompanying vitritis
      c. cataracts
   2. Systemic findings:
      a. cutaneous vesicular eruption
      b. mucosal ulceration
         1) hepatitis
         2) pneumonia
         3) disseminated intravascular coagulation (DIC)

C. Histopathology:
   1. Intranuclear inclusions in infected cells
   2. Necrotizing retinitis
   3. EM—virus particles may be seen

D. Evaluation:
   1. Clinical examination
   2. Cultures from corneal scrapings or vesicles
   3. Serologic testing not helpful

E. Treatment:
   1. IV acyclovir or vidarabine for systemic involvement

2. Herpetic keratitis—trifluorothymidine vidarabine, idoxiuridine (IDU) solution topically
3. Blepharoconjunctivitis—topical acyclovir to prophylaxis against corneal involvement
4. Prevention: Cesarean section for all deliveries in the presence of active genital lesions, no later than 4 hours after rupture of membranes to prevent retrograde infection

XII. SYPHILIS

A. Caused by Treponema pallidum following maternal spirochetemia
   1. Primary acquired disease contracted after 16 weeks; nearly all fetuses acquire disease
   2. Often fatal to fetus if mother acquires infection before 16 weeks
B. Clinical Features:
   1. Ocular findings:
      a. chorioretinitis—commonly in the periphery with areas of pigment mottling and in severe cases with extensive pigmentary changes resembling retinitis pigmentosa; salt and pepper granularity
      b. interstitial keratitis—10 to 40% of untreated congenital syphilis, commonly 5 to 20 years of age
      c. diffuse or sectoral corneal edema
      d. decreased vision because of corneal scarring and ghost vessels
      e. bilateral in 80%
      f. rarely—anterior uveitis, glaucoma, optic atrophy
   2. Systemic findings: develop during the first few months
      a. skeletal abnormalities including metaphyseal abnormalities or periostitis
      b. rhinitis
      c. maculopapular rash
      d. hepatosplenomegaly with jaundice, pneumonia, and anemia
   3. Late findings: sensorineural hearing loss, dental abnormalities
      a. Hutchinson's triad—widely spaced, peg-shaped teeth; eighth nerve deafness; and interstitial keratitis
      b. facial features—saddle nose, short maxilla, linear scars called "rhagades" around body orifices
C. Evaluation:
   1. Dark-field examination of exudate from skin lesions
   2. VDRL and FTA-ABS but neither differentiates maternal from fetal antibodies

3. Fetal IgM-FTA-ABS is strong evidence of congenital infection

D. Treatment:
   1. Parenteral aqueous penicillin G 50,000 units/kg qd for 10 to 14 days

XIII. OPTIC NERVE ABNORMALITIES

A. **Congenital Optic Pit:** usually unilateral, affecting the inferior temporal quadrant; often covered by a gray veil of tissue; has been associated with serous retinal detachments in the second or third decades of life

B. **Optic Disc Coloboma:** unilateral or bilateral abnormality of closure of fetal fissure of the embryonic optic cup; mild inferior deformity of the optic cup, deep excavation or severe deformity with enlargement of the peripapillary area with a deep central excavation crossed over by blood vessels and glial tissue; vision range from normal to no light perception; may produce various visual field defects. May be isolated or part of a chorioretinal coloboma.

C. **Morning Glory Syndrome:** unilaterally enlarged and excavated disc with a central core of glial tissue occupying the position of the cup, and a disc surrounded by a raised ring of subretinal pigmented tissue; spoke-like radiation of vessels; poor vision; retinal detachment may occur. Associated with unilateral high myopia and structural defects of the cranium.

D. **Tilted Disc (Fuchs' Coloboma):** often bilateral, the disc is tilted inferiorly with a scleral crescent, nasal turning of the temporal retinal vessels, and hypopigmentation of the inferonasal fundus. Associated with high myopia, astigmatism, and field defects which correspond to the area of ectasia, particularly in the upper temporal field giving bitemporal defects; mildly reduced vision (up to 20/50 commonly).

E. **Optic Nerve Hypoplasia:** unilateral or bilateral, disc is smaller than usual, often with a white or yellow halo and pigment on the inner and outer portion of this halo (double ring sign); vision is often poor; various field defects seen; afferent pupillary defect present if unilateral. Strabismus, nystagmus, or amblyopia may occur. Associated with aniridia, De-Morsier syndrome (septo-optic dysplasia), pituitary or hypothalamic disorders, fetal alcohol syndrome, microphthalmos, maternal ingestion of LSD or anticonvulsants, and maternal diabetes. Patients should have neuroradiologic imaging to rule out CNS anomalies, and a pediatric endocrinology evaluation.

F. **Myelinated Nerve Fibers:** congenital, white, flame-shaped patches, usually adjacent to the disc; enlarged blind spot; bilateral in 20%; vision is good unless macula involved. Affects females more than males. Associated with optic nerve coloboma, hyaloid remnants, myopia, and amblyopia; may occur as part of a syndrome of unilateral extensive myelinated nerve fibers, high myopia, and amblyopia.

G. **Melanocytoma:** benign melanotic lesion, often inferiorly; usually in dark-skinned races; normal vision

H. **Optic Disc Drusen:** congenital, often familial; 70% bilateral; absent optic cup with multiple opalescent refractile bodies which autofluoresce; retinal vessels not obscured; increased prominence with age; may produce visual field defects. Histopathology reveals hyaline-positive calcium bodies on the disc.

I. **Bergmeister's Papilla:** remnant of glial sheath of hyaloid artery, normal vision

XIV. CRANIOFACIAL DISORDERS

A. **Treacher Collins Syndrome (Mandibulofacial Dysostosis):** maxillary hypoplasia, downward displacement of lateral canthi, notching of outer third of the lower lids with lack of lashes medial to the notch; often misdirected lashes; deafness and ear anomalies may occur; autosomal dominant with variable expression.

B. **Goldenhar Syndrome (Oculoauriculovertebral Dysplasia):** epibulbar corneal dermoids; orbital lipodermoids usually in the inferotemporal quadrant; bilateral in 25%; upper eyelid coloboma; preauricular skin tags. Vertebral anomalies include fused cervical vertebrae, hemivertebrae, spina bifida, and occipitalization of the atlas. Limbal dermoids amenable to local excision if causing astigmatism and anisometropic amblyopia or if impinging on the visual axis—partial lamellar keratectomy; orbital lipodermoids should not be treated surgically.

C. **Hallerman-Streiff-Francois Syndrome (Oculomandibulofacial Dyscephaly):** mandibular hypoplasia, beak nose, and bilateral cataracts that mature rapidly in infancy, but may resorb spontaneously; often associated with microphthalmia and microcornea; glaucoma occasionally occurs; all cases sporadic.

D. **Craniosynostosis (e.g., Crouzon and Apert Syndrome):** premature closure of the cranial sutures, may be complicated by hydrocephalus with increased ICP leading to optic atrophy; wide spectrum of skull shapes including markedly shallow orbits with prominent globes at risk for corneal exposure; V patterns with exotropia common; amblyopia common; midface hypoplasia, hypertelorism (increased separation of the bony orbits), oral or dental problems, and respiratory difficulties and syndactyly may be seen. Usually autosomal dominant. May be associated with systemic disorders. Treatment includes lubrication of the corneas, tarsorrhaphy, reconstructive surgery; strabismus surgery should be delayed until after reconstruction.

E. **Waardenburg Syndrome:** autosomal dominant, lateral displacement of the inner canthi and lacrimal puncta, confluent eyebrows, heterochromia irides, congenital bilateral sensorineural deafness, white forelocks, and fundus hypopigmentation.

F. **Fetal Alcohol Syndrome (FAS):** malformations related to alcohol abuse during pregnancy, short palpebral fissures with increased distance between the medial canthi (telecanthus) most frequent, thin vermillion border of the upper lip, long flat philtrum, epicanthal folds, mental retardation varying in degree, small birth weight, abnormalities of the cardiovascular and skeletal system, strabismus occurring in 50% of patients with FAS. Visual acuity often reduced secondary to high myopia, microphthalmia, or mesenchymal dysgenesis (e.g., Peter's anomaly). Most serious ophthalmic malformations are hypoplasia of the optic nerve head (48%) and increased tortuosity of the retinal vasculature, may be unilateral or bilateral.

XV. LEUKOCORIA (WHITE PUPIL)

A. Differential Diagnosis:
1. Retinoblastoma
2. Cataract
3. Retinal detachment
4. Severe posterior uveitis
5. Retinopathy of prematurity (ROP)
6. Persistent hyperplastic primary vitreous (PHPV)
7. Retinal dysplasia (Norrie's disease)
8. Coats' disease
9. Toxocariasis
10. Colobomas
11. Congenital retinal folds
12. Vitreous hemorrhage
13. Congenital cataract
    a. a leading cause of blindness in children due to severe amblyopia
B. Epidemiology:

    1. One third are inherited, usually autosomal dominant

    2. One third are associated with disease syndromes

    3. One third are due to undetermined causes

C. Clinical Features:

    1. Nystagmus is a sign of poor vision

    2. Monocular infantile cataracts are usually not metabolic in origin

    3. Affected eye may be smaller than nonaffected eye in unilateral cases

    4. Associated ocular abnormalities—congenital defects of cornea, iris, pupil, glaucoma

    5. Associated metabolic disorders: galactosemia, galactokinase deficiency, G6PD deficiency and others

    6. Syndromes with associated cataracts: Lowe, Alport, Cockayne, Stickler, incontinentia pigmenti, Hallerman-Streiff, Rubinstein-Taybi syndrome

    7. Iatrogenic cataracts associated with topical steroids and ionizing radiation

    8. Genetic associations—trisomy 13, 18, or 21

    9. Trauma—must be ruled out, especially in cases of possible child abuse

    10. Types of cataracts:

        a. anterior polar—small (<1–2 mm), nonprogressive; excellent visual prognosis

        b. lamellar—opacification peripheral to Y sutures with clear nucleus; usually bilateral and >5 mm; considered acquired and progressive. Prognosis very good; surgery not required or performed late

        c. nuclear—congenital, dense, >3 mm, associated with microphthalmos; autosomal dominant. Prognosis fair to poor

        d. posterior lenticonus—congenital defect of the posterior lens capsule with opacity; usually acquired in infancy and progressive. Prognosis is excellent with surgery

        e. cataract associated with PHPV—microphthalmic eye, often with secondary glaucoma

    11. Miscellaneous lens abnormalities:

        a. Spherophakia—smaller than normal lens, bilateral; may sublux and cause glaucoma

        b. Ectopia lentis—bilateral, usually autosomal dominant; lens dislocates superotemporally, usually congenital but may sublux later in life; associated with glaucoma. Treatment includes correction of refractive error, mydriasis if edge of lens in pupillary axis, surgical lentectomy.

      c. Ectopia lentis et pupillae—slit/oval pupil, bilateral, autosomal recessive; subluxed lens may be cataractous; may be associated with glaucoma. Treatment often requires correction of refractive error alone.

D. Evaluation:
  1. If bilateral—urinalysis for reducing substances and amino acids
  2. VDRL
  3. Serum calcium and phosphorus
  4. Rule out TORCHS infection

E. Treatment:
  1. Dilation of pupil (palliative until surgery)
  2. Timing of surgery should be individualized depending on the extent of the cataract, age, and status of the patient—earlier surgery is preferred in most cases
  3. Surgery—small limbal incision, anterior capsulotomy, remove lens with a phacoemulsification hand-piece on aspiration only, or with a vitreous cutting instrument; posterior capsulotomy or capsulectomy with anterior vitrectomy should be performed since posterior capsule opacification almost always occurs; in older children, the posterior capsule may be left intact and opened with a YAG laser if necessary
  4. Visual prognosis better for binocular than monocular cataracts

XVI. COATS' DISEASE

A. Retinal vascular disorder resulting in yellow subretinal exudates from abnormal telangiectatic vessels and aneur-ysmal dilation; predilection for macula. Males affected more often than females; usually unilateral. Age at diagnosis 8 to 10 years, but cases in young infants have been reported.

B. Diagnosis:
  1. Fluorescein angiography and angioscopy

C. Treatment:
  1. Ablate abnormal vessels with cryotherapy or photocoagulation

D. Prognosis:
  1. Poor if fovea detached; 50% untreated patients will progress to exudative retinal detachment and subretinal fibrosis, and glaucoma; 70% of treated patients will remain stable or improve.

XVII. TOXOCARIASIS

A. Nematode infection (Toxocara canis) causing a white, dome-shaped retinal granuloma, vitreous cells with traction bands and occasionally an exudative detachment and cyclitic membrane. Rarely bilateral or multifocal, usually diagnosed around 8 years of age.
   1. Contracted by ingestion of dirt contaminated with dog feces or from eating improperly cleaned vegetables; larvae invade intestinal walls, disseminate to liver, lung, and eyes with a predilection for the retina where they migrate and cause inflammation, hemorrhage, and necrosis.
B. Histopathology:
   1. Eosinophilic granuloma with giant cells, epithelioid cells, fibrin, and lymphocytes
C. Diagnosis:
   1. Serum ELISA test for toxocara
D. Treatment:
   1. Topical and/or periocular steroids
   2. Thiabendazole
   3. Vitrectomy—rarely
E. Prognosis:
   1. Depends on location of granuloma

XVIII. NONACCIDENTAL INJURY

A. Two million children are abused each year—injuries to the eye may be evident in up to 40% of nonaccidentally injured children. Mandatory reporting laws of suspected child abuse exist in all 50 states.
   1. Ocular findings presenting signs of abuse in 5% of patients.
   2. Most common ophthalmic finding is extensive intraocular hemorrhage, often with intracranial bleeding; subconjunctival, retinal, preretinal, or vitreous hemorrhages may occur. Shaken baby syndrome (retinal hemorrhages and cotton-wool spots) occurs after violent shaking, direct eye, head, or chest trauma, or choking.
B. Pathogenesis:
   1. Increased pressure in retinal veins secondary to increased intracranial pressure; increased intrathoracic pressure due to squeezing; vitreoretinal traction secondary to repetitive shaking, usually without evidence of external trauma
C. Differential Diagnosis:
   1. Birth trauma, bleeding disorders, acute leukemia, anemia, sepsis, and CPR (uncommon, usually not

extensive). Intraretinal hemorrhages extremely rare in children sustaining head trauma from other causes.

D. Treatment:

1. Vitrectomy indicated for vitreous hemorrhage if ERG intact

E. Prognosis:

1. High mortality; neurologic impairment and visual loss may be mild or severe

XIX. INHERITED METABOLIC DISORDERS

A. Mucopolysaccharidoses (MPS): deficiencies of enzymes responsible for the turnover of mucopolysaccharides, with abnormal tissue accumulation. All but Hunter syndrome are autosomal recessive (X-linked).

1. **MPS-I-H (Hurler syndrome):** corneal clouding, retinal pigmentary degeneration, and optic atrophy; associated with glaucoma
2. **MPS-I-S (Scheie syndrome):** corneal clouding and pigmentary retinal degeneration
3. **MPS-II (Hunter syndrome):** no or mild corneal clouding, retinal pigment degeneration, and optic atrophy
4. **MPS-III (Sanfilippo syndrome):** no corneal clouding, retinal pigmentary degeneration, and optic atrophy
5. **MPS-IV (Morquio syndrome):** corneal clouding, no retinal pigmentary degeneration, optic atrophy reported
6. **MPS-VI (Maroteaux-Lamy syndrome):** prominent corneal clouding, optic atrophy rare, no retinal degeneration (MPS-VI-A, mild; MPS-VI-B, severe)
7. **MPS-VII (Sly syndrome):** mild corneal clouding
8. In summary, corneal clouding is prominent in MPS I-H and I-S and is less severe in MPS-IV, VI, and VII. Pigmentary degeneration of the retina occurs in MPS-I-H, I-S, II, and III, but not in IV or VI.
9. Optic nerve head swelling and subsequent atrophy occurs in all types except VIB.

B. Lipidoses

1. Enzyme deficiencies that interfere with normal hydrolysis of certain sphingolipids, which therefore accumulate in the CNS, viscera, or both. All autosomal recessive except Fabry's disease (X-linked recessive).

   a. **Tay-Sachs disease (G_{M2} gangliosidosis type I):** 65 to 80% are of Ashkenazic Jewish ancestry; infants develop normally until 6 or 7 months. Cherry-red spot seen in the macula as early as

2 months, deficiency of hexosaminidase A with accumulation of GM2 ganglioside in the ganglion cells of the retina. Mental retardation, deafness, blindness secondary to optic atrophy, dementia, nystagmus, ophthalmoplegia, and spasticity caused by accumulation in gray matter. Cherry-red spot fades as the ganglion cells die with resulting optic atrophy; blind by 18 months and dead by 3 years of age.

b. **Sandhoff disease (G_{M2} gangliosidosis type II):** deficiency of hexosaminidase A and B with resultant accumulation of both globoside and G_{M2} ganglioside, cherry-red spot.

c. **G_{M2} type III:** partial hexosaminidase A deficiency; no cherry-red spot, RPE degeneration/retinopathy, and optic atrophy occur late

d. **Niemann-Pick disease Type A (infantile):** sphingomyelinase deficiency with resultant accumulation of sphingomyelin and cholesterol in the viscera and brain with severe retardation, slight corneal clouding, and brown anterior lens capsule discoloration, cherry-red spot, nystagmus, and blindness. Lifespan 2 to 3 years.

e. **Krabbe's disease (globoid cell leukodystrophy):** deficiency of beta-galactosidase and accumulation of galactocerebroside; early progressive CNS degeneration, optic atrophy with blindness and nystagmus. No cherry-red spot. Lifespan 2 years.

f. **Gaucher's disease:** deficiency of B-galactosidase with accumulation of glucocerebroside in the viscera and probably the CNS; paralytic strabismus, pingueculae, conjunctival pigmentation, RPE degeneration. Autosomal recessive.

g. **Fabry's disease (Angiokeratoma corporis diffusum universale):** deficiency of alphagalactosidase A; normal intelligence; angiokeratomas on the trunk; lipid accumulates in blood vessels and may cause severe renal disease and cerebrovascular disease; most striking ophthalmic finding is whorl-like corneal epithelial opacity radiating out in curved lines from a point just inferior to the center of the cornea; kinky conjunctival and retinal vessels; spoke-like cataract. Heterozygous female carriers usually manifest ocular findings but have much less severe systemic involvement.

C. Mucolipidoses

1. Overlap between the mucopolysaccharidoses and the sphingolipidoses. All are autosomal recessive.

2. **G_{M1} gangliosidosis:** corneal clouding; facial and skeletal dysmorphism; high myopia; esotropia; usually have a cherry-red spot and optic atrophy; deficiency of lysosomal betagalactosidase with accumulation of keratin sulfate and G_{M1} ganglioside.

3. **Metachromatic leukodystrophy:** rare cause of corneal clouding; commonly have macular pigmentary changes, cherry-red spot with optic atrophy, and blindness. Deficiency of arylsulfatase A.

D. Aminoacidurias

1. Most are autosomal recessive

2. **Homocystinuria:** deficiency of cystathione synthetase; associated with subluxed lenses (ectopia lentis) which are often cataractous; myopia; retinal detachment; glaucoma; and optic atrophy. Usually mentally retarded; prone to development of arterial and venous thromboses; with general anesthesia, may be helped with pyridoxine.

3. **Cystinosis:** lysosomal transport defect leads to accumulation of cysteine crystals in the cornea, photophobia; also deposited in the choroid and conjunctiva; degenerative pigmentary changes in the retinal periphery. Leads to renal failure.

4. **Lowe syndrome (oculocerebrorenal syndrome):** X-linked recessive, due to unknown enzyme deficiency or defect in amino acid transport; eye involvement is severe and leads to cataract, microphakia, and congenital glaucoma due either to malformation of the angle or to subluxed lenses

5. **Zellweger syndrome (cerebrohepatorenal syndrome):** enzyme deficiency unknown; characteristic hypoplasia of the superior orbital rim with flat brow, peripheral retinal pigmentation (leopard spots), cataracts, glaucoma, and congenital optic nerve hypoplasia. Life expectancy is less than one year.

6. **Galactosemia:** deficiency of galactose-1-phosphate uridyl transferase; accumulation of galactose causes cataracts in infancy and can be reversed in early stages by a galactose-free diet; autosomal recessive

7. **Galactokinase deficiency:** no systemic manifestations; cataracts form when child is exposed to galactose and reversible if treated with a galactose-free diet. Autosomal recessive.

XX. CHROMOSOMAL ABNORMALITIES

A. **Trisomy 21 (Down Syndrome):** incidence—1:672 to 1:1000; ocular findings include upward slanting palpebral fissures, hypertelorism, chronic blepharitis, cicatricial ectropion, esotropia, myopia, cataracts, Brushfield's spots, keratoconus, optic atrophy

B. **Trisomy 13 (Patau Syndrome):** incidence—1:4000 to 1:14,500, 75% die by 6 months of age; severe CNS anomalies (holoprosencephaly characteristic); ocular findings include hypertelorism, epicanthal folds, microphthalmos, uveal colobomas, retinal dysplasia, cataracts, corneal opacities, optic nerve hypoplasia, persistent hyperplastic primary vitreous (PHPV)

C. **Trisomy 18 (Edwards' Syndrome):** incidence—1:5000, females affected more than males, 90% die within the first year; low birth weight, mental retardation, failure to thrive; ocular findings include epicanthal folds, blepharophimosis, ptosis, hypertelorism, corneal opacities, microphthalmos, congenital glaucoma, uveal colobomas, cataracts

D. **Short Arm 11 Deletion (11p13) Syndrome:** mental retardation, Wilm's tumor, aniridia, glaucoma, foveal hypoplasia, nystagmus, ptosis, corneal pannus, optic nerve hypoplasia, cataract

E. **Long Arm 13 Deletion (13q14) Syndrome:** mental retardation, microcephaly, ambiguous genitalia, hand and foot anomalies; ocular findings include retinoblastoma (3 to 7% of patients with retinoblastoma), hypertelorism, microphthalmos, epicanthus, coloboma, cataract

F. **Cri du Chat (5p) Syndrome:** severe mental retardation, hypoplastic larynx, congenital heart defects; ocular findings include hypertelorism, epicanthus, antimongoloid slant, strabismus (exotropia), iris coloboma, and myopia

G. **Turner Syndrome (XO):** affected patients develop as females with short stature, absence of secondary sexual characteristics, and sterility; ocular findings include antimongoloid slant, epicanthus, ptosis, strabismus, nystagmus, blue sclera, eccentric pupils, cataract, coloboma, retinitis-pigmentosa-like fundus

Essentials of Eye Care, edited by Rohit Varma.
Lippincott–Raven Publishers,
Philadelphia © 1997.

6

Cornea/External Disease

I. BLEPHARITIS

A. Staphylococcal
   1. Clinical features:
      a. most common chronic and infectious external disease
      b. classic clinical sign is the fibrin collarette
      c. can be asymptomatic or can cause irritation, burning, redness of lids and/or conjunctiva
   2. Treatment:
      a. mainstay is lid hygiene; includes light rubbing with a cotton-tipped applicator, cotton swab, or washcloth; drop of baby shampoo or commercial mild detergent scrubs may or may not be necessary
      b. antibiotic ointment should be applied twice daily for several weeks, and then intermittently when necessary; bacitracin, sulfa, or erythromycin

B. Seborrheic
   1. Clinical features:
      a. similar to staphylococcal; however, scurf is seen at the base of the eyelashes
      b. usually associated with seborrhea on other areas of the face, scalp, or skin
   2. Treatment:
      a. lid hygiene
      b. occasional mild steroid ointment may be necessary in severe cases

C. Demodex
   1. Clinical features:
      a. similar to staphylococcal disease
      b. sleeve surrounding the base of the lashes is the predominant feature; created by the hair follicle mites (Demodex folliculorum) and sebacious gland mites (Demodex brevis)
   2. Treatment:
      a. lid scrubs, bland ointment applied to the lid margins

  b. manual debridement of the mites when possible
D. Rosacea
  1. Clinical features:
    a. acne-like disease with meibomian gland dysfunction
    b. affects the eyelids, as well as the skin of the nose, cheeks, and forehead
    c. most common in Caucasians over 30 years of age
    d. erythema, telangiectasias, papules, and pustules present
    e. chronic changes include rhinophyma, and meibomian gland scarring, recurrent chalazia, chronic conjunctival erythema, and dilated limbal vessels
    f. punctate keratopathy and subepithelial infiltrates can occur, rarely progressing to ulceration
  2. Treatment:
    a. lid hygiene
    b. topical corticosteroids (fluorometholone 0.1% or prednisone 1/8%) can suppress inflammation
    c. topical antibiotics are often necessary for the associated staphylococcal blepharitis; oral tetracycline (250 mg po qid) or doxycycline (100 mg po bid) alter the meibomian gland dysfunction, as well as provide antibiotic function. Topical metronidazole (0.75%) is used for the manifestations of rosacea on the skin; however, no ophthalmic preparation is currently available.
E. Angular
  1. Clinical features:
    a. lateral canthal angle of the eyes are inflamed, ulcerated, and with mucopurulent discharge
    b. most often caused by species of Moraxella (gram-negative diplobacilli)
  2. Treatment:
    a. sensitive to erythromycin ointment; other useful antibiotics include penicillin, neomycin
    b. variable sensitivity to gentamicin or tobramycin

II. TUMORS OF THE EYELIDS
  A. Epithelial Tumors (Benign)
    1. Papilloma
      a. clinical features:
        1) characteristic lobulated, cauliflower-type appearance of varying size
        2) any lesion with multilobulated growths with a central vascular core, often caused by the human papilloma virus in young patients
      b. pathology:

            1) benign, hyperkeratosis, parakeratosis, and epidermalization surrounding vascular cores
    c. diagnosis:
            1) excisional biopsy when irritating or cosmetically displeasing
  2. Keratoacanthoma
    a. clinical features:
            1) rapidly developing (6 to 8 weeks) tumor which is round and has a central umbilicated core
    b. pathology:
            1) marked acanthosis, hyperkeratosis, and dyskeratosis; dysplasia is absent
    c. diagnosis:
            1) clinical appearance
    d. treatment:
            1) excisional biopsy
            2) often undergo spontaneous regression after several months
  3. Seborrheic keratosis
    a. epidemiology:
            1) common cutaneous tumor in the elderly
            2) inheritance is autosomal dominant
    b. clinical features:
            1) mild elevation, plaque-like tumor with light pigmentation
            2) appears "stuck onto the skin"
    c. pathology:
            1) benign proliferation of epidermal basal cells with keratin cysts
            2) no dysplasia present
            3) no dermal involvement
            4) inflammation absent
    d. diagnosis:
            1) clinical appearance
    e. treatment:
            1) simple excisional biopsy
  4. Epidermal inclusion cyst
    a. clinical features:
            1) smooth, round epidermal mass
            2) dermal tumor
    b. pathology:
            1) squamous epidermal cells are trapped between the cutaneous surface, as a result of trauma
    c. diagnosis:
            1) clinical appearance
    d. treatment:
            1) simple excisional biopsy
  5. Molluscum contagiosum
    a. epidemiology:
            1) viral infection involving the epidermis

      b. clinical feature:
         1) elevated nodule with a central core (umbilicated lesion)
         2) similar to keratoacanthoma though smaller and less rapid growth
         3) associated with a toxic allergic follicular conjunctivitis
      c. pathology:
         1) benign acanthosis with numerous intracytoplasmic inclusion bodies in the central core
      d. diagnosis:
         1) clinical appearance
      e. treatment:
         1) excisional biopsy
   6. Verruca vulgaris (wart)
      a. epidemiology:
         1) cutaneous wart is caused by human papilloma virus
      b. clinical features:
         1) papilloma with hyperkeratosis
         2) moderate pigmentation may be present
      c. pathology:
         1) hyperkeratosis, parakeratosis, acanthosis
      d. diagnosis:
         1) clinical appearance
      e. treatment:
         1) excisional biopsy
         2) must be complete or viral seeding and recurrences can occur
         3) often left untreated, because most disappear spontaneously within a few months
B. Premalignant Tumors
   1. Actinic keratosis
      a. epidemiology:
         1) appear on exposed areas of the skin of older people
         2) excessive exposure to the sun is a risk factor
      b. clinical features:
         1) often multiple with cutaneous horns frequently present
         2) develop into squamous cell carcinoma in 25% of patients
      c. pathology:
         1) chronic inflammation of the dermis with hyperkeratosis, acanthosis, and dysplastic areas
      d. diagnosis:
         1) based on clinical appearance
      e. treatment:
         1) excision
C. Malignant Tumors

1. Basal cell carcinoma
   a. epidemiology:
      1) most common malignancy of the eyelid
   b. clinical features:
      1) begins as small ulcerated nodule with slow growth; other growth patterns are possible including nodular types, fibrosis, with subclinical, finger-like extensions
      2) progressively invasive and destructive locally
      3) metastases are rare
   c. pathology:
      1) malignant proliferation of epidermal basal cells
      2) variety of growth patterns (See pathology text for in-depth discussion.)
   d. diagnosis:
      1) clinical appearance and high index of suspicion
      2) diagnostic and excisional biopsies are imperative
      3) margins of the tumor can be difficult to ascertain and recurrences following excision are common
      4) close cooperation between the surgeon and pathologist essential
   e. treatment:
      1) excision with close monitoring of the margins
      2) alternative or adjunctive therapy: cryotherapy, chemotherapy, or radiation
2. Squamous cell carcinoma
   a. epidemiology:
      1) accounts for only 5% of malignant lid margin tumors; has a poorer prognosis than basal cell carcinoma
   b. clinical features:
      1) more common on the upper eyelid, but can appear anywhere in the periorbital region
      2) grows slowly, but can metastasize to lymph nodes or remote organs
      3) can display prominent hyperkeratosis on lid margins
   c. pathology:
      1) severe dysplasia of all epidermal layers
      2) intraepidermal keratin pearls present
   d. diagnosis:
      1) clinical appearance along with pathologic specimen investigation
   e. treatment:
      1) excision, radiation therapy, chemotherapy necessary in metastatic disease

D. Glandular Tumors

   1. Sebaceous cell carcinoma

   a. epidemiology:

   1) more common in the eyelids than anywhere else in the body

   2) overall mortality rate of at least 20% despite treatment, due to metastatic disease

   b. clinical features:

   1) often misdiagnosed as chronic blepharoconjunctivitis or recurrent chalazion

   2) variable clinical appearance

   3) can be multifocal and associated with inflammation

   c. pathology:

   1) most arise from meibomian glands

   2) tumor cells are variable in appearance; may have pagetoid change

   3) highly dysplastic and anaplastic

   4) stains for lipids are important in this disease, but must be performed on frozen sections because preservation for permanent sections dissolves the fats

   d. diagnosis:

   1) based on clinical suspicion and histopathologic examination

   2) any suspicious chronic blepharoconjunctivitis or recurrence of chalazions should be examined in this manner

   e. treatment:

   1) wide excision is necessary, occasionally with adjunctive radiotherapy

   2) extensive reconstructive surgery is often necessary

E. Nevi and Melanoma

   1. Nevus

   a. epidemiology:

   1) congenital hematomas consisting of modified melanocytes

   2) pigmentation increases with age, but all are present at birth

   b. clinical appearance:

   1) may be flat or elevated, sessile or pedunculated, with varying pigment

   2) location of nevus cells vary, which is important clinically

   a) junctional nevi: have cells in the deep epidermis and along the epidermal interface; may transform into malignancies

      b) intradermal nevi: inactive with rare possibility to transform into malignancy

      c) compound nevi: transitional form, showing features of both junctional and intradermal nevi; rarely transform into malignancy

      d) blue nevi: located deeply in the dermis; pigment from birth onwards; flat and benign

      e) nevis of ota: diffuse congenital blue nevus of the periocular skin; most common in Asian or African-American patients; malignant transformation is rare

  2. Melanoma

    a. epidemiology:

      1) less common than melanoma of other sites

      2) can arise from preexisting junctional or compound nevi

      3) steadily increasing incidence recently

    b. clinical features:

      1) growth can be very rapid, but variable

    c. pathology:

      1) multinucleated tumor giant cells and increased mitotic activity is common

      2) inflammatory cells may be present

      3) tumor cells are highly anaplastic

    d. diagnosis:

      1) clinical appearance and histopathologic studies

    e. treatment:

      1) prognosis depends on depth of vertical invasion at time of surgical removal

      2) essential wide surgical excision with histopathologic examination of margins

      3) regional lymph node dissection should be included when evidence of vascular and lymphatic involvement is present

F. Vascular Tumors

  1. Capillary hemangioma

    a. epidemiology:

      1) often present at birth

      2) accounts for 10% of all orbital tumors in children

      3) begin within the first five years of life and spontaneously regress

    b. clinical appearance:

      1) generally solitary, bright red, and smooth

      2) appear suddenly and often increase in size when the child cries

      3) complications include occlusion amblyopia when the lesion obstructs the visual axis

         4) may result in astigmatism by compression of the globe by the tumor

   c. pathology:

         1) composed of proliferating capillaries consisting of endothelial cells and pericytes

   d. diagnosis:

         1) clinical appearance with histopathologic confirmation

   e. treatment:

         1) lesions involute within the first few years of life

         2) intralesional injections of corticosteroids may be useful

         3) surgical removal is rarely indicated

2. Cavernous hemangioma

   a. clinical feature:

         1) characteristic feature of Sturge-Weber syndrome (encephalotrigeminal angiomatosis)

         2) characteristic facial "port-wine stain"

   b. diagnosis:

         1) clinical appearance

   c. treatment:

         1) moderate success is being reported with argon laser therapy to the skin lesion

         2) control the associated glaucoma with medications

3. Kaposi's sarcoma

   a. epidemiology:

         1) classic form of the disease is rarely found

         2) mainly in Central Africa

         3) most commonly been found in patients with AIDS

   b. clinical features:

         1) tumor presents as a red or purple subepidermal nodule

         2) varies in size

         3) numerous proliferating capillaries, vascular endothelial cells, and atypical fibroblasts

         4) looks like a form of malignant granulation tissue

   c. diagnosis:

         1) clinical appearance

   d. treatment:

         1) excision with or without adjunctive chemotherapy

   e. prognosis:

         1) poor, with many AIDS patients having died as a result of this disease

G. Xanthomatous Tumors

  1. Xanthelasma

   a. epidemiology:

        1) often presents in elderly patients
        2) seems to be some association with hypercho-
           lesterolemia, but many xanthelasmas are idio-
           pathic
     b. clinical features:
        1) yellow plaque just beneath the epidermis any-
           where in the periorbital region
     c. pathology:
        1) benign histiocytic tumor with no inflammation
        2) no malignant potential
        3) cells filled with cholesterol and other lipids
     d. diagnosis:
        1) clinical appearance with histopathologic con-
           firmation
     e. treatment:
        1) excisional biopsy
  2. Juvenile xanthogranuloma
     a. epidemiology:
        1) benign tumor in infants and young children
     b. clinical features:
        1) multiple lesions in the periorbital region and
           on the iris
        2) smooth, round tumors; orange in color
        3) spontaneous hyphemas can occur
     c. pathology:
        1) shows lipid-filled histiocytes with many Tou-
           ton giant cells
        2) large amount of vascularization
     d. diagnosis:
        1) clinical appearance
     e. treatment:
        1) juvenile xanthogranulomas resolve sponta-
           neously
H. Inflammatory Lesions
  1. Chalazion
     a. epidemiology:
        1) chronic granuloma from obstructed Zeiss or
           meibomian glands
        2) appears in patients of all ages, races, and sexes
     b. clinical features:
        1) nodule that arises on either eyelid
        2) can have an acute onset on either the posterior
           or anterior aspect of the lid
        3) when the gland becomes obstructed, the
           trapped sebaceous material extrudes into adja-
           cent tissues and creates chronic lipo-granulo-
           matous inflammation
        4) disappears in weeks to months when the ex-
           truded material gets slowly resorbed
        5) small amount of scar tissue may remain

    c. pathology:
      1) zonular granulomatous inflammation
      2) giant cells are present
    d. diagnosis:
      1) clinical appearance
    e. treatment:
      1) most chalazia are sterile
      2) lid hygiene and antibiotic ointment may be of some value. Otherwise hot compresses and patience are the mainstay of therapy.
      3) resolve spontaneously over time
      4) if the nodule persists, injection of corticosteroids (triamcinolone acetate) is sometimes useful to decrease its size
      5) simple incision and thorough curettage
      6) persistent, recurrent chalazia should be examined for sebaceous cell carcinoma

  2. Pyogenic granuloma
    a. epidemiology:
      1) occurs after injury or trauma and may be thought of as exuberant healing
    b. clinical features:
      1) raised vascular pedunculated tumor with moderate amounts of mucopurulent exudate
      2) often involutes spontaneously
      3) may develop after trauma or other injury, including chalazia or chemical burns
    c. pathology:
      1) lesion is a misnomer as it is neither pyogenic nor granulomatous
      2) consists of granulation tissue
      3) noninfectious and granulomas not present
    d. diagnosis:
      1) clinical appearance with histopathologic confirmation
    e. treatment:
      1) often spontaneous involution (topical corticosteroids may enhance involution)
      2) excisional biopsy is curative

III. CONJUNCTIVITIS
  A. Infectious
    1. Bacterial conjunctivitis
      a. hyperacute conjunctivitis
        1) pathology:
          a) most commonly *Neisseria gonorrhoeae* or *Neisseria meningitidis* (gram-negative diplococci)—occurs in the child as an infection from the maternal genital tract and in adults by inoculation from infected genitalia

      b) ophthalmia neonatorum is *Neisseria conjunctivitis* of the newborn. This becomes symptomatic 2 to 4 days after birth. Diagnosis is clinical, but conjunctival cultures are necessary.

  2) clinical features:

     a) characterized by marked purulence, lid edema, erythema, and chemosis

     b) preauricular lymphadenopathy often present

     c) can lead to keratitis and perforation if untreated

  3) treatment:

     a) requires systemic antibiotic therapy. These patients should probably be admitted. Adult therapy is 10 million units of aqueous crystalline penicillin G IV qd for five days. Since penicillinase-producing organisms are increasingly frequent, the preferred treatment is either with ceftriaxone 1 gm/day, cefoxitin 1 gm/day, or 0.5 grams of cefotaxime qid for seven days. Neonates and children should be given 50,000 units per kilogram per day of IV crystalline penicillin G in two divided doses for seven days or ceftriaxone 25 to 50 mg/kg/ day IV for seven days.

     b) adults with penicillin allergy are treated with 500 mg of tetracycline po qid for a week. Pregnant women should receive 500 mg of erythromycin po qid for seven days. The tetracycline also treats the often accompanying chlamydial infection. Neonates with gonococcal disease should also be treated for chlamydial disease with erythromycin 50 mg/kg/day for 14 days.

     c) topical bacitracin ointments may be instilled in the involved eye every 2 to 4 hours until resolution

     d) irrigation of the conjunctiva with normal saline, to remove the mucopurulent debris and virulence factors, is also recommended

b. acute conjunctivitis

  1) pathology:

     a) *Streptococcus pneumoniae, Staphylococcus,* and *Hemophilus* are the most common causative organisms

  2) clinical features:

     a) acute bilateral mucopurulent conjunctivitis

     b) occasional small subconjunctival hemorrhages present

    3) treatment:

        a) clinical suspicion alone is often enough to begin therapy, but conjunctival cultures are very helpful for isolating specific bacteria and determining sensitivity to antibiotics

        b) often self-limiting infection, but antibiotics can shorten the time course of infection

        c) antibiotic eyedrops should be instilled every 3 to 4 hours with antibiotic ointment at bedtime or ointment instilled qid

        d) treatment should be for 5 to 7 days

        e) broad spectrum antibiotics such as 10% sulfa drops should be considered. Neosporin is effective, but due to the high incidence of neomycin allergy, secondary symptoms can arise. Polymyxin B-trimethoprim combination may be effective and well-tolerated. Fluoroquinolones are effective, but should be reserved for clinically severe conjunctivitis. The aminoglycosides are also a broad spectrum, but also cause toxicity and local hypersensitivity.

        f) erythromycin also works well

  c. chronic conjunctivitis

    1) clinical features:

        a) often occurs with chronic blepharitis or meibomianitis and presents with chronic, red eyes with burning, itching, and mild mucopurulent discharge

    2) pathology:

        a) organisms include *Staphylococcus aureus, Moraxella lacunata, Pseudomonas, Proteus*

    3) diagnosis:

        a) very important to obtain material for conjunctival cultures for these chronic conditions

        b) specific antibiotic therapy can be tailored pending the culture results

    4) treatment:

        a) daily intensive lid hygiene is the mainstay of therapy

        b) five minutes of hot compresses and lid massage

        c) cotton-tip applicators can be used to physically debride the lid margins

        d) numerous topical antibiotics are available, including sulfa, Neosporin, and erythromycin

          e) oral tetracycline is often useful in controlling abnormal meibomian function

          f) in cases where inflammatory reaction of the eyelids is also responsible for the conjunctivitis, combination antibiotic/steroid preparations are effective, but should not be used more than 3 to 4 weeks due to potential side effects from prolonged steroid application

2. Viral conjunctivitis
   a. adenoviral conjunctivitis
      1) epidemiology:
         a) highly contagious in epidemic or sporadic cases
         b) frequent hand washing, use of separate towels, and eating and drinking utensils
         c) avoid direct contact with people as much as possible. Physicians should be careful not to spread infection to other patients.
         d) virus has been known to stay alive on instruments, doorknobs, and tabletops for several weeks
      2) clinical features:
         a) can produce a broad range of findings, from mild injection of the conjunctiva lasting 3 to 4 days to a severe follicular keratoconjunctivitis with visual disturbance
         b) three syndromes:
            i. mild follicular conjunctivitis—serotypes 1, 2, 3, 4
            ii. pharyngoconjunctival fever—serotypes 3, 7
            iii. severe epidemic keratoconjunctivitis—serotypes 5, 8, 19, 37
         c) acute onset of red eyes with watery discharge
         d) follicular reactions in the inferior conjunctival fornices
         e) mild subconjunctival hemorrhages or membranes
         f) secondary keratitis can occasionally occur; these are fortunately transitory and rarely cause permanent visual problems
      3) diagnosis:
         a) clinical
            i. viral cultures are sometimes unreliable and time consuming, but are helpful in epidemic outbreaks and assist in ruling out herpetic infection
      4) treatment:

    a) usually only supportive. Antiviral agents have not been proven to be effective

    b) frank discussion of the natural history of the disease with the patient is important

    c) he/she should be told that the disease is highly contagious, but is always self-limited and rarely results in chronic visual problems

    d) cold compresses and artificial tears can be applied for comfort

    e) corticosteroid drops are not recommended except in cases of severe membrane formation or disabling subepithelial infiltrates with a high occupational demand. These drops suppress the inflammatory response, but do not seem to shorten the course of the disease. Controversy exists on whether the secondary keratitis is worsened by the chronic use of topical steroids.

b. herpes simplex virus (HSV)

  1) epidemiology:

    a) conjunctivitis may be a manifestation of primary ocular involvement with HSV

    b) HSV ocular involvement presents as blepharo-conjunctivitis in 54% of cases

    c) occurs in immunocompromised subjects

    d) humans are the only natural host of this virus

    e) type 1 herpes simplex virus is the type that is usually involved in the ocular disease; type 2 HSV usually causes genital disease and neonatal ocular disease as the neonate passes through the infected birth canal

    f) it is therefore important to explain to the adult ocular herpes patient that his/her ocular disease is not sexually transmitted

    g) by age 5, up to 60% of all individuals have been infected with type 1 HSV; by age 60, 97% of all individuals have been infected; less than 1% of these present as ocular disease

  2) clinical features:

    a) follicular conjunctivitis can be present

    b) usually an associated cutaneous vesicle or pustule

    c) probable preauricular nodes

    d) corneal involvement may follow the conjunctivitis

  3) diagnosis:

    a) clinical features

    b) in cases of doubt, herpes virus cultures can be performed

        4) treatment:

            a) self-limiting

            b) topical antiviral agents are recommended for the primary involvement, especially when the cornea is infected

            c) pharmacologic options include:

                i. Trifluridine 1% (Viroptic) 1 drop five times daily

                ii. Idoxuridine (IDU) 0.1% drops every hour during the day

                iii. IDU 0.5% ointment five times a day. Oral acyclovir in immunosuppressed individuals with severe skin and conjunctival involvement should be considered.

            d) must be used for approximately 1 week.

                i. When a favorable response has been seen, the medication is rapidly tapered.

3. Chlamydial conjunctivitis

    a. hyperendemic blinding trachoma

        1) epidemiology:

            a) disease of the underdeveloped societies with poor hygienic conditions

            b) most often seen in the Middle East and Africa, where it remains a major reason for blindness

            c) epidemic among some American Indian tribes

            d) sporadic cases appear occasionally in the United States

        2) clinical features:

            a) four clinical stages (WHO) based according to severity:

                i. Stage I consists of immature follicles on the upper palpebral conjunctiva with no scars

                ii. Stage II consists of mature follicles on the upper palpebral conjunctiva with no scars

                iii. Stage III consists of follicles and scarring of the upper tarsal conjunctiva

                iv. Stage IV consists of inactive trachoma with extensive scarring

            b) progressive cicatrization results in entropion, trichiasis, corneal scarring, opacification, and blindness

        3) treatment:

            a) improved facial hygiene—face washing with water

    b) topical tetracycline, erythromycin, or sulf-acetamide ointment

    c) oral administration of any of these is curative

    d) medications must be continued for at least 2 months

    e) single dose administration of systemic macrolides (Azithromycin, Clarithromycin) may be curative

b. adult inclusion conjunctivitis

  1) epidemiology:

    a) associated with sexually transmitted chlamydial disease

    b) eye is involved by direct or indirect contact with genital secretions

    c) transmission through inadequately chlorinated swimming pools has been published

    d) ocular involvement occurs 1 to 2 weeks following exposure

    e) often occurs in adults and in adolescence

    f) subacute or chronic in nature, with patients presenting with symptoms of at least 6 months

  2) clinical features:

    a) follicular conjunctivitis present with nontender preauricular adenopathy

    b) no membranes appear

    c) in contrast to newborn inclusion conjunctivitis (inclusion blennorrhea), mild mucopurulent discharge may be present

  3) diagnosis:

    a) should be based on clinical suspicion

    b) difficult to obtain chlamydial cultures; however, can reinforce your clinical diagnosis

  4) treatment:

    a) treatment of choice for adults is doxycycline 100 mg po bid for 7 days or oral tetracycline 500 mg tid for 3 weeks or oral erythromycin 250 mg qid for 3 weeks

    b) the patient and his/her sexual partner must be examined and treated

    c) erythromycin may be prescribed to children, or pregnant or lactating women

c. inclusion blennorrhea

  1) clinical features:

    a) inclusion conjunctivitis of the newborn

    b) can cause less follicular response, more mucopurulent discharge, and can present with inflammatory membranes as opposed to chlamydial infection in the adult

        2) treatment:

            a) topical and systemic erythromycin therapy

B. Noninfectious Conjunctivitis

  1. Toxic

    a. clinical features:

      1) often presents with patient currently using ocular medication

      2) usually a history of "pink eye" in the recent past

      3) may note that the eye transiently got better, but worsened despite continued usage of medication

      4) examination will reveal a follicular and papillary response

      5) chemosis may be present

      6) no preauricular node present

    b. treatment:

      1) eliminate the suspected offending medication

      2) mild ocular lubricants and rarely topical corticosteroids may be necessary to help with comfort

    c. diagnosis:

      1) cultures are negative or may have normal flora present

      2) cold compresses can occasionally alleviate discomfort

  2. Contact lens associated

    a. clinical features:

      1) can develop ocular irritation with redness, itching, and mucoid discharge

      2) corneal involvement can involve punctate staining and limbal vascularization

      3) characteristic papillae on the upper tarsal conjunctiva

      4) "giant papillae" can occur as a more severe form of this disease; greater than 1 millimeter in diameter

      5) soft contact lenses are primarily responsible, but reactions to solutions or other unknown factors can be responsible for this disease

    b. diagnosis:

      1) clinical, based on contact lens wearing history

    c. treatment:

      1) ideally, discontinuation of contact lens usage is curative; however, patients are not usually willing to do this. If the specific offending agent can be isolated, the avoidance of this can relieve the patient of the symptoms.

      2) trial of stopping various offending agents is recommended (e.g., changing the contact lens solution); specific contact lens type may be changed next

    3) pharmacology therapy includes inhibition of mast cell degranulation; Alomide (lodoxamide) or Crolom (cromolyn sodium) and a short course of mild topical corticosteroid for severe inflammation

3. Hay fever conjunctivitis
  a. clinical features:
    1) occurs with other systemic manifestations of hay fever
    2) eyelids swell, with itching, conjunctival chemosis and erythema, and watery discharge
  b. diagnosis:
    1) clinical, often in association with systemic manifestations of hay fever, such as allergic rhinitis, urticaria, or asthma
  c. treatment:
    1) numerous topical antihistamine drops are available
    2) formulations are often made in conjunction with vasoconstricting agents
    3) cold compresses
    4) oral antihistamine drugs

4. Vernal conjunctivitis
  a. clinical features:
    1) hyperemia and chemosis of the conjunctiva
    2) itching lids and occasionally edematous
    3) photophobia and a mucous discharge
    4) diffuse papillary hypertrophy on tarsal conjunctival surface
    5) papillae can coalesce into giant papillae
    6) "limbal vernal" conjunctivitis presents with limbal papillae and micropannus; more common in young male African-American patients
    7) focal collections of eosinophils may be seen at the limbus (Horner-Trantas dots)
    8) in severe cases, a "shield ulcer" develops on the cornea in a characteristic oval shape
  b. treatment:
    1) mast cell degranulation inhibitors, Alomide (lodoxamide) and Crolom (cromolyn sodium) are effective
    2) because of their mode of action, relief of symptoms may take up to 2 weeks
    3) cold compresses and topical vasoconstricting drops
    4) topical corticosteroid drops work well for this disease; should be used sparingly due to side effects with prolonged administration

IV. INFECTIOUS KERATITIS

A. Bacterial Keratitis
1. Epidemiology:
   a. risk factors associated with bacterial keratitis include:
      1) corneal injury—physical or chemical
      2) contact lens wear; overnight use of contact lenses and extended wear contact lenses carry a higher risk
      3) prolonged use of topical corticosteroids
      4) prior corneal disease such as bullous keratopathy
      5) lid abnormalities such as trichiasis, lagophthalmos, entropion
      6) dry eyes
      7) systemic conditions such as extensive burns, systemic immunosuppression, chronic alcoholism, severe malnutrition
2. Clinical features:
   a. ulceration of corneal epithelium
   b. corneal stromal infiltration in an area lacking epithelium
   c. surrounding edema and striae of the cornea
   d. endothelial fibrin plaque may be present
   e. cell and flare and/or a hypopyon in the anterior chamber may be associated with corneal infection
   f. may be central or peripheral
   g. can be caused by any of a large number of microorganisms
   h. peripheral ulcers are usually staphylococcal, and are often associated with a concurrent blepharoconjunctivitis
   i. possible predisposing factors include ocular environment, focal or systemic abnormalities, and status of the host defense system
   j. clinical characteristics of an infection caused by a specific organism are well documented in the literature. However, it is not usually possible to make this determination by clinical exam alone
   k. obtaining material for culture in suspected infectious keratitis is essential to identify causative organisms and to determine antimicrobial susceptibility
   l. typically, gram-positive organisms tend to produce discrete focal infections. Gram-negative bacteria (e.g., Pseudomonas) create a highly destructive keratitis with more necrosis and suppurative exudate.

3. Diagnosis:
   a. corneal scrapings with a sterile #15 Bard-Parker blade or a flame-sterilized platinum kimura spatula must be taken for culture; done after instillation of topical anesthesia; obtain as much material as possible, especially from the margins and deep edges of the infected area
   b. scrapings should be cultured on several media, including blood agar (for common bacteria), chocolate agar (for Neisseria and Hemophilus species), Sabouraud's agar (for fungi), thioglycolate broth (for anaerobic and aerobic bacteria). In cases where Nocardia or Mycobacteria species are suspected, the Löwenstein-Jensen medium should be used.
   c. Gram, Giemsa, and acid-fast stains should be performed
4. Treatment:
   a. start broad spectrum topical antibiotic therapy at frequent intervals, changing to specific therapy when culture/susceptibility reports return
   b. should be intensive and closely supervised and observed to prevent progression
   c. specific initial antibiotic therapy should be guided by results of the Gram stain from the corneal scraping
   d. one possible initial therapy for broad spectrum coverage is cefazolin 50 mg/ml, and tobramycin 14 mg/ml; initially given every 15 to 30 minutes for the first 24 hours
   e. can be tapered as clinical improvement occurs
   f. antibiotic preparations are not commercially available. Therefore, they must be fortified by the local or hospital pharmacy. The formulas for preparation of these fortified antibiotic eyedrops are well described in the literature.
   g. patients should be admitted to the hospital for initial therapy since the necessity for frequent instillation of eye drops necessitates nursing help.
   h. in the community, corneal ulcers are now being treated on an outpatient basis with the commercially available ophthalmic preparation of ciprofloxacin (Ciloxan) or ofloxacin (Ocuflox). Results have generally been good for small ulcers, usually gram-positive in origin. Concerns exist, however, for resistant strains of streptococci, anaerobes, enterococci.
   i. The efficacy of subconjunctival instillation of antibiotics is controversial, especially with good

compliance of the topical regimen. In cases when compliance with topical therapy is in doubt, subconjunctival therapy should include 100 mg of cefazolin and 40 mg of gentamicin. The injection should be given every 12 to 24 hours depending on the severity of the infection and the subsequent culture results.

j. systemic antibiotics have not proven to add benefit for bacterial keratitis except in cases with marked stromal thinning and impending perforation

k. steroid therapy is most controversial in the management of bacterial keratitis. It is unwise to use steroids until at least 1 to 2 days of antibiotic treatment has been completed. Low-dose topical steroids may diminish the inflammatory reaction in the cornea once the infection has been brought under control. In fact, the secondary inflammation in the cornea is often as big a problem as the infection itself in causing visual loss.

B. Herpes Simplex Viral Keratitis
1. Epidemiology
   a. viral keratitis is primarily herpes simplex virus disease, though other viral infections are possible (including herpes zoster virus, Epstein-Barr virus, adenovirus, and coxsackie virus)
   b. HSV keratitis is the most common cause of corneal blindness in the western hemisphere (up to half a million cases diagnosed in the U.S. annually)
   c. 0.5 to 1.5 cases of HSV keratitis/1000 population
   d. bilateral HSV involvement in 12% of cases
   e. in adults, over 85% of ocular isolates are HSV1
   f. in neonates, 80% of HSV infection by HSV2; HSV2 corneal disease more severe than HSV1
   g. herpetic keratitis may be the third most common cause for penetrating keratoplasty
   h. clinically manifest disease begins 3 to 9 days after exposure
   i. primarily ocular infection with herpes simplex includes conjunctivitis
   j. recurrent HSV disease in the cornea can occur in four forms:
      1) epithelial keratitis
      2) disciform stromal keratitis
      3) necrotizing stromal keratitis
      4) stromal keratouveitis
2. Epithelial keratitis:
   a. epidemiology
      1) 63% of initial ocular HSV episodes are epithelial keratitis
   b. clinical features:

       1) marked by a typical dendritic epithelial defect, with overhanging margins of swollen epithelial cells

       2) shape may also be ameboid, punctate, or stellate

       3) edges of the epithelial defect stain with rose bengal, and the bed stains with fluorescein

       4) stroma is not involved initially

       5) stromal edema and subepithelial infiltrates may appear after a week

       6) corneal hypesthesia is variable

  c. treatment:

       1) often heals spontaneously

       2) treatment options include simple minimal wiping debridement and topical antiviral agents

       3) benefits of antiviral usage should be weighed against the toxic effects of the medication

       4) prolonged treatment causes delayed epithelial healing. A short course, therefore, is all that is usually necessary.

       5) options include:

          a) Viroptic (trifluridine) 1 drop five times daily

          b) IDU ointment five times daily

          c) IDU solution every hour during the day with ointment at night

       6) after the dendrites have healed, most cornea have no residual scars; may see hazy, subepithelial scars ("ghost dendrites"); may or may not cause visual acuity changes

3. Disciform stromal keratitis

  a. epidemiology:

       1) precise pathogenesis not known

       2) why some patients have disciform keratitis following dendritic epitheliitis and others do not is unclear; multiple factors may play a role, including virus strains subtyped, host defense factors, and environmental factors

  b. clinical features:

       1) a descriptive term initially used before the advent of modern diagnostic techniques

       2) thought to represent a cell-mediated immune response to herpes virus antigens, though virus particles have been seen in the stroma in certain studies

       3) stromal edema usually marked with striae present

       4) keratic precipitates and cell and flare in the anterior chamber may be present

       5) ocular hypo- or hypertension is also common

6) corneal hypesthesia, the concurrent or previous presence of dendrites, and the history of prior herpetic disease are also associated

c. treatment:
1) corticosteroids are indicated for suppression of edema and inflammation
2) ophthalmologists debate the treatment regimen, so clinical judgment is required
3) Prednisolone acetate or phosphate 1% 6 to 8 times a day is a common beginning point
4) concomitant prophylactic antiviral usage is also controversial. Many clinicians use trifluridine 1% drops 3 to 4 times a day.
5) oral acyclovir (200 to 400 mg five times a day) is also used by many ophthalmologists
6) tapering of the steroid drops should be slow, up to several months
7) premature discontinuance causes rebound inflammation

4. Necrotizing stromal keratitis
a. epidemiology:
1) patients often have had many prior attacks of herpetic disease in the eye
b. clinical features:
1) necrotic, white, opaque, and heavily infiltrated appearing lesions
2) vascularized cornea present
3) occasional thinning or perforation is possible
4) exact pathogenesis not known. Many doctors believe that it is caused by direct viral infection of the stroma, with the resulting immune process causing the visible clinical signs.
c. treatment:
1) much controversy surrounds the treatment
2) corticosteroid drops may suppress inflammation, but may enhance viral replication. Therefore, commonly, corticosteroids are given concomitantly with prophylactic antiviral agents; slow taper may take many months and up to a few years to complete.

5. Keratouveitis
a. epidemiology:
1) occurs in patients with or without active keratitis
2) etiology is unknown; viral particles have been isolated from the aqueous humor; an immune inflammatory component is also postulated
b. clinical features:
1) iritis may be focal or diffuse

        a) focal iritis—focal corneal edema, keratic precipitates, cell and flare in the anterior chamber, scattered areas of hyperemic and swollen iris, localized posterior synechiae

        b) diffuse iritis—3+ to 4+ cell and flare, sterile hypopyon, fibrin in anterior chamber, secondary elevated intraocular pressure

    c. treatment:

        1) manage mild disease with cycloplegics only

        2) if inflammation uncontrolled, use topical corticosteroids

        3) role of oral acyclovir (200 mg five times a day for 2 to 3 weeks) is unclear; it is suggested that oral acyclovir may prevent chronic recurrent episodes of HSV epithelial keratitis

C. Herpes Zoster Keratitis

  1. epidemiology:

    a. occurs in primary and secondary form

    b. acute infection is primary disease commonly known as chicken pox

    c. virus remains latent in a dorsal root ganglion

    d. secondary disease characterized by reeruption of the virus distributed over the sensory dermatome innervated by the affected ganglion

    e. both characterized by the vesicular skin lesions

    f. ophthalmic involvement usually presents with a combination of one or more of the following:

        1) conjunctivitis

        2) scleritis

        3) keratitis

        4) uveitis

        5) glaucoma

    g. rarely extraocular muscles, choroid, or optic nerve may be involved

  2. Conjunctivitis

    a. clinical features:

        1) occurs in the majority of cases

        2) follicular conjunctival inflammation present with preauricular adenopathy

        3) sclera can be diffusely inflamed and may leave scleral thinning upon resolution

  3. Keratitis

    a. clinical features:

        1) cornea may develop superficial, geographic, or dendritic keratitis resembling herpes simplex

        2) smaller and less branching dendrites

        3) coarse dendrites, with dull, irregular staining; appear as "painted on"

        4) disciform keratitis is also possible; this may occur in any layer of the stroma

        5) corneal thinning may occur with corneal perforation as a rare complication

4. Uveitis

  a. clinical features:

      1) frequent occurrence

      2) independent of corneal inflammation

      3) presents with keratic precipitates on the posterior cornea

      4) cell and flare, with occasional hypopyon

      5) synechia and occasional secondary glaucoma can result

      6) sector atrophy of the iris is often seen after resolution

5. Glaucoma

  a. clinical features:

      1) usually acutely secondary to uveitis

      2) chronic glaucoma after resolution is due to the anterior synechia that may have formed

  b. diagnosis:

      1) clinician should have no problem in differentiating herpes zoster from herpes simplex

      2) characteristic dermatomal distribution of vesicular eruption on the skin is present

      3) often severe neuralgia from the acute swelling and inflammation during the early phase of the disease

      4) prolonged and severe pain sometimes occurs for years after the cutaneous lesions have healed (postherpetic neuralgia)

      5) other features differentiating herpes zoster from herpes simplex include: coarser, blunter dendrites, iris atrophy, and unilaterality

  c. treatment:

      1) high dose of systemic antiviral acyclovir appears to decrease iris progression and pain (600 to 800 mg po five times a day for 2 weeks is recommended)

      2) if uveitis or stromal inflammation is present, prednisone 1% drops qid may be necessary

      3) topical antibiotics should be used if ulcerative keratitis is present

      4) of grave concern are epithelial defects and corneal melting. Because of the hypoesthesia often present, care should be taken to protect the ocular surface. This includes daily lubrication, antibiotics, and close observation.

      5) cycloplegics should be used to control pain and prevent posterior and anterior synechiae

6) use of systemic steroids for postherpetic neuralgia is controversial

7) upon resolution of inflammation, corneas that are scarred by herpes zoster receive corneal transplants, though long-term prognosis for these grafts is only fair

D. Fungal Keratitis

1. Epidemiology:

   a. incidence of fungal keratitis is increasing, partially because of better recognition and laboratory abilities; increased use of corticosteroids and immunosuppressive drugs may play a role

   b. different organisms are predominant in different geographical areas. Yeast species are more common in northern latitudes, whereas filamentous fungi predominate in the southern U.S.

2. Clinical features:

   a. opportunistic organisms often infecting a previously traumatized cornea, as well as following contact with plant or vegetable matter

   b. usually slowly progressing, but may manifest in 1 to 2 days following trauma especially with organic materials

   c. granular infiltrates with a dirty gray color

   d. minimal stromal inflammation

   e. feathery appearing infiltrate with irregular margins

   f. frequently present immune rings

   g. decreasing conjunctival hyperemia, cell, flare, and hypopyon as the disease progresses

   h. produces a completely opaque cornea with severe infections, with features similar to severe bacterial keratitis

   i. necrosis and perforation may follow

3. Pathology:

   a. Two major classifications of fungi are responsible: the filamentous type (the molds), and the yeasts, and also a diphasic group of organisms that have both yeast and filamentous phases.

      1) the yeast consist primarily of *Candida* species; unicellular, oval organisms that reproduce by budding

      2) filamentous fungi are multicellular that produce long branching hyphae; hyphae may or may not be septate. Examples: *Fusarium, Aspergillis, Acremonium, Mucor,* and *Penicillium.* Diphasic organisms include *Blastomyces, Coccidioides,* and *Histoplasma.*

   b. often mimics other corneal diseases which may lead to improper treatment and secondary progression of the fungal infection

      c. may occur in a variety of clinical settings and have different presentations

      d. stains and cultures are essential to make the diagnosis accurately. Gram and Giemsa stains can be examined for yeast or hyphae. Other useful stains include Gomori's methenamine silver stain and periodic acid-Schiff stain.

      e. cultures may be on blood agar at room temperature or Sabouraud's agar or brain-heart infusion with gentamicin

      f. the majority of organisms and fungal keratitis may grow within a week. However, several instances have been documented where two weeks have been necessary for organisms to grow.

   4. Treatment:

      a. natamycin 5% is the only commercially available and FDA-approved antifungal agent

      b. none of the presently available antifungal agents are ideal for fungal keratitis. Problems include resistant organisms, low solubility of medication in solution, and local ocular toxicity.

      c. amphotericin B (0.5 to 10 mg/ml) applied every hour has been the mainstay of therapy against *Candida* and *Aspergillis* species

      d. natamycin 50 mg/ml suspension is active against a variety of filamentous fungi, especially *Fusarium* species

      e. both agents cause ocular surface toxicity, especially the amphotericin B solution, which causes the toxicity due to the vehicle that holds it in solution

      f. other drugs are available and are being investigated for their efficacy against fungal keratitis. In severe fungal keratitis, systemic treatment with oral flucytosine is recommended.

      g. aqueous humor levels are high after oral administration of this medication

E. Parasitic Keratitis

   1. Common causes of blindness in many third-world countries

      a. leishmaniasis is found throughout the Middle East, Africa, India, and Central and South America

      b. onchocerciasis, one of the four leading causes of blindness worldwide, is found in Africa, Mexico, and Central and South America

      c. in the United States, *Acanthamoeba* is the most common parasite causing keratitis

   2. Acanthamoeba keratitis

      a. epidemiology:

    1) five species have been reported to cause keratitis: *A. castellani, A. culbertsoni, A. hatchetti, A. polyphaga, A. rhysodes*

    2) found in soil, fresh water, salt water, and air

    3) present in swimming pools, bottled and tap water, homemade saline solutions, air conditioning units, and contact lens cases and solutions; 85% of *Acanthamoeba* keratitis cases occur in contact lens wearers

    4) the life cycle consists of two stages: a trophozoite stage and a cyst stage

    5) the trophozoite is mobile, and in unfavorable environmental conditions, it encysts

    6) the cyst form of *Acanthamoeba* is highly resistant to heat, cold, and extremes of pH, and can exist for months to years in such harsh conditions

    7) infections result from exposure to large numbers of organisms through a break in the ocular surface

  b. clinical features:

    1) young, healthy individuals, history of direct contact of the eye with contaminated fluid

    2) infection usually unilateral with severe pain out of proportion to findings

    3) recurrent corneal erosions with pseudodendrites

    4) classic appearance is a stromal ring infiltrate, but presentation can vary widely

    5) mild anterior chamber reaction, rarely creating a hypopyon

    6) chronic and progressive infection

    7) often delay in diagnosis and misdiagnosed as herpes

    8) concurrent scleritis often present

    9) negative routine cultures

  c. diagnosis:

    1) difficult, often missed because of weeks and months of therapy

    2) fruitless search for other causative organisms

    3) calcafluor white or acridine orange stains are sensitive stains for detection of *Acanthamoeba* organisms. Fluorescent microscope is needed.

    4) nonnutrient agar plate coated with *E. coli* needed for culturing. Plates therefore must be prepared ahead of time

    5) contact lenses and cases cultured for contact lens wearers

    d. treatment:
        1) controversial
        2) no ideal treatment
        3) includes topical polyhexamethylene biguanide 0.2% or chlorhexidine gluconate 0.2% combined with propamidine isethionate (Brolene) or hexamidine every hour while awake, polymyxin B sulfate, neomycin sulfate, and gramicidin drops (Neosporin) every hour while awake, and oral itraconazole or fluconazole
        4) topical corticosteroid use is controversial
        5) penetrating keratoplasty may be necessary, but should be avoided while active inflammation is present
        6) reported recurrence of the infection in grafts

V. IMMUNOLOGIC DISEASES OF THE CONJUNCTIVA AND CORNEA

  A. Allergic Conjunctivitis (see Chapter 14)
  B. Vernal Conjunctivitis (see Chapter 14)
  C. Giant Papillary Conjunctivitis (see Chapter 14)
  D. Cicatricial Pemphigoid
    1. Epidemiology:
      a. presumed autoimmune disorder of unknown etiology
      b. probably Type II hypersensitivity reaction
    2. Clinical features:
      a. chronic bilateral disease of the elderly
      b. repeated mild ulceration early on
      c. with progression, the fornices shorten with symblepharon formation
      d. severely destructed ocular surface with further scarring, loss of goblet cells, and decreased mucin and aqueous
      e. corneal surface damaged due to an abnormal tear film
      f. secondary trichiasis and occasional exposure keratopathy, leading to keratinization, ulceration, vascularization, and possible perforation
    3. Pathology:
      a. numerous conjunctival changes present
      b. chronic inflammation with decrease in goblet cells
      c. deposition of immunoglobulins along the basement membrane of the conjunctival epithelium
    4. Diagnosis:
      a. based on clinical findings
      b. conjunctival biopsies with immunopathologic studies
      c. temporary conjunctival inflammation from biopsy

 5. Treatment:
  a. difficult, and often ineffective
  b. various studies differ widely in recommended treatments
  c. options: high dose systemic corticosteroids, cyclophosphamide, azathioprine, or cyclosporine
  d. topical treatment: aggressive artificial tears and ointments
  e. avoid eyelid or conjunctival surgery due to secondary reactivation of the disease
E. Stevens-Johnson Syndrome (Erythema Multiforme Major)
 1. Epidemiology:
  a. occurs usually secondary to infections, drug reactions, or spontaneously (idiopathic)
 2. Clinical features:
  a. primarily a cutaneous and mucosal eruption of erythematous macules, papules, and vesicles
  b. healing of the skin occurs within weeks, ocular involvement presents as severe bilateral conjunctivitis of varying severity with up to half of patients experiencing permanent visual sequelae
  c. conjunctival inflammation frequently results in cicatrization
  d. symblephara, entropion, trichiasis, and tear film abnormalities with varying degrees of corneal scarring and vascularization
  e. similar to cicatricial pemphigoid in appearance
 3. Pathology:
  a. inflammation of the subepithelial layers of the conjunctiva with subsequent fibrosis
  b. many potential etiologic agents
  c. commonly associated drugs include sulfa drugs, various antibiotics, anticonvulsants, and antiinflammatory agents
  d. infectious agents include most commonly streptococci, but can include others including herpes simplex and mycoplasma
 4. Diagnosis:
  a. based on history and clinical features
 5. Treatment:
  a. difficult
  b. acutely, systemic corticosteroids can lessen the inflammatory stage
  c. ocular surface treatment should include topical lubrication to protect the corneal surface and correction of eyelid abnormalities
  d. corneal transplants have a poor prognosis
F. Connective Tissue Diseases
 1. Rheumatoid arthritis

     a. clinical features:
       1) most common systemic vasculitic disorder to involve the ocular surface
       2) keratoconjunctivitis sicca, scleritis, and rarely keratitis occur
       3) development of scleritis portends poor prognosis. Studies show most of these patients will die within five years without aggressive treatment.
       4) corneal involvement is most often due to K-sicca
       5) may lead to corneal thinning and perforation. This can occur in the perilimbal region and extends centrally.
     b. pathology:
       1) pathogenesis is not clear; possibilities include immunologic responses to unknown antigens and genetic susceptibility
     c. treatment:
       1) imperative
       2) ocular lubricants are necessary for the secondary aqueous tear layer insufficiency
       3) topical corticosteroids should be avoided in cases of corneal melting
       4) for corneal melting, gluing (with a cyanoacrylate adhesive), or lamellar or penetrating keratoplasty may be necessary
       5) surgery should be avoided if possible while active inflammation exists
  2. Sjögren's syndrome
     a. epidemiology:
       1) multisystem disease primarily in middle-aged women, but can be seen in both sexes at all ages
       2) can be associated with other autoimmune disorders
     b. clinical features:
       1) keratoconjunctivitis sicca is most common ocular presentation
       2) peripheral corneal changes may occur including stromal infiltrates
     c. pathology:
       1) autoimmune disease of unknown etiology
     d. treatment:
       1) lubricating agents on ocular surface
       2) punctal occlusion and bandage contact lenses
       3) short-term therapy with topical corticosteroids for peripheral infiltrates; avoid if melting occurs
  3. Systemic lupus erythematosus (SLE)

       a. epidemiology:
          1) multisystem autoimmune disorder
       b. clinical features:
          1) ocular complications occur in all levels including keratoconjunctivitis sicca, episcleritis, keratitis, corneal ulceration, uveitis, and retinal vasculitis
       c. treatment:
          1) systemic treatment is imperative
          2) topical corticosteroids are often useful, except in cases of corneal melting

    4. Other vasculitides: polyarteritis nodosa, Wegener's granulomatosis, scleroderma (multisystem autoimmune disorders)
       a. clinical features:
          1) ocular involvement includes keratoconjunctivitis sicca and inflammation of various layers of the globe
       b. treatment:
          1) treatment of ocular involvement is dependent on adequate therapy of the systemic disease
          2) topical lubrication is essential
          3) topical steroids may occasionally be of benefit (unless melting is present)

G. Corneal Melts
    1. Rheumatoid arthritis
      (see above)
    2. Terrien's marginal degeneration
       a. epidemiology:
          1) quiet, slowly progressive thinning of peripheral cornea of unknown etiology
       b. clinical features:
          1) thinning is usually superior and spreads circumferentially
          2) inferior cornea is rarely involved
          3) epithelium intact
          4) fine vascular pannus crosses the area of stromal thinning up to the relatively steep central wall of the gutter
          5) lipid line appears at the leading edge of the pannus
          6) perforation is rare, but astigmatism develops from corneal thinning
       c. pathology:
          1) histiocytes are predominant on microscopic examination
       d. diagnosis:
          1) infectious ulceration must be eliminated with corneal scrapings and culture

 2) systemic workup for immunologic disorders should be undertaken
 3) diagnosis of exclusion
 e. treatment:
 1) symptoms of mild irritation may need to be treated with lubrication
 2) lamellar or full thickness corneal-scleral grafting may be required for severe thinning
H. Mooren's Ulcer
  1. Epidemiology:
   a. rare, idiopathic, noninfectious ulceration of the peripheral cornea
   b. two clinical types categorized, one more malignant than the other
  2. Clinical features:
   a. typically affects adult males
   b. begins as a peripheral corneal infiltrate and progresses following the limbus, classically inferiorly, with ulceration
   c. usually no clear zone between the ulcer and limbus
   d. central margin of the ulcer has a characteristic overhanging edge of intact epithelium
   e. adjacent sclera is characteristically inflamed
   f. perforation is common, especially in the malignant form of Mooren's ulcer
   g. healing occurs with conjunctival and scleral vessels growing into the ulcer bed
  3. Pathology:
   a. autoimmune disease with all types of inflammatory cells present
  4. Diagnosis:
   a. based on clinical appearance and lack of positive cultures or lid margin disease
  5. Treatment:
   a. often frustrating and ineffective
   b. topical steroids may be of use in the limited subtype of Mooren's ulcer; not useful in the malignant type
   c. systemic corticosteroids are controversial
   d. systemic immunosuppressive agents are occasionally helpful (azathioprine, cyclophosphamide, methotrexate, or cyclosporine)
  6. Surgical treatment:
   a. includes resection of adjacent conjunctival tissue
   b. for perforation, lamellar or penetrating keratoplasties may be necessary if cyanoacrylate glue application is inadequate
   c. reports of patch graft involvement in the disease process

d. a vascularized, thinned, and scarred cornea is left after the inflammation with often diminished visual acuity

VI. CORNEAL DYSTROPHIES

A. Epithelial Corneal Dystrophies

1. Epithelial basement membrane dystrophy—also called Map-Dot-Fingerprint Dystrophy and Cogan's Microcystic Dystrophy
   a. epidemiology:
      1) probable autosomal dominant inheritance
      2) onset early adulthood and middle age
   b. clinical features:
      1) bilateral and symmetric
      2) presenting symptoms: transient blurred vision; mild early morning irritation; painful recurrent erosions
      3) biomicroscopic findings: gray patches, microcysts, and/or thin concentric lines in central epithelium
      4) clinical course: recurrent erosions common; even minor trauma may cause a major epithelial breakdown with impaired subsequent healing
   c. pathogenesis:
      1) abnormality of epithelial turnover, maturation, and production of basement membrane with abnormal adhesion complexes (hemidesmosomes, anchoring fibrils)
      2) intraepithelial microcysts (dots) represent intraepithelial spaces with debris of degenerated epithelial cells; subepithelial ridges (fingerprints) and geographic opacities (maps) represent thickened multilaminar strips of epithelial basement membrane with some extension into the abnormal epithelium
   d. diagnosis:
      1) based on clinical presentation
   e. treatment:
      1) conservative treatment consists of lubricants, hypertonic saline, patching, and bandage soft contact lens
      2) epithelial debridement, superficial keratectomy, phototherapeutic keratectomy, and anterior stromal puncture may be necessary
2. Meesman's Dystrophy—also called Hereditary Juvenile Epithelial Dystrophy
   a. epidemiology:
      1) autosomal dominant inheritance
      2) may be evident in first few months of life

      b. clinical features:
- **1)** bilateral and symmetric
- **2)** presenting symptoms: foreign body sensation and mildly decreased visual acuity
- **3)** biomicroscopic findings: tiny epithelial cysts seen as clear to gray-white punctate opacities located mostly in the interpalpebral zone of the cornea but may extend to limbus; cysts are uniform size and shape and a few may stain with fluorescein; thickened epithelium and basement membrane
- **4)** clinical course: recurrent erosions

      c. pathogenesis:
- **1)** cysts are accumulations of degenerated cellular material and basement membrane-like debris surrounded by adjacent cells; cells contain periodic acid Schiff (PAS)-positive material and a dense intracellular substance of unknown composition ("peculiar substance")

      d. diagnosis:
- **1)** based on clinical presentation

      e. treatment:
- **1)** conservative treatment consists of lubricants and patching

  3. Reis-Bückler's dystrophy

      a. epidemiology:
- **1)** autosomal dominant inheritance
- **2)** onset first to second decade

      b. clinical features:
- **1)** bilateral and symmetric
- **2)** presenting symptoms: pain and decreased vision
- **3)** biomicroscopic findings: irregular epithelium with diffuse, irregular, patchy geographic opacities at the level of Bowman's layer
- **4)** clinical course: recurrent erosions; central opacities develop as a diffuse superficial stromal haze

      c. pathogenesis:
- **1)** destruction of Bowman's membrane and its replacement by fibrillar material

      d. diagnosis:
- **1)** based on clinical presentation

      e. treatment:
- **1)** superficial keratectomy, phototherapeutic keratectomy; it recurs in the corneal transplant following penetrating keratoplasty

B. Stromal Corneal Dystrophies

  1. Central cloudy dystrophy (Francois)

      a. epidemiology:
          1) autosomal dominant inheritance
      b. clinical features:
          1) bilateral and symmetric
          2) presenting symptoms: often asymptomatic; vision may be mildly affected
          3) biomicroscopic findings: axial posterior cloudy stromal opacities with clear intervening stroma
          4) clinical course: nonprogressive
      c. diagnosis:
          1) based on clinical presentation
      d. treatment:
          1) no therapy is required

2. Central crystalline dystrophy (Schnyder)
      a. epidemiology:
          1) autosomal dominant inheritance
          2) onset age 1 year
      b. clinical features:
          1) bilateral and symmetric
          2) presenting symptoms: decreased vision
          3) biomicroscopic findings: tiny yellow-white anterior stromal crystals; dense arcus; limbal girdle of Vogt
          4) clinical course: diffuse stromal haze may develop
      c. pathogenesis:
          1) the abnormal deposits are composed of neutral fats and cholesterol
      d. diagnosis
          1) based on clinical presentation
          2) some patients exhibit hypercholesterolemia, xanthelasma, genu valgum
      e. treatment:
          1) penetrating keratoplasty
          2) if superficial, consider phototherapeutic keratectomy

3. Congenital hereditary stromal dystrophy
      a. epidemiology:
          1) autosomal dominant inheritance
          2) onset at birth
      b. clinical features:
          1) bilateral and symmetric
          2) biomicroscopic findings: flaky or feathery clouding of the stroma; both the peripheral and central cornea are affected, especially the central cornea
          3) clinical course: nonprogressive
      c. pathogenesis:

            1) possibly a disorder in collagen fibrogenesis
      d. diagnosis:
            1) based on clinical presentation
      e. treatment:
            1) not usually necessary
    4. Fleck dystrophy (Francois-Neetens)
      a. epidemiology:
            1) autosomal dominant inheritance
            2) onset possibly at birth
            3) rare
      b. clinical features:
            1) bilateral and symmetric
            2) presenting symptoms: asymptomatic
            3) biomicroscopic findings: subtle grayish specks
               present in all layers of the cornea; some appear
               as rings with relatively less opacified centers
            4) clinical course: nonprogressive
      c. pathogenesis:
            1) abnormal keratocytes which contain a fibrillo-
               granular substance with intracytoplasmic vac-
               uoles
      d. diagnosis:
            1) based on clinical presentation
      e. treatment:
            1) not necessary
    5. Granular dystrophy
      a. epidemiology:
            1) autosomal dominant inheritance
            2) onset early adolescence
      b. clinical features:
            1) bilateral and symmetric
            2) presenting symptoms: minimal inflammation
               and irritation
            3) biomicroscopic findings: discrete, white, focal
               granular deposits resembling bread crumbs
               that are confined to the anterior stroma and do
               not extend to the periphery; there are interven-
               ing clear zones
            4) clinical course: slowly progressive; the lesion
               may extend more posteriorly in the stroma
               with time; recurrent erosions
      c. pathogenesis:
            1) the abnormal deposits are composed of hyaline
            2) Masson's trichrome stain: bright red
            3) PAS negative
      d. diagnosis:
            1) based on clinical presentation
      e. treatment:
            1) superficial keratectomy, phototherapeutic ker-
               atectomy, penetrating keratoplasty

    6. Lattice dystrophy

      a. epidemiology:

         1) autosomal dominant inheritance

         2) onset first decade

      b. clinical features:

         1) bilateral and symmetric

         2) presenting symptoms: painful recurrent erosions and decreased vision

         3) biomicroscopic findings: grayish linear, branching, thread-like opacities with intervening clear areas; more involved centrally

         4) clinical course: recurrent erosions common; stromal haze develops

      c. pathogenesis:

         1) the abnormal deposits are composed of amyloid

         2) congo red: positive

         3) crystal violet: metachromasia

         4) thioflavin-T: fluorescence

         5) birefringence and dichroism

         6) PAS positive

      d. diagnosis:

         1) based on clinical presentation

         2) there are several types of lattice dystrophy:

            a) lattice corneal dystrophy type I: described above; onset less than 10 years of age; visual acuity markedly impaired by age 40 to 60 years; no systemic amyloidosis

            b) lattice corneal dystrophy type II (Meretoja Syndrome): onset greater than 20 years of age; visual acuity usually good until after age 65 years; evidence of systemic amyloidosis; autosomal dominant inheritance; mask-like facial expression, blepharochalasis, floppy ears, protruding lips; cranial and peripheral nerve palsies; dry itchy and lax skin with amyloid deposits; corneal involvement characterized by thick and radially oriented lines; episodic corneal erosions common

            c) lattice corneal dystrophy type III: onset greater than 40 years of age; visual acuity impaired after age 60 years; no evidence of systemic amyloidosis; possible autosomal recessive inheritance; corneal involvement characterized by thick lines; no recurrent erosions

            d) familial subepithelial amyloidosis: onset less than 20 years of age; visual acuity markedly impaired by age 10 to 30 years; no evidence of systemic amyloidosis; autosomal recessive inheritance; corneal involvement characterized by multiple prom-inent subepithelial nodules; no recurrent erosions

  e) polymorphic stromal dystrophy: axial polymorphic star and snowflake shaped and branching filamentous stromal opacities in the posterior stroma; intervening stroma is clear; visual acuity not markedly affected; the late appearance of the linear opacities, the lack of progression, and the apparent nonfamilial pattern help to distinguish this condition from lattice dystrophy

  f) gelatinous droplike dystrophy: possibly autosomal recessive inheritance; presents early in life; milky white gelatinous mulberry-like elevated lesion of the epithelium and anterior stroma; mounds of amyloid between the epithelium and Bowman's layer as well as deposits in the deeper stroma; the type of corneal amyloid may be different from that found in lattice dystrophy

e. treatment:
  1) penetrating keratoplasty

7. Macular dystrophy
  a. epidemiology:
    1) autosomal recessive inheritance
    2) onset first decade
    3) rare
  b. clinical features:
    1) bilateral and symmetric
    2) presenting symptoms: decreased vision
    3) biomicroscopic findings: focal gray-white opacities in the superficial stroma with indefinite edges; intervening stroma is not clear; endothelial guttata
    4) clinical course: progression to full stromal thickness and to corneal periphery with time
  c. pathogenesis:
    1) the abnormal deposits are composed of keratin sulfate-like glycosaminoglycans (acid mucopolysaccharide)
    2) colloidal iron: positive
    3) alcian blue: positive
    4) PAS positive
  d. diagnosis:
    1) based on clinical presentation
  e. treatment:
    1) penetrating keratoplasty
8. Posterior mosaic crocodile shagreen

     a. epidemiology:
       1) probable autosomal dominant inheritance
     b. clinical features:
       1) bilateral and symmetric
       2) presenting symptoms: asymptomatic
       3) biomicroscopic findings: small, gray, polygonal patches of various sizes, separated by dark regions, at the level of Descemet's membrane
       4) clinical course: nonprogressive
     c. pathogenesis:
       1) the grayish opacities correspond with sawtooth-like configurations of the corneal collagen lamellae
     d. diagnosis:
       1) based on clinical presentation
     e. treatment:
       1) not necessary

C. Endothelial Corneal Dystrophies
  1. Congenital hereditary endothelial dystrophy
     a. there are two types: an autosomal recessive form (type I) and an autosomal dominant form (type II)
       1) type I
         epidemiology:
         a) autosomal recessive inheritance
         b) onset at birth
         c) more common than autosomal dominant form
       2) clinical features:
         a) bilateral and symmetric
         b) presenting symptoms: decreased visual acuity; no pain, photophobia, or tearing
         c) biomicroscopic findings: profound epithelial and stromal edema (congenital corneal clouding); nystagmus common
         d) clinical course: nonprogressive
       3) type II
         epidemiology:
         a) autosomal dominant inheritance
         b) onset 1 to 2 years
       4) clinical features:
         a) bilateral and symmetric
         b) presenting symptoms: decreased vision, pain, photophobia, tearing
         c) biomicroscopic findings: blue-gray ground glass opacification (corneal clouding); nystagmus absent
         d) clinical course: slowly progressive
       5) pathogenesis:

           a) enlarged stromal collagen fibrils suggest primary developmental abnormality of keratocytes and endothelium

           b) histopathology: long-standing edema results in basal epithelial cell swelling, basement membrane thickening and disruption, and irregularity of Bowman's membrane with pannus formation; Descemet's membrane may be thinned (to 3μ) or thickened (to 40μ) (normal thickness is 3 to 5μ in neonates and 8 to 10μ in adults)

      6) diagnosis:

           a) based on clinical presentation

      7) treatment:

           a) may require penetrating keratoplasty

2. Fuchs' dystrophy

   a. epidemiology:

      1) females > males

      2) onset fifth to sixth decade

      3) frequently autosomal dominant inheritance

   b. clinical features:

      1) bilateral

      2) presenting symptoms: decreased vision, foreign body sensation, pain upon awakening

      3) biomicroscopic findings: corneal guttata give a beaten metal appearance to Descemet's membrane, usually in the axial area; brown pigment may be seen at the level of the guttata (pigment phagocytized by endothelium); axial edema is present and this may spread peripherally

      4) clinical course: stromal edema may progress to involve the epithelium, resulting in microbullous elevations and eventually bullous keratopathy, these blisters may rupture, the course of the dystrophy may be accelerated after cataract extraction or other intraocular surgery

   c. pathogenesis:

      1) corneal guttata in the periphery may be seen in young patients, these are termed Hassall-Henle bodies; these are of no clinical significance. If these become more numerous and centrally located, they may portend functional compromise of the endothelial cells such that the barrier and pump functions become insufficient; the condition is termed Fuchs' dystrophy when stromal edema occurs, and this may be followed by epithelial edema and bullous keratopathy

      2) progressive deterioration of endothelium; as endothelial cells undergo attrition, the surviv-

ing cell population must enlarge and spread to
maintain an intact monolayer

   3) histopathology: diffuse thickening of Descemet's membrane (often to 20µ or more) with
   posteriorly projecting excrescences, corresponding to clinically apparent guttata

   d. diagnosis:
   1) based on clinical presentation
   2) pachymetry: the normal corneal thickness is
   0.52 to 0.56 mm; in Fuchs' dystrophy it may
   increase to 1 mm
   3) specular microscopy

   e. treatment:
   1) conservative treatment consists of lubricants,
   occlusion, bandage soft contact lens
   2) penetrating keratoplasty may ultimately be
   necessary

3. Posterior polymorphous dystrophy
   a. epidemiology:
   1) autosomal dominant inheritance
   b. clinical features:
   1) bilateral
   2) biomicroscopic findings: polymorphous opacities, some of them vesicular or annular with
   surrounding halos, at the level of Descemet's
   membrane
   3) clinical course: stationary or slowly progressive; patients usually retain normal vision;
   rarely, endothelial decompensation occurs
   with resultant stromal edema
   c. pathogenesis:
   1) endothelium may be multilayered and it acquires epithelial characteristics such as
   desmosomes and tonofilaments; the endothelium may migrate over the trabecular meshwork and the iris
   d. diagnosis:
   1) based on clinical presentation
   2) specular microscopy
   e. treatment:
   1) penetrating keratoplasty rarely necessary

VII. CORNEAL DEGENERATIONS

   A. Band Keratopathy
   1. Epidemiology:
      a. conditions associated with band keratopathy include the following:
      1) ocular disease
         a) chronic uveitis (juvenile rheumatoid arthritis)

          b) prolonged glaucoma
          c) long-standing corneal edema
          d) phthisis bulbi
          e) spheroid degeneration
      2) toxic and mercury vapors
      3) hypercalcemia
          a) sarcoidosis
          b) hyperparathyroidism
          c) multiple myeloma
          d) vitamin D toxicity
          e) metastatic disease
      4) noncalcific band keratopathy (urate deposits)

2. Clinical features:

    a. unilateral or bilateral

    b. presenting symptoms: asymptomatic or may result in severe visual loss

    c. biomicroscopic findings: white deposits in the epithelial basement membrane, Bowman's layer, and the superficial stroma confined to the interpalpebral fissure area; the lucid interval separates the calcific band from the limbus; small defects in the band are usually present

    d. clinical course: usually slowly progressive

3. Pathogenesis:

    a. band keratopathy results from localized ocular inflammation or systemic disease

    b. hydroxyapatite deposits of calcium carbonate accumulate in the epithelial basement membrane, Bowman's layer, and the superficial stroma

    c. basophilic staining of the basement membrane of the epithelium is present; this is followed by involvement of Bowman's layer with calcium deposition and eventual fragmentation

    d. band keratopathy may also result from deposition of urates in the cornea; these are usually brown instead of white, which is seen in calcific band keratopathy

4. Diagnosis:

    a. based on clinical presentation

5. Treatment:

    a. superficial keratectomy with the application of the calcium-binding agent ethylenediaminetetraacetic acid (EDTA) may be indicated in cases with visual loss

B. Corneal Arcus

    1. Epidemiology:

        a. juvenile form: arcus juvenilis; may be associated with abnormalities in serum lipids

        b. adult form: arcus senilis

   c. more common in African-Americans

  2. Clinical features:

   a. bilateral and symmetric

   b. presenting symptoms: asymptomatic

   c. biomicroscopic findings: whitish ring of the peripheral cornea separated from limbus by a clear zone; the outer border is sharp and the inner border is indistinct

   d. clinical course: arcus usually begins inferior and superiorly, and eventually encircles the peripheral cornea

  3. Pathogenesis:

   a. paralimbal stromal accumulation of cholesterol esters, triglycerides, and phospholipids; these deposits appear wedge-shaped, being most prominent near Bowman's layer and Descemet's membrane

  4. Diagnosis:

   a. based on clinical presentation

  5. Treatment:

   a. none

 C. Keratoconus

  1. Epidemiology:

   a. onset adolescence

   b. usually sporadic but some cases are familial with an autosomal dominant pattern with incomplete penetrance and variable expressivity

  2. Clinical features:

   a. bilateral but asymmetric

   b. presenting symptoms: subtle irregular astigmatism

   c. biomicroscopic findings: central or paracentral corneal thinning with protrusion of the apex; bulging of the lower lid may occur in downgaze due to the protruding apex of the cone (Munson's sign); vertical stress lines (Vogt's striae) may be present in the deep stroma; a brown iron line may be present deep in the epithelium and Bowman's layer at the base of the cone (Fleischer's ring)

   d. clinical course: acute hydrops may occur when Descemet's membrane is ruptured spontaneously resulting in sudden profound corneal edema and decreased vision; this heals spontaneously in 6 to 10 weeks with resultant stromal scarring

  3. Pathogenesis:

   a. a noninflammatory condition

   b. occurs in association with several ocular and systemic diseases; atopic dermatitis, or a history of eye(lid) rubbing, Down syndrome, Marfan's syndrome

       c. histopathology: focal disruption of Bowman's layer which is replaced in affected areas with keratocytes and collagen; the epithelium is irregular and has abnormal basement membrane in areas where Bowman's layer is destroyed; healing of acute hydrops shows Descemet's membrane to have retracted as scrolls and new Descemet's membrane being deposited by migrating endothelium

    4. Diagnosis:

       a. based on clinical presentation

    5. Treatment:

       a. initial treatment consists of astigmatic spectacle correction or rapid gas permeable or hard contact lens

       b. penetrating keratoplasty may be necessary and is highly successful

D. Keratoglobus

    1. Similar to keratoconus except that the cornea is uniformly thinned, particularly peripherally; the corneal deformation is globular rather than conical; rupture of Descemet's membrane may rarely occur; may be associated with Ehlers-Danlos syndrome; minor trauma may result in rupture of the globe

E. Pellucid Marginal Degeneration

    1. Similar to keratoconus except that the inferior cornea is particularly thinned such that the normal cornea protrudes above the inferior thinned area

F. Mooren's Ulcer

    1. Epidemiology:

       a. males > females

       b. older patients: a benign form; usually unilateral; responsive to treatment

       c. younger patients: severe ocular disease; progressive; bilateral

       d. young Nigerians exhibit a particularly severe form of Mooren's ulcer, with rapid progression to perforation and marked involvement of the limbal sclera in a necrotizing process

    2. Clinical features:

       a. unilateral or bilateral (25% bilateral)

       b. presenting symptoms: usually presents with pain and redness

       c. biomicroscopic findings: peripheral corneal ulceration; usually begins in intrapalpebral area and spreads circumferentially, then centrally; the leading edge of the ulcerative process often undermines the more central corneal stroma

       d. clinical course: may progress to corneal perforation

    3. Pathogenesis:

       a. necrosis of collagen tissue with vessels and chronic inflammatory cells in the adjacent limbal margin; polymorphonuclear leukocytes intensely infiltrate the zone of active ulceration

       b. autoimmunity may play a role

    4. Diagnosis:

       a. based on clinical presentation

    5. Treatment:

       a. conjunctival resection adjacent to the ulcer may be beneficial

       b. perforation may occur following the use of topical steroids

       c. tissue adhesive and lamellar grafting may be necessary if perforation occurs

       d. systemic immunosuppression may be necessary in patients with progressive bilateral disease

G. Pinguecula

    1. Epidemiology:

       a. an age-related degeneration associated with ultraviolet and general environmental exposure

    2. Clinical features:

       a. unilateral or bilateral

       b. biomicroscopic findings: raised, cream-colored, white, or chalky lesion of the conjunctiva adjacent to the limbs and within the palpebral fissure

       c. clinical course: may become inflamed (pingueculitis)

    3. Pathogenesis:

       a. may represent elastotic degeneration of the substantia propria of the conjunctiva

    4. Diagnosis:

       a. based on clinical presentation

    5. Treatment:

       a. treatment is generally not indicated

H. Pterygium

    1. Epidemiology:

       a. an age-related degeneration associated with ultraviolet and general environmental exposure

    2. Clinical features:

       a. unilateral or bilateral

       b. biomicroscopic findings: triangular, fibrovascular connective tissue overgrowth of bulbar conjunctiva onto cornea; horizontally located in interpalpebral fissure on either nasal or temporal side of cornea; may have pigmented iron line (Stocker's line) in advance of the pterygium

       c. clinical course: may progress slowly toward axial cornea; indications of activity are corneal epithelial irregularity, opacification of Bowman's layer,

and prominence of active blood vessels and inflammation
3. Pathogenesis:
    a. subepithelial tissue exhibits elastotic degeneration of collagen, resulting from breakdown of the collagen and destruction of Bowman's membrane; the subepithelial material stains for elastin but is not sensitive to elastase
4. Diagnosis:
    a. based on clinical presentation
5. Treatment:
    a. conservative treatment is recommended
    b. excision is indicated if the visual axis is threatened or if extreme irritation occurs
    c. recurrences may occur within several weeks; recurrences occur in up to 40% of cases
    d. the recurrence rate is reduced if surgery is followed by beta irradiation with strontium 90
    e. treatment with autologous conjunctival transplantation reduces recurrence to 5%
    f. adjunctive treatment with mitomycin C may be beneficial; should be used with caution as cases of scleral necrosis have been reported following the use of mitomycin C
I. Salzmann's Nodular Degeneration
  1. Epidemiology:
      a. occurs in patients with long-standing keratitis, especially phlyctenular disease, trachoma, and interstitial keratitis
  2. Clinical features:
      a. unilateral and bilateral
      b. presenting symptoms: usually asymptomatic but may cause decreased vision and recurrent erosions
      c. biomicroscopic findings: multiple bluish-white superficial corneal nodules usually in a circular configuration in the paracentral cornea; may be present at the end of pannus vessels
      d. clinical course: may be slowly progressive
  3. Pathogenesis:
      a. nodules represent focal areas of subepithelial fibrocellular avascular pannus, replacing Bowman's layer and superimposed on normal stroma
      b. a noninflammatory degeneration
  4. Diagnosis:
      a. based on clinical presentation
  5. Treatment:
      a. superficial keratectomy occasionally necessary
      b. lamellar or penetrating keratoplasty rarely necessary

J. Spheroid Degeneration

  1. Also called climatic droplet keratopathy, keratinoid degeneration, Labrador keratopathy, and chronic actinic keratopathy

  2. Epidemiology:

    a. an age-related degeneration associated with ultraviolet and general environmental exposure

    b. males > females

  3. Clinical features:

    a. usually bilateral

    b. presenting symptoms: usually asymptomatic but may cause mild irritation

    c. biomicroscopic findings: yellow, oily appearing subepithelial droplets within the interpalpebral fissure, generally beginning at the periphery; these droplets may replace Bowman's layer or may lie deeper; lattice-like lines may be seen in the stroma

    d. clinical course: may be slowly progressive

  4. Pathogenesis:

    a. probably related to elastotic degeneration of collagen; the lesions appear to develop from extracellular material deposited on collagen fibrils; amyloid deposition can be seen histologically

  5. Diagnosis:

    a. based on clinical presentation

  6. Treatment:

    a. superficial keratectomy may occasionally be indicated

K. Terrien's Marginal Degeneration

  1. Epidemiology:

    a. males 75%

    b. usually occurs in young patients

  2. Clinical features:

    a. usually bilateral, although often asymmetric

    b. presenting symptoms: induced corneal astigmatism, ocular irritation

    c. biomicroscopic findings: peripheral corneal thinning which begins superiorly as a marginal opacification and spreads circumferentially; stromal thinning and ectasia develop; the epithelium is intact; there is a lucid zone between the advancing edge and the limbus; the central wall is steep and the peripheral edge is gradual; a yellow border of lipid is typically present at the advancing edge; a fine vascular pannus may traverse the furrow

    d. clinical course: progressive astigmatism; spontaneous perforation is rare; minor trauma may result in rupture

      3. Pathogenesis:
        a. noninflammatory
      4. Diagnosis:
        a. based on clinical presentation
      5. Treatment:
        a. tectonic grafting is occasionally necessary to prevent or to repair perforation of thinned areas

VIII. TUMORS OF THE CONJUNCTIVA AND CORNEA

  A. Congenital Tumors
    1. Dermoids
      a. epidemiology:
        1) congenital choristoma which is sporadic and nonhereditary
        2) consist of displaced embryonic tissue that was supposed to be skin
      b. clinical features:
        1) smooth, round lesions that occur anywhere on the globe
        2) most commonly on the inferotemporal limbus
        3) often accompanying dermoids are anomalies of the ear and vertebral anomalies
        4) this triad is called Goldenhar's syndrome (oculo-auriculo-vertebral syndrome)
        5) composed of fibrous and fatty tissue covered by conjunctival epithelium
        6) called dermolipomas when fatty tissue is prominent
        7) accessory structures of skin, such as hair follicles, hairs, and sebaceous glands may be present
      c. diagnosis:
        1) based on clinical features
      d. treatment:
        1) excision is difficult, since these lesions may extend deep into underlying tissues
        2) cosmesis from excision may be worse than the original lesion itself
        3) elevated portion is often shaved flush with the sclera/limbus
  B. Epithelial Tumors
    1. Papilloma—Please see the discussion on papilloma under the Tumor of the Eyelid section. The same discussion applies here.
    2. Malignant tumors
      a. Malignancies of the conjunctival and corneal epithelium are similar to those of the cervix (cervical intraepithelial neoplasia, CIN). This designation is used for conjunctival and corneal epithelial neoplasia as well. The degree of malignancy has been divided into four categories:

      1) benign

      2) premalignant

      3) locally malignant (carcinoma in situ)

      4) frank malignancy (squamous cell carcinoma)

b. CIN is a term applied only to intraepithelial malignancy. Once the basement membrane of the epithelium is disturbed by the neoplastic cells, it is called squamous cell carcinoma.

c. benign and premalignant

      1) epidemiology:

          a) usually a disease of older people, often associated with exposure to sun or radiation

      2) clinical features:

          a) premalignant lesions characterized by gelatinous thickening of the epithelium with abnormal vascularization

          b) often seen at the limbus, but can spread to any other area of the conjunctiva

      3) pathology:

          a) acanthosis with possible moderate dysplasia is present

          b) with dysplasia, hypokeratosis, parakeratosis, and dyskeratosis

      4) treatment:

          a) excisional biopsy

          b) cryotherapy to the margins of the excision can destroy abnormal cells that are left behind

d. carcinoma in situ (CIS)

      1) clinical features:

          a) similar to precancerous lesions

      2) pathology:

          a) severe dysplasia and anaplasia throughout the entire thickness of the epithelium without disturbing the epithelial basement membrane

      3) treatment:

          a) complete excisional biopsy with cryotherapy

e. squamous cell carcinoma

      1) clinical features:

          a) may appear identical to carcinoma in situ

          b) invasion can be massive with progressive growth

          c) much more common than metastasis

          d) deaths are rare

      2) treatment

          a) complete local excision when possible. This may require dissection into deeper layers

          b) extensive invasion requires orbital exenteration, with adjunctive radiation therapy

C. Melanocytic Tumors
   1. Nevus
      a. Nevi of the eyelids have been discussed in the previous section of Tumors of the Eyelid. The conjunctival subepithelial nevus is equivalent to the dermal nevus of the eyelid. One important feature of the nevus is the frequent appearance of epithelial inclusion cysts within the nevi. These cysts are filled with mucin by goblet cells. Pigmentation of conjunctival nevi is variable. Malignant transformation is rare, but these nevi should be observed.
   2. Congenital ocular melanocytosis
      a. equivalent to the blue nevus of the skin, and occurs on the episclera and sclera
      b. often associated with increased pigmentation of the uveal tract
      c. clinical features:
         1) multiple slate gray patches are seen in the sclera or episclera
         2) unilateral, rare malignant transformation
   3. Primary acquired melanosis (PAM)
      a. epidemiology:
         1) acquired pigmentation of the conjunctiva appearing in middle age
         2) should be differentiated from acquired racial melanosis that appears in darker pigmented patients
         3) malignant transformation occurs in a third of patients with PAM
         4) characterized by subepithelial invasion of atypical melanocytes
         5) clinically typified by nodularity
      b. treatment:
         1) excisional biopsy upon appearance of nodularity, otherwise, closely monitored
D. Malignant Melanoma of Conjunctiva
   1. Epidemiology:
      a. better prognosis than cutaneous melanoma, but certainly can cause death
   2. Clinical features:
      a. pigmentation is variable with increased vascularity
      b. nodular appearance is common
      c. published reports indicate that 40% of conjunctiva melanomas arise from nevi with a mortality rate of 20%
      d. 30% of melanomas arise from PAM with a 40% mortality rate

      e. 30% of melanomas arise *de novo* with a mortality rate of 40%

   3. Pathology:

      a. subepithelial presence of atypical melanocytes with rare invasion to deeper structures

      b. metastasis is common

   4. Treatment:

      a. excisional biopsy should be done

      b. if malignancy is seen, local excision with cryotherapy is required

      c. for intraocular or orbital invasion, enucleation or exenteration is occasionally required

E. Lymphoid Tumors

   1. Benign reactive lymphoid hyperplasia

      a. clinical features:

         1) benign accumulation of various lymphoid cells presents as a salmon-colored epithelial tumor

      b. pathology:

         1) benign lymphoid lesions are polymorphous, with large and small lymphocytes, histiocytes, neutrophils, eosinophils, and plasma cells

         2) highly vascularized and contain lymphoid follicles

      c. treatment:

         1) general, medical consultation is advisable to rule out systemic lymphoma

         2) often resolve spontaneously, but may be treated with local excision

         3) topical steroids

         4) radiation treatment

   2. Malignancy

      a. clinical features:

         1) same as benign lymphoid hyperplasias

         2) can occur in conjunction with systemic lymphoma

      b. pathology:

         1) typically have monotonous and benign-appearing lymphocytes

         2) usually monoclonal

         3) vascularity is much less than benign lesions

      c. treatment:

         1) excisional biopsy, with local radiation therapy or systemic chemotherapy for systemic disease

         2) internist should be involved for systemic care

Essentials of Eye Care, edited by Rohit Varma.
Lippincott–Raven Publishers,
Philadelphia © 1997.

7

Glaucoma

I. PRIMARY OPEN ANGLE GLAUCOMA (POAG)

A. Elevation of intraocular pressure (IOP) accompanied by characteristic optic nerve damage and/or visual field loss, in the setting of open iridocorneal angle and the absence of a secondary etiology
Epidemiology

B. Most common form of glaucoma in US—overall prevalence 0.5 to 1.6%; prevalence among whites over age 40 approximately 1.7%; among African-Americans over age 40, prevalence approximately 5.6% (Baltimore Eye Survey data). POAG is the leading cause of irreversible blindness in African-Americans in the U.S. Age-adjusted blindness from glaucoma in African-Americans is 6.6 times that in Caucasians. It is estimated that glaucoma leads to blindness in a total of 12,000 new cases every year.

C. Multifactorial inheritance: a juvenile form of ocular hypertension/open angle glaucoma has been linked to the long arm of chromosome 1 (1q21-1q31).

  1. Risk factors

    a. intraocular pressure: The higher the intraocular pressure, the higher the prevalence of glaucoma. Additionally, the risk of developing glaucoma increases from a relative risk of 1.0 at IOPs of less than 16 to a relative risk of 4.0 at IOPs of 20 to 23, to a relative risk of 10.5 at IOPs of $24 mm Hg.

    b. race: POAG is 3 to 4 times more prevalent in African-Americans than in Caucasians. POAG is also thought to develop approximately 10 years earlier on average in African-Americans than in Caucasians. POAG is also believed to be more severe in African-Americans than in Caucasians.

    c. age: The incidence of visual field defects is approximately seven times greater in individuals over the age of 60 compared to individuals under 40 years of age over a 13-year period. Among both black and white persons aged 80 and over, there is a two- to tenfold higher prevalence of POAG compared to persons 40 to 49 years of age.

    d. family history: The association of glaucoma with a family history of a sibling with glaucoma is higher (relative risk 3.69) than with a family history of glaucoma in parents (relative risk 2.17) or in children (relative risk 1.12).

  2. The evidence to support a pathogenetic association among myopia, diabetes mellitus, and systemic hypertension is weak at best.

D. Clinical

  1. Insidious onset, slowly progressive, painless, central visual acuity affected late in course

  2. Usually bilateral, may be asymmetric

  3. Signs—elevated IOP, open angles by gonioscopic exam, increased cup-to-disc ratio, inter-eye asymmetry in C/D of 0.2 or more, asymmetry of superior versus inferior neuroretinal rim, optic disc hemorrhage, nerve fiber layer defects, visual field loss by kinetic or static perimetry. The most important sign of glaucomatous optic nerve damage is progressive glaucomatous changes in the optic disc or nerve fiber layer and or progressive glaucomatous visual field loss.

  4. Course—optic nerve changes: development of nerve fiber layer defects in the superior and inferior arcuate regions, progressive cupping at the superior and inferior poles of the optic disc, development of notches in the neural rim; the patterns of visual field loss may include nasal steps, temporal wedge loss, arcuate scotomas, paracentral scotomas, hemifield altitudinal defects, central islands of vision only (tunnel visual fields), and temporal islands. It is important to correlate visual field changes with optic disc changes when possible.

E. Pathology

  1. Mechanism of glaucomatous optic nerve damage is not clearly defined—theories include direct compression of optic nerve fibers against lamina cribrosa, vascular compromise with subsequent ischemic damage to the axons

  2. Histopathology—normal depth and width of anterior chamber angle; thickened trabecular beams, narrow intertrabecular spaces, decreased cellularity of trabecular meshwork; selective loss of retinal ganglion cells and thinning of the nerve fiber layer especially in the peripapillary region; optic nerve atrophy characterized by backward bowing and compression of lamina cribrosa, and enlarged, excavated optic cup. The superior and inferior poles of optic nerve are most susceptible to glaucomatous damage.

F. Diagnosis
   1. Serial measurements of IOP
   2. Confirmation of normal, open, anterior chamber angles
   3. Evaluation of the optic nerve for signs of glaucomatous damage
   4. Visual field examination—superior and inferior poles of optic nerve most susceptible to glaucomatous damage resulting in paracentral scotomas, arcuate scotomas, arcuate defects, temporal wedge, or nasal step
   5. Evidence of optic nerve damage or visual field loss is essential for a diagnosis of POAG. IOP >21 mm Hg in and of itself is not sufficient for a diagnosis of POAG.
   6. Differential diagnosis includes secondary causes of glaucoma and anterior ischemic optic neuropathy.

G. Treatment
   1. Initiated when IOP high enough to cause optic nerve damage or visual field loss or risk of damage is too high; IOP >30 mm Hg generally an indication for therapy; IOPs 21 to 30 mm Hg may be treated if there are other associated risk factors, IOPs below 21 may need to be lowered if there is progressive damage at that IOP; the greater the existing damage to optic nerve, the lower the IOP should be to avoid further visual loss; therapy stepped up if progression of disc damage with visual field loss occurs under treatment regimen
   2. Medical
      a. adrenergic agonists—(epinephrine hydrochloride 0.25%, 0.5%, 1%, 2%—Glaucon and Epifrin; epinephrine borate 0.25%, 0.5%, 1%, 2%—Epinal, Eppy/N; epinephrine bitartarate 2%—Epitrate; dipivefrin 0.1%—Propine, apraclonidine hydrochloride 0.5%, 1%—Iopidine). α-adrenergic receptor stimulation constricts blood vessels in the ciliary processes and thus reduces aqueous production and β-adrenergic receptor stimulation increases conventional and uveoscleral outflow; minimal effects on accommodation; most common ocular side ef-

fects are conjunctival hyperemia follicular conjunctivitis, adrenochrome deposits; aphakic and pseudophakic patients at risk for epinephrine maculopathy (reversible). Dipivefrin is a prodrug form of epinephrine. Hydrolytic enzymes in the corneal stroma cleave dipivefrin and release epinephrine into the anterior chamber. Dipivefrin has a lower incidence of side effects compared with epinephrine. Apraclonidine is a selective α_2-adrenergic receptor agonist that suppresses aqueous humor production by vasoconstriction of ciliary body blood vessels and by lowering episcleral venous pressure. Side effects include allergic blepharoconjunctivitis, lid retraction, dry mouth and/or nose, bradycardia, and hypotension.

b. β-adrenergic blockers—(timolol maleate 0.25%, 0.5%—Timoptic; levobunolol hydrochloride 0.25%, 0.5%—Betagan; betaxolol 0.25%, 0.5%,—Betoptic-S and Betoptic; metipranolol 0.3%,—OptiPranolol; carteolol 1%,—Ocupress) lower IOP by reducing aqueous production, effects additive in combination with miotics and carbonic anhydrase inhibitors; ocular and systemic side effects—difficulty breathing, impotence, lethargy, mood changes, bradycardia, and hypotension. Topical timolol increases serum triglyceride levels and lowers high density lipoprotein levels. Carteolol does not alter plasma lipid profiles. Selective β-1 antagonists (betaxolol) indicated for patients with pulmonary disease.

c. parasympathomimetic agents—(pilocarpine hydrochloride 0.25%, 0.5%, 1%, 2%, 3%, 4%, 5%, 6%, 8%, 10%—Adsorbocarpine, Isopto Carpine, Pilocar, Pilocel; Ocusert 20μg/hr, 40μg/hr; Pilopine HS gel; Carbachol 0.75%, 1.5%, 2.25%, 3%; demecarium bromide 0.125%, 0.25%—echothiophate iodide 0.03%, 0.06%, 0.125%, 0.25%—Phospholine Iodide; Diisopropyl fluorophosphate 0.025% gel, 0.1%—Floropryl) stimulate motor endplates similar to acetylcholine (direct acting, e.g., pilocarpine and carbachol) or inhibit acetylcholinesterase (indirect acting, e.g., demecarium, echothiophate); they reduce IOP by causing contraction of ciliary muscle and putting traction on the scleral spur and trabecular meshwork and thus opening the trabecular meshwork; the aqueous outflow is increased; ocular and systemic side effects include fluctuating myopia and ciliary spasm, reduced vision in low illumination, retinal detachment, increased salivation, diarrhea, nausea, vomiting, dizziness, hypotension, cataractogenesis, formation of iris cysts, and increased inflammation by increasing the permeability of the blood-aqueous barrier.

d. carbonic anhydrase inhibitors (CAIs)—topical (dorazolamide 2%—TrusOpt) and systemic (acetazolamide—Diamox, methazolamide—Neptazane, dichlorphenamide—Daranide) reduce aqueous formation by inhibiting carbonic anhydrase in the ciliary body (topical CAIs and systemic CAIs) and by producing generalized acidosis (systemic CAIs only); adverse effects of dorazolamide include bitter taste, burning, blurred vision, itching, headaches, vertigo, fatigue; side effects of the systemic CAIs include depression, fatigue, lethargy, malaise, anorexia, weight loss, paresthesias, kidney stones, rarely aplastic anemia; all CAIs contraindicated in patients with sulfa allergy; use of both systemic and topical CAIs simultaneously is not recommended.

e. prostaglandins—(latanoprost 0.005%) a prostaglandin F2a analogue lowers IOP by increasing uveoscleral outflow; once a day usage may increase patient compliance; side effects include burning, increased irreversible iris pigmentation of blue/ green irides and corneal epithelial erosions

f. hyperosmotic agents—(oral glycerol—Glyrol, Osmoglyn, oral isosorbide—Ismotic, intravenous mannitol—Osmitrol, intravenous urea—Urevert, Ureaphil) lower IOP by increasing blood osmolality and increasing the blood-ocular osmotic gradient; this draws water from the vitreous cavity through the retinal and uveal vasculature; the reduction in vitreous volume also allows the iris-lens plane to move posteriorly and thus deepens the anterior chamber; the effectiveness is primarily dependent on a rapid rate of administration; systemic side effects include headache, mental confusion, hyperglycemia, congestive heart failure, subdural hemorrhage. Glycerol—unpalatable sweet taste that leads to nausea and vomiting; isosorbide recommended for use in diabetic patients over glycerol since it is not metabolized and has no caloric value; mannitol—administer with caution in renal patients as it may not be cleared efficiently and may cause acute oliguric renal failure, congestive heart failure, acidosis; urea—extravasation may produce thrombophlebitis and skin necrosis.

3. Argon laser trabeculoplasty (ALT) (see Chapter 15)
4. Trabeculectomy (see Chapter 15)
5. Ciliodestructive procedures (see Chapter 15)
6. Drainage devices (see Chapter 15)
7. Laser suture lysis (see Chapter 15)

H. Glaucoma suspect
1. Patient with positive family history, elevated IOP, optic disc or visual field changes suspicious for glaucomatous damage
2. Most common finding is ocular hypertension (IOP >21 mm Hg)—found in 4 to 7% patients over age 40, 0.5 to 1.0% per year develop visual field loss over 5 to 20 years
3. Diagnosis—must rule out glaucomatous optic disc or visual field damage; progressive cupping, asymmetric cupping, disc hemorrhages, nerve fiber layer loss
4. Management—select and treat those patients at greatest risk of glaucomatous damage; level of IOP, suspicious-appearing optic disc, family history of glaucoma, increasing age, myopia, central retinal vein occlusion (CRVO), diabetes mellitus, systemic vascular disease; also consider desires of patient, reliability of visual fields, compliance with follow-up, and ability to examine the optic nerve
   a. patients not treated should be followed closely and treatment initiated if patient develops reproducible visual field defects, acquired enlargement of optic cup, loss of nerve fiber layer, or acquired peripapillary atrophy
   b. if one eye requires treatment, treat both as risk for progression to fellow, untreated eyes is 29% over 5 years

II. PRIMARY ANGLE CLOSURE GLAUCOMA

A. Epidemiology
1. Less common than POAG in Caucasians and African-Americans, compared with Asians; prevalence increases with age

    2. Less common in African-Americans than Caucasians; more likely to be chronic in African-Americans

    3. Hereditary influence, but family history does not predict risk of future attacks

    4. Peak incidence age 55 to 70 years, rare prior to age 45, but may be seen at any age

    5. Risk factors
        a. highest prevalence in Eskimos and Asians
        b. lens intumescence in older patients predisposing factor
        c. typically associated with hyperopia
        d. fellow eye of eye with acute angle closure glaucoma has 40 to 80% chance of developing an acute attack of angle closure over 5 to 10 years

B. Clinical Features

    1. Symptoms—intermittent attacks of acute angle closure characterized by dull pain around the eye, mildly blurred vision, halos around lights, lacrimation, nausea and vomiting; attacks tend to occur at the same time of day and last half an hour; subacute angle closure characterized by increased severity, frequency, and duration of attacks; chronic angle closure has minimal symptoms

    2. Signs (of acute attack)—markedly elevated IOP, conjunctival hyperemia, corneal edema, mid-dilated, nonreactive pupil, shallow peripheral anterior chamber with anterior bowing midperipheral iris, inflammatory anterior chamber reaction, optic nerve head may appear hyperemic, CRVO may occur; visual field may exhibit generalized constriction (may normalize); hallmark is narrow angle by gonioscopic exam

    3. Course—intermittent attacks initially benign and may cause no damage, but may progress into acute angle closure glaucoma; may also lead to formation of peripheral anterior synechiae resulting in chronic angle closure glaucoma
        a. subacute attacks can produce severe damage without inflammation
        b. acute attacks may terminate spontaneously
        c. chronic angle closure produces elevated IOP without symptoms resulting in glaucomatous cupping and visual field defects; often develop peripheral anterior synechiae (PAS); iris appears to insert anteriorly

C. Pathology

    1. Pupillary block results in impeded movement of aqueous from posterior to anterior chamber through the pupil leading to elevated posterior chamber pressure; peripheral iris pushed forward covering trabecular meshwork and closing angle—if IOP is not elevated, PAS will form leading to chronic angle closure glaucoma

2. Histopathology—shallow anterior chamber, abnormal configuration of anterior chamber angle, peripheral anterior synechiae; corneal edema; necrosis of lens epithelium (glaucomoflecken); ischemic atrophy of sectors of iris; retinal and optic nerve atrophy similar to that seen in POAG

D. Diagnosis
1. History—symptoms related to intermittent angle closure attacks, medication, activity preceding attack
2. Exam—slit-lamp and gonioscopic examination of both eyes
   a. evaluation of anterior chamber depth
      1) aim penlight from temporal edge of cornea—will illuminate entire iris if anterior chamber deep and iris flat; if anterior chamber (AC) shallow centrally, nasal iris will not be illuminated
      2) compare thickness of corneal slit beam to AC depth
      3) gonioscopic examination must demonstrate closed anterior chamber angle; fellow eye should be examined for narrow/occludable angle, especially if corneal edema prohibits adequate evaluation of involved eye
      4) provocative testing—place patient in dark room in prone position for 1–2 hours and look for elevation in IOP of 8–10 mm Hg

E. Treatment
1. Attempt to open angle and lower IOP—topical beta blockers and apraclonidine, oral hyperosmotic agents; 4% pilocarpine every 5 minutes times 4, then every 15 minutes times 4, then every hour times 4; topical steroids to decrease inflammation; topical glycerin to decrease corneal edema; indentation gonioscopy; flattens peripheral iris
2. Laser iridectomy treatment of choice—relieves pupillary block preventing iris from being pushed forward over trabecular meshwork
3. Argon laser—0.1 second duration, 50 micron, 1000 mW; complications include lens opacity, acute rise in IOP, transient or persistent iritis, early closure of iridectomy, corneal and retinal burns

4. Nd:YAG laser—5 to 10 millijoules; requires less energy and fewer pulses; complications include corneal burns, anterior lens capsule disruption, bleeding, postoperative IOP spike, inflammation, closure of iridectomy site
5. Surgical iridectomy indicated if laser PI cannot be performed—cloudy cornea, flat anterior chamber, poor patient cooperation
6. Postoperatively, continue medical therapy if IOP still elevated; topical steroids until inflammation clears; future pupillary dilation to determine if angle still occludable
7. If angle remains closed after patent PI—angle closure glaucoma without pupillary block:
   a. plateau iris—tends to occur in younger, myopic patients; anatomic configuration in which iris root angulates forward resulting in obstruction of trabecular meshwork by iris after pupillary dilatation, iris surface appears flat and central AC deep; may have component of pupillary block and be relieved by PI
   b. intumescent or dislocated lens—lens extraction indicated
   c. malignant glaucoma—anterior chamber uniformly shallow, not relieved by patent PI

III. ANIRIDIA

A. Bilateral, near-total absence of the irides
B. Epidemiology
   1. May be associated with congenital cataracts, foveal hypoplasia, nystagmus, corneal pannus, glaucoma, and decreased vision; predominantly iris defects with normal visual acuity; associated with genitourinary abnormalities such as Wilms' tumor; associated with mental retardation
   2. Occurs in 1/50,000 live births
   3. Autosomal dominant transmission in most cases due to mutation in the homeobox-containing PAX-6 gene; sporadic cases more often associated with Wilms' tumor (20%) and deletion on chromosome 11; occasional patients with autosomal recessive inheritance, particularly those with associated mental retardation
   4. Incidence of associated glaucoma highly variable (range, 6–75% reported), main cause of progressive visual loss
   5. Onset of glaucoma usually in preadolescent or early adult years, but may be congenital

C. Clinical
1. Symptoms—photophobia, decreased visual acuity
2. Signs—pendular nystagmus; visual acuity <20/100 in better eye in 86%; high refractive errors, amblyopia, and strabismus; corneal pannus and peripheral opacity, may advance centrally; iris appears as rudimentary stump although may have only mild iris hypoplasia; persistent iris strands, persistent tunica vasculosa lentis and pupillary displacement; lenticular opacities may be present, which can progress to become visually significant by third decade; foveal hypoplasia common; optic nerve hypoplasia; anisometropic or strabismic amblyopia may develop
3. Anterior chamber angle open although some patients have congenital anomalies of the angle; as patient ages, iris stump begins to overlie trabecular meshwork
4. Course—progressive visual loss due to corneal opacities, cataract formation, and angle closure glaucoma; prognosis for glaucoma better if develops in second to third decade

D. Pathology
1. Iris stroma hypoplastic, incomplete cleavage of angle or angle closure secondary to PAS, thinning of corneal Bowman's layer with vascular pannus, lens opacification; trabecular meshwork and Schlemm's canal may be absent; angle closure glaucoma develops secondary to progressive apposition of rudimentary stump of iris to trabecular meshwork; hypoplastic macula

E. Diagnosis
1. Based on examination, family history
2. Differential diagnosis:
   a. other isolated anterior segment anomalies (Axenfeld-Rieger syndrome, Peter's anomaly, anterior segment mesenchymal dysgenesis)
   b. other systemic disorders associated with aniridia: Gillespie syndrome; aniridia with absent patellae

F. Treatment
1. Genetic counseling—thorough family history; systemic evaluation with periodic renal ultrasound; banded chromosome analysis (linkage analysis if large family), mutation analysis of the PAX-6 gene; ocular examination of patient, parents, and other relatives
2. Photophobia—tinted or iris contact lens, tinted spectacle shades

    3. Correction of refractive errors, treatment of amblyopia and strabismus

    4. Glaucoma:

        a. medical therapy safest—miotics to increase outflow facility, beta blockers and CAIs; medical treatment usually fails with time

        b. surgical—goniotomy or trabeculotomy; trabeculectomy may accelerate cataract and is associated with an increased risk of vitreous loss; aqueous shunting devices and cycloablation may be effective

IV. AXENFELD-RIEGER SYNDROME

Developmental arrest late in gestation of neural crest derived structures

A. Types

    1. Posterior embryotoxon—anteriorly displaced and prominent Schwalbe's line

    2. Axenfeld's anomaly—posterior embryotoxon with iridocorneal adhesions

    3. Rieger's anomaly—iris atrophy with or without Axenfeld's anomaly

    4. Rieger's syndrome—Rieger's anomaly with facial, dental, periumbilical, and other abnormalities

B. Epidemiology

    1. Inheritance—autosomal dominant, rarely associated with chromosomal abnormalities; no sex predilection

    2. Usually diagnosed in infancy or childhood but may be diagnosed in later life

    3. Frequently associated with secondary glaucoma (>50% by age 20, 10 to 15% patients per decade after age 20); most commonly appears in childhood or young adulthood

C. Clinical

    1. Symptoms—tearing and photophobia in infants with glaucoma; decreased vision in older patients

    2. Signs—typically bilateral

        a. cornea: prominent, anteriorly displaced Schwalbe's line, occasionally abnormal size or shape

        b. anterior chamber angle: iridocorneal adhesions, posterior insertion of peripheral iris obscuring scleral spur; high insertion of peripheral iris more pronounced in eye with glaucoma

        c. iris: may have isolated peripheral abnormalities, stromal thinning, or marked iris atrophy with hole or pseudohole formation, corectopia, and ectropion uveae; occasionally central iris changes may progress with increased thinning and hole formation

    d. extraocular: absent or cone-shaped abnormal teeth and facial bones, maxillary hypoplasia, hypertelorism, telecanthus, broad flat nose, redundancy of periumbilical skin

D. Pathology

  1. Histopathology—prominent, anteriorly displaced Schwalbe's line; tissue strands attaching peripheral iris to corneoscleral junction (anterior and/or posterior to Schwalbe's line); iris peripheral to these iridocorneal adhesions inserts into posterior aspect of trabecular meshwork; iris stroma thin or absent, holes may involve pigment epithelium; trabecular meshwork composed of attenuated lamellae

E. Diagnosis

  1. Differential diagnosis:

    a. iridocorneal endothelial syndrome (ICE)—unilateral, corneal endothelial abnormalities, no family history, onset in young adulthood

    b. posterior polymorphous dystrophy—disorder of corneal endothelium, may have iris changes

    c. aniridia

    d. oculodentodigital dysplasia—may have iris hypoplasia, microcornea, and glaucoma

    e. ectopia lentis et pupillae—autosomal recessive, bilateral, normal angle

    f. congenital ectropion uveae—iris pigment epithelium on stroma, may have iris hypoplasia, angle defects, microphthalmia, and glaucoma

    g. Peter's anomaly

    h. congenital iris hypoplasia—iris defects without anterior chamber angle defects or other ocular anomalies; also associated with juvenile onset glaucoma and autosomal dominant inheritance

F. Treatment

  1. Genetic counseling

  2. Detection and control of glaucoma, may appear in infancy to middle age; patients with positive family history should be followed closely for development of glaucoma; all family members should be examined

  3. Medical treatment—beta blockers, CAIs; miotics usually ineffective

  4. Laser—not effective

   5. Surgery—trabeculectomy procedure of choice if IOP not controlled

V. PETER'S ANOMALY

A. Congenital central corneal leukoma with defect in posterior stroma and Descemet's membrane centrally, with variable degrees of irido-lenticulo-corneal adhesions

B. Epidemiology

   1. Most cases isolated; minority associated with various chromosomal abnormalities; families with autosomal recessive inheritance pattern reported; may present as part of well-delineated clinical syndromes

   2. Glaucoma occurs in majority of patients, often present at birth

C. Clinical

   1. Central corneal opacity at birth

   2. Two-thirds bilateral

   3. Signs:

   a. cornea—ground glass appearance with epithelial stippling secondary to corneal edema; well demarcated central defect in Descemet's membrane and corneal endothelium with thinning and opacification of overlying stroma; peripheral cornea usually clear

   b. iris—iridocorneal adhesions

   c. angle—trabeculodysgenesis common, various angle anomalies; glaucoma occurs in 50 to 70%

   d. lens—keratolenticular adhesions may occur; may be associated with anterior polar cataracts

   4. Often associated with systemic abnormalities

D. Pathology

   1. May represent intrauterine keratitis or incomplete separation of lens vesicle from surface ectoderm

   2. Histopathology—corneal epithelium edematous and disorganized; Bowman's layer thinned, may be replaced by pannus, absent for central 3 to 4 mm; stromal edema, histiocytic cells with residual bodies in stroma but no inflammatory cells; crater-like defect in posterior stroma or fibrous scar; centrally, endothelium and Descemet's membrane attenuated or absent; strands of iris to edges of defect

   3. Anterior chamber angle may have PAS, phagocytosed pigment in endothelium, developmental abnormalities such as Axenfeld-Rieger syndrome, or absent Schlemm's canal

E. Diagnosis

1. Exam under anesthesia, measurement of IOP, A and B scan ultrasonography, ERG
2. Differential diagnosis—congenital glaucoma, mucopolysaccharidoses, birth trauma, congenital hereditary endothelial dystrophy, perforated corneal ulcer with iris incarceration, posterior keratoconus

F. Treatment
   1. Early penetrating keratoplasty (PK) with or without cataract extraction to prevent amblyopia—successful in 20 to 50%
   2. Elevated intraocular pressure—topical therapy with oral acetazolamide 5 to 15 mg/kg/day in four divided doses; may require surgery—trabeculectomy (often fails), prosthetic drainage devices, cyclodestructive procedure
   3. Optical iridectomy if peripheral cornea clear and leukoma well circumscribed
   4. Unilateral cases associated with severe amblyopia
   5. >50% patients no light perception (NLP) due to glaucomatous optic nerve damage

VI. GLAUCOMA ASSOCIATED WITH INCREASED EPISCLERAL PRESSURE

A. Pathophysiology
   1. Episcleral pressure is a component of the normal IOP, thus intraocular pressure rises proportionate to episcleral venous pressure. Typically, angle is open and outflow facility is normal. However, increased venous pressure in the vortex veins may lead to congestion and edema of choroid, which causes forward displacement of lens-iris-diaphragm and angle closure glaucoma. Ocular ischemia may lead to rubeosis iridis and neovascular glaucoma.

B. Clinical
   1. Dilated and tortuous episcleral vessels
      a. unilateral: Sturge-Weber syndrome, orbital varices, carotid-cavernous fistula
      b. bilateral: superior vena cava syndrome, carotid-cavernous fistula, Sturge-Weber syndrome
   2. Angle usually open, may see blood in Schlemm's canal
   3. Rarely leads to decreased ocular perfusion, neovascular glaucoma

VII. STURGE-WEBER SYNDROME

A. Encephalotrigeminal angiomatosis

B. Epidemiology
  1. Thought to be autosomal dominant with incomplete penetrance
  2. Present at birth
  3. Glaucoma—one third of patients, usually those whose hemangioma involves the lid, tarsus, or conjunctiva; develops ipsilateral to lesion; 60% congenital onset, 40% adult onset—the earlier it's diagnosed, the more severe

C. Clinical
  1. Unilateral facial cutaneous angioma (nevus flammeus) in region of the first and second divisions of the fifth cranial nerve, usually involving supraorbital region
  2. Bilateral in 10 to 30%
  3. Facial hypertrophy in region of lesion common
  4. Associated with ipsilateral meningeal racemose hemangioma—exhibits progressive calcification, may result in mental deficiency (60%) and seizures (85%)
  5. May have localized or diffuse visceral angiomas
  6. Ocular—hemangioma of lid, episclera, iris, ciliary body; iris heterochromia 7 to 8%; scleral melanosis; tortuous retinal vessels; choroidal hemangiomas (40%) which may lead to exudative retinal detachment; occasionally uveal involvement will be diffuse

D. Pathology
  1. Etiology of glaucoma
    a. developmental anomalies of anterior chamber angle—poorly developed scleral spur, thickened uveal meshwork, anterior insertion of iris root, incomplete development of Schlemm's canal (similar to aging changes)
    b. forward displacement of iris secondary to choroidal or subretinal hemorrhage—leads to PAS, iris neovascularization, and angle closure
    c. increased episcleral pressure secondary to hemangioma
  2. Histopathology—dilated, thin-walled capillaries in dermis and subcutaneous tissue
  3. Choroidal cavernous hemangioma—thin-walled blood-filled sinuses lined by single layer of epithelium

E. Treatment
  1. Medical treatment if buphthalmos is not apparent—beta blockers, CAIs if outflow normal; mi-

otics and epinephrine if outflow decreased; most patients respond poorly

2. Laser—ALT ineffective
3. Surgery—filtration surgery indicated if glaucoma not controlled by medical therapy; complicated by higher risk expulsive choroidal hemorrhage and choroidal effusion—prophylactic posterior sclerotomy sometimes recommended
4. If conventional glaucoma surgery fails, cilioablation may be attempted
5. Neovascular glaucoma—poor prognosis for surgical intervention, may respond to panretinal photocoagulation (PRP)

VIII. CAROTID-CAVERNOUS FISTULA

A. Fistula between carotid artery and cavernous sinus
B. Epidemiology
   1. Risk factors—trauma, surgery
C. Clinical
   1. Symptoms—audible bruit; pulsating exophthalmos; diplopia; blurred vision; orbital pain
   2. Signs—elevated IOP (60 to 70% of patients) with large ocular pulse pressure; conjunctival and orbital vessel engorgement; ophthalmoplegia; initially outflow facility normal; some patients may develop ischemic ocular necrosis due to elevated ocular venous pressure and decreased arterial pressure—may lead to retinal and iris neovascularization and neovascular glaucoma
   3. 18% will close spontaneously, 43% will improve, no change in 33%
D. Pathology
   1. Elevated IOP secondary to increased episcleral venous pressure
E. Diagnosis
   1. Carotid angiography—reveals fistula
   2. Low ophthalmic artery pressure
   3. Large IOP pulsations
   4. Dilated ocular veins
F. Treatment
   1. Conservative approach especially if mild, as many will improve or resolve
   2. Surgical intervention indicated for secondary glaucoma or ischemic ocular necrosis—complicated by cerebral vascular accident and ocular ischemia, complication risk may be decreased by transvascular surgical approach

IX. IRIDOCORNEAL ENDOTHELIAL SYNDROMES

A. Types: "lumpers" classify these as one disease whereas the "splitters" classify these as three separate diseases
  1. Chandler's syndrome—abnormality of corneal endothelium
  2. Cogan-Reese syndrome—essential iris atrophy with pigmented iris nodules (nevi)
  3. Essential iris atrophy (EIA)—extreme atrophy of iris with hole formation

B. Epidemiology
  1. No systemic associations
  2. Recognized early to middle adulthood
  3. Women involved more often than men

C. Clinical
  1. Almost always unilateral
  2. Symptoms—patients may note changes in the iris, decrease in vision, pain secondary to corneal edema
  3. Signs
     a. cornea: hammered silver appearance of posterior cornea; variable degrees of corneal edema; pleiomorphic endothelial cell size and shape
     b. angle: PAS common; aqueous outflow obstructed by membrane over trabecular meshwork by synechial closure; progressive angle closure occurs with development of glaucoma
     c. iris: EIA—marked iris atrophy, variable degrees of corectopia and ectropion uveae, iris hole formation in area being stretched or "melting" iris holes
        1) Chandler's syndrome—minimal corectopia, mild iris atrophy
        2) Cogan-Reese syndrome/iris nevus syndrome—variable iris atrophy, pigmented iris stromal nodules

D. Pathology
  1. Histopathology—disorder of corneal endothelium, with varying degrees of endothelialization of angle and anterior iris surface
  2. Cellular membrane consisting of endothelial cells and Descemet's-like membrane extending from peripheral cornea—may cover angle or be associated with PAS; similar membrane found on anterior iris surface, most often in quadrant toward which pupil distorted
  3. Secondary glaucoma thought to occur due to cellular membrane

E. Diagnosis
  1. Differential diagnosis:
     a. corneal endothelial disorders—posterior polymorphous dystrophy, Fuchs' endothelial syndrome
     b. Axenfeld-Rieger syndrome
     c. aniridia
     d. iridoschisis
     e. nodular lesions of iris—melanosis, neurofibromatosis, sarcoidosis
F. Treatment
  1. Medical—beta blockers, CAIs to decrease aqueous production
  2. Laser—ALT not effective
  3. Surgery—trabeculectomy often effective, late failures occur secondary to endothelialization of bleb
  4. PK indicated for advanced corneal edema after IOP controlled

X. PIGMENT DISPERSION SYNDROME

A. Pigment deposition on corneal endothelium, trabecular meshwork, and lens periphery
B. Epidemiology
  1. Familial predisposition—both autosomal dominant and autosomal recessive inheritance reported
  2. Pigment dispersion syndrome affects Caucasians more than African-Americans and Asians, women and men in equal proportion, males at increased risk to develop elevated IOP
  3. Glaucoma develops in 25 to 50%; time between diagnosis of pigment dispersion syndrome and onset of glaucoma 12 to 20 years
  4. Characteristically affects young myopic males between 20 and 50 years old; age of affected women slightly higher (40 to 50 years)
  5. The higher the myopia, the younger the age of developing glaucoma
C. Clinical
  1. Occasionally presents with symptoms of halos and blurred vision
  2. Bilateral condition, often asymmetric
  3. Associated with moderate myopia
  4. Ocular findings:
     a. cornea—endothelial pigment in central vertical band (Krukenberg spindle), although may be more diffuse

  b. anterior chamber and angle—AC tends to be deep, angle open with homogenous band of hyperpigmentation on trabecular meshwork, ring of pigment on Schwalbe's line (Sampoloesi's line)

  c. iris—spoke-like loss of iris pigment epithelium resulting in peripheral transillumination defects; deposition of pigment on iris surface

  d. lens—pigment deposited on lens capsule (Scheie stripe)

  5. Progressive glaucoma associated with active pigment deposition; occasionally course will stabilize or decrease in severity with age

D. Pathology

  1. Presumably, contact between zonular packets and iris contributes to iris pigment released

  2. Pigment accumulates in cells and spaces of trabecular meshwork; cells phagocytose pigment—IOP normal or slightly increased; eventually trabecular beams degenerate, leading to uncontrolled pigmentary glaucoma

  3. Histopathology—pigment granules and cellular debris in trabecular meshwork (intra- and extracellularly), phagocytosed pigment in and on endothelial cells of cornea, focal loss of iris pigment epithelium

E. Diagnosis

  1. Differential diagnosis—uveitis, pigment dispersion secondary to intraocular melanoma, cysts of iris and ciliary body, postoperative pigment liberation particularly after posterior chamber intraocular lens (IOL), aging changes

F. Treatment

  1. Miotics effective, but poorly tolerated in younger patients; beta blockers and CAIs also effective

  2. Laser—effective in lowering IOP, but short-term only; laser iridectomy proposed as means of minimizing posterior bowing of iris and possibly decreasing pigment release from the iris

  3. Surgery—same indications as used in POAG

XI. PSEUDOEXFOLIATION SYNDROME

A. Characterized by deposition of fibrillar material in the anterior segment

B. Epidemiology

  1. No clear familial tendency

  2. In the U.S., increased prevalence with age from 0.6% among patients aged 50 years, to 7.9% among patients aged 80 years

    3. Glaucoma occurs more frequently in eyes with pseudoexfoliation syndrome than those without (prevalence glaucoma 7% in U.S.)

    4. Pseudoexfoliation syndrome without glaucoma—women involved more than men

    5. Pseudoexfoliation syndrome with glaucoma—affects both sexes equally; increased incidence with age, but younger age of onset than patients with pseudoexfoliation syndrome without glaucoma

C. Clinical

  1. Unilateral or bilateral, often becomes bilateral with time

  2. Ocular findings:

    a. cornea—flakes of exfoliative material on endothelium, small amount of pigment inferiorly, decreased number of endothelial cells

    b. iris—flakes of exfoliative material on pupillary margin, fine pigment on iris surface, transillumination defects at pupillary margin, iridodonesis and posterior synechiae may occur

    c. anterior chamber—pigment dispersion after mydriasis may be seen, irregular pigment in trabecular meshwork prominent aspect (early finding), pigment in Schwalbe's line may be found, angle usually open, but may be narrowed secondary to zonular weakness and anterior movement of lens-iris diaphragm

    d. lens—exfoliative material on anterior lens surface diagnostic, occurs in characteristic pattern with translucent central disc and granular girdle in periphery, separated by clear zone; exfoliative material on zonules, phacodonesis, subluxation or dislocation of lens

    e. IOP—mean IOP in normotensive eyes with exfoliation syndrome higher than that of normal population; elevation in IOP, glaucomatous optic nerve damage, and visual field loss greater in patients with exfoliation syndrome than patients with POAG and more often require surgery

D. Pathology

  1. Exfoliative material thought to arise from multiple sources (lens capsule, nonpigmented ciliary epithelium, iris pigment epithelium) as part of a generalized basement membrane disorder

  2. Glaucoma thought to be secondary to obstruction of flow through trabecular meshwork by fibrillar material, dysfunction of trabecular endothelial

cells, and/or concomitant POAG; pupillary block and angle closure glaucoma may occasionally occur

3. Histopathology—fibrillar material found in and on lens epithelium and capsule, pupillary margin, ciliary epithelium, iris pigment epithelium, iris stroma and blood vessels, and subconjunctival tissue

4. Histochemically, material resembles amyloid

5. Electron microscopy reveals fibrillogranular, basement membrane-like material, 30 nm diameter

E. Diagnosis

1. Examination of anterior segment and pupillary border, especially after dilation, gonioscopy, transillumination, and measurement of IOP

2. Iris angiography demonstrates abnormalities of iris vessels and leakage

3. Differential diagnosis

a. pigmentary dispersion syndrome

b. true exfoliation of lens capsule secondary to heat exposure

c. iritis with pigment dispersion in trabecular meshwork and posterior synechiae

d. toxic exfoliation due to iridocyclitis or foreign body

e. Fuchs' heterochromic iridocyclitis

f. pigment dispersion secondary to surgery or intraocular tumor

F. Treatment

1. Medical therapy attempted initially, patients often resistant—beta blockers, epinephrine compounds, miotics, CAIs

2. Laser—often very effective, but associated with late, abrupt rise in IOP

3. Surgery—results comparable to those for POAG, no unusual complications

4. Cataract extraction—does not improve IOP control, increased rate of complications including capsular rupture, lens dislocation, zonular dialysis, insufficient mydriasis

XII. STEROID-INDUCED GLAUCOMA

A. Minority of general population develops increased IOP with long-term topical, systemic, or periocular steroids—"steroid responders."

B. Epidemiology

1. Patients at increased risk to develop increased IOP when treated with steroids—patients with di-

abetes mellitus, first-degree relatives of steroid responders, high myopes

2. Latent period and magnitude of elevation in IOP proportionate to dose, potency, frequency, and rate of administration, as well as dependent on presence of other ocular or systemic disease; elevation in IOP associated with systemic steroids may occur weeks to years after initiation of therapy; elevated IOP associated with periocular steroids most persistent after depo-steroids

3. Occasionally, endogenous corticosteroids (for example, steroid-producing tumors) may cause elevated IOP

C. Clinical
   1. Symptoms—children may develop tearing, photophobia, and blepharospasm
   2. Signs
      a. children: corneal clouding, buphthalmos, breaks in Descemet's membrane, increased IOP, increased C/D
      b. adults: increased C/D, glaucomatous visual field loss with normal IOP and outflow or with uncontrolled open-angle glaucoma
   3. Associated ocular side effects of steroids—posterior subcapsular cataract, ptosis, mydriasis, atrophy of lid skin, ocular infection, corneal ulceration, uveitis

D. Pathology
   1. Mechanism of glaucoma—decreased outflow facility by affecting glycosaminoglycan (GAG) metabolism, accumulation of GAGs in trabecular meshwork, inhibition of phagocytosis of foreign material by trabecular endothelial cells, inhibition of synthesis of prostaglandins that modulate IOP
   2. Histopathology—increased density of meshwork and thinning of endothelial lining of Schlemm's canal

E. Diagnosis
   1. Discontinuation of glucocorticoids—monitor IOP for decrease after several days; if IOP remains elevated, steroids may have unmasked POAG
   2. Diagnosis difficult if steroids used to treat ocular disease that may also cause increased IOP

F. Treatment
   1. Obtain baseline ophthalmological examination
   2. Check IOP 2 to 3 weeks after initiating steroid therapy, then every 2 to 3 weeks for first few months, then every 2 to 3 months thereafter; if glaucoma develops, discontinue steroids

3. If unable to discontinue steroids, change to less potent drug
4. May require treatment with topical or systemic antiglaucoma medications
5. Elevated IOP after periocular steroids often requires medical therapy—if IOP not controlled and vision threatened, removal of residual steroid material may be indicated
6. Occasionally may require filtration surgery for progressive optic nerve damage and visual field loss
7. ALT not effective for this condition

XIII. UVEITIC GLAUCOMA

A. Uveitis often causes hyposecretion of aqueous; aqueous outflow channels may be obstructed by swelling or dysfunction of trabecular sheets or endothelial cells, or by accumulation of inflammatory material in channels; therapy involves controlling inflammation, dilatation of pupil, antiglaucoma treatment—beta blockers, CAIs, and hyperosmotic agents, laser peripheral iridectomy for pupillary block, surgery (may require anti-metabolites to increase chance of success)

B. Fuchs' Heterochromic Iridocyclitis
   1. Epidemiology
      a. approximately 2% of all cases of uveitis
      b. onset in third to fourth decade, males and females affected equally
   2. Clinical
      a. often insidious when chronic and mild, patients may experience pain, irritation, photophobia, minimal redness, heterochromia
      b. characteristic triad of heterochromia, cyclitis, and cataract; cyclitis usually mild and chronic, posterior synechiae rare; keratic precipitates (KP) characteristically small, round or stellate, never confluent, with fine filaments between them; anterior vitreous opacities; cataract frequently a late sign and may progress rapidly
      c. glaucoma occurs in 5 to 13% in unilateral cases, 25 to 33% in bilateral cases, angle open but there may be fine blood vessels in angle, rubeosis iridis may also develop
   3. Pathology
      a. histopathology—degenerative changes in iris consisting of decreased number of stromal

melanocytes, degeneration of iris pigment epithelium, thickening and hyalinization of iris blood vessels, lymphocytes and plasma cells in trabecular meshwork, patchy rubeosis

4. Diagnosis
    a. differential diagnosis
        1) uveitis of other causes
        2) glaucomatocyclitic crisis
        3) essential iris atrophy
5. Treatment
    a. steroids ineffective
    b. medical treatment of glaucoma—often refractory, filtration surgery often required

C. Glaucomatocyclitic Crisis (Posner-Schlossman Syndrome)
1. Epidemiology
    a. patients usually aged 20 to 50 years, rare beyond age 60 years
    b. may be associated with POAG—IOP may be elevated between attacks
2. Clinical
    a. symptoms: recurrent attacks of unilateral blurred vision, halos, slight discomfort
    b. signs:
        1) mild cyclitis with trace cell and flare, slight decrease in vision, elevated IOP (40 to 60 mm Hg), angle open, few KP, corneal edema, heterochromia rare; absence of posterior synechiae, hyperemia, pigmented KP, or PAS
        2) attacks last several hours to several weeks
        3) between attacks, IOP normal
        4) visual fields and optic discs appear normal unless associated with POAG
3. Pathology
    a. etiology unknown—theorized to be allergic; trabeculitis; increased prostaglandins which may alter aqueous-blood permeability resulting in elevated IOP
4. Diagnosis
    a. normal IOP, visual fields, and optic discs with episodic, unilateral glaucoma
    b. negative provocative test
    c. normal outflow facility
    d. differential diagnosis:
        acute angle closure glaucoma
        uveitic glaucoma
        Fuchs' heterochromic cyclitis
5. Treatment

    a. attack usually subsides without treatment; if IOP markedly elevated, may treat with CAIs, beta blockers, epinephrine compounds—no therapy needed between attacks

    b. topical steroids will decrease inflammation but may cause elevation in IOP

        1) indocin (75 to 150 mg/day) reported to decrease IOP faster than antiglaucoma therapy

        2) surgical intervention for glaucomatocyclitic crises will not prevent recurrence, but may prevent elevation of IOP during attacks

XIV. MALIGNANT GLAUCOMA

A. Postoperative shallowing or flattening of anterior chamber with increased IOP

B. Epidemiology

  1. Most commonly occurs as a complication of surgery for angle closure glaucoma, occasionally after lens extraction

  2. Chance of developing malignant glaucoma greatest in eyes in which some of the angle is closed at the time of surgery—not related to type of procedure or IOP prior to surgery; opposite eye at increased risk of developing malignant glaucoma

C. Clinical

  1. Onset occurs during surgery or any time after surgery, even months later (may be related to discontinuation of cycloplegics or initiation of miotics)

  2. Markedly elevated IOP with shallow or flat anterior chamber, in the presence of a patent laser or surgical peripheral iridectomy

D. Pathology

  1. Diversion of aqueous posteriorly into, behind, or beside vitreous cavity by unknown mechanism—may be secondary to relative block of anterior movement of aqueous by junction of ciliary processes, lens equator, and anterior vitreous face

E. Diagnosis

  1. Based on clinical characteristics, response to medical therapy, surgical confirmation:

    not relieved by peripheral iridectomy

    no fluid in suprachoroidal space when sclerotomy performed

  2. Differential diagnosis:

    choroidal separation

         pupillary block
         suprachoroidal hemorrhage

F. Treatment

  1. Medical:

    a. mydriatic/cycloplegic drops—atropine 1% and phenylephrine 2.5% or 10% every 4 to 6 hours for indefinite period; add CAIs and/or hyperosmotic agents if malignant glaucoma not relieved

    b. continue treatment for 4 or 5 days or until anterior chamber reforms and IOP is lowered, then taper treatment over several days but maintain patient on cycloplegics/mydriatics indefinitely

    c. 50% patients relieved by medical treatment

G. Laser:

  1. If medical therapy not effective, may attempt to shrink ciliary processes with argon laser through peripheral iridectomy—300 to 1000 mw, 0.1 to 0.2 seconds duration, 100 to 200 micron spot size

  2. In aphakics, Nd:YAG laser hyaloidotomy to disrupt vitreous face may be successful

H. Surgical: diagnostic confirmation and definitive therapy if others fail, must confirm presence of patent iridectomy preoperatively and perform laser or surgical PI if any question of patency arises

  1. Vitreous surgery for malignant glaucoma—a pars plana vitrectomy can be performed if medical and laser therapy fails to lower the IOP

    a. postoperative care—atropine 1% for weeks to months, topical steroids until inflammation resolves

    b. complications—choroidal separation, cataract, recurrence of malignant glaucoma (manage with medical therapy, reoperate if necessary)

I. Treatment of the fellow eye: laser iridectomy prior to intraocular surgery, perform at two sites in case one closes; avoid miotics; if patient develops angle closure glaucoma in this eye, treat with laser PI, mydriatics/cycloplegics; if surgical iridectomy required, treat with atropine and full medical regimen as for malignant glaucoma postoperatively

XV. TRAUMATIC GLAUCOMA

A. Angle Recession Glaucoma

  1. Epidemiology

      a. occurs after blunt trauma to the anterior segment, incidence 2 to 10%

      b. risk of glaucoma proportional to severity and extent of angle recession, especially if more than 270° of the angle involved

      c. eyes that develop angle recession glaucoma may be predisposed as up to 50% of fellow eyes may develop increased IOP

  2. Clinical

      a. monocular open angle glaucoma which may occur years after blunt trauma

  3. Pathology

      a. glaucoma results from outflow obstruction due to direct damage to trabecular meshwork or due to endothelial proliferation from cornea over iridocorneal layer; may also result from cyclodialysis which leads to poor perfusion of trabecular meshwork and hypotony— if cleft closes, IOP elevates, may improve spontaneously with time

      b. histopathology—tear through ciliary body between longitudinal and circular muscle layers, cyclodialysis cleft (focal separation of ciliary body from its attachment to scleral spur); collapse and scarring of trabecular sheets

  4. Diagnosis

      a. gonioscopic examination reveals irregular widening of ciliary body band, absence of ciliary processes, increased prominence of scleral spur, torn iris processes; cyclodialysis appears as a deep angle recess with gap between sclera and ciliary body

  5. Treatment

      a. medical—suppression of aqueous outflow by beta blockers, CAIs, hyperosmotic agents; often poorly responsive

      b. laser—poor chance of success

      c. surgery—trabeculectomy

B. Hyphema

  1. Epidemiology

      a. usually occurs after blunt trauma, may be complicated by corneal blood staining, elevated intraocular pressure, recurrent bleed

      b. glaucoma more commonly occurs after rebleed

      c. risk of glaucoma generally related to the size of the hyphema

       d. significantly increased risk of glaucoma after hyphema in patients with sickling hemoglobinopathies; optic nerves in these patients much more sensitive to increased IOP

  2. Clinical

     a. decreased visual acuity after blunt trauma

     b. IOP usually normal or slightly increased initially, often less than normal for first 5 days

     c. if rebleed occurs, patients may experience pain and nausea secondary to total hyphema and acute glaucoma

  3. Pathology

     a. mechanism of glaucoma is obstruction of trabecular meshwork by RBCs, inflammatory cells and blood products, occasionally pupillary block may develop secondary to clot

     b. as IOP increases, bleeding decreases and clot forms; clot lysis and retraction occurs 2 to 4 days postinjury, highest risk for rebleed within 5 to 7 days of injury

  4. Treatment

     a. hyphema treated with bed rest, aminocaproic acid or oral steroids, cycloplegics, topical steroids

     b. elevated IOP treated with beta blockers, CAIs, hyperosmotic agents

     c. indications for surgery—early blood staining of cornea, unremitting pain, patient with sickling hemoglobinopathy, increased IOP

     d. optimal time of intervention is 4 days

     e. surgery—AC paracentesis, irrigation with balanced salt solution (BSS) or fibrinolytic agents; evacuation of clot if necessary; iridectomy if total hyphema with pupillary block; if IOP remains uncontrolled, trabeculectomy may be indicated

C. Subluxated Lens

  1. causes elevated IOP due to relative pupillary block:

     a. dislocated lens may fall into AC—requires early surgery to prevent corneal decompensation

     b. rupture of zonules may lead to vitreous herniation anteriorly, pushing iris forward

     c. lens incarceration into pupil

  2. symptoms worsened by miosis, may be relieved by dilation

  3. Treatment

     a. lensectomy and vitrectomy should be done early to prevent formation of PAS

XVI. GHOST CELL GLAUCOMA

A. Transient secondary glaucoma resulting from obstruction of trabecular meshwork by degenerated erythrocytes, usually after vitreous hemorrhage

B. Epidemiology

    1. Typically transient, but may last many months

    2. History of vitreous hemorrhage usually secondary to trauma, surgery, or primary retinal disease; history of disruption of anterior hyaloid face—cataract extraction, vitrectomy, trauma; rarely, defect occurs spontaneously, with no history of disruption of the vitreous face

C. Clinical

    1. Elevated IOP associated with khaki-colored cells in anterior chamber, may also be found in trabecular meshwork; pseudohypopyon may occur; may be associated with pain, corneal edema, ghost cells scattered on endothelium; khaki-colored cells and clumped hemoglobin in vitreous

    2. Generally self-limited, resolves as hemorrhage clears

D. Pathology

    1. Degenerated RBCs appear as red, biconcave, pliable cells—converted to khaki-colored, spherical, hollow, less pliable cells; ghost cells remain for several months, do not adhere to each other or vitreous strands and may move anteriorly

    2. During conversion, intracellular hemoglobin lost into extracellular vitreous space where it forms accumulations that adhere to vitreous strand; does not leave vitreous cavity

    3. If anterior hyaloid face disrupted, ghost cells may move into anterior chamber where they can obstruct trabecular meshwork

    4. Three scenarios of ghost cell glaucoma after cataract surgery with disruption of anterior hyaloid face:

        a. early—hyphema after cataract extraction which extends into vitreous space, elevation of IOP initially secondary to hemorrhage, resolves but then recurs 2 to 6 weeks postoperatively with ghost cells in anterior chamber

        b. preoperative bleed—patient has vitreous hemorrhage prior to cataract extraction, elevation in IOP within days

        c. late—patient develops vitreous hemorrhage subsequent to cataract extraction, ghost cells pass into anterior chamber

E. Diagnosis
   1. Anterior chamber aspiration, usually combined with irrigation—examine fluid with phase contrast microscopy for ghost cells with Heinz bodies, occasionally macrophages, no inflammatory cells, no extracellular hemoglobin clumps
   2. Differential diagnosis:
      a. neovascular glaucoma
      b. hemosiderotic glaucoma (seen years after injury, no ghost cells, chronic)
      c. inflammatory glaucoma
      d. hemolytic glaucoma (hemoglobin-laden macrophages in AC and blocking trabecular meshwork)
F. Treatment
   1. Medical—preferred as glaucoma usually self-limited—beta blockers, CAIs
   2. Surgical—if IOP markedly and persistently elevated—anterior chamber irrigation, vitrectomy if washout ineffective

XVII. GLAUCOMA AFTER CATARACT SURGERY

A. Epidemiology
   1. May develop immediately after cataract surgery or weeks to months later
   2. Onset may be acute or insidious
B. Clinical Features
   1. Patients may experience pain, decreased vision secondary to corneal edema
   2. May be associated with open or closed anterior chamber angle
   3. Open angle:
      a. exacerbation of POAG—diagnosis of exclusion, usually self-limited, cataract extraction does not affect efficacy of preoperative ALT, but may lead to 50% loss or reduction of filtering blebs
      b. transient, early, IOP rise may occur in the immediate postoperative period secondary to tight wound closure, plasmoid aqueous obstruction of trabecular meshwork, edema at site of incision blocking aqueous outflow; usually no treatment required unless severe pain or integrity of wound threatened; may be prevented by prophylactic beta blocker or CAI
      c. zonulytic glaucoma—occurs 2 to 5 days post-intracapsular cataract extraction (ICCE) when alpha-chymotrypsin used; may be prevented by judicious use of zonulytic agents; usually

abates after 48 to 72 hours; beta blockers and CAIs effective

d. viscoelastic agents may increase IOP by mechanical obstruction of trabecular meshwork, IOP more severely elevated in eyes with pre-existing outflow impairment; begins within 24 hours, resolves after 48 to 72 hours; reduce risk by aspirating material from anterior chamber at the end of surgery; prophylactic treatment with beta blockers, adrenergic agonists, miotic agents

e. vitreous in anterior chamber secondary to spontaneous or traumatic rupture of anterior hyaloid face, rare after extracapsular cataract extraction (ECCE), elevation in IOP occurs weeks to months after surgery, secondary to obstruction of trabecular meshwork by vitreous; may be accompanied by inflammation; treated with mydriatics, medical therapy similar to that for POAG

f. hyphema—may be spontaneous (early) or secondary to neovascularization across wound site (late); usually asymptomatic, may cause pain if IOP markedly increased; if anterior vitreous face has been disrupted, may lead to vitreous hemorrhage and subsequent ghost cell glaucoma; usually self-limited, treat with beta blockers, CAIs, hyperosmotic agents only if corneal blood staining occurs or IOP threatens wound integrity or visual field loss; surgical therapy only if medical therapy fails to control IOP—anterior chamber washout, laser coagulation of wound neovascularization

g. uveitic glaucoma

h. steroid-induced glaucoma

i. lens-particle glaucoma—lens cortex remnants in anterior chamber obstruct trabecular meshwork directly and by inciting inflammatory reaction; marked inflammatory response with white KP; medical treatment of glaucoma usually effective with topical steroids; glaucoma resolves as lens material reabsorbed; surgery to remove cortical remnants indicated if medical therapy fails to control IOP

j. ghost cell glaucoma

k. epithelial ingrowth/fibrous downgrowth—late complication

    l. glaucoma associated with pseudophakia—lens-induced uveitis or hyphema, or uveitis glaucoma hyphema (UGH) syndrome

    m. Nd:YAG laser capsulotomy—elevated IOP occurs in 39 to 95% of patients, increased incidence in eyes with preexisting glaucoma; occurs 1 to 2 hours posttreatment; usually self-limited but may be persistent; prophylactic treatment with apraclonidine, beta blockers, pilocarpine

  4. Closed angle:

    a. pupillary block: patients may experience decreased vision, pain, or be asymptomatic; anterior chamber often shallow, pupil mid-dilated and nonreactive, elevated IOP, cornea clear or edematous, angle closed by gonioscopy; accompanied by adhesions between hyaloid face, lens capsule, or lens optic and iris; most common cause of angle closure after cataract extraction (incidence 1 to 7% after ICCE); usually occurs in immediate postoperative period; predisposing factors include wound leak with flat anterior chamber, iridectomy which is incomplete, too anterior, or included in iris prolapse, persistence of lens remnants, air or vitreous in anterior chamber, eyes with rubeosis iridis, uveitis, or posterior vitreous detachment

C. Pathology

  1. Open angle—angle obstructed by vitreous, blood and blood products, inflammation, lens cortex remnants, epithelial downgrowth

  2. Closed angle—iris pushed forward against trabecular meshwork by air, vitreous, lens remnants

D. Diagnosis

  1. Based on exam, etiology important to differentiate as treatment differs for each

E. Treatment

  1. Medical—cholinesterase inhibitors, epinephrine compounds, beta blockers, CAIs, and hyperosmotic agents all can be utilized; mydriatics (breaks adhesions between anterior hyaloid and posterior capsule and iris), miotics if pupil already dilated or if iridectomy blocked or pulled into iris prolapse; topical steroids to prevent iridovitreal adhesions; beta blockers or CAIs to decrease aqueous production if wound leak present

2. Laser—peripheral iridotomy for pupillary block; ALT is indicated only if preexisting POAG is present; it is successful in 50% of cases

3. Surgery—rarely required; anterior chamber paracentesis may temporize; trabeculectomy successful 32 to 92%, less successful after ICCE than ECCE; aphakic eyes at increased risk of suprachoroidal hemorrhage especially in myopic eyes; success rate increased by postoperative steroids or antimetabolites; tube implant or cyclocryotherapy indicated if conventional surgery fails; complications of cyclocryotherapy include phthisis, anterior segment necrosis, prolonged inflammation, macular edema

XVIII. EPITHELIAL PROLIFERATION AND GLAUCOMA

A. Usually occurs after anterior segment surgery

B. Pearl Tumors

1. Pearly cysts on iris surface, unconnected to surgical wound; small, grow slowly, associated with mild inflammation, usually have minimal sequelae

C. Epithelial Cysts

1. Epidemiology
   a. more common than epithelial ingrowth after trauma or cataract surgery
   b. greatest risk factor is poorly closed wound, especially with iris, lens, or vitreous incarcerated into wound

2. Clinical
   a. translucent/gray cysts which connect to wound, occasionally in posterior chamber
   b. associated with pupillary distortion, iridocyclitis, glaucoma, occlusion of visual axis secondary to growth of cyst (indication for treatment)

3. Pathology
   a. epithelial cysts enter anterior chamber as a loop, expands in a balloon fashion, may convert to sheet-like growth after surgical intervention
   b. histopathology—one or more layers of squamous or cuboidal cells, occasionally goblet cells, posterior layers may be pigmented; cyst cavity filled with serous proteins, mucin, cholesterol, keratin debris, degenerating cells

    c. electron microscopy—epithelial cells with thin basal lamina, desmosomes, tonofilaments, and apical microvilli

  4. Diagnosis

    a. history of trauma or surgery

    b. evidence of cystic nature by transillumination, tremulousness, lack of vascularity on iris fluorescein angiogram, inflammation accompanying growth, location on iris surface

  5. Treatment

    a. antiglaucoma and anti-inflammatory medication to temporize

    b. surgical intervention indicated if cyst grows, causes significant glaucoma or iritis, or interferes with vision

      1) wide surgical excision with or without diathermy or cryotherapy

      2) if cysts adherent to anterior segment structures, collapse cysts by aspiration, peel away from cornea; cysts may be frozen if small; if larger, excise iris and vitreous adherent to cyst with vitrectomy instruments, then freeze

    c. complications—corneal edema, recurrence as sheet-like epithelial ingrowth

D. Epithelial Ingrowth

  1. Epidemiology

    a. incidence 0.2 to 1.1% after cataract surgery, penetrating keratoplasty, or glaucoma surgery; equal incidence after ICCE and ECCE

    b. predisposing factors—complicated surgery, incarceration of tissue in wound leading to wound gape, postoperative hypotony, apposition of iris to wound leading to PAS, presence of fistula or bleb in one third of cases, chronic inflammation

    c. hypotony, inflammation, and shallowing of anterior chamber predispose to formation of PAS and glaucoma

  2. Clinical

    a. symptoms—tearing, dull aching pain, occasionally photophobia, blurred vision

    b. signs:

      1) conjunctival hyperemia; persistent inflammation; wound gape, bleb, or fistula formation; occasionally band keratopathy present

      2) corneal edema overlying posterior corneal membrane which is demarcated by gray line (best seen by retroillumination)—gray line rarely extends inferiorly past midcornea, may have scalloped edge with focal thickening, not associated with keratic precipitates

3) anterior chamber cell and flare variable

4) gonioscopy—iris, lens cortex, lens capsule incarcerated into wound; epithelium along suture tracts or lining inner opening of bleb or fistula; PAS common

5) epithelium grows more rapidly over iris and ciliary body than cornea, obscuring iris details, pupillary distortion, pupillary membrane in advanced cases

3. Pathology

   a. breakdown of blood-aqueous barrier in hypotonus/inflamed eyes allows entrance of serum-borne growth factors which support epithelial proliferation

   b. glaucoma occurs secondary to formation of PAS; chronic inflammation may lead to trabeculitis and decreased aqueous outflow; proliferation of epithelium covers trabecular meshwork and the false angle created by PAS—may contract and lead to angle closure glaucoma; proliferation of epithelium over pupil may lead to pupillary block

   c. histopathology—one to eight layers of nonkeratinized stratified squamous epithelium over posterior cornea, lining angle, and over iris, extending deep into surgical wound; epithelium thicker over trabecular meshwork and iris, thinner over vitreous and ciliary body, occasionally giant cells present

      1) iris, lens capsule, or vitreous incarcerated into wound

      2) neovascularization of deep corneal stroma, especially near wound

      3) gray line—multicellular thicker layer of cells at advancing edge of epithelial sheet

      4) chronic inflammatory cell infiltrate seen in episclera, iris, ciliary body; cystoid macular edema in cases of long-standing inflammation

      5) exfoliated epithelial cells and macrophages may plug trabecular meshwork—meshwork beneath epithelium becomes sclerosed and necrotic

   d. electron microscopy—multilayers of squamous epithelium with surface microvilli,

wide intercellular borders, occasional desmosomes, multiple intracellular tonofilaments, basal cells with dense granules attached to basal layer; subepithelial connective tissue layer
4. Diagnosis
   a. Seidel test with pressure on globe to detect microcysts, bleb, fistula
   b. specular microscopy—detect sharp border between corneal endothelial cells and epithelial growth
   c. argon laser photocoagulation (100 mw, 0.1 second duration, 500 micron spot size)—aim laser at iris surface in areas suspected of epithelial coverage; if fluffy white lesion results, epithelium has been burned as compared to well demarcated iris burn
   d. for histologic confirmation—iris biopsy, anterior chamber curettage, aqueous aspiration, diagnostic vitrectomy
   e. differential diagnosis:
      1) reduplicated Descemet's membrane in eyes with iridocyclitis
      2) fibrous ingrowth—very slow growth and vascularity
      3) vitreocorneal adhesions—corneal edema
      4) detachment of Descemet's membrane
5. Treatment
   a. surgical extirpation—photocoagulation performed preoperatively to delineate extent of iris involvement, placing 500 micron spots along advancing edge; fixation sutures placed under each rectus muscle and a conjunctival incision is created; if a fistula is discovered, it is excised or closed with a conjunctival flap; if no fistula is discovered, the anterior chamber is entered posterior to the original surgical wound and the involved iris, ciliary body, and vitreous is excised; involved cornea is frozen or scraped
      1) complications—persistent corneal edema, glaucoma, hypotony, phthisis, need for subsequent enucleation
      2) prognosis—approximately 25% of patients reported to have final visual acuity better than 20/50; younger patients tend to do better than older patients; worse prognosis if eyes retain fistulae after surgical repair

XIX. CONGENITAL GLAUCOMA

A. Improper development of the eye's aqueous outflow system

B. Epidemiology
1. Incidence 1/12,500, 65% patients male, 60 to 80% cases bilateral
2. 60% patients diagnosed in first 6 months, 80 to 90% patients present in the first year of life
3. Glaucoma may be primary congenital (50 to 70% of cases), associated with other ocular or systemic congenital anomalies, or secondary to other ocular disease
4. Primary congenital glaucoma may occur in families in autosomal recessive inheritance pattern (10% cases) with incomplete penetrance (40 to 80%); risk to subsequent children of same parents having glaucoma if 2 children have disease is 25% (most likely autosomal recessive inheritance)
5. Prognosis for control of IOP worse for glaucoma associated with developmental anomalies of the cornea

C. Clinical
1. Symptoms—epiphora, photophobia, blepharospasm
2. Signs—enlarged corneal diameter, corneal haze or edema, Haab's striae (vertical tears in Descemet's membrane), axial myopia, and buphthalmos; elevated IOP; ophthalmoscopy reveals an increased C/D—partly due to loss of nerve fibers, partly due to stretching of the scleral canal and posterior bowing of the lamina cribrosa (latter one reversible); gonioscopy may reveal normal anterior chamber structures and angle (isolated trabeculodysgenesis), abnormal insertion of the iris flatly into trabecular meshwork at or anterior to scleral spur, or angle anomalies associated with anomalous anterior and or posterior segment structures
3. Prognosis—worse outcome if present at birth (<50% better than 20/200 vision) or diagnosed after age 24 months; amblyopia secondary to corneal edema and scarring, strabismus, anisometropia, cataract; poor vision secondary to optic nerve atrophy

D. Pathology
1. Normal embryogenesis—anterior iris meets corneal endothelium at 5 months gestation to form peripheral anterior chamber with trabecular meshwork posteriorly; trabecular meshwork be-

comes exposed to anterior chamber as angle recess deepens and moves posteriorly, iris inserts into angle posterior to scleral spur

2. Histopathology—iris and ciliary body appear like those in an eye that is at 7 or 8 months gestation—fail to recede posteriorly such that iris insertion and anterior ciliary body overlap the posterior portion of the trabecular meshwork; thickened trabecular beams and uveal meshwork; late—PAS may be seen, degeneration of iris root and trabecular band, loss of Schlemm's canal, atrophic ciliary body, thinned retina and choroid

E. Diagnosis

1. Examination under anesthesia almost always required—most anesthetic agents lower IOP except ketamine which has a minimal effect on IOP

2. Diagnosis based on clinical evaluation including measurement of IOP, corneal diameter, gonioscopy, and ophthalmoscopy, must rule out associated systemic or ocular anomalies

3. Differential diagnosis:
   a. cornea:
      1) megalocornea—no signs of glaucoma, 90% male, sex-linked inheritance
      2) sclerocornea—associated with high myopia and exophthalmos
      3) metabolic disease—corneal haze (e.g., cystinosis, Hurler's syndromes, mucopolysaccharidoses)
      4) posterior polymorphous dystrophy—occasionally in infants
      5) CHED—similar by exam, normal IOP
      6) corneal inflammatory disease
      7) birth trauma/forceps injury
   b. epiphora/photophobia
      1) nasolacrimal duct obstruction
      2) superficial corneal dystrophies—Meesman's and Reis-Buckler's dystrophies
   c. optic nerve abnormalities
      1) congenital malformations—pits, colobomata, optic nerve hypoplasia
      2) axial myopia—tilted disc, scleral crescent
      3) physiologically enlarged optic cups

F. Treatment

1. Surgery is primary therapy, often with high success rate and low complication rate, should be performed to prevent permanent compression of and adhesion of trabecular sheets; first operation has highest chance of success

2. Preoperative medical treatment: a topical beta-blocker, pilocarpine 1 to 2% every 6 hours, acetazolamide 5 to 15 mg/kg every 6 to 8 hours for short term
3. Surgery
    a. trabeculotomy—a limbal based 7-mm conjunctival incision is created and dissected down to sclera; a partial thickness scleral flap is created 3 mm posterior to cornea; a radial incision is made across the scleral-limbal junction until blood or aqueous is noted at the lateral wall; Schlemm's canal is identified and a probe is placed into the canal and rotated anteriorly into the anterior chamber; procedure repeated, entering Schlemm's canal from other side of the flap; the scleral flap is closed with three interrupted 9-0 or 10-0 nylon sutures and the conjunctival incision is closed with a running 8-0 vicryl suture; postoperatively, patient treated with miotics and an antibiotic-steroid drop qid for 1 to 2 weeks
    b. Advantage of trabeculotomy is that it may be performed in eyes with cloudy cornea; 80 to 90% success rate; complications—hyphema, tears in Descemet's membrane, cyclodialysis, iridodialysis, difficulty locating Schlemm's canal, synechiae, staphyloma formation
    c. examination under anesthesia (EUA) performed 4 to 6 weeks postoperatively, then in 3 to 4 months, then every 6 months for 1 year, then annually; may be repeated
    d. goniotomy—more straightforward approach, does not disturb conjunctiva, only incises trabecular tissues, requires clear cornea
    e. trabeculectomy—if 360° goniotomy or trabeculotomy fail, success rate may be increased by use of adjuvant anti-metabolites
    f. synthetic drains—Molteno, Baerveldt, Ahmed, or Krupin valve implant may be promising
    g. cyclodestructive procedures—used when repetitive surgery has failed
4. Signs of progression include recurrence of corneal clouding, increased axial length, and increased C/D

XX. NEOVASCULAR GLAUCOMA

A. Epidemiology

1. Most cases of rubeosis iridis secondary to hypoxic disease of the retina:
    a. rubeosis iridis occurs in 1 to 17% of diabetic eyes; 33 to 64% occurs in eyes with proliferative diabetic retinopathy (PDR); one third of cases of neovascular glaucoma seen in diabetic eyes
    b. one third of patients with rubeosis iridis have diabetic retinopathy (risk increased in aphakic patients) and 28% have central retinal vein occlusion; neovascular glaucoma occurs in 30% of patients with CRVO; 58 to 86% of patients with ischemic CRVO; 4% of patients with nonischemic CRVO; onset usually 3 to 4 months after CRVO
2. May also be associated with retinal detachment, uveitis, and carotid occlusive disease
3. Younger patients often have associated hypertension or cardiovascular disease, older patients often have associated ocular hypertension or POAG

B. Clinical
1. Symptoms—acute onset of pain secondary to increased IOP, decreased vision secondary to corneal edema, conjunctival hyperemia
2. Signs—initially, tufts of new vessels at pupillary margin, although in dark irides may first be seen in the angle; neovascularization progresses over the iris surface, extending from iris root across ciliary body and arborizing over trabecular meshwork; in later stages, fibrovascular membrane over angle contracts, pulling iris root into angle and causing ectropion uvea and intractable glaucoma due to angle closure; hyphema may also occur

C. Pathology
1. Ischemic retina thought to liberate angiogenic factors that diffuse forward—lens and vitreous may serve as partial barriers to diffusion of such substances
2. New vessels arise from arteries of iris and ciliary body—thin walled, with irregular endothelium and pericytes and open junctions between endothelial cells; fibrous membranes develop along vessels; vessels cross scleral spur into trabecular meshwork and branch, intertwining with other vessels and forming localized anterior synechiae—angle closure

D. Diagnosis
1. Clinical signs, evidence of retinal disease; if CRVO, fluorescein angiography and electroretino-

gram (ERG) to distinguish ischemic from non-ischemic
   2. Iris angiography—abnormal leaking vessels of iris
   3. Differential diagnosis:
       a. acute narrow angle glaucoma
       b. Fuchs' heterochromic iridocyclitis
       c. ICE syndrome
       d. uveitic glaucoma
E. Treatment
   1. Most patients respond poorly to therapy—prevention is best
   2. Treat glaucoma with medical agents—beta blockers, CAIs, hyperosmotic agents
   3. Treat rubeosis iridis with atropine and topical steroids to temporize
   4. Panretinal photocoagulation should be performed as soon as possible, panretinal cryotherapy if media cloudy—neovascularization of angle regresses in several days to several weeks
   5. If glaucoma persists and not controlled—filtering surgery if eye has favorable visual potential (success rate improved if neovascularization has regressed); if poor visual potential—cyclocryotherapy or laser endophotocoagulation of ciliary body, drainage implants
   6. Technique for Molteno implant—the implant consists of a silicone tube that connects to the upper surface of an acrylic plate (12 mm diameter); a fornix-based conjunctival flap is created in the superonasal or superotemporal quadrant, dissected to expose equator; the plate is sutured to the sclera in subTenon's space with 8-0 silk sutures, 9 to 10 mm posterior to limbus; a rectangular, partial thickness scleral flap is dissected at the limbus; the tube is laid radially across the scleral flap, excess tube is cut off such that the tube overlies the limbus by 2 mm; the anterior chamber is entered parallel to the iris with a 21-gauge needle and the tube is inserted into the anterior chamber through this tract and secured with a 9-0 or 10-0 nylon suture; a scleral patch graft may be sutured over the silicone tube; the scleral flap is then sutured with 9-0 or 10-0 sutures and Tenon's capsule and the conjunctiva are sutured to the limbus; absorbable or releasable sutures may be placed around the internal or external portions of the tube and the suture may be cut later with a knife or laser

      a. success rate 50 to 94% in eyes with neovascular glaucoma, other types of secondary glaucoma, and eyes with prior filtration failure

      b. complications—persistent flat anterior chamber and delayed suprachoroidal hemorrhage associated with one stage procedure; uncontrolled IOP for 4 to 6 weeks in two stage procedure; conjunctival erosion with exposure of implant

XXI. NORMAL TENSION GLAUCOMA

A. Glaucomatous optic disc and visual field changes in the setting of "normal" intraocular pressure (IOP below 21 mm Hg). It is considered as a continuum of POAG in which a significant but smaller proportion of individuals develop visual field loss at IOPs below 21 mm Hg.

B. Epidemiology

    1. Prevalence of glaucomatous optic disc damage in eyes with normal intraocular pressure unknown—from the Baltimore Eye Survey, 50% of patients with glaucomatous optic disc and visual field changes had IOP less than 21 mm Hg on one measurement, and 33% had IOP less than 21 mm Hg on two measurements

    2. No clear familial predisposition, but POAG and glaucoma with normal IOP have been found within families

    3. Higher frequency of vasospastic disorders in patients with normal tension glaucoma—migraine headache, Raynaud's phenomenon; also associated with hematologic abnormalities such as increased blood and plasma viscosity, hypercoagulability, and hypercholesterolemia

C. Clinical

    1. Asymptomatic until severe visual loss ensues

    2. IOP—less than 21 mm Hg, mean plus two standard deviations for nonglaucomatous eyes

    3. Angle—normal, open

    4. Optic disc—similar appearance as in POAG, may have greater degree of thinning of neuroretinal rim, especially inferiorly and temporally; more commonly associated with acquired pits, and peripapillary crescents; optic disc hemorrhage more likely to be a sign of POAG

    5. Visual field defects—no clear distinction from the changes found in POAG, may be more likely to find focal, deep defects closer to fixation as compared to the changes found in POAG

6. Tends to present at more advanced stage than eyes with POAG

7. When IOP statistically normal but asymmetric, more severe damage in eye with consistently higher IOP

D. Pathology

1. Optic nerves of individuals with normal tension glaucoma more sensitive than nonglaucomatous eyes to factors which cause glaucomatous damage—possibly related to blood supply to optic nerve, connective tissue support, and/or the axons of the ganglion cells

2. Controversy exists on whether this is a primary optic neuropathy or a variant of POAG

E. Diagnosis

1. Careful examination of the optic disc most important as this will raise suspicion of glaucomatous damage

2. POAG associated with elevated IOP often mistaken for normal tension glaucoma as IOP may be statistically normal at the time of patient's visit—repetitive IOP measurements over the course of a day and on several different days necessary; systemic medications may obscure elevated IOP

3. Chronic narrow angle glaucoma—may have intermittent elevations of IOP

4. Traumatic glaucoma—may have resolved, leaving glaucomatous damage

5. Steroid-induced glaucoma

6. Congenital disc anomalies, especially large discs with large cups, optic disc drusen

7. Ischemic/compressive optic neuropathies—occasionally causes cupping; must rule out causes of optic disc ischemia such as anemia, heart disease, syphilis, vasculitis, carotid occlusive disease

F. Treatment

1. No treatment proven effective, but methods of lowering IOP pursued—identical to those used for POAG; goal should be IOP as low as possible (8 to 12 mm Hg)

2. Medical—topical medications, CAIs

3. Laser—ALT sometimes effective in reducing IOP

4. Surgery—filtration surgery if optic neuropathy is progressive despite above interventions

XXII. HYPOTONY

A. Statistically defined as IOP less than 6.5 mm Hg

B. Epidemiology

    1. Occurs secondary to other ocular or systemic diseases, surgery, or trauma—iridocyclitis, retinal detachment, vascular occlusive disease, wound leak, excessive filtration after glaucoma filtering surgery (usually self-limited), cyclodialysis, ciliochoroidal detachment, scleral rupture or perforation, hyperosmolarity, myotonic dystrophy. The most common cause is overfiltration following filtration surgery with an antifibrotic agent.

C. Clinical

    1. Reduced IOP, may lead to visual loss; may also be associated with photophobia; may progress to phthisis

    2. Clinical findings:

        a. wound leak—low and diffuse filtering bleb, microcystic subepithelial conjunctival changes, positive Seidel test, profound hypotony

        b. iridocyclitis—aqueous cell and flare, mild hypotony

        c. cyclodialysis—separation of ciliary body from scleral spur often after trauma, cataract surgery, or intentionally as a treatment for glaucoma; profound hypotony, cyclodialysis cleft on gonioscopic examination

        d. ciliochoroidal detachment—may be cause or consequence of hypotony; aqueous flare, profound hypotony, suprachoroidal effusion

        e. retinal detachment—rhegmatogenous retinal detachment associated with mild hypotony, level of hypotony related to extent of detachment

        f. miscellaneous—hyperosmotic state can cause bilateral hypotony, readily reversible (dehydration, hyperglycemia, uremia, systemic acidosis); myotonic dystrophy also causes mild bilateral hypotony (usually not clinically significant) possibly secondary to atrophic ciliary muscle; vascular occlusive disease—carotid occlusive disease, temporal arteritis, CRVO

D. Pathology

    1. Hypotony may result from external leakage of fluid, reduced aqueous humor flow secondary to inflammation, and/or enhanced uveoscleral flow; hypotony may lead to modest breakdown of blood-ocular barrier, which in turn leads to hyposecretion and creates a vicious cycle of hypotony

    2. Increased transudation of fluid from vessel walls and breakdown of blood-ocular barrier with leakage of protein have deleterious effects on the eye—edema of optic disc and macula; if prolonged, cataract formation, permanent macular changes, and phthisis bulbi may ensue

    3. Histopathology—generalized edema of uvea, retina, optic nerve; proteinaceous fluid in suprachoroidal space

E. Diagnosis

    1. History—trauma or surgery

    2. Seidel test

    3. Gonioscopic evaluation for cyclodialysis cleft

    4. Ophthalmoscopy to evaluate for retinal or ciliochoroidal detachment

    5. Ultrasonography or CT scanning may be required if posterior view is poor, exploratory surgery may also be required for diagnosis (see later)

F. Treatment

    1. Correct underlying abnormality—may require surgical intervention

    2. No medical treatment for hypotony per se

    3. Injection of autologous blood into bleb

    4. Surgical exploration—to examine for wound leak, cyclodialysis cleft, or suprachoroidal effusion; release of ciliary body traction from cyclitic membrane or lenticular remnants may dramatically reverse hypotony

Essentials of Eye Care, edited by Rohit Varma.
Lippincott–Raven Publishers,
Philadelphia © 1997.

8

Uveitis

I. EPISCLERITIS

A. Epidemiology:
1. No gender predilection
2. Age 20 to 60 years
B. Clinical Features:
1. Unilateral 67%
2. Two types of episcleritis:
   a. simple: ocular irritation, painless; episcleral injection and edema; no tenderness after administration of topical anesthetic; phenylephrine blanches episcleral vessels; diffuse 1/3, sectoral 2/3; ocular complications rare; 2/3 recurrent
   b. nodular: in addition to findings in simple scleritis, episcleral nodules are present; these are mobile since they are within the episclera
C. Diagnosis:
1. Based on clinical presentation
2. Rarely associated with systemic disease
D. Treatment:
1. Topical fluorometholone (FML)
2. Observation
3. Oral nonsteroidal anti-inflammatory medications, if topical therapy ineffective

II. SCLERITIS

A. Epidemiology:
1. More common in females than in males
2. Age 20 to 60 years
B. Clinical features:
1. Unilateral or bilateral
2. Three types of anterior scleritis:
   a. diffuse: 40% of cases; most benign form; presents with redness, pain, tenderness; scleral vessels appear engorged and bluish-red with

249

overlying edema; phenylephrine blanches conjunctival and episcleral vessels but not deep scleral vessels; conjunctival and episcleral vessels are mobile while scleral vessels are not; globe is tender even after administration of topical anesthetic

   b. nodular: 45% of cases; in addition to findings of diffuse scleritis, deep red nodules are present; the overlying conjunctiva and episclera are mobile while the nodules are not; multiple nodules are present in 40%; episcleritis is also often present

   c. necrotizing: 15% of cases; two types:

      1) without inflammation (scleromalacia perforans): painless; gray-blue patches of progressive scleral thinning; bulging staphylomas may develop; most patients have longstanding rheumatoid arthritis

      2) with inflammation: painful; the most destructive form; avascularity of an area of episcleral tissue overlying or adjacent to the area of scleral edema is a sign that necrotizing disease is present; 40% experience loss of vision; need intensive and prompt treatment; 20% of patients die within 8 years of autoimmune disease

C. Diagnosis:

   1. Based on clinical presentation

   2. Usually there is an associated episcleritis

   3. 46% associated with systemic disease:

      a. infections: herpes zoster, herpes simplex, syphilis

      b. autoimmune diseases: rheumatoid arthritis (most commonly associated disease), vasculitis (Wegener's granulomatosis, polyarteritis nodosa, lupus), inflammatory bowel disease (ulcerative colitis, Crohn's disease), relapsing polychondritis

D. Treatment:

   1. Complications of scleritis include keratitis, uveitis, and scleral thinning

   2. Topical steroids and cycloplegics

   3. Nonsteroidal anti-inflammatory agents (indomethacin 50 mg po tid)

   4. May require systemic steroids (oral or intravenous)

   5. Necrotizing scleritis may occasionally require immunosuppressive drugs

III. ANKYLOSING SPONDYLITIS

A. Epidemiology:
  1. Males 90%
  2. Age 20 to 30 years most common, but wide range at onset
  3. Ocular involvement occurs in up to 25% of patients with ankylosing spondylitis (usually occurs after the onset of back disease; there is no correlation with the severity of the spondylitis)
  4. 88% of patients with ankylosing spondylitis are HLA-B27 positive (HLA-B27 is positive in up to 6% of normals)

B. Clinical features:
  1. Unilateral at any one time; eventually bilateral in 80% but this involvement is rarely simultaneous
  2. Presenting symptoms: pain, redness, and photophobia
  3. Biomicroscopic findings: acute anterior nongranulomatous uveitis; fine keratic precipitates; fibrinous aqueous; severe cases may develop hypopyon
  4. Ophthalmoscopic findings: usually normal; occasional vitreous cell
  5. Clinical course: acute episodes last 2 to 6 weeks; may develop secondary glaucoma, cataract, posterior synechiae, cystoid macular edema; recurrences are common; permanent loss of vision is rare

C. Systemic involvement:
  1. Rheumatologic manifestations: lower back pain and stiffness after inactivity; improvement with exercise and prone positioning; insidious onset; persistence greater than 3 months; loss of normal lordosis; limited chest expansion
  2. Cardiovascular manifestations: 5% develop aortitis

D. Diagnosis:
  1. Physical examination shows spine and joint limitation
  2. Sacroiliac joint x-rays show sclerosis, narrowing, ligamentous ossification, squaring of vertebral bodies, and spinal fusion
  3. HLA-B27 positive
  4. Rheumatoid factor negative

E. Treatment:
  1. Ocular involvement treated with mydriatics, cycloplegics, intensive topical steroids, occasionally periocular steroids, and systemic steroids

      2. Systemic involvement treated with indomethacin and physical therapy

      3. Rheumatology and cardiology consultation

IV. REITER'S SYNDROME

A. Epidemiology:
    1. Males
    2. 20 to 40 years
    3. 85 to 95% of patients with Reiter's syndrome are HLA-B27 positive (HLA-B27 positive in 6% of normals)

B. Clinical features:
    1. Presenting symptoms: itching, pain, redness, photophobia
    2. Biomicroscopic findings: papillary conjunctivitis with hyperemia and mucopurulent discharge, occasionally peripheral corneal infiltrates, acute anterior nongranulomatous uveitis with fine keratic precipitates
    3. Ophthalmoscopic findings: usually normal, occasional vitreous cell
    4. Clinical course: primary attack is severe, most recurrent attacks are not; secondary complications including glaucoma and cataract are uncommon

C. Systemic involvement:
    1. Rheumatologic manifestations: asymmetric oligo arthritis typically involving knees, ankles, feet, and wrists; sacroiliitis occurs in 70%; onset within 4 weeks of episode of urethritis/diarrhea
    2. Genitourinary/gastrointestinal manifestations: Reiter's syndrome occurs after an episode of nongonococcal urethritis (chlamydia, ureaplasma) or gram-negative dysentery (shigella, salmonella, yersinia)
    3. Dermatologic manifestations: keratoderma blennorrhagica (vesicles, pustules, hyperkeratosis on palms and soles or genitals) in 8%; mucosal lesions of mouth/ genitals in 25%; balanitis circinata of penis; subungual hyperkeratosis

D. Diagnosis:
    1. Sacroiliac joint x-rays
    2. HLA-B27 positive
    3. Rheumatoid factor negative

E. Treatment:
    1. Topical steroids, occasional periocular steroids
    2. Genitourinary/gastrointestinal infection treated with antibiotics

    3. Rheumatologic, genitourinary/gastrointestinal, dermatologic consultation

V. INFLAMMATORY BOWEL DISEASE

    1. Crohn's disease
    2. Ulcerative colitis

A. Epidemiology:
    1. Age 20 to 40 years
    2. Acute anterior uveitis occurs in 5 to 10% of patients with Crohn's disease and in 5% of patients of ulcerative colitis

B. Clinical features:
    1. Unilateral or bilateral
    2. Presenting symptoms: pain, redness, photophobia
    3. Biomicroscopic findings: acute anterior nongranulomatous uveitis, fine keratic precipitates; fibrinous aqueous; patients with Crohn's disease may also develop episcleritis, scleritis, peripheral corneal infiltrates, and optic neuritis (if sclerouveitis occurs these patients are usually HLA-B27 negative, have no sacroiliitis, and have rheumatoid arthritis)
    4. Ophthalmoscopic findings: usually normal; patients with Crohn's disease rarely have choroidal infiltrates, papillitis, serous retinal detachment, retinal vasculitis
    5. Clinical course: the acute anterior uveitis is usually recurrent and does not result in significant loss of vision

C. Systemic involvement:
    1. Rheumatologic manifestations: sacroiliitis occurs in 20%
    2. Gastrointestinal manifestations: chronic intermittent diarrhea; patients with Crohn's disease may also have perirectal fistulas and abscesses

D. Diagnosis:
    1. HLA-B27 positive

E. Treatment:
    1. Topical steroids
    2. Rheumatologic and gastrointestinal consultation

VI. PSORIATIC ARTHRITIS

A. Epidemiology:
    1. More common in males than in females
    2. Age 20 to 40 years

B. Clinical features:
    1. Presenting symptoms: pain, redness, photophobia

   2. Biomicroscopic findings: acute anterior nongran-
      ulomatous uveitis, fine keratic precipitates
   3. Ophthalmoscopic findings: usually normal
C. Systemic involvement:
   1. Rheumatologic manifestations: arthritis character-
      ized by terminal phalangeal joint inflammation;
      sacroiliitis in 20%
   2. Dermatologic manifestations: psoriasis, typically
      with ungual involvement
D. Diagnosis:
   1. HLA-B27 positive
   2. Rheumatoid factor negative
E. Treatment:
   1. Topical steroids
   2. Rheumatologic and dermatologic consultation

VII. JUVENILE RHEUMATOID ARTHRITIS

A. Epidemiology:
   1. More common in females than in males
   2. Age 2 to 8 years
   3. Three types of juvenile rheumatoid arthritis:
      a. Still's disease: a severe systemic illness consist-
         ing of fever, large joint involvement, spleno-
         megaly, and lymphadenopathy; rare ocular dis-
         ease
      b. polyarticular: fever, lymphadenopathy, irido-
         cyclitis
      c. pauciarticular (monoarticular, oligoarticular):
         severe iridocyclitis
B. Clinical features:
   1. Usually bilateral
   2. Presenting symptoms: insidious onset; no con-
      junctival injection; painless; later, patients pre-
      sent with decreased vision
   3. Biomicroscopic findings: aqueous nongranuloma-
      tous cell and flare, small keratic precipitates
   4. Ophthalmoscopic findings: vitritis
   5. Clinical course: many patients develop band ker-
      atopathy, dense posterior synechiae with bound
      down pupil, cataract and glaucoma which result
      in severe visual loss
C. Diagnosis:
   1. Antinuclear antibody (ANA) positive (in 80% of
      patients who develop iridocyclitis but negative in
      patients without iridocyclitis)
   2. Rheumatoid factor negative
   3. Erythrocyte sedimentation rate (ESR) elevated
D. Treatment:

1. If severe anterior segment inflammation, topical steroids and cycloplegics; avoid overuse of topical steroids as long-term use is often necessary, which can lead to cataract and glaucoma
2. Sub-Tenon's or systemic steroids may be necessary
3. Immunosuppressives rarely used
4. Band keratopathy removed with chelating agents such as ethylenediaminetetraacetic acid (EDTA)
5. Glaucoma managed with nonmiotic medical therapy
6. Cataract surgery has guarded prognosis; IOL placement is contraindicated; vitrectomy may be required to control postoperative inflammation
7. Pediatric and rheumatologic consultation

VIII. FUCHS' HETEROCHROMIC IRIDOCYCLITIS

A. Epidemiology:
   1. No gender predilection
   2. Age 40 years, range 20 to 60 years
B. Clinical features:
   1. Unilateral 85%
   2. Presenting symptoms: none—no pain or redness
   3. Biomicroscopic findings: iris heterochromia in which the involved eye is lighter in color (most easily recognized in blue-eyed patients); loss of iris rugae; iris nodules; low-grade aqueous cell and flare; fine gray-white keratic precipitates involve both upper and lower cornea and have characteristic stellate appearance with filaments extending between larger deposits; occasional angle vessels seen on gonioscopy; posterior subcapsular cataract
   4. Ophthalmoscopic findings: usually normal, occasional vitreous cell, rarely cystoid macular edema
   5. Clinical course: vision may be decreased due to cataract; glaucoma may develop and is often refractory to medical therapy
C. Pathogenesis:
   1. Histopathology: iris and ciliary body have diffuse mononuclear cell infiltrate consisting of lymphocytes and plasma cells; iris has decreased number of pigment cells in the anterior border layer, stroma, and iris pigment epithelium; keratic precipitates consist of monocytes, lymphocytes, and plasma cells
   2. Etiology unknown: possible immunologic mechanism and possible association with Toxoplasma chorioretinitis

D. Diagnosis:
    1. Differential diagnosis of iris heterochromia: iris nevus, iris malignant melanoma, ocular melanocytosis, metallic siderosis, iris atrophy, Horner's syndrome

E. Treatment:
    1. Topical steroids may transiently decrease anterior chamber inflammation but little effect on overall course of disease
    2. Cataract extraction if visually significant
    3. Glaucoma may be treated with medical therapy, laser, or trabeculectomy

IX. LENS-INDUCED UVEITIS

A. Epidemiology:
    1. Rare, sporadic condition related to disruption of lens integrity, usually by surgery or trauma
    2. No known age, sex, or race predilection

B. Clinical features:
    1. Phacoanaphylaxis: immune-mediated inflammatory response occurring after injury to lens capsule; usually of acute onset with development of granulomatous anterior uveitis with mutton-fat keratic precipitates, iris synechiae, iris congestion, cell and flare; posterior segment lesions uncommon unless concomitant sympathetic ophthalmia; milder non-granulomatous forms of inflammation may occur (e.g., after extracapsular cataract extraction—phacotoxic/phacoallergic)
    2. Phacolysis: not inflammatory; leakage of liquified lens protein through intact lens capsule resulting in secondary glaucoma; occurs with hypermature cataract, rarely in persistent hyperplastic primary vitreous (PHPV)

C. Pathology:
    1. Phacoanaphylaxis: zonal granulomatous inflammation centered around lens material with neutrophils in apposition to lens, middle zone of pallisading macrophages/multinucleated giant cells, and outer layer of lymphoid cells, plasma cells, macrophages, and fibroblasts; can be accompanied by sympathetic uveitis
    2. Phacolysis: macrophages with swollen cytoplasm containing PAS-positive granules

D. Diagnosis:
    1. Phacoanaphylaxis: clinical diagnosis based on identification of ruptured lens capsule/retained lens material in an eye with (granulomatous)

uveitis; confirmed on histopathologic examination of lens material

   2. Phacolysis: based on identification of hypermature lens in an eye with markedly elevated intraocular pressure (IOP), and no inflammation; confirmed by aspiration of aqueous or vitreous demonstrating swollen macrophages

E. Treatment:

   1. In both phacoanaphylactic uveitis and phacolytic glaucoma, definitive treatment is meticulous removal of entire lens/lens remnants; nonspecific medical therapy to control uveitis (e.g., corticosteroids) and glaucoma (e.g., beta blockers) is indicated especially prior to intraocular surgery

X. BEHCET'S DISEASE

A. Epidemiology:

   1. Most commonly occurs in Mediterranean countries and the Far East
   2. More common in males than in females
   3. 90% of males and 70% of females with Behcet's disease develop ocular disease
   4. Age 20 to 40 years

B. Clinical features:

   1. Bilateral in 80%
   2. Presenting symptoms: pain, photophobia, blurred vision
   3. Biomicroscopic findings: conjunctival and ciliary injection, aqueous cell and flare, fine keratic precipitates, small transient hypopyon (present in 20 to 30% of patients)
   4. Ophthalmoscopic findings: vitritis, occlusive vasculitis (arteritis and phlebitis), attenuation of retinal vessels, retinal hemorrhages, macular edema, focal retinal necrosis, optic nerve edema from ischemic optic neuropathy
   5. Clinical course: multiple remissions and exacerbations; posterior synechiae, cataract, secondary glaucoma, macular edema; hemorrhagic infarction of retina and optic nerve (optic nerve pallor) may develop; severe visual loss usually results; 25% develop central nervous system symptoms (stroke, cranial nerve palsies, confusional states) and patients may die from central nervous system involvement
   6. Systemic involvement:
      a. major criteria

>
> 1) aphthous stomatitis: multiple, tender, aphthous ulcers of the mucous membranes of the mouth
> 2) genital ulceration: tender ulcers occur in both males and females
> 3) skin involvement: erythema nodosum, subcutaneous thrombophlebitis, cutaneous hypersensitivity
> b. minor criteria
> 1) joint involvement: polyarthritis and arthralgias develop in 60% of patients, usually involving wrists and ankles; gastrointestinal lesions, central nervous system involvement, vascular lesions

C. Pathogenesis:
1. Autoimmunity plays a role: associated with HLA-B5, subset Bw51; microbial etiology also possible
2. Histopathology: necrotizing obliterative vasculitis affecting both arteries and veins of all sizes

D. Diagnosis:
1. Behcetine skin test: skin is punctured with a sterile needle; a pustule forms within a few minutes (a nonspecific test)
2. Fluoroscein angiography (FA): profuse leakage of dye from affected retinal vessels and optic nerve; no well-defined foveal avascular zone
3. Four types of Behcet's disease:
   a. complete: all four major criteria (ocular, oral, genital, dermatologic)
   b. incomplete: three major criteria or ocular disease plus one other major criterion
   c. suspect: two major criteria
   d. possible: one major criterion
4. Neurologic and dermatologic consultation

E. Treatment:
1. Acute anterior segment inflammation: topical steroids ± periocular sub-Tenon's steroids
2. Posterior segment involvement: systemic steroids (prednisone 1.0 to 1.5 mg/kg/day) in conjunction with immunosuppressive therapy; the steroids act immediately and then are gradually tapered until the immunosuppressive drugs take effect
3. Cytotoxic agents:
   a. chlorambucil: 6 to 10 mg/day, up to 15 to 20 mg/day may induce remission in up to 80% of patients; several side effects; takes 6 weeks to produce results
   b. cyclophosphamide: for cases refractory to chlorambucil

    c. azathioprine

    d. cyclosporine: 5 to 7 mg/kg/day

       1) patients are often maintained on these medications for several years

XI. INTERMEDIATE UVEITIS

Also known as pars planitis, peripheral uveitis, chronic cyclitis

A. Epidemiology:
1. Young adults and children
2. 10% to 15% of all uveitis patients; 20% of children with uveitis
3. No gender predilection
4. No associated systemic disease in majority; 15% associated with multiple sclerosis

B. Clinical features:
1. Bilateral 80%, may be asymmetric
2. Presenting signs: floaters, decreased vision
3. Biomicroscopic findings: occasional mild anterior chamber inflammation with small white keratic precipitates and few posterior synechiae; cataracts may develop
4. Ophthalmoscopic findings: marked vitritis with vitreous opacities ("snowballs") inferiorly; pars plana exudate ("snowbank") inferiorly (which may be vascularized); peripheral periphlebitis; cystoid macular edema; 5% develop peripheral neovascularization and/or disc neovascularization
5. Clinical course: unpredictable; 10% gradual improvement and self-limited; 60% prolonged course without exacerbation; 30% chronic smoldering course with exacerbation; decreased vision usually due to cystoid macular edema, may occasionally be due to cataract, neovascularization with vitreous hemorrhage, traction retinal detachment, rhegmatogenous retinal detachment

C. Pathology:
1. Etiology unknown; possible autoimmune reaction against inner retinal or vitreal antigen or immune reaction against infectious agent; possible immunogenetic predisposition since pars planitis associated with certain HLA types (especially HLA-DR2)
2. Fibrovascular condensation of vitreous base with chronic inflammatory cell infiltration in advanced cases

D. Diagnosis:

   1. Differential: sarcoidosis, Lyme disease, toxocariasis
   2. FA: documents cystoid macular edema when present
E. Treatment:
   1. No treatment if vision greater than or equal to 20/40
   2. Periocular steroids (40 mg methylprednisolone q month; triamcinolone acetonide can also be used): for unilateral less than or equal to 20/40 (from cystoid macular edema [CME])
   3. Oral steroids (1 mg/kg/d prednisone times 2 weeks with slow taper): for bilateral less than or equal to 20/40 (from CME)
   4. Cryotherapy to peripheral snowbank: for vascularized pars plana exudate
   5. Pars plana vitrectomy: for persistent inflammation, vitreous hemorrhage, or traction retinal detachment
   6. Systemic immunosuppressives (cyclophosphamide): for resistant cases
   7. Cataract extraction with posterior chamber intraocular lens implantation and control of postoperative inflammation can yield good results (greater than or equal to 20/40) in 50 to 80%

XII. ACUTE RETINAL NECROSIS

Necrotizing viral infection characterized by vitritis, retinitis, and retinal vasculitis

A. Epidemiology:
   1. Age 20 to 60 years, but may occur at any age
   2. Slightly more common in males
   3. Most patients immunocompetent; recently increasingly seen in immunocompromised
B. Clinical features:
   1. One-third bilateral acute retinal necrosis (BARN); second eye involvement usually delayed several weeks
   2. Presenting symptoms: floaters, blurry vision (especially peripherally), occasional pain and foreign body sensation
   3. Biomicroscopic findings: conjunctival injection and chemosis; elevated IOP common; anterior chamber granulomatous inflammation with keratic precipitates; hypopyon and posterior synechiae very rare
   4. Ophthalmoscopic findings: vitritis; necrotizing, confluent, peripheral retinitis with well-defined

border between necrotic (white) and normal areas; retinal occlusive vasculitis with arteries more involved than veins; disc edema with optic neuritis

5. Clinical course: retinal detachment (characterized by large, multiple, posterior retinal holes) develops in 50 to 75%

C. Pathology:

1. Herpes virus etiology suggested by clinical features (acute retinal necrosis may occasionally be seen in conjunction with primary or recurrent herpes simplex virus or varicella zoster virus infection [meningio-encephalitis, cutaneous herpetic vesicles, cutaneous zoster, acute varicella infection]), and by pathologic examination (herpes virus particles demonstrated in vitreous and retina)

D. Diagnosis:

1. FA: "cut-off" sign highly suggestive
2. CT/MRI: enlarged optic nerve sheaths
3. Lumbar puncture: CSF pleocytosis
4. Diagnostic vitrectomy/endoretinal biopsy: eosinophilic intranuclear inclusions (diagnosis is clinical and invasive procedure rarely needed)
5. Differential: CMV retinitis, syphilis, toxoplasmosis, Behcet's disease, sarcoid, endophthalmitis

E. Treatment:

1. Acyclovir: 500 mg/m^2 q 8 hours ×5 to 10 days; then 400 to 600 mg po 5×/d ×6 weeks
2. Steroids: 60 mg prednisone po q day with a tapering dose
3. Antithrombic therapy: oral aspirin may have a possible benefit
4. Prophylactic confluent laser posterior to areas of retinitis: may decrease development of retinal detachment
5. Scleral buckle and vitrectomy: when retinal detachment develops

XIII. CYTOMEGALOVIRUS (CMV) RETINITIS

A. Epidemiology:

1. Congenital CMV (rare)
2. In adults, occurs almost exclusively in immune deficient individuals
3. Incidence of CMV retinitis in patients without AIDS is low (e.g., estimated 1% of renal transplant patients)

   4. Most common ocular opportunistic infection in AIDS patients, with incidence between 16 and 40%
   5. In the setting of AIDS, CMV retinitis occurs almost exclusively in patients with CD4+ counts less than 50 cells/mm^3, CD8+ reduced to 280 cells/mm^3, and CD4+/CD8+ ratio reduced to .05

B. Clinical features:
   1. Occasionally, CMV retinitis is a presenting opportunistic infection in AIDS
   2. Presenting symptoms: floaters, decreased vision, photopsia, metamorphopsia
   3. Anterior segment findings: trace inflammation including fine keratic precipitates, cell and flare, anterior vitreous cells
   4. Posterior segment findings: hemorrhagic retinal necrosis often in a wedge-shaped configuration surrounding retinal blood vessels with base oriented towards retinal periphery; "pizza pie" fundus, "crumbled cheese and ketchup" retinal necrosis
   5. Additional fundus findings: serous macular/retinal detachment, papillitis
   6. Visual loss in CMV retinitis—causes include macular or optic nerve infection, macular serous exudation, retinal detachment
   7. Clinical course: without AIDS, spontaneous remission if immune deficiency/suppression reversed; with AIDS, untreated CMV—inexorable progression to blindness (average rate = 25 microns/day, maximum rate = 165 microns/day toward fovea), if not receiving systemic therapy, bilateral (second eye) involvement eventually develops in 80%; complex rhegmatogenous retinal detachment occurs in 25% to 50% of treated patients related to total area of retinal involvement; CMV treated with systemic agents—greater than 90% remission (see below), if reactivated, slow progression (average rate with IV ganciclovir = 12 microns/day, maximum rate = 25 microns/ day toward fovea)

C. Pathology:
   1. Full thickness retinal and retinal pigment epithelial necrosis, infected cytomegalic cells show intranuclear (Cowdry A) and intracytoplasmic inclusions, adjacent areas of round cell and occasionally neutrophilic infiltrates; retinal vascular occlusion present

D. Diagnosis:
   1. Differential: progressive outer retinal necrosis (PORN) due to herpes simplex/zoster infection, toxoplasmosis, candida and other fungal infections, cotton wool spots/HIV retinopathy (early); other posterior segment infections are usually choroidal
   2. Diagnosis is clinical based on fundus findings, rarely corroborated by results of polymerase chain reaction of ocular fluids or histopathologic analysis of chorioretinal biopsy; in patients without AIDS, positive systemic cultures for CMV provide supportive evidence
E. Treatment:
   1. In patients without AIDS, CMV retinitis usually responds well to reduction of immune suppression therapy; if this is not possible, treatment with systemic antiviral agents is indicated for active retinitis (see below)
   2. Intravenous: induction with ganciclovir, foscarnet, or cidofovir followed by long-term maintenance therapy, drug treatment typically administered by an infectious disease specialist guided by information on disease activity provided by ophthalmologist typically on a monthly basis; fundus photographs useful in monitoring active borders/disease activity; initial response rate >90%, relapse inevitable, average at 3 to 4 months and usually responsive to reinduction; however, relapses become more frequent, necessitating a change in antiviral agent or combination (ganciclovir and foscarnet) IV therapy
      a. IV therapy advantages: provides protection/ treatment of CMV infection of other organs including contralateral eye, useful in bilateral disease
      b. disadvantages: ganciclovir and foscarnet require indwelling intravenous catheter, repeated administration, long infusion time, very expensive. Cidofovir must be given with oral probenecid
      c. side effects: ganciclovir—bone marrow suppression (responds well to bone marrow stimulating factors); foscarnet—nausea with drug administration, nephrotoxicity with electrolyte imbalance, cystitis; cidofovir—nephrotoxicity, probenecid-related rash, nausea, fever
   3. Oral: oral ganciclovir is effective against CMV retinitis but less efficacious than IV administered

ganciclovir; closer follow-up than with IV administered ganciclovir required

4. Intravitreal: intraocular injection of ganciclovir or foscarnet effectively controls CMV retinitis; indicated in patients unable to tolerate systemically administered antiviral therapy, when delay in receiving treatment for macula-threatening lesions is anticipated, or occasionally as an adjunct; when long-term therapy is required, repeated injections typically at weekly intervals are required due to the short half-life after single intravitreal injection; ganciclovir implant should be considered in this situation (see below)

   a. procedure: using topical anesthetic, eye aseptically prepped, TB syringe with 30 gauge needle used to inject 0.05 to 0.1 ml of drug solution through superior temporal pars plana, 4 mm posterior to limbus, done under direct visualization using the illumination of the indirect ophthalmoscope without a condensing lens, eye pressure adjusted afterwards with paracentesis if necessary to establish blood flow through central retinal artery, topical antibiotic drops for 24 hours after injection; ganciclovir prepared (by qualified pharmacist) in concentration 0.2 mg to 1 mg per 0.1 ml, foscarnet prepared in concentration 1.2 to 2.4 mg per 0.1 ml (for injection of 0.1 ml)

5. Sustained-release ganciclovir implants: FDA approved for treatment of CMV retinitis in AIDS patients; most appropriate as a first-line therapy in unilateral CMV retinitis along with systemic antiviral therapy (e.g., oral ganciclovir) for treatment of systemic CMV and prophylaxis against CMV retinitis in second eye, effective for approximately 6 months with reactivation of CMV after 210 days

   a. procedure: 5 mm circumferential scleral incision is made 4 mm posterior to the limbus in the inferotemporal quadrant, pars plana incision made with MVR blade and extended for full length of scleral incision (entry incision through pars plana should be confirmed by direct visualization), prolapsed vitreous excised 6 limited mechanical vitrectomy, implant with double-armed 8-0 nylon suture preplaced 0.5 mm from the trimmed end of the tab is positioned in the vitreous with the drug depot facing anteriorly, sclera closed with tab of the implant secured in the wound, position of the

implant confirmed with indirect ophthalmoscopy and eye reformed with pars plana injection of balanced salt solution

b. implant advantages: single administration, efficacy against CMV retinitis appears superior to
systemic antiviral therapy, long effect (6
months), no need for indwelling catheter

c. disadvantages: risk of intraocular surgery, temporary decrease in vision lasting 2 to 4 weeks
due to astigmatism, early increase in incidence
of retinal detachment (though not necessarily
increased overall), no protection against second eye or nonocular CMV, need for new implants after 6 months

6. Other investigational agents include intravitreous
cidofovir, monoclonal antibodies against CMV
(MSL-109) and mRNA antisense drugs (ISIS 2922)

7. CMV retinal detachment: most CMV-related retinal detachments involve multiple breaks in atrophic retina; additionally, vitreous pathology may
be evident; except in cases of straightforward
rhegmatogenous retinal detachment, vitreoretinal
surgery with silicone oil tamponade is indicated
for CMV-related retinal detachments in AIDS patients (see retinal detachment chapter); greater
than 85% anatomic success with visual prognosis
related to extent of preoperative detachment, extent of retinitis/optic atrophy

XIV. TOXOPLASMOSIS

A. Epidemiology:

1. 30 to 50% of all posterior uveitis

2. 20 to 70% of the population has positive serology
(depends on age)

3. Four types of infection:

a. acquired infection in adult: asymptomatic in
85%, self-limited flu-like disease in 15%, occasionally results in ocular disease

b. infection in immunocompromised host: may
be acquired or may be a reactivation of congenitally acquired infection; encephalitis, pneu-
monitis, myocarditis, and ocular disease may
develop

c. transplacental fetal infection (congenital): cerebral calcifications, seizures, hydocephalus,
microcephaly, organomegaly, rash, fever, and
ocular disease (retinochoroiditis of posterior
pole, bilateral in 80%); if pregnant woman ac-

quires the infection in the first or second trimester, infection in the infant is rare but severe; if infection is acquired during the third trimester, involvement in the infant is common but subclinical

d. reactivation of congenitally acquired infection: this results in the typical ocular disease described below

B. Clinical features:
1. Unilateral
2. Presenting symptoms: floaters, blurred vision, +1- redness and photophobia
3. Biomicroscopic findings: initially the anterior segment is quiet; later, granulomatous inflammation and increased intraocular pressure may develop
4. Ophthalmoscopic findings: vitreous opacities, chorioretinal scar with adjacent focal necrotizing retinitis (white-yellow, slightly raised, fluffy lesion) usually in posterior pole; adjacent venous and arterial sheathing; occasionally papillitis and white peripapillary lesion develops; there are three types of ophthalmoscopic presentations:
   a. large destructive lesion (>1 disc diameter)
   b. punctate inner retinal lesion
   c. punctate outer retinal lesions (rare)
5. Clinical course: small peripheral lesions heal spontaneously in 3 weeks to 6 months; larger active lesions enlarge for 1 to 2 weeks, then fade over months leaving an atrophic chorioretinal scar with pigmented borders; the sclera can be seen through the scar when the choroid has been involved; other complications include secondary glaucoma, cystoid macular edema, optic atrophy, choroidal neovascularization, and retinal detachment

C. Pathogenesis:
1. Toxoplasma gondii is a cat intestinal parasite; sporozoites (oocysts) are shed in cat feces and ingested by rodents and birds; cats acquire the infection by eating infected rodents and birds; bradyzoites are tissue cysts that may exist in cats or other mammals (pig, sheep, cattle); humans become infected by ingesting raw or undercooked meats containing tissue cysts or vegetables containing oocysts; tissue cysts are responsible for latent infection since they remain viable for the life of the host; bradyzoites transform into tachyzoites; tachyzoites are the invasive form of the or-

ganism and can cross the placenta to infect the fetus

    2. Histopathology: cysts and tachyzoites in inner retina; retinal necrosis with sharp borders

D. Diagnosis:

    1. FA: staining in area of retinochoroiditis; focal areas of nonperfusion may be present in active lesions; retinal vessels demonstrate dye leakage when vasculitis is present

    2. Sabin-Feldman dye test: serum is incubated with live organisms; measures mostly IgG and IgM

    3. Indirect fluorescent antibody test: detects IgG and IgM

    4. ELISA: detects IgG and IgM

    5. Differential: CMV retinitis, rubella, acute retinal necrosis, syphilis, Candida, histoplasmosis (outer retinal toxoplasmosis may appear similar to acute multifocal placoid pigment epitheliopathy (AMPPE) and serpiginous choroiditis)

E. Treatment:

    1. Not all lesions need to be treated; factors that usually warrant treatment include active lesions within the temporal arcades or within 1 disc area of the optic disc, lesions causing a decrease in visual acuity and lesions that have caused moderate or severe vitritis; factors that occasionally warrant treatment include lesions >1 dd in size, multifocal lesions, and lesions outside the temporal arcades

    2. Pyrimethamine (Daraprim) loading dose 100 to 200 mg, followed by 25 to 50 mg/day 2 6 weeks; sulfadiazine loading dose 75 mg/kg up to 4 gm, followed by 100 mg/kg/day up to 8 gm per day in 4 divided doses; folinic acid (Leukovorin) 5 to 10 mg 3 to 5 times per week to prevent leukopenia and thrombocytopenia associated with pyrimethamine usage

    3. Monitor for leukopenia and thrombocytopenia weekly

    4. Oral corticosteroids may be added; prednisone 20 to 40 mg/day may be started 1 to 2 days after antimicrobial therapy

    5. Other drugs: clindamycin 300 to 600 mg 3 to 4 times a day (may be added to other medications or may be used to substitute for pyrimethamine in patients with bone marrow toxicity or to substitute for sulfadiazine in patients with sulfa allergy); pseudomembranous colitis is a potential complication

6. In immunocompromised patients: preexisting retinal scars may not be present; in patients with toxoplasmosis lesions without adjacent chorioretinal scars, consider HIV testing; rule out CMV retinitis; treat with same medications in immunocompromised patients but prolonged treatment with at least one antimicrobial agent may be necessary since recurrences are common; consider an imaging study to rule out coexisting central nervous system toxoplasmosis (approximately 50% of patients with AIDS and ocular toxoplasmosis have CNS toxoplasmosis)

XV. TOXOCARIASIS

A. Epidemiology:
1. More common in males than in females
2. Average age 7 years, range 2 to 40 years
B. Clinical features:
1. Unilateral
2. Presenting symptoms: photophobia, redness, leukocoria, strabismus
3. Biomicroscopic findings: mild anterior chamber cell/flare and cataract in cases with endophthalmitis
4. Ophthalmoscopic findings—three types of ophthalmoscopic presentations:
   a. endophthalmitis: age 2 to 9 years; severe vitritis, occasionally cyclitic membrane, possible retinal detachment, no fundus details visible
   b. macular chorioretinal granuloma: age 6 to 14 years; mild vitritis; macular granuloma with overlying serous retinal detachment
   c. peripheral chorioretinal granuloma: age 6 to 40 years; mild vitritis; macular heterotopia (resulting in pseudoexotropia) with traction band from posterior pole to peripheral granuloma
5. Systemic involvement: 2% of patients with ocular disease have visceral larval migrans (a systemic disease involving fever, hepatosplenomegaly, and eosinophilia)
C. Pathogenesis:
1. Histopathology: eosinophilic abscess surrounding Toxocara larva
2. Toxocara canis is a dog intestinal parasite; dogs acquire the organism by ingesting ova; ova mature into larvae which then migrate to the lungs via the bloodstream; larvae migrate up the trachea to be reingested; ova can then be produced which are

shed in the feces; humans acquire the organism by ingesting ova, usually from contaminated soil or from direct contact with puppies; these mature into larvae and migrate throughout the body (including the eye) via the bloodstream; no ova are produced in humans

D. Diagnosis:
1. Usually based on clinical presentation
2. ELISA of undiluted serum or intraocular fluid

E. Treatment:
1. Thiabendazole and diethylcarbamazine not usually beneficial, and the death of the larvae can increase intraocular inflammation
2. Topical or systemic steroids may be useful if the inflammation is severe
3. Surgery is limited to patients with traction retinal detachment

XVI. SYPHILIS

A. Epidemiology:
1. Uncommon etiology for uveitis, estimates range between 0.6 and 4.6% of cases
2. Populations at risk: children (congenital), sexually active adults, elderly (incompletely treated, tertiary); routine serologic testing for marriage licenses/prenatal care has almost eliminated congenital cases
3. Occurrence parallels incidence of sexually transmitted diseases (STD) in population; decline related to effective antibiotic therapy (penicillin), with a reported recent rise in the male homosexual population

B. Clinical features:
1. Uveitic syndrome(s), typically bilateral
2. Presenting signs: decreased vision, irritation, red eye
3. Congenital: eye findings seen in late childhood, acute interstitial keratitis/keratouveitis; late stage with corneal ghost vessels, opacification; fundus with "salt-and-pepper" retinal pigment epithelium (RPE) changes, optic atrophy, pseudo-retinitis pigmentosa
4. Acquired STD: anterior segment—chronic steroid-resistant iridocyclitis, iris papules and roseolae noted in classic cases; posterior segment—acute chorioretinitis with multiple large, creamy, placoid choroidal infiltrates often associated with pa-

pillitis, vasculitis, serous exudation and (pan) uveitis

5. Clinical course: congenital—quiescent/stable at presentation without active keratitis/chorioretinitis, occasionally penetrating keratoplasty required for progressive corneal opacification (noninfectious); acquired STD—acute presentation with severe inflammatory signs generally seen in recently acquired or reactivated syphilis with markedly elevated serologies, often in late secondary/early latent stage of infection; these cases show correspondingly dramatic improvement with systemic therapy for syphilis; chronic presentation with steroid-resistant iridocyclitis often seen in elderly individuals with low titers and equivocal findings supporting active tertiary syphilis; correspondingly less dramatic/no response to systemic therapy

C. Pathology:
1. *T. Pallidum* found throughout the eye in syphilitic fetuses; identification/recovery of organisms from intraocular fluids and ocular tissues from children or adults reported but rare/difficult; acute interstitial keratitis—organisms rarely identified, secondary inflammatory/immune complex reaction with predominantly lymphocytes and plasma cells

D. Diagnosis:
1. Tissue diagnosis rare in intact eyes, identification of spirochetes on dark field examination of aqueous fluid difficult and unreliable; diagnosis usually presumptive based on 1) corroborative findings of systemic syphilis infection (dark field examination of skin lesions, positive serology, CSF), and 2) local, ocular response to a specific therapy for syphilis; systemic corticosteroids may give a false positive result by nonspecific treatment of inflammation; however, may be necessary to manage acute Jarisch-Herxheimer reaction; in equivocal cases (low titer, previous treatment), treatment administered both for possible therapeutic benefit and to eliminate syphilis as possible etiology; all cases with diagnosis of syphilitic uveitis should be evaluated and treated for neurosyphilis

2. Serologic testing—by 40 days after infection, reagin tests (RPR, VDRL) have high sensitivity, specific treponemal tests (FTA-ABS, MHA-TP) almost 100% sensitive; titers of reagin tests decline sig-

nificantly with treatment and in tertiary/latent syphilis while specific treponemal tests usually remain positive; in neurosyphilis, CSF usually shows positive reagin titers and/or pleocytosis; rare cases of seronegativity with both reagin and specific treponemal test in latent syphilis/altered immunity (AIDS)

3. Differential diagnosis: idiopathic uveitis, sarcoidosis, toxocariasis, toxoplasmosis, lymphogranuloma venereum, tuberculosis, fungal choroiditis, idiopathic central serous chorioretinopathy, metastatic choroidal tumor, APMPPE, retinitis pigmentosa, multifocal choroiditis

E. Treatment:

1. Because syphilis is treatable, therapeutic trial should be strongly considered in uveitis cases with equivocal diagnosis

2. With diagnosis of syphilitis uveitis, treat aggressively as for neurosyphilis (not as for recent acquired infection with normal CSF); treatment monitored by serology and CSF response

3. Aqueous penicillin G 12 to 24 million units IV/day divided doses for 10 days followed by benzathine penicillin G 2.4 million units IM/weekly for 3 weeks; in penicillin-allergic patients, doxycycline 200 mg po bid for 3 weeks; consultation with an infectious disease/internal medicine specialist is advisable

4. Recurrent disease may occur in individuals due to inadequate treatment (pre-antibiotic) and/or altered immunity (AIDS)

XVII. TUBERCULOUS UVEITIS (TB)

A. Epidemiology:

1. Thought at one time to be a common (presumptive) etiology for posterior uveitis, recently estimated to account for approximately 0.2% of all cases; presumably, incidence will rise with recent tuberculosis epidemic

2. Occurs in populations at risk for TB exposure (therefore less common in children), no known sex predilection

3. Usually occurs without overt systemic disease versus positive PPD/CXR

B. Clinical features:

1. Often unilateral or bilateral with significant asymmetry

2. Presenting signs: decreased vision, 6 irritation, red eye
3. Ocular manifestations: include conjunctival, corneal, uveal, retinal, choroidal, and orbital disease; rarely found as the presenting sign of systemic tuberculosis
4. Anterior segment: phlyctenular conjunctivitis; sclerokeratitis; interstitial keratitis; granulomatous iritis with iris infiltration, Busacca, and Koeppe nodules
5. Posterior segment: necrotizing retinitis with periphlebitis, tuberculous granuloma, exudative retinal detachment; other variants include "Eale's disease," miliary choroiditis, chronic subacute panuveitis (endophthalmitis), optic neuritis; choroidal involvement is most frequent posterior segment finding
6. Clinical course (untreated): chronic steroid-resistant uveitis, progressive multifocal choroiditis/necrotizing retinitis, exudative choroidal/retinal detachment

C. Pathology:
1. Acid-fast bacilli; tuberculoma containing epithelioid cells, lymphocytes, and Langhans giant cells, tissue disruption due to release of lytic enzymes; hypersensitivity reaction with immune complex deposition a possible but unproven mechanism of recurrent iritis
   a. Endophthalmitis limited to atypical/avian strains

D. Diagnosis:
1. Tissue diagnosis rare in intact eyes; diagnosis usually presumptive based on 1) corroborative findings of systemic TB infection (recovery of acid-fast bacilli, positive PPD, chest x-ray; or culture; and 2) local, ocular response to specific anti-TB chemotherapy; isoniazid therapeutic test consists of the administration of 300 mg of oral isoniazid daily for 3 weeks, positive test equals marked improvement of signs (note placebo effect with mood-elevating properties of isoniazid); note that intermediate PPD usually strongly positive unless patient immune suppressed; systemic corticosteroids may give a false positive result by nonspecific treatment of inflammation
2. Differential diagnosis: idiopathic uveitis, sarcoidosis, toxocariasis, toxoplasmosis, lymphogranuloma venereum, syphilis, fungal choroiditis, idiopathic central serous chorioretinopathy, meta-

static choroidal tumor; trial of antituberculous medication may be warranted in equivocal cases

E. Treatment:

1. Specific antiTB therapy: current therapeutic recommendations include combination therapy with INH and rifampin for 9 months supplemented in the initial phase by an additional agent such as ethambutol; adult dose—INH 5 to 10 mg/kg up to 300 mg; rifampin 10 to 20 mg/kg up to 600 mg; prompt response often encountered (1 to 2 weeks); significant toxicities include hepatitis (INH), optic neuropathy (ethambutol)—consultation with an infectious disease/internal medicine specialist warranted

2. Nonspecific therapy: anti-inflammatory regimen with topical and systemic corticosteroids useful in controlling uveitic activity; note that systemic immune suppression can cause activation of TB unless there is concomitant use of specific antiTB therapy; systemic corticosteroids can cause diagnostic confusion by nonspecific anti-inflammatory activity versus therapeutic response to antiTB regimen

XVIII. LYME DISEASE

A. Epidemiology:

1. Occurs after infection with the spirochete Borrelia burgdorferi; acquired via a tick bite (Ixodes dammini, Ixodus pacificus); endemic areas are northern United States, particularly the Northeast

B. Clinical features:

1. Divided into three stages:

   a. stage I
      1) occurs within 1 month of infection
      2) constitutional symptoms: headache, stiff neck, malaise, myalgias, arthralgias, fever
      3) ocular manifestations: follicular conjunctivitis
      4) dermatologic manifestations: erythema chronicum migrans (an erythematous rash at the site of the tick bite with central clearing)

   b. stage II
      1) occurs 1 to 4 months after infection
      2) represents spirochete dissemination
      3) ocular manifestations: keratitis, iritis with keratic precipitates and posterior synechiae,

intermediate uveitis, vitritis, panophthalmitis, optic neuritis

4) neurologic manifestations: facial nerve palsy, encephalitis, meningitis

5) musculoskeletal manifestations: arthritis, tendonitis, joint effusions

6) cardiac manifestations: myocarditis, heart block

   c. stage III

1) occurs at 5 or more months after infection

2) ocular manifestations: keratitis

3) neurologic manifestations: chronic meningitis

4) musculoskeletal manifestations: chronic arthritis

5) dermatologic manifestations: chronic atrophic changes

6) pulmonary manifestations: adult respiratory distress syndrome

C. Diagnosis:

1. Lyme immunofluorescent antibody (this cross-reacts with FTA)

2. ELISA: detects IgM and IgG (IgM is absent in Stage I)

D. Treatment:

1. Systemic oral antibiotics (tetracycline, erythromycin, or penicillin)

2. Systemic intravenous antibiotics for neurologic involvement (ceftriaxone or penicillin)

XIX. FUNGAL RETINITIS: CANDIDA CHORIORETINITIS/ENDOPHTHALMITIS

A. Epidemiology:

1. Two different manifestations of intraocular Candida infection

   a. chorioretinitis: ocular involvement limited to choroid 6 overlying retina

   b. endophthalmitis: chorioretinitis with inflammation which extends into the vitreous resulting in vitreous abscess

2. Patients who are critically ill, immunosuppressed, or have chronic indwelling catheters (alcoholism, malignancy, hemodialysis, recent surgery, pharmacologic immunosuppression, injection drug use, prolonged antibiotic use, hyperalimentation, intravenous catheters)

3. Candidal organisms are the most common pathogen causing endogenous endophthalmitis

    4. Ocular involvement commonly seen when positive blood cultures are present (documented candidemia)

B. Clinical features:

    1. Presenting signs/symptoms: asymptomatic (chorioretinitis): blurred vision, floaters, pain, photophobia (endophthalmitis)

    2. Biomicroscopic findings: normal (chorioretinitis); conjunctival hyperemia, aqueous cell and flare, occasional hypopyon, posterior synechiae, vitritis (endophthalmitis)

    3. Ophthalmoscopic findings: one or more white or pale-colored choroidal infiltrates (300m diameter) with indistinct borders; intraretinal hemorrhages, and cotton-wool spots also occasionally present (chorioretinitis); one or more large white fluffy vitreous abscesses located solely within the vitreous or extending from the underlying retina (endophthalmitis)

C. Pathology:

    1. Candida albicans and Candida tropicalis (budding yeasts)

    2. Hematogenous dissemination (Candidemia) from nonocular site results in endogenous endophthalmitis

    3. Organisms first seen in choroid, then invade subretinal space and retina, and ultimately involve the vitreous

D. Diagnosis:

    1. Diagnosis of chorioretinitis and some cases of endophthalmitis are presumed (appropriate clinical setting ± positive blood cultures for Candida)

    2. In cases of suspected endophthalmitis, vitreous biopsy with culture (Sabouraud's medium) and histopathologic examination (Giemsa stain) establishes the diagnosis

E. Treatment:

    1. Candidemia (i.e., positive blood culture): thorough medical evaluation to search for evidence of visceral organ involvement including dilated fundus exam; if no ocular involvement, IV amphotericin B (2 weeks)

    2. Chorioretinitis: if blood cultures negative, observe lesions for signs of progression and treat if progression is observed; if blood cultures positive, IV amphotericin B (4 weeks)

    3. Endophthalmitis: if no other systemic involvement, vitrectomy and intravitreal amphotericin B (5 micrograms); if eye and systemic involvement, vitrectomy, intravitreal and intravenous amphotericin B; if high risk surgical patient, omit vitrectomy but administer intravitreal amphotericin B at bedside (when performing vitrectomy, it is essential that the vitreous abscess be isolated and sent for stains and cultures)

XX. ACUTE MULTIFOCAL PLACOID PIGMENT EPITHELIOPATHY (AMPPE)

A. Epidemiology:
1. More common in females than in males
2. Average age 25 years, range 20 to 50 years
3. Often there is a preceding flu-like illness
B. Clinical features:
1. Usually bilateral
2. Presenting symptoms: acute onset of central or paracentral visual loss; presenting visual acuity may be as low as count fingers
3. Biomicroscopic findings: possible mild anterior chamber inflammation
4. Ophthalmoscopic findings: mild vitritis; multiple flat, pale lesions in the posterior pole, approximately 1/2 disc diameter in size, at the level of the retinal pigment epithelium or choriocapillaris; well circumscribed
5. Clinical course: spontaneous resolution in 2 to 3 weeks; hyperpigmentation may develop in 7 to 10 days; eventually discrete pigment epithelial scars develop; visual recovery to 20/30 occurs in 95% of patients; recurrences are rare
6. Systemic involvement: case reports have described patients with cerebral vasculitis, headache, cerebrospinal fluid pleocytosis, neurologic deficits, dysacousis, tinnitus
C. Pathogenesis:
1. Possible viral etiology
2. The choriocapillaris may be the area of primary involvement; the lesions may represent occluded terminal choroidal arterioles and the early hypofluorescence may represent choroidal filling defects
3. The retinal pigment epithelial cell may be secondarily involved, with its cytoplasm becoming sufficiently cloudy that it blocks background choroidal fluorescence; this later absorbs fluorescence due to breakdown of the blood retinal barrier
D. Diagnosis:

1. FA: initially the lesions are hypofluorescent; in the late phases the lesions are diffusely hyperfluorescent (staining); in inactive resolved cases there is early transmission of the background fluorescence through the areas of retinal pigment epithelial atrophy
2. Indocyanine green angiography (ICG): active disease—profound segmental choroidal perfusion abnormalities; inactive disease—return of choroidal perfusion

E. Treatment:
1. A self-limited disease; treatment does not appear to be indicated in most cases
2. Steroids have been used if the fovea is compromised and visual acuity is poor, although the effect of such treatment on the course of the disease is unknown

XXI. MULTIPLE EVANESCENT WHITE DOT SYNDROME (MEWDS)

A. Epidemiology:
1. Age 15 to 45 years (average 26 years)
2. 80% female
3. No racial predilection
B. Clinical features:
1. Unilateral 90% (if bilateral, one eye is asymptomatic and has 20/20 vision)
2. Presenting signs/symptoms: acute onset decreased vision (20/20 to 20/400), dark spots in peripheral field, photopsia, 20% have preceding flu-like illness, 6 APD
3. Biomicroscopic findings: occasional mild iritis
4. Ophthalmoscopic findings: posterior vitreous cell, discrete white spots, 100–200m diameter, deep retina or RPE, most concentrated at posterior pole and perifoveal region, migratory (spots disappear in several days); foveal RPE granularity; may have mild blurring of disc margin and perivascular sheathing
5. Clinical course: spontaneous recovery of vision 3 to 10 weeks, disappearance of spots; foveal granularity persists; subjective symptoms of photopsia and dim vision persist; enlarged blind spot may persist; very rarely recurrent
C. Pathology:
1. Viral etiology possible
D. Diagnosis:

1. Differential: AMPPE (larger fundus lesions, bilateral, hypofluorescent early with late staining on FA); acute retinal pigment epitheliitis (perifoveal clusters of dark spots surrounded by hypopigmented halos, central blockage with surrounding hyperfluorescence on FA); birdshot retinochoroidopathy (older age, bilateral, chronic, vitritis); multifocal choroiditis with panuveitis (bilateral, overlying serous detachment, occasional choroidal neovascularization, vitritis, lesions develop pigment over time, early hyperfluorescence with late staining on FA)
2. VF: variable findings; usually enlarged blind spot but may be normal or show generalized depression; degree of field loss is striking when compared to retinal/disc findings
3. FA: white spots show early punctate hyperfluorescence (clusters of hyperfluorescent dots); late staining of spots and disc
4. ERG: reversible decreased a-wave and early receptor potential amplitudes

E. Treatment:
   1. None

XXII. MULTIFOCAL CHOROIDITIS AND PANUVEITIS

Several entities are probably variants of this condition: punctate inner choroidopathy (PIC), recurrent multifocal choroiditis, chorioretinopathy with anterior uveitis, and multifocal choroiditis with progressive subretinal fibrosis

A. Epidemiology:
   1. More common in females than in males
   2. Age 20 to 40 years
   3. Myopes
B. Clinical features:
   1. Bilateral
   2. Presenting symptoms: decreased vision, scotomas, photopsias
   3. Biomicroscopic findings: aqueous cells and flare
   4. Ophthalmoscopic findings: vitritis; multiple, small (50 to 500m), round, gray or yellow spots in the posterior pole and/or periphery; may have associated focal serous detachment overlying the acute lesions; may have mild disc edema and/or peripapillary atrophy
   5. Clinical course: the lesions evolve into multiple punched-out spots at the level of the retinal pig-

ment epithelium or inner choroid; the central portion of the spots becomes hypopigmented with a rim of hyperpigmentation; the focal serous detachments resolve; cystoid macular edema may develop; choroidal neovascularization occurs frequently

C. Pathogenesis:
   1. Some investigators have described an association with Epstein-Barr virus but others were unable to reproduce these findings
D. Diagnosis:
   1. FA: acute lesions show early blockage and late staining; chronic lesions exhibit window defects
   2. VF: may show enlarged blind spot
   3. Differential: presumed ocular histoplasmosis syndrome (no vitritis or active lesions, larger lesions), birdshot retinochoroidopathy (older patients, lesions larger and deeper, nyctalopia, ERG changes), MEWDS (no punched-out lesions, unilateral)
E. Treatment:
   1. Periocular and systemic steroids may suppress the inflammation and possibly cause resolution of choroidal neovascularization; no effect on subretinal fibrosis

XXIII. BIRDSHOT RETINOCHOROIDOPATHY

Also called vitiliginous choroiditis
A. Epidemiology:
   1. age greater than 40 years (mean 50 years)
   2. females 70%
B. Clinical features:
   1. Bilateral 80%
   2. Presenting symptoms: gradual blurring of vision, floaters, nyctalopia, decreased color vision
   3. Biomicroscopic findings: mild nongranulomatous iritis with fine KP in 25%, diffuse vitritis
   4. Ophthalmoscopic findings: multiple, post-equatorial, de-pigmented or cream-colored spots at the level of the outer retina, RPE and inner choroid; lesions are ovoid with ill-defined borders, 500 to 1500m, often radially oriented, not associated with hyperpigmentation; occasional disc edema
   5. Clinical course: a chronic disease with exacerbations and remissions; decreased acuity develops secondary to CME and epiretinal membrane formation; optic atrophy and attenuated/sheathed retinal vessels develop; occasional serous retinal

detachment (RD) and choroidal neovascular membranes (CNVM)

C. Pathology:
  1. Autoimmunity plays a role: associated with HLA-A29 in 80 to 96% (present in 7% of normals); 92% of patients have a strong cell-mediated immune response to retinal S-antigen and IRBP (interstitial retinoid binding protein)

D. Diagnosis:
  1. FA: vascular incompetence results in dye leakage from vessels and cystoid macular edema. The birdshot lesions show only mild hyperfluorescence and staining in the late phase.
  2. ERG: reduced or extinguished
  3. Differential: VKH, sympathetic ophthalmia, reticulum cell sarcoma, sarcoidosis, tuberculosis, syphilis, intermediate uveitis, AMPPE, MEWDS, multifocal choroiditis and panuveitis

E. Treatment:
  1. Sub-Tenon triamcinolone (40 mg/ml) when CME or severe inflammation is present
  2. Oral prednisone (1 mg/kg/d): only 15% achieve good clinical response
  3. Cyclosporine (2 to 5 mg/kg/d)

XXIV. SERPIGINOUS CHOROIDITIS

Also called geographic/helicoid peripapillary choroidopathy

A. Epidemiology:
  1. More common in males than in females
  2. Age 30 to 70 years

B. Clinical features:
  1. Bilateral but disease activity usually not simultaneous
  2. Presenting symptoms: blurred vision
  3. Biomicroscopic findings: usually normal but may have aqueous cell and vitritis
  4. Ophthalmoscopic findings: acute lesions consist of peripapillary or macular gray geographic areas; peripapillary lesions may represent multiple confluent old scars and finger-like projections; acute lesions last weeks to months and result in scarring characterized by pigmentary loss or hyperplastic mottling of the retinal pigment epithelium, and variable atrophy of the choriocapillaris and large choroidal vessels
  5. Clinical course: multiple recurrences at intervals of months to years; new lesions are usually con-

tiguous with previous scars and spread centrifugally from the disc, often toward the macula; choroidal neovascularization occurs in 13 to 25% of eyes; occasionally results in serous detachment of retina or RPE, retinal vasculitis, disc or retinal neovascularization

C. Pathogenesis:
  1. Autoimmunity plays a role as there is an increased prevalence of HLA-B7
  2. Inflammatory etiology likely, either due to an autoimmune disease and/or an infectious agent
  3. Histopathology: atrophy of choriocapillaris, photoreceptors, and retinal pigment epithelium in affected areas; fibrocellular scars line the inner portion of Bruch's membrane in regions of atrophy; choroidal lymphocytic infiltrate, most prominent at the borders of retinal pigment epithelial atrophy
  4. Swollen retinal pigment epithelial cells or choriocapillaris nonperfusion results in early hypofluorescence of active lesions

D. Diagnosis:
  1. FA: active lesions show early hypofluorescence; spotty hyperfluorescence and hyperfluorescence at the borders may be present and there is late staining; inactive scars show mottled hyperfluorescence due to pigment clumping, and some late staining
  2. VF: small central or paracentral scotomas
  3. ERG: decreased in advanced disease
  4. EOG: normal
  5. Differential: AMPPE (both have outer retinal yellow-white lesions with early hypofluorescence on fluorescein angiography; AMPPE lesions resolve in 7 to 14 days and recurrences are uncommon more than several months after disease onset, scarring is limited to pigment mottling, choroidal atrophy not prominent, visual recovery is common even with foveal involvement, younger patients, simultaneous bilateral onset of disease, rare choroidal neovascularization); toxoplasmosis (both have recurrent lesions beginning at margins of inactive scar; toxoplasma lesions have marked vitritis, occur throughout the fundus and exhibit greater atrophy)

E. Treatment:
  1. Choroidal neovascularization treated with photocoagulation; some show spontaneous regression

2. Periocular and systemic steroids (prednisone 60 to 80 mg/day) may hasten resolution of active lesions and decrease frequency of recurrences
3. Triple therapy (prednisone, azathioprine, cyclosporine) may be necessary; some feel immunosuppression with cyclosporine or cyclophosphamide alone is as effective

XXV. SARCOIDOSIS

A. Epidemiology:
   1. Ratio of African-American to white = 10 : 1
   2. More common in females than in males
   3. Age 20 to 50 years
   4. 15 to 25% of patients with sarcoidosis develop ocular disease
B. Clinical features:
   1. Usually bilateral
   2. Presenting symptoms: pain, photophobia, redness, decreased vision, floaters
   3. Biomicroscopic findings: lacrimal gland enlargement, keratoconjunctivitis sicca, conjunctival nodules, aqueous cell and flare with small or large keratic precipitates (large KP appear mutton fat), iris nodules (Koeppe and Busacca), loss of iris crypts
   4. Ophthalmoscopic findings: posterior segment involvement in 25% of cases of ocular sarcoid; vitritis with inferior snowballs (frequently occurs in chains, called "string of pearls"); retinal vasculitis with diffuse or focal venous sheathing (when severe may resemble candle wax drippings, called "taches de bougie," large yellowish nodular deposits along the veins); peripheral neovascularization or disc neovascularization; disc edema; granulomas of the disc, retina, or choroid (when large have associated serous retinal detachment)
   5. Clinical course: band keratopathy (secondary to chronic uveitis or to hypercalcemia), posterior synechiae, cataract, glaucoma may develop
   6. Systemic involvement:
      a. pulmonary manifestations: intrathoracic involvement is the most common manifestation (90% of patients); CXR shows bilateral hilar adenopathy without pulmonary infiltration (65%), hilar adenopathy with pulmonary infiltration (22%), or pulmonary infiltration with fibrosis but without hilar adenopathy (13%)

      b. reticuloendothelial manifestations: extrapulmonary lymph nodes and/or spleen involvement (22 to 37% of patients)

      c. dermatologic manifestations: erythema nodosum, lupus pernio, maculopapular rashes (12 to 27% of patients)

      d. neurosarcoidosis: facial nerve palsy, meningitis, space occupying (2 to 7% of patients)

C. Pathogenesis:

  1. Etiology unknown; familial studies and HLA typing suggest a possible genetic predisposition; infectious agents may play a role

D. Diagnosis:

  1. FA: vascular staining and leakage, disc leakage, macular edema

  2. Tissue biopsy demonstrates noncaseating granuloma (conjunctival nodule; lacrimal gland, especially if enlarged or positive Gallium scan; however, may result in dry eye)

  3. Chest x-ray shows symmetric hilar lymphadenopathy

  4. Pulmonary function tests may be abnormal

  5. Angiotensin converting enzyme elevated (produced by macrophages and epithelioid cells in the granuloma)

  6. Lysozyme elevated

  7. Gallium scan shows increased uptake in lacrimal and parotid glands

  8. Increased serum calcium in 10 to 15% and hypercalciuria

  9. Anergy on skin testing (50%)

E. Treatment:

  1. Anterior segment inflammation: frequent topical steroids and cycloplegics

  2. Posterior segment involvement: periocular steroids to the more affected eye

  3. Systemic disease and/or posterior segment involvement: systemic steroids

  4. Retinal/disc neovascularization: panretinal photocoagulation

XXVI. VOGT-KOYANAGI-HARADA SYNDROME

A. Epidemiology:

  1. No gender predilection

  2. Age 20 to 50 years

  3. More common in heavily pigmented people, typically Asians, Native Americans, and African-Americans

B. Clinical features:
1. Bilateral
2. Presenting symptoms: pain, redness, photophobia, decreased vision
3. Biomicroscopic findings: granulomatous inflammation with mutton fat keratic precipitates, iris nodules, posterior synechiae, decreased intraocular pressure, perilimbal vitiligo (Sugiuras' sign)
4. Ophthalmoscopic findings: vitritis, disc hyperemia and edema, choroiditis with exudative retinal detachment, peripheral yellow nodules at the level of the choroid
5. Clinical course: cataracts, secondary glaucoma, iris and angle neovascularization, retinal and optic nerve neovascularization, areas of depigmentation and clumping of pigment in the fundus produces a "sunset glow"; retinal detachment resolves in 2 to 3 months and anterior chamber inflammation may persist despite therapy
6. Systemic involvement:
   a. ear involvement: tinnitus and vertigo may occur 1 to 2 weeks prior to eye disease; dysacousia and high frequency hearing loss may develop in 75% of patients
   b. meningeal involvement: neck stiffness, headache, and cerebrospinal fluid pleocytosis may occur 1 to 2 weeks prior to eye disease; encephalitis, cranial nerve palsies, hemiparesis, aphasia, and psychosis may develop
   c. skin involvement: alopecia, poliosis, vitiligo, and skin and hair sensitivity to touch
C. Pathogenesis:
1. Autoimmunity may play a role; increased HLA-DR4
2. Viral etiology also possible
3. Histopathology: thickened choroid (especially choriocapillaris) with infiltration of macrophages, lymphocytes, epithelioid cells, and plasma cells; Dalen-Fuchs' nodules are composed of epithelioid cells and are located between the retinal pigment epithelium and Bruch's membrane
D. Diagnosis:
1. FA: patchy delay of choroidal perfusion; multiple pinpoint areas of leakage at the level of the RPE; these can be associated with serous retinal detachment; later phases may show large confluent areas of leakage and disc leakeage
E. Treatment:

1. Steroids (prednisone 1.0 to 1.5 mg/kg/day); may require long-term treatment
2. Cyclosporine may be used alone or in combination with steroids; renal toxicity
3. Chlorambucil may be useful in some cases; systemic toxicity

XXVII. SYMPATHETIC OPHTHALMIA

A. Epidemiology:
   1. Occurs in patients with a history of penetrating trauma or intraocular surgery
   2. No gender, racial, or age predilection except as related to trauma
   3. Interval between penetrating injury to one eye (exciting eye) and the development of inflammation in the fellow eye (sympathizing eye) usually varies from 2 weeks to 1 year (65% within first 2 months and 80% within 3 months)

B. Clinical features:
   1. Bilateral
   2. Presenting symptoms: photophobia, redness, accommodative difficulties
   3. Biomicroscopic findings: granulomatous inflammation with mutton fat keratic precipitates and aqueous cell and flare
   4. Ophthalmoscopic findings: vitritis; isolated or confluent patches of yellow-white choroidal infiltrates; Dalen-Fuchs' nodules (small, discrete, yellowish infiltrates at the level of the RPE, most concentrated and largest in the periphery)
   5. Clinical course: posterior synechiae, cataract, glaucoma, rubeosis, papillitis, optic atrophy, exudative retinal detachment, chorioretinal scarring, eventually leads to phthisis if untreated; 65% of treated eyes return to 20/60 or better

C. Pathogenesis:
   1. Penetrating injury, especially with prolapse of intraocular tissue, removes intraocular antigen from usual immune privileged site; the immune system initiates an immunopathogenic process targeting the eye, primarily the uveal tract; the inciting antigen is unknown but may be retinal S antigen isolated from photoreceptor membranes, rhodopsin, and interphotoreceptor retinoid binding protein
   2. Histopathology: thickened choroid (sparing of choriocapillaris) with infiltration of macrophages, lymphocytes, and epithelial cells (paucity of plasma cells); Dalen-Fuchs' nodules are com-

posed of epithelioid cells and are located between
the retinal pigment epithelium and Bruch's membrane (these are present histopathologically in 25
to 40% of cases)

D. Diagnosis:

1. FA: multiple early hyperfluorescent sites of
   choroidal leakage (these correspond to Dalen-
   Fuchs' nodules); less commonly, there may be
   early hypofluorescent lesions (similar to AMPPE);
   optic nerve head may demonstrate late leakage

E. Treatment:

1. Enucleation soon after injury, before sensitization
   can develop (usually within 2 weeks)
2. Once inflammation develops in sympathizing eye,
   enucleation of traumatized eye will usually not affect visual outcome in the uninjured eye
3. Topical and systemic corticosteroids (prednisone
   1 to 2 mg/kg/day) are effective in improving visual
   outcome and in preventing recurrences
4. Immunosuppressive drugs may be useful in severe cases (chlorambucil, azathioprine, methotrexate, cyclosporine, cyclophosphamide); severe
   toxicity may result with these medications

Essentials of Eye Care, edited by Rohit Varma.
Lippincott–Raven Publishers,
Philadelphia © 1997.

9

Retina

I. DIABETIC RETINOPATHY

A. Epidemiology

1. One of four most frequent causes of new blindness in the United States
2. Leading cause of blindness in patients 20 to 64 years of age
3. 25% of diabetic population has some retinopathy
4. 5% have severe retinopathy (proliferative)
5. 50% of patients with proliferative diabetic retinopathy progress to legal blindness without treatment
6. With current treatment protocols legal blindness reduced to 5%
7. Duration of diabetes and retinopathy
   a. diagnosis prior to age 30:
   1) duration < 5 years
      a) 17% with some retinopathy
      b) macular edema uncommon
      c) proliferative changes rare
   2) duration > 15 years
      a) 98% with retinopathy
      b) macular edema 29%
      c) proliferative changes 29%
   b. diagnosis after age 30:
   1) duration < 5 years
      a) 29% with some retinopathy
      b) macular edema uncommon
      c) proliferative changes 2%
   2) duration > 15 years
      a) 78% with some retinopathy
      b) macular edema 28%
      c) proliferative changes 16%
8. Proliferative diabetic retinopathy is associated with increased incidence of:
   a. stroke

   b. coronary artery occlusion
   c. amputation of lower extremity
   d. premature death
9. Systemic risk factors for development and progression of diabetes:
   a. elevated blood sugar
   b. hypertension
   c. pregnancy
   d. proteinuria
   e. elevated serum lipids

B. Clinical Features
   1. Classification
      a. nonproliferative diabetic retinopathy (background retinopathy, and preproliferative changes)—changes confined to the retina
      b. proliferative diabetic retinopathy
        1) abnormal new blood vessels grow out of the retina onto the posterior vitreous
        2) abnormal new vessels that grow on the anterior iris surface (rubeosis irides)
   2. History
      a. determine:
        1) length of diabetes
        2) age of onset
        3) insulin dependency
        4) blood glucose control
        5) whether pregnant
      b. symptoms
        1) variable depending on specific diabetic pathology
          a) acute loss of vision; vitreous hemorrhage, rhegmatogenous retinal detachments
          b) gradual loss of vision; macular edema, traction detachments, retinal ischemia, cataracts
          c) red painful eye; rubeosis irides
   3. Signs
      a. nonproliferative
        1) microaneurysms:
          a) small saccular or fusiform areas of capillary dilatation
          b) appear as red dots 75 to 100 microns in size
          c) leak fluid, lipid, protein
        2) intraretinal hemorrhage:
          a) dot: small, round, located in deeper retina

       b) blot: larger, irregular, flame shaped, represents blood in nerve fiber layer

   3) hard exudates:
- **a)** lipoprotein deposit in outer plexiform layer
- **b)** waxy appearance, sharp borders
- **c)** may form a circinate ring

   4) macular edema:
- **a)** greatest cause of visual impairment
- **b)** focal or diffuse serous exudation from microaneurysms or areas of abnormal capillaries
- **c)** leads to thickening of the retina

   5) clinically significant macular edema (CSME):
- **a)** retinal thickening at or within 500 microns of the foveal center
- **b)** hard exudates at or within 500 microns of the foveal center associated with thickening of the adjacent retina
- **c)** retinal thickening at least one disc area in extent, any part of which is within one disc diameter of the foveal center

   6) fluorescein angiogram: early hyperfluorescence (microaneurysms) with late leakage, may be cystic

   7) natural history of macular edema:
- **a)** at 3 years without treatment, 32% with moderate visual loss (doubling of visual angle)
- **b)** at 3 years without treatment, 5% experienced moderate visual gain

   8) differential diagnosis
- **a)** hypertension
- **b)** vein occlusion
- **c)** pseudophakic, aphakic (Irvine-Gass)
- **d)** posterior uveitis
- **e)** retinitis pigmentosa

b. preproliferative

   1) progressive capillary closure and retinal ischemia

   2) eyes with advanced preproliferative retinopathy have a 50% chance of developing neovascularization in 1 year, and 6% develop high risk proliferative diabetic retinopathy in 5 years

   3) followup exams needed every 3 months when preproliferative changes present

      4) venous beading: irregular constrictions and dilatations of lumen

      5) nerve fiber infarcts (soft exudates, cotton-wool spots)
- **a)** focal infarcts result in swelling of axons
- **b)** opaque white area in nerve fiber layer
- **c)** blocked fluorescence on fluorescein angiography

      6) intraretinal microvascular abnormalities (IRMA):
- **a)** shunt vessels
- **b)** enlarged hypercellular capillaries adjacent to occluded capillaries
- **c)** mild leakage on fluoroscein angiography ischemic maculopathy
- **d)** closure of foveal capillaries
- **e)** enlargement of foveal avascular zone
- **f)** area devoid of capillaries on angiography

      7) differential diagnosis: disorders with intraretinal hemorrhage, cotton-wool spots, and/or microaneurysms:
- **a)** hypertension
- **b)** vein occlusion (branch, central)
- **c)** collagen vascular disease
- **d)** hyperviscosity syndrome
- **e)** sickle cell disease
- **f)** ocular ischemia
- **g)** sarcoidosis
- **h)** valsalva retinopathy
- **i)** HIV/AIS
- **j)** papilledema
- **k)** Purtscher's

c. proliferative (PDR)

      1) changes no longer confined to the retina

      2) abnormal vessels grow onto the posterior surface of the vitreous and on the iris

      3) optic disc neovascularization (NVD)
- **a)** neovascular vessels on or within one disc diameter of the nerve head

      4) retinal neovascularization elsewhere (NVE)
- **a)** frequently along the arcades
- **b)** more than one disc diameter

      5) high risk characteristics (Diabetic Retinopathy Study [DRS] criteria) equals three or more of the following:
- **a)** presence of any neovascularization (NVD, NVE)

        b) NVD

        c) moderate to severe new vessels: NVD > 1/3 of disc area (standard photo 10A) and/or NVE ≥ 1/2 disc area

        d) vitreous and/or preretinal hemorrhage

    6) iris neovascularization

        a) new vessel seen on slit lamp first at pupillary margin

        b) continued growth over trabecular meshwork will lead to angle closure and glaucoma

        c) gonioscopy will reveal anterior synechia and neovascular vessels over the TM (trabecular meshwork)

    7) natural history of proliferative diabetic retinopathy (PDR)

        a) neovascular tufts continue to grow in size and extent with increasing fibrosis

        b) vitreoretinal adhesion form

        c) subsequent contraction of the vitreous can cause:

            i. vitreous hemorrhage

            ii. traction retinal detachments

            iii. retinal breaks and rhegmatogenous retinal detachments

            iv. macular distortion

        d) 5-year risk of severe visual loss (acuity < 5/200)

            i. 1 or 2 risk characteristics—26%

            ii. high risk characteristic—50%

    8) differential diagnosis of retinal neovascularization:

        a) branch retinal vein occlusion (BRVO), central retinal vein occlusion (CRVO)

        b) sickle cell retinopathy

        c) retinopathy of prematurity (ROP)

        d) inflammatory disorders

        e) Eales' disease

        f) intraocular tumors

        g) ocular ischemic syndrome

        h) sarcoidosis

    9) differential diagnosis of iris neovascularization:

        a) congenital

        b) inflammatory

        c) aging

        d) other causes of retinal ischemia

C. Pathology/Pathogenesis

1. A disease of retinal vasculature
2. Hyperglycemia and/or genetic predisposition leads to vascular changes
   a. hyperglycemia leads to production of sugar alcohol (sorbitol) which may alter metabolism in retinal pericytes
   b. hyperglycemia may lead to nonenzymatic glycation of proteins with altered function
   c. hyperglycemia may directly affect genetic material
3. Principal pathologic changes:
   a. basement membrane thickening
   b. endothelial proliferation
   c. loss of pericytes
   d. capillary closure
   e. microaneurysm formation
   f. neovascularization
4. Secondary pathologic changes:
   a. retinal edema; outer plexiform may be cystic
   b. exudates; PAS-positive lipoprotein in outer plexiform layer with associated lipid-laden macrophages
   c. cotton-wool spots; 10 to 20 micron accumulations of axoplasmic organelles (cytoid bodies)
   d. hemorrhage: dot-outer plexiform; blot-nerve fiber layer
   e. preretinal—between internal limiting membrane (ILM) and vitreous
   f. traction; cystic degeneration, retinoschisis, retinal detachment

Pathogenesis of neovascularization

capillary closure
↓
retinal nonperfusion
↓
production of vasoproliferative substance
(angiogenic factor)
↓
neovascularization (NVD, NVE, iris)
↙   ↓   ↘
rubeotic glaucoma   vitreous hemorrhage   retinal detachment
(traction,
rhegmatogenous)

D. Diagnosis
   1. Ophthalmoscopy

   a. 90 diopter lens; useful for detection of pro-liferative changes
   b. fundus contact lens; essential for detection of macular edema, 10% of CSME will be missed with 90 diopter lens. To detect retinal thickening:
      1) use thin slit beam
      2) bright illumination
      3) fundus contact lens
      4) narrow angle (10 to 20 degrees) between slit beam and microscope
2. Fluorescein angiography
   a. to classify macular edema as diffuse or focal, not for diagnosis (ophthalmoscopy)
   b. to identify microaneurysm and associated leakage prior to treatment
   c. to help distinguish CSME from pseudophakic macular edema

CSME:	Pseudophakic:
no disc leakage (unless NVD)	disc leakage
leakage often from micro-aneurysms	leakage from perifoveal capillary bed
late leakage rarely in petalloid pattern	late leakage often in petalloid pattern

   d. to identify areas of nonperfusion, and diagnose ischemic maculopathy
   e. to identify neovascularization when the media is not clear (vitreous hemorrhage or cataract)
3. Iris angiography
   a. not more helpful for diagnosis than careful clinical exam
   b. may have some use in gauging clinical course
4. Fundus photography
   a. routine 30 or 60 degree photos should be obtained to:
      1) serve as adjunct to careful fundus examination
      2) document progression of disease
      3) aid in following progress of treatment
      4) extremely useful if patient examined by different physician on followup
5. Ultrasound B-scan

        a. use to rule out retinal detachment when media not clear

E. Treatment

    1. Systemic

        a. strong evidence that tight control of glycemia will reduce the risk of retinopathy, nephropathy, and neuropathy

        b. Diabetes Control and Complications Trial (DCCT)

        c. tight control prevented or delayed onset of diabetic retinopathy and slowed progression

        d. if no retinopathy at baseline; reduced risk of developing retinopathy by 76%

        e. if mild retinopathy at baseline; slowed progression by 54% and reduced development of PDR by 47%

        f. early treatment diabetic retinopathy study (ETDRS) demonstrated that aspirin 650 mg QD did not prevent the development of high risk PDR or increase the risk of vitreous hemorrhage

    2. Laser therapy: see chapter 15

    3. Cryotherapy in proliferative diabetic retinopathy

        a. indications:

            1) proliferation despite full PRP (panretinal photocoagulation)

            2) media opacity (cataract, hemorrhage)

        b. methods:

            1) retrobulbar or general anesthesia

            2) 360 degree peritomy

            3) approximately 10 applications in each quadrant

            4) place at 9, 11, 13 millimeters posterior to limbus in each quadrant

            5) obtain white retinal burn observed with indirect ophthalmoscopy if possible

        c. results:

            1) no randomized prospective controlled study has been done to date

        d. complications:

            1) iritis

            2) cataract

            3) cystoid macular edema

            4) epiretinal membrane formation

            5) retinal detachment

            6) increased intraocular pressure

            7) iris atrophy

8) vitreous, suprachoroidal hemorrhage
4. Vitrectomy in the treatment of diabetic retinopathy
  a. indications
    1) severe nonclearing vitreous hemorrhage
      a) Diabetic Retinopathy Vitrectomy Study (DRVS) demonstrated role for early vitrectomy (1 to 4 months) in type I insulin diabetics with presenting vision worse than 20/800: 36% of patients who underwent early vitrectomy had a visual acuity of 20/40 or better; only 12% of patients who deferred vitrectomy for 12 months had a visual acuity of 20/40 or better.
      b) type II patients generally wait until 6 months
      c) may consider early vitrectomy if fellow eye has poor vision or there is bilateral vitreous hemorrhage
      d) up to 1/3 of diabetic patients undergoing vitrectomy for nonclearing vitreous hemorrhage may result in NLP vision
    2) traction retinal detachment involving the macula
      a) only if recent detachment (few months old)
      b) rate of extramacular progression to involve the macula is approximately 15% per year
      c) if detached greater than 6 months, very poor prognosis for visual return
      d) anatomic success reported at 65% to 80% at 6 months followup
      e) improved visual acuity 26 to 65%
    3) combined tractional and rhegmatogenous retinal detachment
      a) look for holes, hydration lines in the inner retina
      b) surgery as soon as possible
      c) goal is to relieve traction and seal breaks
      d) better prognosis if macula on and no rubeosis present
      e) advanced active proliferative disease
        i. often a type I diabetic
        ii. vitreous hemorrhage may preclude laser photocoagulation

        iii. proliferation may not respond to laser photocoagulation

        iv. must have some useful vision preoperatively

        v. DRVS demonstrated; early vitrectomy 44% with better than or equal to 20/40 conventional treatment 28% with better than or equal to 20/40 with poor outcome was similar in each group

        vi. goal is to remove vitreous, fibrovascular tissue, and perform endolaser

b. Other less common indications

    1) dense premacular hemorrhage

    2) ghost cell glaucoma

        a) degenerated red cells from vitreous hemorrhage, blocks trabecular meshwork causing increased intraocular hemorrhage

        b) if IOP uncontrolled despite medical treatment consider vitrectomy

    3) rubeosis irides in patient with dense vitreous hemorrhage

        a) must remove vitreous and perform endolaser

        b) alternative is cryotherapy

        c) may also consider laser to ciliary body

    4) macular edema associated with premacular traction

        a) uncommon cause of macular edema in diabetics

        b) consider in recalcitrant cases of CSME

II. RETINAL ARTERIAL OCCLUSIVE DISEASE

A. Central retinal artery occlusion (CRAO); accounts for 57% of arterial occlusions

B. Epidemiology

    1. Age 60s

    2. More common in males than in females

    3. May have a history of amaurosis fugax

    4. Associated systemic conditions: hypertension (66%), diabetes (25%), cardiac valvular disease (25%), giant cell arteritis (2%)

C. Clinical Features

    1. Presenting symptoms: sudden, severe, painless, unilateral visual loss

    2. VA: count fingers to light perception

     3. Afferent pupillary defect may appear immediately

     4. Biomicroscopic findings: normal unless rubeosis develops

     5. Ophthalmoscopic findings: may be normal during the first hour; subsequently, the posterior pole becomes opaque and edematous except at the foveola producing a cherry red spot (orange reflex from underlying RPE and choroid beneath the thin foveola stands out in contrast to the surrounding opaque retina); arteries are thinned, show segmentation or "boxcarring" of the blood column, or are nonperfused; emboli can be seen in 20% of cases

     6. Clinical course: within 4 to 6 weeks, the opacification resolves, the arteries remain thinned and the disc becomes pale; iris neovascularization develops in 15 to 20%, disc neovascularization in less than 5%; decreased survival (56% mortality over 9 years versus 27% in controls) in cases where emboli are seen

D. Pathogenesis

     1. Etiologies include thrombosis, embolization, and vasculitis

     2. Emboli seen in 20% and include glistening yellow cholesterol emboli (Hollenhorst plaque) from carotid arteries; calcium, fibrin-platelet, and vegetations from cardiac valves; talc or steroids from injections; and fat, amniotic fluid, or tumors

     3. Vasculitis (giant cell arteritis) accounts for 2% of cases

     4. In patients under 30 years of age, etiologies include migraine, coagulation abnormalities, trauma, cardiac abnormalities, sickling hemoglobinopathies

E. Diagnosis

     1. Fluorescein angiogram (FA): delay in retinal arterial filling and arteriovenous transit times; late staining of disc; arteries reopen with time, and the angiogram may revert to normal

     2. Electroretinogram (ERG): decreased b-wave

F. Treatment

     1. If less than 24 hours duration: anterior chamber paracentesis (topical anesthetic, 25-gauge or smaller needle, remove 0.1 to 0.4 cc), intravenous acetazolamide (decrease in intraocular pressure may move the obstructing embolus distally), ocular massage (digital pressure 10

seconds, sudden release), inhalation of carbogen (95% O_2, 5% CO_2 mixture: CO_2 vasodilates and high O_2 concentration may increase diffusion from choroidal circulation)

2. Must initiate systemic workup (including erythrocyte sedimentation rate [ESR] if no emboli are seen to rule out giant cell arteritis: if giant cell arteritis (GCA) present, initiate immediate high dose corticosteroids) and a search for embolic sources

3. Branch Retinal Artery Occlusion (BRAO): accounts for 38% of arterial occlusions; 90% involve temporal arteries (nasal occlusions may be asymptomatic); 80% improve to 20/40 or better; neovascularization is rare; ocular therapeutic measures generally are not undertaken; workup is the same as for CRAO

4. Cilioretinal Artery Occlusion: accounts for 5% of arterial occlusions; cilioretinal artery is present in 15 to 30% of patients; 90% of eyes with isolated cilioretinal artery occlusions improve to 20/40 or better (CRAO may occur with cilioretinal artery sparing: the prognosis is better than for CRAO without sparing)

5. Ophthalmic Artery Occlusion: may present similarly to CRAO but some features help distinguish (visual acuity no light perception, cherry red spot may be absent, retinal opacification severe, late pigmentary disturbance common, optic atrophy severe, FA: compromised retinal and choroidal flow, ERG: decreased a- and b-waves)

III. CENTRAL RETINAL VEIN OCCLUSION

A. Epidemiology
   1. Age 60s; 90% are more than 50 years old
   2. Slight male preponderance
   3. Occasionally seen in young adults: termed "papillophlebitis"
   4. Associated systemic conditions: hypertension, diabetes, cardiovascular disease; 40% have preexisting glaucoma or develop glaucoma during followup

B. Clinical Features
   1. Presenting signs/symptoms: asymptomatic or sudden painless visual loss
   2. Visual acuity 20/20—hand motion (20/100 or worse usually indicates ischemic)

3. Afferent pupillary defect present in all ischemic and many nonischemic
4. Biomicroscopic findings: rubeosis may develop
5. Ophthalmoscopic findings: dilation and tortuosity of retinal veins; intraretinal hemorrhages radiating from optic disc and extending into periphery in all quadrants; cotton-wool spots; retinal and optic disc edema; these findings are striking in full-blown cases and subtle in mild cases; ischemic central retinal vein occlusion typically has more hemorrhages and cotton-wool spots
6. Clinical course: subclassified as nonischemic (partial, perfused, incomplete) versus ischemic (complete, hemorrhagic) as determined by fluorescein angiography; ischemic defined as ten or more disc areas of retinal nonperfusion; nonischemic usually resolves without significant sequelae but some progress to ischemic; ischemic may develop NVD/NVE/rubeosis and neovascular glaucoma; both nonischemic and ischemic may develop macular edema; over time, retinal hemorrhages decrease, venous dilation and tortuosity diminishes, and disc edema regresses; disc collaterals (optociliary shunt vessels) may develop (these are larger caliber vessels than seen in neovascularization and do not leak on fluorescein angiography); some eyes with extensive retinal hemorrhage cannot be categorized at the initial evaluation; eyes in this indeterminate category must be followed closely until the perfusion status is determined; papillophlebitis is similar to nonischemic in that complete or nearly complete recovery usually occurs

C. Pathology
1. Thrombus formation in the central retinal vein in the region of the lamina cribrosa with secondary endothelial cell proliferation and inflammation
2. Decreased vision due to macular edema, foveal hemorrhage, or foveal ischemia and occasionally due to vitreous hemorrhage
3. Macular edema results from leakage of perifoveal capillaries secondary to hydrostatic stress and ischemia (usually cystoid)
4. Ischemia stimulates neovascularization

D. Diagnosis

1. FA: prolonged arteriovenous transit time, blocked fluorescence by hemorrhage, venous wall staining, retinal nonperfusion, diffuse or petalloid pattern of macular edema
2. ERG: prolonged b-wave implicit time; reduced b-wave amplitude; decreased b:a-wave ratio

E. Treatment
   1. Grid photocoagulation not shown to be beneficial for macular edema in most patients
   2. Panretinal photocoagulation beneficial for ischemic vein occlusions after onset of neovascularization
   3. Panretinal photocoagulation is indicated for retinal, optic disc, or iris neovascularization

IV. BRANCH RETINAL VEIN OCCLUSION (BRVO)

A. Epidemiology
   1. Associated with systemic hypertension
   2. 60 to 70 years old
   3. No gender predilection
B. Clinical Features
   1. 90% unilateral
   2. Presenting symptoms: sudden onset blurred vision (if macula is involved) or field defect; may be asymptomatic
   3. Biomicroscopic findings: normal unless iris neovascularization develops
   4. Ophthalmoscopic findings: segmentally distributed intraretinal hemorrhage and cotton-wool spots along the distribution of a retinal vein; if this involves a major retinal vein, one quadrant is involved; if the occlusion is at the optic nerve head, two quadrants will be involved (hemiretinal vein occlusion); visual loss may occur and is due to macular edema, foveal hemorrhage, or macular ischemia
   5. Clinical course: collateral vessels that cross the temporal raphe may develop; macular edema may develop and can decrease vision; neovascularization of the disc, retina, or iris may develop which can result in peripheral traction retinal detachment and/or vitreous hemorrhage; patients with greater than five disc diameters of capillary nonperfusion are at high risk for retinal neovascularization; if visual loss is due to capillary nonperfusion, there will be no recovery; if visual loss is due only to foveal hemorrhage, vision may recover; if visual

loss is due to macular edema, improvement may occur either spontaneously or after photocoagulation

C. Pathogenesis

    1. Branch retinal vein occlusion always occurs at the site of an arteriovenous crossing

D. Diagnosis

    1. FA: in the acute phase there is blocked fluorescence by the intraretinal hemorrhage; may need to wait for reabsorption of hemorrhage to evaluate nonperfusion status. In the chronic phase, capillary nonperfusion, dilatation of capillaries, microaneurysms, collateral vessel formation (vein to vein channels around blockage site which may become tortuous), macular edema, and neovascularization may be detected; collateral vessels do not leak fluorescein while neovascularization does.

E. Treatment

    1. Systemic blood pressure control

    2. Macular edema: branch retinal vein occlusion study has demonstrated that argon laser photocoagulation is helpful in reducing visual loss from macular edema in patients who meet eligibility criteria (fluorescein proven macular edema involving the fovea, absorption of intraretinal hemorrhage, branch retinal vein occlusion of 3 to 18 months duration, no diabetic retinopathy, vision 20/40 or worse after refraction, visual loss not due to macular nonperfusion or foveal hemorrhage) and who are treated according to protocol (photocoagulation applied in grid pattern throughout the leaking area on fluorescein angiography, not within the foveal avascular zone, not outside the major arcades); after 3-year followup, 63% of treated eyes gained two or more lines of vision, as compared with 36% of control or untreated eyes

    3. Neovascularization: branch retinal vein occlusion study has defined greater than five disc diameters of capillary nonperfusion, as assessed by fluorescein angiography, as a risk factor for the development of retinal neovascularization; 40% of these patients will develop neovascularization; 60% of the patients who develop neovascularization (24% of total patients) will develop vitreous hemorrhage; laser photocoagulation should be applied only after neovascularization develops; peripheral scatter photocoagulation is applied to the areas of nonperfusion, at least two disc diameters from the fovea and at least out to the equator; in patients who develop neovascularization, the risk of vitreous hemorrhage is reduced from 60% to 30% (from 24% to 12% of total patients)

V. RETINOPATHY OF PREMATURITY

A. Epidemiology
  1. Occurs almost exclusively in premature infants with gestational age less than 33 weeks and birth weight less than 1500 grams; incidence of development of ROP and of unfavorable outcome strongly related to birth weight (e.g., less than 750 gms—90% develop any ROP/16% threshold ROP; 1000 to 1250 gms—45% develop any ROP/2% threshold ROP)
  2. Other prognostic factors related to the development of threshold ROP (but not to unfavorable outcome) include gestational age (19% decrease with each additional week), race (64% lower in African-Americans), and multiple births (40% lower in singletons)
B. Clinical Features
  1. More than 80% bilateral symmetry
  2. Presenting signs: ROP should be detected on routine screening examination; first examination for premature infants under 1500 gms at 4 to 6 weeks, over 1500 gms at 6 to 8 weeks, sequential followup at 2-week intervals until retina fully vascularized/ROP regressed, at least every week if prethreshold; infants rarely first present with regressed or late "cicatricial" ROP (retrolental fibroplasia) typically when ROP screening has not been performed; in such cases, decreased vision, leukocoria, and/or strabismus noted by parents or pediatrician
  3. Ophthalmoscopic findings: goal—identify "threshold" ROP = Stage 3 ROP in zone 1 or 2 totalling 5 or more contiguous/8 cumulative clock hours with "Plus+" disease present; "prethreshold" = zone 1—any stage ROP, zone 2—stage 2+ or 3 ROP, zone 2—stage 3+ less than 5 hours
  4. ROP zones:

    a. zone 1—a circle centered on the disc with radius two times the distance from the disc to the fovea; when using a 28 diopter condensing lens for indirect ophthalmoscopy, the radius is contained within the viewing field of the lens

    b. zone 2—a circle outside zone 1 bounded nasally by the ora serrata and temporally by the equator

    c. zone 3—the residual crescent of temporal retina outside zone 2

5. ROP stages:
    a. stage 1 - demarcation line (vascular—avascular retina);
    b. stage 2 - ridge (height and width);
    c. stage 3 - ridge with extraretinal fibrovascular proliferation;
    d. stage 4 - subtotal retinal detachment (RD); 4A—macula-on, 4B—macula-off;
    e. stage 5 - total RD (open/closed, anterior/posterior funnel)

6. ROP extent: circumferential extent (in clock hours) of ROP for the entire 360 degrees of peripheral retina, specifying whether ROP is contiguous or noncontiguous

7. "Plus" disease: engorgement of veins/tortuosity of arterioles apparent when viewing the disc-macula by indirect ophthalmoscopy; if these changes exist only outside the posterior pole, not Plus disease

8. ROP summary diagnosis:
    a. look at posterior pole, determine presence/absence of Plus disease
    b. look at nasal retina, determine zone of ROP; if nasal retina not vascularized, zone 1 or 2 disease is present, if vascularized, check for zone 3 disease (scleral depress)
    c. determine stage and circumferential extent
    d. each eye scored by worst stage, most posterior zone, extent, and presence/absence of Plus disease

9. Regressed ROP: abnormal vasculature (nondichotomous branching), myopia, lattice-like changes, pigment migration, macular RPE changes, vitreoretinal traction (vascular straightening, macular heterotopia, disc dragging), fibrotic ridge, traction/rhegmatogenous retinal detachment; infants with mild/regressing ROP should be reevaluated at 1 to 3 months

to confirm ROP status, evaluate for other abnormalities (e.g., strabismus)

10. Clinical course: threshold typically develops around 10 weeks after birth and retinal detachment within 1 to 2 weeks of term; at threshold—51% of untreated eyes progress to an unfavorable anatomic/visual outcome (e.g., retinal detachment, macular fold) versus 31% of treated eyes; with zone 1 threshold disease, 95% of eyes progress to an unfavorable anatomic outcome (75% with treatment, but not a statistically significant difference)

C. Pathology
1. Vasoproliferative process occurring at the juncture between vascular and avascular retina; proliferating vanguard cells form demarcation line, proliferating rearguard forms the ridge (spindle cell proliferation)
2. A disease of immature retinal vasculature; though pronounced/prolonged hyperoxia can stimulate ROP in immature retinas, ROP can develop without elevated PaO_2

D. Diagnosis
1. Differential (cicatricial ROP): unilateral—persistent hyperplastic primary vitreous toxocariasis, trauma; bilateral—familial exudative vitreoretinopathy; diagnosis usually straightforward based on history of prematurity, low birth weight, bilateral symmetry, lack of inflammation, characteristic retinal findings

E. Treatment
1. Based on diagnosis of threshold disease
2. Screening techniques: dilate with two sets cyclomydril drops q5min (0.2% cyclopentolate/1.0% phenylephrine); trained assistant to monitor premie; binocular indirect ophthalmoscope with 20, 28, 30 diopter lens; (Alfonso) lid speculum, scleral depressor, topical anesthetic, irrigating solution
3. Cryotherapy/laser: when threshold ROP identified, cryotherapy/indirect laser photocoagulation performed within 72 hours; retinal cryotherapy and laser photocoagulation appear to be of comparable efficacy in treating threshold disease
4. Cryotherapy/laser technique:
   a. preoperative—NPO, premedication, pupillary dilation

    b. operative—local or general anesthesia (ICU/OR) with appropriate monitoring; contiguous, nonoverlapping applications to all avascular retina anterior to ridge with no treatment applied to ridge

      1) cryotherapy—appropriate cryoprobe tip used, treat until sudden whitening, conjunctival incision if necessary; advantages—can use with impaired media; disadvantages—postoperative edema/inflammation, difficulty treating posterior disease, harder to control applications, retinal hemorrhage; systemic complications include bradycardia, respiratory arrest, arrhythmia, transient hypoxia

      2) laser—argon or diode with indirect ophthalmoscope delivery system; peripheral scatter/PRP-type applications (often more than 1000/eye); advantages—less ocular manipulation, easy to see applications, easier (and probably more effective) treatment of posterior/zone 1 disease; disadvantages—(non)port-ability of some (larger) laser systems, unable to treat through impaired media, risk of cataract, hyphema

   c. postoperative—homatropine 2% drops qd/bid for 5 days, topical antibiotics if conjunctival incision

5. Retreatment with cryo/laser: indicated within 2 weeks if significant areas of untreated avascular retina remain and Plus disease with progression of extraretinal proliferation exists

6. Treatment of Stage 4 ROP: careful examination to determine if retinal detachments are exudative or tractional; exudative detachment may resolve with treatment of neovascularization; traction retinal detachment threatening (4A) or involving (4B) the macula may respond to encircling scleral buckling procedure; lens-sparing vitrectomy may be indicated for detachment caused by tractional membranes in the posterior pole

7. Treatment of Stage 5 ROP: controversial due to the poor functional outcomes in most series regardless of treatment; not indicated in asymmetric disease (one eye with functional vision and stable anatomy); vitreoretinal surgery by

ROP specialist may be cautiously considered after careful discussion/informed consent

8. Late complications of ROP: including retinal detachment, cataract, glaucoma, should be monitored and treated according to standard techniques

VI. HYPERTENSIVE RETINOPATHY

A. Epidemiology
   1. Patients with severe acute hypertension or chronic systemic hypertension
B. Clinical Features and Pathogenesis
   1. Biomicroscopic features: normal
   2. Ophthalmoscopic features:
      a. chronic hypertension: initially there is local or generalized vasoconstriction of arterioles—this results in focal arteriolar narrowing, cotton-wool spots, and areas of capillary nonperfusion (seen only on fluorescein angiography); with prolonged hypertension, there is disruption of the blood-retinal barrier—leakage of plasma and formed blood elements results in intraretinal flame and splinter hemorrhages and exudates; with prolonged hypertension there is also thickening of the walls of the arterioles due to endothelial hyperplasia, intimal hyalinization, and medial hypertrophy (arteriolar sclerosis)—this results in copper-wire arterioles (broader and duller light reflex), silver-wire arterioles (no blood column seen), and arteriovenous crossing changes (AV nicking, deviation of vein, venous banking, and right-angled crossings); with prolonged severe hypertension, proliferative retinopathy may develop, which is characterized by retinal neovascularization and vitreous hemorrhage
      b. severe acute hypertension: hypertensive choroidopathy may develop due to fibrinoid necrosis of choroidal arterioles and occlusion of choriocapillaris—this results in focal areas of opaque retinal pigment epithelium which leak fluorescein acutely and appear as pigmented spots with a hypopigmented halo when healed (Elschnig spots) and focal areas of exudative neurosensory detachment; with severe acute hyperten-

sion, optic nerve head edema may develop (malignant hypertension); associated findings in patients with hypertensive retinopathy include branch retinal vein occlusion, retinal arterial macroaneurysm, and anterior ischemic optic neuropathy

C. Diagnosis

    1. Based on ophthalmoscopic findings in patients with acute or chronic systemic hypertension

D. Treatment

    1. Panretinal photocoagulation is indicated in proliferative hypertensive retinopathy

    2. Blood pressure control is indicated in any patient with ophthalmologic manifestations of hypertension

VII. RETINAL ARTERIAL MACROANEURYSM

A. Epidemiology

    1. Age 60 years

    2. Ratio of females to males is 3:1

    3. 75% of patients have history of hypertension

B. Clinical Features

    1. 10% bilateral; 20% have multiple aneurysms in one eye

    2. Presenting symptoms: often asymptomatic but may present with sudden visual loss from rupture of the aneurysm and resultant hemorrhage; gradual visual loss may occur if macular edema occurs

    3. Biomicroscopic findings: normal

    4. Ophthalmoscopic findings: 100 to 250 m diameter fusiform or saccular dilatation of retinal artery, usually at bifurcation site or at AV crossing; most often found along superotemporal arcade (this location is most likely to produce symptoms); lipid exudate may surround the aneurysm and/or involve the fovea; hemorrhage may occur in the subretinal space, within the retina and the subinternal limiting membrane space, in the retrohyaloid space, and/or in the vitreous; the retinal arterial macroaneurysm may be hidden by the overlying hemorrhage; as hemorrhage resorbs an epiretinal membrane may develop

    5. Clinical course: the aneurysms may involute; hemorrhage may occur; macular edema may occur; epiretinal membrane may develop

C. Diagnosis
1. FA: usually there is immediate and uniform filling of the arterial macroaneurysm; partial filling may occur if partial involution or thrombosis has occurred; the surrounding area often has microaneurysms and capillary non-perfusion; leakage from the retinal arterial macroaneurysm is common and macular edema may be seen

D. Treatment
1. In cases with macular edema, focal treatment of the lesion with photocoagulation may be beneficial

VIII. RADIATION RETINOPATHY

A. Epidemiology
1. History of radiotherapy or radiation exposure to the eye(s)
2. Depends on total dose delivered (retinopathy usually develops at 3,000 to 3,500 rad [30 to 35 Gy]), the volume of retina irradiated, and the fractionation scheme (usually daily fractions are 200 to 300 rad)
3. Patients with preexisting diabetic retinopathy and patients receiving certain chemotherapeutic agents (5-fluorouracil) have a lower threshold for the development of radiation retinopathy

B. Clinical Features
1. Presenting symptoms: gradual blurring of vision, floaters (if vitreous hemorrhage present)
2. Biomicroscopic findings: iris neovascularization (in advanced cases)
3. Ophthalmoscopic findings: cotton-wool spots, microaneurysms, retinal hemorrhages, exudates, retinal neovascularization, perivascular sheathing, macular edema, disc pallor, disc edema, disc neovascularization; may result in vitreous hemorrhage and neovascular glaucoma; rarely results in central retinal artery occlusion, central retinal vein occlusion, subretinal neovascularization
4. Clinical course: develops months to years (usually 12 to 18 months) after exposure to radiation, slowly progressive

C. Pathology
1. Alteration in structure and permeability of retinal and optic nerve blood vessels

2. Preferential damage to inner retinal layers
3. Occlusion of retinal and optic nerve arterioles with thickening of the vessel walls by fibrillar and hyaline material, capillary damage consisting of focal loss of capillary endothelial cells and pericytes, intraretinal exudation, outer plexiform and inner nuclear cystic changes, ganglion cell loss

D. Diagnosis

1. FA: retinal vascular occlusion, capillary telangiectasia, capillary nonperfusion
2. Differential: diabetic retinopathy (severe fibrovascular proliferation much less common in radiation retinopathy), multiple branch vein occlusions or branch retinal artery occlusions, retinal telangiectasia

E. Treatment

1. Macular capillary nonperfusion is not reversible; panretinal photocoagulation is indicated for neovascularization; cystoid macular edema may benefit from focal treatment

IX. HEMOGLOBINOPATHIES

A. Types

1. Hemoglobin A—normal hemoglobin
2. Hemoglobin S—(sickle hemoglobin)—substitution of valine for glutamic acid at 6th position of beta chain
3. Hemoglobin C—substitution of lysine for glutamic acid at 6th position of beta chain
4. Thalassemia—inadequate normal globin chain synthesis

B. Epidemiology

1. AS (sickle trait): in 8% of U.S. African-American population; these patients experience morbidity only in severe hypoxic conditions
2. AC: 2.5% of U.S. African-American population
3. SS (sickle cell disease): 0.3% of U.S. African-American population; chronic anemia; intravascular sickling causes sludging in microvascular circulation with frequent sickle crises; systemic symptoms/signs include painful joints, abdominal pain, dyspnea, stroke, bone infarcts, aseptic necrosis of the femoral head, fish-mouth vertebrae, bacterial infection
4. SC (double heterozygote): 0.1% of U.S. African-American population; mild anemia

with few sickle crises; most severe ocular findings

5. S thal (double heterozygote): 0.03% of U.S. African-American population

C. Clinical Features

1. Biomicroscopic findings: conjunctival comma-shaped capillaries (occlusion on both ends results in stagnant column of blood); iris sector atrophy (occlusion in iris circulation)

2. Ophthalmoscopic findings:

   a. stage I—background retinopathy:
      1) peripheral arteriolar occlusion
      2) salmon patch hemorrhage; round or oval hemorrhage with sharp borders; flat or dome shaped; 1/4 to 1 disc diameter in size; located in sensory retina; initially bright red, fades to red-orange; due to sudden occlusion, infarction, and blow-out of arteriole
      3) irridescent spot; a retinoschisis cavity that contains refractile copper-colored granules (hemosiderin laden macrophages); these may appear where salmon patch hemorrhages have reabsorbed
      4) black sunburst: circular black chorioretinal scar with stellate or spiculate borders; 1/2 to 2 disc diameters in size; usually peripheral; due to RPE hypertrophy, hyperplasia, and migration

   b. stage II: arteriovenous anastomoses at border of perfused and nonperfused retina

   c. stage III: retinal neovascularization (proliferative sickle retinopathy) in a sea fan configuration (resembles marine invertebrate Gorgonia flabellum); may be flat but usually elevated into the vitreous

   d. stage IV: vitreous hemorrhage; due to bleeding neovascular tissue; most common in SC disease

   e. stage V: retinal detachment; can be traction and/or rhegmatogenous

3. Other posterior segment findings include macular depression sign (dark circle adjacent to macula with bright central reflex; atrophy and thinning of retina due to capillary occlusion), sickle disc sign (comma-shaped capillaries similar to conjunctival findings), and angioid streaks (present in 6% of SS patients)

D. Diagnosis

1. FA: in proliferative sickle retinopathy, fluorescein angiogram demonstrates hyperfluorescence from the neovascular sea fans
2. Fluorescein angioscopy: for patients with vitreous hemorrhage in whom fundus angiography cannot be performed (because of media opacity) or for patients in whom fluorescein angiography does not demonstrate leakage (because of extreme peripheral location); fluorescein angioscopy involves fundus indirect ophthalmoscopy using a blue light after fluorescein has been injected to visualize the leaking sea fans

E. Treatment
   1. Proliferative sickle retinopathy:
      a. feeder vessel photocoagulation: direct treatment of the feeding arteriole and subsequently the draining vein; heavy treatment is needed which results in frequent complications (especially chorioretinal neovascularization and retinal detachment)
      b. scatter photocoagulation: similar to diabetic PRP but only the area immediately around the sea fan is treated
   2. Vitreous hemorrhage: may require vitrectomy if nonclearing
   3. Retinal detachment: scleral buckle and/or vitrectomy, depending on the degree of traction
   4. Surgical procedures in sickle patients: consider the risk of anterior segment ischemia (strabismus surgery, scleral buckling surgery) and the risk of optic nerve infarction (any procedure that transiently elevates IOP); exchange transfusion to obtain greater than 50% hemoglobin A and hematocrit greater than 35% may help reduce risks; however, this is currently less commonly performed due to the risks of transfusion-related infections; intraoperative and postoperative supplemental oxygen may reduce the risks; avoid sympathomimetics (epinephrine) and carbonic anhydrase inhibitors (diamox)
   5. Hyphema in sickle patients: sickled erythrocytes occlude the trabecular meshwork and cause elevated intraocular pressure; may result in optic nerve infarction; obtain hemoglobin electrophoresis in any African-American patient with hyphema; early paracentesis is performed if IOP increases above 25 mm Hg for any 24-hour period

X. COATS' DISEASE

A. Definition
   1. Idiopathic retinal vascular disorder; telangiectatic and aneurysmal retinal vessels with progressive intraretinal and subretinal exudation
   2. Leber's miliary aneurysms: early or nonprogressive form with similar vascular lesions but without subretinal exudation

B. Epidemiology
   1. Age 4 to 10 years, but may become clinically evident at any age
   2. 85% male
   3. Nonfamilial
   4. Juvenile form: no associated systemic disease; adult form: frequently associated with hypercholesterolemia

C. Clinical Features
   1. Unilateral 80%
   2. Presenting signs: leukocoria, strabismus, decreased vision
   3. Ophthalmoscopic findings: retinal vascular anomalies consist of telangiectasia, aneurysms, venous dilation, and capillary nonperfusion; most pronounced in temporal quadrants; retinal exudate may be mild (minimal intraretinal lipid) or severe (massive intraretinal and subretinal yellow exudate with exudative RD); may see refractile particles (cholesterol) and blood in subretinal space; advanced cases may have neovascular glaucoma, spontaneous hyphema, or total RD appearing as white retrolental mass
   4. Clinical course: generally progressive; severity and rate of progression greater in patients under age 4

D. Pathology
   1. Accumulation of serum and blood products within and under retina due to leakage of abnormal vessels
   2. Many eyes enucleated for suspected retinoblastoma
   3. Gross: total RD with thick subretinal fluid that contains yellow refractile particles and occasionally blood
   4. Histopathology: subretinal fluid contains cholesterol clefts and macrophages with ingested lipid and pigment

E. Diagnosis
   1. FA: telangiectasia, aneurysms, and beading showing early and persistent leakage; areas of capillary nonperfusion
   2. B scan: useful in advanced cases; echographic features of RD with particulate echoes in subretinal space, no distinct tumor demonstrated
   3. Differential: juvenile form—differential for leukocoria and/or strabismus (retinoblastoma, ROP, PHPV, congenital cataract, toxocariasis, FEV, angiomatosis retinae); adult form—diabetes, BRVO, juxtafoveal telangiectasis, tumors accompanied by exudate, any vasculopathy that produces an exudate
F. Treatment
   1. Close observation for limited lesions that do not threaten macular vision
   2. Photocoagulation (FA-guided) if macular exudate present and retina not elevated by exudate; xenon, argon blue-green, argon green, dye yellow; treat leaking lesions directly; 200 to 500μ spot size; vascular closure documented by FA with retreatment as indicated
   3. Cryopexy if lesions too peripheral for laser or if exudative RD; freeze-refreeze technique
   4. Untreated eyes: 75% deteriorate, 25% stabilize; eyes treated with laser or cryo: 25% deteriorate, 50% stabilize, 25% improve
   5. Diathermy used as alternative to cryo
   6. Scleral buckling and/or subretinal fluid drainage may be used if RD present

XI. PARAFOVEAL TELANGIECTASIS

A. Group 1A: unilateral congenital parafoveal telangiectasis

   A condition of microaneurysmal and saccular dilation and capillary nonperfusion of parafoveal capillaries; often accompanied by right angled venules draining the telangiectatic capillary bed
   1. Epidemiology
      a. males
      b. age 40 years
   2. Clinical features
      a. VA: 20/25 to 20/40
      b. ophthalmoscopic features: temporal half of macula involved, one to two disc areas in

size, equal areas superior and inferior to horizontal raphe involved

   c. clinical course: visual loss due to macular edema and exudation; spontaneous resolution may occur; however, some cases improve with laser

B. Group 1B: unilateral idiopathic parafoveal telangiectasis

   1. Epidemiology

      a. males

      b. age 40 years

   2. Clinical features

      a. VA: 20/25

      b. ophthalmoscopic features: capillary telangiectasis confined to one clock hour at the edge of the foveal avascular zone; may have hard exudates

C. Group 2: bilateral acquired parafoveal telangiectasis

   1. Epidemiology

      a. no gender predilection

      b. age 50 to 60 years

      c. most common parafoveal telangiectasis; possibly familial

   2. Clinical features

      a. bilateral and symmetric

      b. VA: 20/30

      c. ophthalmoscopic features: usually temporal to foveal but may involve entire perifoveal capillary network; minimal macular edema without exudation; right angle venules commonly seen; occasional superficial glistening dots in perifoveal area; may see yellow lesion in center of foveal avascular zone in deep retinal or subretinal space

      d. clinical course: many patients develop hyperplastic retinal pigment epithelium along the right angled venules; rarely develop choroidal neovascularization with acute visual loss

D. Group 3: bilateral idiopathic perifoveal telangiectasis and capillary obliteration

   1. Epidemiology

      a. age 50 years

      b. very rare

   2. Clinical features

      a. severe visual loss

      b. ophthalmoscopic features: disc pallor in addition to retinal vascular changes

3. Pathogenesis
   a. unknown
   b. histopathology: narrowed capillaries, localized endothelial defects in temporal parafoveal region, degeneration of pericytes with accumulation of lipid, and capillary walls with presence of multilaminar basement membrane (changes similar to diabetic retinopathy)
   c. there is a possible association with diabetes; some patients have abnormal glucose tolerance test
4. Diagnosis
   a. FA: telangiectasis of retinal capillaries and microaneurysms; leakage from the telangiectasis and microaneurysms
   b. differential: diabetic retinopathy, branch retinal vein occlusion, radiation retinopathy, age-related macular degeneration, adult onset foveomacular pigment epithelial dystrophy (if yellow macular lesion is present)
5. Treatment
   a. some cases have improved following photocoagulation; however, photocoagulation is not generally recommended

XII. AGE-RELATED MACULAR DEGENERATION (SENILE MACULAR DEGENERATION)

A. Epidemiology
   1. Prevalence
      a. leading cause of new blindness in the United States in persons over 65 years of age
      b. of all new cases of blindness, 14% accounted for by age-related macular degeneration (AMD)
      c. age-related macular degeneration is present in 9% of people over 52 years of age and in 25 to 33% of people over 75 years of age
      d. atrophic (nonneovascular, dry) AMD accounts for 85% of all eyes with AMD
      e. neovascular AMD (exudative AMD, wet) accounts for 90% of severe visual loss associated with AMD (vision less than 20/200)
      f. neovascular AMD is much more common in whites than in African-Americans
      g. neovascular AMD is slightly more common in females than in males

   2. Risk factors:
      a. age
      b. family history
      c. hyperopia
   3. Other possible risk factors:
      a. light colored irides
      b. history of cardiovascular disease
      c. cumulative lifetime exposure to visible light
      d. smoking (males)
      e. decreased hand grip strength
B. Clinical Features:
   1. History:
      a. onset of symptoms usually in sixth or seventh decade
      b. gradual visual loss (months to years), or acute visual loss (choroidal neovascular membrane [CNV])
      c. metamorphopsia (distortion)
      d. paracentral scotoma
      e. often asymptomatic or noticed only when closing less affected eye
      f. may complain of difficulty reading
      g. rarely complain of changes in Amsler grid testing
   2. Clinical Signs:
      a. drusen
         1) hard drusen
            a) small, less than 64 nanometers
            b) represent lipodized RPE
            c) are of questionable significance in the pathogenesis of age-related macular degeneration
         2) soft drusen
            a) larger, more ill-defined with amorphous borders
            b) may become confluent
            c) found in 26% of people in the ages of 70 to 79 with confluent aspects in approximately 17% of the patients in this age group.
            d) represents significant risk factors for the development of choroidal neovascular AMD
         3) Ophthalmoscopy: yellow round spots at the level at the RPE found near the center of the macula
         4) Angiography
            a) hard drusen: transient staining with early hyperfluorescence

   b) soft and confluent drusen: accumulate fluorescein becoming increasingly hyperfluorescent in later phases

b. RPE abnormalities

   1) focal hyperpigmentation or reticular clumps of pigment representing hyperplastic RPE on fluorescein angiography presents as blocked fluorescence

   2) atrophy area of loss of retinal pigment epithelium, overlying photoreceptors, and choriocapillaris

   3) ophthalmoscopy:

   a) often circular to oval

   b) well-circumscribed margins

   c) can be unifocal or multifocal

   d) usually one disc diameter within the macular center

   e) range in size from 200 to 5,300 microns

   f) atrophy may be slowly progressive and can become geographic

   4) angiography: atrophic areas demonstrate "window defects" with early visualization of the choroidal circulation and early hyperfluorescence without increasing intensity with time

c. pigment epithelial detachments

   1) detachment or elevation of the RPE

   2) in patients under 55 years, prognosis is good, generally not associated with CNV

   3) in patients over 55 years, prognosis is worse, 33% present with or develop CNV

   4) ophthalmoscopy: (use fundus contact lens) uni- or multifocal elevations of the retinal pigment epithelium and overlying retina. May contain areas of hyperplastic RPE and hemorrhage.

   5) angiography:

   a) classic serous pigment epithelial detachment (PED): uniform bright hyperfluorescence in early phase with smooth contours by midphase and little leakage into the overlying neurosensory detachment

   b) drusenoid detachments: (extensive area of confluent drusen) fluoresces faintly during transit and does not progress to bright fluorescence in later phases. Usually more irregular, smaller, and more shallow than serous or fibrovascular RPE detachments

c) fibrovascular PED: (associated with CNV, a subset of occult CNV). Slow filling with a stippled appearance to the RPE and later pooling of fluorescein into the neurosensory retinal detachment.

d. the RPE: may develop from RPE detachments, rip or tear of the RPE, some are precipitated by photocoagulation. This is seen as a crescent-shaped defect of the RPE with an adjacent area of hyperpigmentation and hemorrhage. On angiography, early hyperfluorescence in the area of the RPE defect with an adjacent area of blocked fluorescence caused by the retracted edge of the RPE or hemorrhage.

e. choroidal neovascularization (CNV)

1) risk factors for development of CNV

a) bilateral soft drusen—approximately 2 to 4% of eyes per year will develop CNV

b) confluent soft drusen

c) presence of disciform scar in fellow eye

d) focal hyperpigmented areas

e) increasing age (greater than 75 years)

2) be suspicious of choroidal neovascularization in any patient over the age of 65 with obvious drusen who complains of metamorphopsia or paracentral scotoma of acute onset

3) ophthalmoscopic findings include:

a) subretinal fluid

b) cystoid macular edema

c) subretinal blood or lipid

d) serous detachments of the neurosensory retina

e) pigment epithelial detachments

f) may visualize choroidal neovascularization as a green/gray subretinal lesion

g) rarely intraretinal hemorrhage or vitreous hemorrhage may be present

h) none of the above are diagnostic; however, if present, one should proceed to fluorescein angiography to diagnose CNV and to determine if a treatable lesion is present

4) angiography
  a) patterns of choroidal neovascular hyperfluorescence
    i. classic choroidal neovascularization; CNV discerned during early transit with a lacy or cartwheel appearance; well-demarcated boundaries in early transit late phase of fluorescein angiography demonstrates leakage with increased intensity of the hyperfluorescence and obscuration of the boundaries of the CNV
    ii. poorly defined choroidal neovascularization; fibrovascular pigment epithelial detachments; irregular elevation of pigment epithelium in early transit; boundaries may be well or poorly demarcated persistent staining or leakage after 10 minutes late leakage of undetermined source; poorly demarcated boundaries; source of leakage cannot be defined in early fluorescein transit
  b) other important angiographic features of choroidal neovascularization
    i. features that obscure boundaries or borders—thick blood, elevated blocked fluorescence secondary to hyperpigmentation or fibrovascular scar, serous detachments of the pigment epithelium
    ii. locations of choroidal neovascularization on fluorescein angiography; extrafoveal—edge at least 200 microns from the foveal center; juxtafoveal—edge of choroidal neovascularization 1 to 199 microns from the foveal center; subfoveal—choroidal neovascularization underlies the foveal center

5) natural history: general progression of choroidal neovascularization to subretinal fibrosis and disciform scarring. Rare report of involution of the choroidal neovascularization.

6) history by location:

   a) extrafoveal—62% of the untreated eyes had six or more lines of visual loss with mean visual acuity 5 years of followup at 20/200 (MPS)

   b) juxtafoveal—58% of the untreated eyes at 5 years had six or more lines of visual acuity loss and a mean visual acuity of 20/200 (MPS)

   c) subfoveal—at 24 months, 37% of eyes lost six or more lines of vision. In patients with 20/100 acuity on presentation, 77% lost greater than four lines of vision and 64% lost six lines by 2 years.

   d) poorly defined—(leakage of undetermined course, occult AMD, fibrovascular PED). Generally involves foveal center on presentation. Average acuity at 28 months is 20/250 with 42% of the eyes with six or more lines of visual acuity loss.

Pathogenesis and Histopathology:

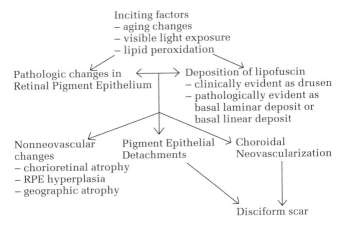

Inciting factors
- aging changes
- visible light exposure
- lipid peroxidation

Pathologic changes in Retinal Pigment Epithelium ⟷ Deposition of lipofuscin
- clinically evident as drusen
- pathologically evident as basal laminar deposit or basal linear deposit

Nonneovascular changes
- chorioretinal atrophy
- RPE hyperplasia
- geographic atrophy

Pigment Epithelial Detachments

Choroidal Neovascularization

Disciform scar

7) defects thought to reside in retinal pigment epithelium

   a) lipofuscin accumulates throughout life. Lipofuscin thought to represent incomplete degradation products derived from phagocytized inner and outer segments of the rods and cones.

b) progressive accumulation of material by the RPE leads to extrusion to Bruch's membrane resulting in:

   i. basal laminar deposits; material mostly composed of widely spaced collagen and located between the plasma membrane and basement membrane of the RPE

   ii. basal linear deposits (diffuse drusen or diffuse thickening of RPE)—this material is located external to the basement membrane of the RPE and consists of granular and vesicular material with foci of widely spaced collagen

   iii. basal linear or basal laminar deposit may result in localized detachments of the RPE and its basement membrane. If localized, represents soft drusen. If larger, represents RPE detachments

c) accumulation of the above products appears to be associated with overlying RPE atrophy with consequential loss of photoreceptors and choriocapillaris

d) the presence of these deposits may also predispose to the development of choroidal neovascularization

e) choroidal neovascularization histopathologically is seen as ingrowth of capillary-like vessels (choroidal in origin) that extend through the outer layer of Bruch's membrane into the sub RPE space. Occasionally, these choroidal vessels may extend into the subretinal space. On average, there are 2.2 defects in Bruch's membrane with associated choroidal neovascularization present in patients with AMD and CNV.

f) these choroidal new vessels leak blood and protein resulting in subretinal lipid, blood, and detachments of the RPE and/or neurosensory retina

g) other pathologic changes include: cystoid macular edema, intraretinal hemorrhage, and rarely, vitreous hemorrhage

    h) the natural course of choroidal new vessels appears to be continued fibrovascular/fibrocellular ingrowth with resultant disciform scarring

    i) disciform scars greater than 0.2 mm in thickness are associated with diffuse loss of surface photoreceptors

C. Diagnosis

  1. Amsler grid testing

    a. in a study of age-related macular degeneration, of patients given an Amsler grid:

      1) only 50% of the patients reported actually using this diagnostic tool

      2) 10% of patients with choroidal neovascularization noted their first symptom while using the Amsler grid

      3) 80% of patients using Amsler grid testing who developed choroidal neovascularization noted a change on the Amsler grid but not the first symptom

  2. Ophthalmoscopy

    a. 20 diopter lens examination or direct ophthalmoscopy may be diagnostic in severe cases. In patients at risk one must examine with 90 or 78 diopter lens. Macular edema or small areas of elevation may only be detected on fundus contact lens examination.

  3. Refraction

    a. when pigment epithelial or neurosensory retinal detachments are present, often patients become more hyperopic

  4. Stereo fundus photography

    a. important tool to follow suspicious lesions. Both eyes should be photographed; 30 degree photos are preferable.

  5. Fluorescein angiography

    a. the gold standard in defining pathologic changes present in age-related macular degeneration. Safe and effective; national survey of 2,430 ophthalmologists using over 221,000 fluorescein angiograms, there was one reported death. Severe reactions included anaphylaxis and hypotension, and were present in only one out of 2,000. Moderate to mild symptoms including nausea, vomiting, and syncope were present in less than 5% of the cases.

b. there is no strong evidence for fetal toxicity; however, it may not be safe for use in pregnant females
c. sodium fluorescein is not cross-reactive in patients with iodine allergy.
d. procedure
　1) recommended use for diagnosis and followup of treatment.
　2) transit eye of most concern but 30 degree views of both maculae should be obtained
　3) in patients with history of minor or moderate reaction, consider pretreatment with 50 mg oral prednisone and 50 mg oral Benadryl the morning of examination
　4) if history of severe reaction, consider anesthesia standby
　5) patient should be informed of rare but potential risks of the fluorescein angiography and should be warned that the fluorescein dye itself may discolor urine for a few hours
6. Indocyanine green (ICG)
　a. experimental
　b. FDA approved with extensive use and history in cardiology
　c. absorptive in fluorescence spectrum, near infrared allowing penetration of ocular pigment and hemorrhage
　d. theoretic enhanced viewing through pigmentation or subretinal hemorrhage
　e. enhanced imaging of choroidal vasculature
　f. ICG angiography may demonstrate abnormalities that are not evident on fluorescein angiography
D. Differential Diagnosis:
　1. Masquerades of age-related macular degeneration: important to recognize as laser photocoagulation is not indicated for these conditions
　　a. basal laminar drusen (cuticular drusen)
　　　1) often present in middle age with pseudovitelliform detachments
　　　2) fluorescein angiography demonstrates early hypofluorescence with progressive staining
　　　3) natural course is spontaneous clearing or slow atrophy
　　　4) normal EOG differentiating from Best's disease

      b. pattern dystrophy (adult vitelliform dystrophy, adult onset foveal pigment epithelial dystrophy, butterfly-shaped pigment dystrophy, reticular dystrophy)

        1) reticular pattern of pigmentation, often symmetric

        2) yellow deposits present in the outer retina

        3) petalloid pattern of hyperpigmentation

      c. central serous chorioretinopathy

        1) only occasionally occurs in patients greater than 65 years of age

        2) multifocal areas of mottled RPE atrophy

        3) absence of drusen

        4) uniform collection of fluid in a sensory retinal space without speckled hyperfluorescence as seen in poorly demarcated areas of leakage in AMD

  2. Conditions associated with choroidal neovascularization other than AMD

      a. myopia

      b. angioid streaks

      c. ocular histoplasmosis

      d. choroidal rupture

      e. Candida endophthalmitis

      f. photocoagulation

      g. idiopathic

      h. optic nerve head drusen

  3. Other conditions associated with subretinal blood, lipid, or fluid other than AMD

      a. microaneurysm

      b. lacquer cracks in pathologic myopia

      c. traumatic choroidal rupture

      d. posterior vitreous detachment

      e. choroidal tumor

      f. central serous chorioretinopathy

      g. inflammatory conditions (i.e., Harada's disease or posterior scleritis)

E. Treatment:

  1. Nonneovascular/atrophic AMD

      a. currently no effective treatment to prevent or halt the progression of age-related macular degeneration

      b. areas of active research:

        1) nutritional (antioxidants)

          a) rationale

            i. light theory suggests that light may lead to activated form of oxygen (free radicals) which cause retinal damage. Theorized role of antioxidants in preventing such damage (vitamin C, vitamin E, glutathione, beta carotene, and selenium)

b) evidence:

   i. analysis of data from the first National Health and Nutrition Examination Surveys (NHANES) found diets with vegetable-rich vitamin A to be protective against age-related macular degeneration

   ii. animals fed vitamin E-deficient diets demonstrate enhanced susceptibility to retinal damage

   iii. vitamin E is a potent antioxidant found in high concentrations in the retina

   iv. Eye Disease Case Control Study found that subjects with high levels of combined vitamin E, selenium, and carotenoid had statistically significant reduced risks of CNV

2) nutrition (zinc)

   a) rationale

      i. high concentration in ocular tissues; zinc has a role in metabolism of proteins and nucleic acids; serves as a cofactor for enzymes such as retinol dehydrogenase and catalase

   b) evidence

      i. a small prospective, randomized, double-masked, controlled trial (N = 151 with AMD) found that 100 mg of zinc by mouth, twice a day, decreased the risk of visual loss of ten letters on the ETDRS chart at 24 months, from 34% to 14%. However, this was a pilot study and has shown diminishing effects with time. Zinc has possible serious side effects, including anemia and worsening of cardiovascular disease. At this time we cannot recommend use of zinc or antioxidants until further larger clinical trials are completed (age-related eye disease study [AREDS])

   2. Low vision rehabilitation

      a. low vision definition: moderate—visual acuity 20/70 to 20/160; severe—20/200 to 20/400; profound—20/500 to 20/1000, near blindness to no light perception

      b. the United States government considers "legal blindness" to be any patient with visual acuity less than 20/200 or field of vision of less than 20 degrees. At these levels patients are eligible for services and benefits, especially tax benefits.

      c. frequent problem with over 3,000,000 patients affected

      d. assessment can be in the ophthalmologist's office or in specialized low vision centers

      e. assessment of the low vision patient should include:

         1) history, including evaluation of patient's goals, motivation, and assessment of general health

         2) specific tasks to consider include reading, television viewing, cooking, taking medicines, ambulation, and recognizing faces

         3) vision and reading assessment should be done under various lighting conditions. Refraction is an often neglected aspect of the low vision assessment and should be done in all patients. Note: use 0.5 and 1.0 diopter, cross cylinders.

         4) rehabilitation planning, taking into consideration motivation, health, and visual status

      f. visual aids; magnifiers, telescopes, videomagnifiers, computer assisted devices, spectacles, proper illumination, large print books

      g. modifying the patient's environment; modifying patient's home, talking books

      h. ambulatory devices, including canes, seeing eye dogs, and telescopes

   3. Neovascular AMD (CNV and PED)

      a. laser photocoagulation under certain conditions does decrease the risk of visual loss. Details of the treatment parameters are given in chapter 15.

      b. rationale for treatment:

1) results of macular photocoagulation studies (MPS):

   a) extrafoveal choroidal neovascularization (classic CNV, plus contiguous blocked fluorescence with posterior border 200 to 250 microns from the fovea)

      i. three-year relative risk of severe visual loss (greater than six lines of visual loss on Bailey-Love chart) no treatment/treatment = 1.4 (i.e., there is a 40% greater risk of severe visual loss in untreated eyes, compared with treated eyes)

      ii. outcome at five years: treated eyes, 48% with six lines or more loss with mean visual acuity of 20/152 (quadrupling of the visual angle); untreated eyes, 62% with six lines or more loss with mean acuity of 20/200

      iii. recurrence rate: 54% at five years

   b) juxtafoveal choroidal neovascularization (posterior border of choroidal neovascularization 1 to 199 microns from the foveal center or if its posterior border is greater than 199 microns, then contiguous blood or blocked fluorescence on the foveal side from 1 to 199 microns from the center of the fovea

      i. outcome at four years: treated eyes: 49% have six or more lines of visual loss, mean visual acuity 20/200; untreated eyes: 58% have six or more lines of visual acuity loss, mean visual acuity 20/250

      ii. recurrence rate: 76% at four years

   c) subfoveal CNV: presence of classic CNV under the foveal center with well-demarcated boundaries and size less than or equal to 3.5 disc areas

      i. outcome at three months: treated eyes—20% lost six or more lines; untreated eyes—11% lost six or more lines

      ii. outcome at 24 months: treated eyes—20% lost six or more lines; untreated eyes—37% lost six or more lines

        iii. persistence or recurrence in 51% of laser treated eyes by 24 months, but was not associated with visual acuity loss

    d) subfoveal recurrence

        i. recurrence of CNV after laser treatment that now involves the foveal center

        ii. boundaries of old treatment and necessary new treatment cannot exceed six disc areas

        iii. at 24 months: treated eyes—average acuity 20/250 with 9% of eyes losing six or more lines

c. surgical removal of choroidal neovascularization rationale:

    1) poor natural history and limited efficacy of laser photocoagulation for subfoveal CNV

    2) many lesions do not meet MPS criteria

    3) frequent recurrences and persistences following laser treatment

    4) laser treatment destroys photoreceptors and RPE

d. procedure:

    1) pars plana vitrectomy with removal of vitreous

    2) retinotomy site is selected usually temporal to fovea

    3) subretinal space is filled with balanced salt solution, creating a localized neurosensory retinal detachment

    4) angle subretinal forceps introduced through retinotomy to grasp and extract neovascular complex

    5) fluid gas exchange and photocoagulation to retinotomy site

e. complications:

    1) loss of RPE

    2) rhegmatogenous retinal detachment

    3) foveal avulsion

    4) retinal tears

    5) submacular hemorrhage

    6) macular pucker

    7) recurrence—33%

f. results:

    1) lesion can be removed but visual results often limited in AMD

    2) review of 52 eyes with AMD and CNV:

a) 2% with visual acuity greater than 20/100; 7% with visual acuity of 20/100; 71% with visual acuity 20/200 to 20/800; 20% with visual acuity less than or equal to count fingers

XIII. CENTRAL SEROUS RETINOPATHY

A. Epidemiology
   1. Males 85%
   2. Age 20 to 50 years, mean 45 years
   3. Possibly more common in patients with type A personality and in patients under stress
B. Clinical Features
   1. Unilateral 70%
   2. Presenting symptoms: decreased vision (20/20 to 20/200, mean 20/30), metamorphopsia, micropsia, dyschromatopsia, central scotoma; occasionally preceded or accompanied by migraine-like headaches
   3. Biomicroscopic findings: normal
   4. Ophthalmoscopic findings: serous macular detachment; may have underlying retinal pigment epithelial detachment (usually < 1/4 dd in size, best seen with retroillumination, beneath superior half of sensory retinal detachment, no underlying choroidal pattern visible, may have pigment clumping on surface); may have grayish deposit at leakage site
   5. Clinical course: heals spontaneously in 4 to 8 weeks; full recovery of vision in 90%; many patients have persistent decreased contrast sensitivity; in some patients the disease does not heal rapidly and becomes chronic (may have yellow deposits on posterior surface of elevated sensory retina, presumably macrophages; may have pigment alteration and/or RPE tract with dependent inferior peripheral serous retinal detachment); 30 to 50% of patients have recurrence; 10% have greater than three recurrences; few develop choroidal neovascular membrane
C. Pathogenesis
   1. Fluid from choriocapillaris reaches subretinal space through a small defect in the retinal pigment epithelium; circulating catecholamines may play a role
D. Diagnosis
   1. FA: one or several leakage points which represent focal RPE defects; most leak within 1 mm

of fovea; 10% leak within the fovea; dye spreads symmetrically to all sides of subretinal blister, spreads slowly and does not extend beyond border; 20% have smoke-stack phenomenon where the dye first ascends superiorly from the leakage site and then spreads laterally to fill the subretinal blister; fellow eye often has evidence of prior disease (window defect); FA may not show a leakage point (leak is outside the macula, usually superiorly; the leak has healed and retinal detachment will resolve); RPE detachment may show blocked fluorescence from pigment on its surface (cruciate or triradiate pattern); in recurrent cases 62% of leakage points occur within 0.5 mm of initial site and 80% occur within 1 mm

E. Treatment
   1. Xenon photocoagulation: treatment of the leakage site may hasten resolution and decrease recurrence; no benefit to final visual acuity
   2. Argon photocoagulation: treatment of the leakage site hastens resolution; no benefit to final visual acuity
   3. Krypton photocoagulation: treatment of the leakage site may decrease recurrence; no benefit to final visual acuity
   4. All forms of treatment have associated complications including the development of choroidal neovascularization

XIV. MACULAR HOLE

A. Epidemiology
   1. Females 70%
   2. Age 50 to 60 years

B. Clinical Features
   1. Unilateral 90%
   2. Presenting symptoms: metamorphopsia, decreased vision (20/100 to 20/400 for full thickness holes), central scotoma
   3. Biomicroscopic features: normal
   4. Ophthalmoscopic features: stages of macular hole:
      a. stage 1A—foveolar detachment: small round yellow spot (250 to 300 m) at foveola
      b. stage 1B—foveal detachment: small round yellow ring at fovea; may have reddish center and radiating striae; yellow hue may be due to greater visibility of xanthophyll; FA

shows faint hyperfluorescence or no abnormality

    c. stage 2—Early Hole: may be eccentric or central: a very small hole that develops at the edge or the center and may enlarge in a can opener fashion; operculum may be attached to the edge

    d. stage 3—Hole: with or without operculum; operculum is suspended on the surface of the posterior hyaloid immediately in front of the hole (if stage 2 Hole was central instead of eccentric, no operculum will be present)

    e. stage 4—Hole: with posterior vitreous detachment; complete posterior vitreous detachment; operculum, if present, is adherent to mobile posterior hyaloid

        1) stages 2, 3, and 4 represent full thickness holes; the retinal pigment epithelium at the base of the hole is intact and usually appears normal initially; with time it may become hyperplastic or atrophic; cystic degeneration at the border of the hole may be present; epiretinal membrane formation surrounding the hole is present in 10 to 20%; cuff of subretinal fluid may encircle the hole creating limited sensory retinal detachment; yellow deposits at the base of the hole represent lipid laden macrophages; size of hole usually 500 m

C. Pathogenesis

    1. Forces exerted by the cortical vitreous on central macula produce anteroposterior and/or tangential traction; macular hole will not develop in an eye with a posterior vitreous detachment

D. Diagnosis

    1. Patient notes a discontinuity in the slit beam as the beam is narrowed and passes over the hole

    2. FA: granular hyperfluorescent window defect at the fovea; surrounding retinal elevation may cause partial blockage of choroidal fluorescence

E. Treatment

    1. Vitrectomy with removal of posterior cortical vitreous and epiretinal membrane stripping followed by intraocular gas injection has recently been shown to result in closure of the hole and improvement in visual acuity; further studies are currently in progress

2. Pseudoholes—lesions that mimic retinal excavation without actual tissue loss: most are seen in association with epiretinal membrane formation with a dehiscence of a portion of the gliotic membrane overlying the macula producing a lesion with a sharp border; FA shows no abnormal fluorescence except for traction induced retinal vascular leakage

3. Macular cysts—an intact inner and outer retinal layer with fluid present intraretinally: cystic spaces in the macula develop from degeneration of Müller cells and eventually progress to liquefactive necrosis of these cells and neuronal degeneration; the smaller cystic spaces collapse and create a large confluent cyst; FA shows late pooling in the cystoid spaces

4. Partial thickness holes
   a. outer lamellar hole: the outer wall of a large macular cyst collapses; may occur after trauma
   b. inner lamellar hole: excavation of the inner layers of the retina but with recognizable retinal tissue at its base

XV. ANGIOID STREAKS

A. Epidemiology

1. 85% of patients with pseudoxanthoma elasticum develop angioid streaks; pseudoxanthoma elasticum is a connective tissue disorder characterized by changes in the skin, cardiovascular system, and eyes; skin changes include hyperelasticity—particularly of the neck, axilla, inguinal, and antecubital areas; cardiovascular changes include hypertension, claudication, premature coronary atherosclerosis, mitral valve prolapse, gastrointestinal and intracranial hemorrhages; inheritance is autosomal recessive; however, some pedigrees are autosomal dominant; the condition is more common in females

2. 10 to 15% of patients with osteitis deformans (Paget's disease of bone) develop angioid streaks; osteitis deformans is a connective tissue disease characterized by bony pain in association with increased alkaline phosphatase and increased urine hydroxyproline; bony x-rays show both lytic and sclerotic areas due to

an increased number of both osteoblasts and osteoclasts; inheritance is autosomal dominant

    3. 6% of patients with sickle cell disease develop angioid streaks

    4. other conditions include familial hyperphosphatemia, metastatic calcification, and possibly Ehlers-Danlos syndrome

B. Clinical Features

    1. Visual acuity normal unless choroidal neovascularization develops

    2. Biomicroscopic findings: normal

    3. Ophthalmoscopic findings: dark reddish lines with a crack-like appearance surround the optic disc and extend radially; these lines are deep, at the level of Bruch's membrane; in patients with pseudoxanthoma elasticum, a speckled appearance to the temporal macula is usually present, termed peau d'orange

    4. Clinical course: choroidal neovascularization develops in association with angioid streaks, presenting with acute visual loss in the presence of subretinal hemorrhage, fluid, or lipid; ultimately, disciform degeneration and hypertrophic scars develop; in patients with angioid streaks, choroidal rupture may develop after relatively minor eye trauma

C. Pathogenesis

    1. Angioid streaks represent visible cracks in Bruch's membrane; Bruch's membrane has five layers, the middle layer being elastic; in these conditions, there are abnormal elastic fibers with secondary calcification, rendering Bruch's membrane brittle and prone to fragmentation

D. Diagnosis

    1. FA: streaks appear hyperfluorescent due to atrophic pigment epithelium at the site of the streaks; FA may show streaks not readily apparent on ophthalmoscopy; if choroidal neovascularization is present, late leakage will be seen

    2. The workup includes skin biopsy, skull x-rays, alkaline phosphatase, calcium, phosphorus, and hemoglobin electrophoresis

    3. The diagnosis can be established in 50% of patients with angioid streaks; 34% pseudoxanthoma elasticum, 10% Paget's disease, 6% sickle cell disease

E. Treatment

1. Laser photocoagulation may be beneficial in treating choroidal neovascularization

XVI. OCULAR HISTOPLASMOSIS SYNDROME

A. Epidemiology
  1. Occurs in endemic areas (Ohio River Valley)
  2. Onset middle age; mean age 43 years
  3. No gender predilection
B. Clinical Features
  1. Bilateral 60%
  2. Presenting symptoms: asymptomatic; if choroidal neovascularization present, metamorphopsia and central scotoma
  3. Biomicroscopic findings: normal, clear vitreous
  4. Ophthalmoscopic findings: peripapillary atrophy; peripheral "histo spots" are characterized by focal healed punched-out chorioretinal scars; may have histo spots in the macula; maculopathy consists of choroidal neovascularization with serous retinal detachment, usually with subretinal hemorrhage and/or lipid
  5. Clinical course: if bilateral macular histo spots and no disciform scar, less than 5% chance of developing choroidal neovascularization in either eye over five years; if bilateral macular histo spots and disciform scar in one eye, 20% chance of developing choroidal neovascularization in the fellow eye in three years; in patients with choroidal neovascularization, 10% of patients develop choroidal neovascularization in fellow eye: after successful treatment of choroidal neovascularization, 30% of patients develop recurrent choroidal neovascularization
C. Pathogenesis
  1. 90% of patients have skin test positivity to histoplasma antigen (versus 50 to 60% of normals)
D. Diagnosis
  1. FA: shows typical features of choroidal neovascularization: early lacy hyperfluorescence with late leakage
E. Treatment
  1. Argon laser photocoagulation is beneficial for extrafoveal (greater than 200 microns from foveal avascular zone) choroidal neovascular membrane; severe visual loss (greater than six

lines) is reduced from 31% to 11% at 1 year and from 45% to 10% at 3 years
   2. Krypton laser photocoagulation is beneficial for juxtafoveal (1 to 199 microns from foveal avascular zone) choroidal neovascular membranes; severe visual loss reduced from 25% to 7% at 1 year and from 26% to 6% at 3 years

XVII. HIGH MYOPIA

   A. Epidemiology
      1. Generally defined as greater than −6 diopters refractive error or greater than 26 mm axial length
      2. Approximately 2% of U.S. population
   B. Clinical Features
      1. Biomicroscopic features: deep anterior chamber
      2. Ophthalmoscopic findings: disc may appear oval with the long axis oriented vertically; if tilted, nasal edge may be raised (supertraction) and temporal side surrounded by concentric area of depigmentation (myopic conus or temporal crescent); temporal crescent is secondary to absent RPE and choroid at the temporal edge (some are white due to visible sclera and some are pigmented due to visible choroid); 10% of crescents surround entire disc; in some cases it may extend to the macula; posterior staphyloma (ectasia involving sclera, choroid, and RPE) may be present and sometimes involves the macula; thinning of RPE and choroid may result in better visibility of larger choroidal vessels; focal areas of atrophy may exist, sometimes with pigment clumping within these areas; peripheral retinal lattice degeneration is present in up to 20% of high myopes
      3. Clinical course: ruptures of Bruch's membrane (lacquer cracks) may develop in the macula and appear as linear or stellate, fine, horizontally oriented lines with pigmented edges; lacquer cracks are present in 4% of high myopes and reduce vision (20/50 to 20/100); lacquer cracks can be associated with macular hemorrhage in the absence of choroidal neovascularization; these hemorrhages are focal, round, deep, and often centered on the fovea; may be associated with sudden decrease in visual acuity which may improve when the hemorrhage

resolves; a dark or black spot (Fuchs' spot) develops in the macula in 5% of high myopes and is associated with visual loss; neovascularization extending from the choroid into the subpigment epithelial space is associated with Fuchs' spot; the subepithelial hemorrhage organizes and combines with proliferating RPE, resulting in a dark spot; choroidal neovascularization develops in 5 to 10% of high myopes and is associated with sudden visual loss; choroidal neovascularization often develops at the site of a lacquer crack; greater than 50% involve the fovea initially; in some patients there is visual improvement after the acute process and a Fuchs' spot is seen as the only sequelae; in others severe visual loss remains; high myopia is a major risk factor for rhegmatogenous retinal detachment, as 35% of nontraumatic retinal detachments occur in high myopes

C. Pathogenesis

    1. Biomechanical theory: the chorioretinal lesions are a consequence of excessive axial elongation; progressive distension of the posterior pole stretches the ocular coats and results in thinning of the sclera, choroid, RPE, and retina as well as temporal crescent

    2. Heredodegenerative theory: the chorioretinal changes are genetically determined

    3. Histopathology: the sclera is thinned with thinning of the collagen bundles; the choroid is thin with a lack of vessels in some areas and a pronounced thinning of the choriocapillaris, the RPE cells appear flatter and larger than usual, Bruch's membrane undergoes thinning, splitting, and rupturing

D. Diagnosis

    1. FA: may help detect lacquer cracks not visible by ophthalmoscopy and appear hyperfluorescent with late fading; the pigment in a Fuchs' spot will block fluorescence; choroidal neovascularization will exhibit late leakage

E. Treatment

    1. Krypton laser photocoagulation of choroidal neovascular membranes has been attempted: the membranes were located 100 to 1,000 microns from the center of the fovea; however, in some patients the fovea is difficult to locate; after two years follow-up, 40% of treated eyes versus 13% of untreated eyes improved two

lines of visual acuity; 40% of treated eyes versus 77% of untreated eyes lost two lines of visual acuity; after five years there was no statistically significant difference in the outcome; late visual loss occurred because of recurrence of choroidal neovascularization in 31% and expansion of the laser scar in 92%

XVIII. STARGARDT'S DISEASE/FUNDUS FLAVIMACULATUS

A. Classification
  1. Stargardt's disease: the macular lesion is prominent and decreased vision occurs at an early age
  2. Fundus flavimaculatus: flecks are prominent and macular involvement occurs late or not at all
  3. Also called juvenile macular degeneration
B. Epidemiology
  1. Onset first to second decade
  2. Autosomal recessive inheritance; some autosomal dominant pedigrees exist
C. Clinical Features
  1. Bilateral, usually symmetric
  2. Presenting symptoms: reduced visual acuity (20/25 to 20/200); early in the disease, reduced vision is out of proportion to ophthalmoscopic findings (markedly reduced vision, minimal findings)
  3. Biomicroscopic findings: normal
  4. Ophthalmoscopic findings: loss of foveal reflex, granular appearance, beaten bronze appearance of fovea; some patients have bullseye maculopathy; yellow flecks at level of RPE may surround macular lesion and extend to periphery; flecks are variable in size, shape, and distribution and may have a fishtail configuration (pisciform); advanced disease may have midperipheral pigmentary changes
  5. Clinical course: rapid progression in first or second decade (usually to 20/200); severe RPE atrophy and/or macular choroidal neovascular membrane may occur
D. Pathology
  1. Excessive lipofuscin within the RPE (prevents visualization of choroidal details on fluorescein angiography); variably shaped RPE cells,

enlarged RPE cells, apical concentration of melanin, basal concentration of PAS-positive material (lipofuscin), subretinal melanolipofuscin concentration (reticular change)

E. Diagnosis
   1. FA: central hyperfluorescence, pericentral window defects, dark choroid; flecks appear either nonfluorescent or show an irregular pattern of fluorescence
   2. ERG: normal; abnormal if extensive peripheral involvement (about 20%); delayed rod dark adaptometry
   3. EOG: normal; abnormal if extensive peripheral involvement (about 20%)
   4. Differential: Best's disease, cone degeneration, x-linked juvenile retinoschisis

F. Treatment
   1. None

XIX. BEST'S VITELLIFORM MACULAR DYSTROPHY

A. Epidemiology
   1. Age of onset usually childhood
   2. Autosomal dominant inheritance

B. Clinical Features
   1. Bilateral and symmetric
   2. Visual acuity mildly reduced (20/30 to 20/50) initially; may decline to 20/200
   3. Biomicroscopic findings: normal
   4. Ophthalmoscopic findings: there is a characteristic evolution of the macular findings; previtelliform = normal fundus; vitelliform = round yellow material at level of RPE, resembles egg yolk, 1 to 5 disc diameters in size; pseudohypopyon = yellow lesion breaks up and settles to resemble a hypopyon, material is in subretinal space; scrambled egg = multiple irregularly shaped yellow deposits in subretinal space; atrophic = reabsorption of yellow material, leaving an oval area of RPE atrophy
   5. Clinical course: vision may occasionally decline markedly due to atrophy and/or choroidal neovascular membrane

C. Pathology
   1. Retinal pigment epithelium and photoreceptor atrophy in central macula

D. Diagnosis

1. FA: blocked fluorescence by yellow material; window defect at area of RPE atrophy; leakage if choroidal neovascular membrane present
2. ERG: normal
3. EOG: markedly decreased (< 1.55) in both clinically affected patients and carriers

E. Treatment
   1. No treatment for macular lesion unassociated with choroidal neovascular membrane; observe closely for signs of choroidal neovascularization

XX. ADULT ONSET FOVEOMACULAR PIGMENT EPITHELIAL DYSTROPHY

Also called foveomacular vitelliform dystrophy, adult type

The most common pattern dystrophy

A. Epidemiology
   1. Onset 30 to 50 years old
   2. Probable autosomal dominant inheritance

B. Clinical Features
   1. Bilateral; may be asymmetric
   2. Presenting symptoms: visually asymptomatic or mild blurring and metamorphopsia in one or both eyes
   3. Biomicroscopic findings: normal
   4. Ophthalmoscopic findings: round to oval, slightly elevated, yellow subretinal lesion often with central pigmentation, 1/3 disc diameter to 1 disc diameter in size, usually symmetric; may have small yellow flecks in paracentral region
   5. Clinical course: visual acuity may deteriorate because of atrophy or choroidal neovascular membrane

C. Pathology
   1. Central foveal pigmentation corresponds histologically to a hyperplastic clump of RPE; the pale yellow rim surrounding the central pigmentation corresponds to dense PAS-positive material underlying thinned atrophic RPE; thickened Bruch's membrane and choriocapillaris; photoreceptor damage overlying the atrophic RPE

D. Diagnosis
   1. FA: nonfluorescent lesion or central blocked fluorescence with a surrounding hyperfluorescent ring; the paracentral small yellow lesions may

be nonfluorescent, show discrete staining, or
have a halo of fluorescence surrounding them
2. EOG: normal to slightly subnormal
3. ERG: normal
4. Differential: age-related macular degeneration,
Best's disease (earlier onset, larger lesion, disruption of lesion with layering of yellow pigment), other pattern dystrophies (butterfly-
shaped pattern dystrophy)
E. Treatment
1. No treatment for macular lesion unassociated
with choroidal neovascular membrane; observe
closely for signs of choroidal neovascularization

XXI. CONE DYSTROPHY

A. Epidemiology
1. Onset first to second decade
2. Usually autosomal dominant inheritance
B. Clinical Features
1. Visual acuity on presentation 20/40 to 20/60;
acuity typically declines to 20/200
2. Presenting symptoms: decreased vision, decreased color vision, photophobia
3. Biomicroscopic findings: normal
4. Ophthalmoscopic findings: visual loss typically precedes macular changes as detected by
ophthalmoscopy: bullseye macular appearance
eventually develops, consisting of a sharply
defined ring of atrophic retinal pigment epithelium surrounding a central homogenous
darker zone
5. Clinical course: disc may become pale and
vessels attenuated; bone spicule pigmentation
may develop; some cases begin as purely cone
dysfunction but develop cone-rod dysfunction
C. Pathogenesis
1. Histopathology: absent outer nuclear layer of
rods and cones and pronounced pigment
changes of the retinal pigment epithelium
D. Diagnosis
1. FA: useful in early stage as ophthalmoscopy
may be normal; FA may show faint central hyperfluorescence; in more advanced cases, a
horizontal ovoid zone of hyperfluorescence
surrounds a nonfluorescent center
2. VF: central or paracentral scotoma

        3. Color vision: in early cone degeneration red-green deficiency predominates; in advanced disease, both red-green and blue-yellow deficiencies are severe

        4. ERG: absent photopic ERG; scotopic ERG normal but may become subnormal with progression

    E. Treatment

        1. None

    F. Related Conditions

        1. Autosomal Recessive Cone Dystrophy: rare; color vision entirely lacking (complete monochromatism) or severely limited (incomplete monochromatism); decreased vision, photophobia, and nystagmus are present

        2. X-linked Blue Cone Monochromatism: decreased vision, photophobia, nystagmus, and myopia are present

XXII. X-LINKED JUVENILE RETINOSCHISIS

    A. Epidemiology

        1. Males (female carriers cannot be identified)

        2. X-linked recessive inheritance

    B. Clinical Features

        1. Onset early childhood, possibly at birth (congenital)

        2. Vision 20/100 to 20/400

        3. Biomicroscopic findings: normal

        4. Ophthalmoscopic findings: foveal radiating retinal folds; 50% also have peripheral retinoschisis, usually inferotemporally; may have dendritiform occluded vessels and vitreous veils

        5. Clinical course: progressive; pigment retinopathy and/or macular atrophy may develop; retinal detachment occurs in 5 to 20%; holes may develop in inner lamina (75%) or outer lamina (13%)

    C. Pathology

        1. Separation between the nerve fiber layer and ganglion cell layer; inner layer may or may not contain blood vessels

    D. Diagnosis

        1. FA: in cases with macular atrophy, there is late central hyperfluorescence; in cases with peripheral neovascularization there is late leakage

        2. ERG: reduced b-wave; normal a-wave

3. EOG: normal
4. VF: central and peripheral scotomata
E. Treatment
1. scleral buckling surgery if retinal detachment develops

XXIII. NORTH CAROLINA MACULAR DYSTROPHY/CENTRAL AREOLAR PIGMENT EPITHELIAL DYSTROPHY

Originally described as separate diseases, these are currently thought to represent the same genetic defect since the two original pedigrees were found to be related

A. Epidemiology
1. Autosomal dominant inheritance
2. Onset in infancy; peak visual loss in teenage years
B. Clinical Features
1. Bilateral, usually symmetric
2. Presenting symptoms: gradual reduction in visual acuity (20/20 to 20/200, median = 20/50)
3. Biomicroscopic features: normal
4. Ophthalmoscopic features: macular drusen; may increase in number and become confluent; normal disc, vessels, and periphery
5. Clinical course: some patients develop atrophy of the choroid, retinal pigment epithelium, and retina with resultant visual loss; some develop choroidal neovascularization with disciform scarring
C. Pathology
1. Unknown
D. Diagnosis
1. ERG: normal
2. EOG: normal
E. Treatment
1. None

XXIV. BASAL LAMINAR DRUSEN

A. Epidemiology
1. Onset early adulthood and midlife (average age 40s)
2. More common in females than in males
3. African-Americans > white

    4. (Basal laminar drusen with pseudovitelliform detachment more common in whites; average age 60s)

B. Clinical Features

    1. Bilateral; often symmetric

    2. Often asymptomatic (basal laminar drusen with pseudovitelliform detachment visual acuity 20/30 to 20/50)

    3. Biomicroscopic findings: normal

    4. Ophthalmoscopic findings: numerous subretinal nodules (drusen) that are small (25 to 75μ), uniformly sized, discreet, round, yellow and sometimes arranged in clusters; some patients develop yellow exudative macular detachment (pseudovitelliform detachment) measuring 0.5 to 1.5 disc diameters); this yellow material may layer within the detachment

    5. Clinical course: 40% develop pseudovitelliform detachment; most of the pseudovitelliform detachments resolve spontaneously; some develop geographic atrophy or choroidal neovascularization

C. Pathology

    1. Retinal pigment epithelial basement membrane (the innermost part of Bruch's membrane) is diffusely thickened with nodularity; the remainder of Bruch's membrane is normal; the drusen are focal areas of pigment epithelial attenuation overlying the nodular thickenings of the basement membrane of the RPE

D. Diagnosis

    1. FA: numerous window defects (even more than the drusen seen by ophthalmoscopy) which give the angiogram a "stars in the sky" or "milky way" appearance; these fluoresce earlier than typical drusen; if pseudovitelliform detachment is present, the yellow subretinal fluid within the exudative detachment blocks early and stains late

    2. ERG: normal

    3. EOG: normal

    4. Differential: age-related macular degeneration (basal laminar drusen, occurs in younger patients, and the drusen are more numerous, smaller, and uniformly sized); Best's disease (basal laminar drusen, normal EOG and the yellow subretinal material stains on angiography); adult onset foveomacular pigment epithelial dystrophy (basal laminar drusen, occurs in younger patients)

   E. Treatment
      1. Photocoagulation is indicated if choroidal neovascularization develops

XXV. BIETTI'S CRYSTALLINE DYSTROPHY

A. Epidemiology
    1. Probable autosomal recessive inheritance
    2. Becomes clinically evident in third decade

B. Clinical Features
    1. Presenting signs/symptoms: nyctalopia and decreased vision
    2. Biomicroscopic findings: very fine corneal crystals in paralimbal anterior stroma, also present in conjunctiva
    3. Ophthalmoscopic findings: yellow-white crystals in all layers of perimacular and peripapillary retina; macula may have irregular pigmentation; RPE and choriocapillaris atrophy; bone spicule pigment in periphery; normal disc and vessels
    4. Clinical course: slowly progressive loss of visual acuity, visual fields, and color vision

C. Pathology
    1. Crystals and lipid inclusions within corneal and conjunctival fibroblasts and, less frequently, in the extracellular space; circulating lymphocytes contain similar crystals and lipid inclusions; retinal histopathology unknown; most likely a systemic metabolic abnormality

D. Diagnosis
    1. FA: discrete areas of hypofluorescence in which medium sized choroidal vessels are apparent, suggesting atrophy or depigmentation of RPE and choriocapillaris atrophy; adjacent areas hyperfluoresce, probably representing RPE atrophy with relatively intact choriocapillaris
    2. ERG: variable (normal to subnormal)

E. Treatment
    1. None

XXVI. OXALOSIS

Multiple diseases which result in accumulation of calcium oxalate crystals in the retina

A. Epidemiology

1. Depends on specific cause
2. Primary oxalosis: hereditary hyperoxaluria
3. Secondary oxalosis: dietary excess; methoxy-fluorane anesthesia; ethylene glycol toxicity, xylitol toxicity; ascorbic acid treatment in chronic renal failure; pyridoxine deficiency; fat malabsorption

B. Clinical Features
  1. Ophthalmoscopic findings: refractile crystals in inner retina along distribution of arteries

C. Pathology
  1. Disease occurs when dietary intake (absorbed by colon) and endogenous production (end product of amino acid and ascorbic acid metabolism) exceeds renal excretion

D. Diagnosis
  1. Differential: cystinosis, tamoxifen, canthaxanthine, Bietti's

E. Treatment
  1. Depends on specific cause

XXVII. RETINITIS PIGMENTOSA AND RELATED DISEASES

A. Syndromes Associated with Retinitis Pigmentosa:
  1. Bassen-Kornzweig syndrome: hereditary abetalipoproteinemia; autosomal recessive disease characterized by absent apolipoprotein B; fat malabsorption, diffuse neuromuscular disease with ataxia, acanthocytosis, and decreased serum cholesterol and triglycerides; ERG can be reversed in early stages with supplemental vitamin A but not in advanced stages
  2. Refsum's disease: accumulation of exogenous phytanic acid; characterized by a peripheral neuropathy, ataxia, increased cerebrospinal fluid protein; some patients have anosmia, hearing deficit, EKG abnormalities, and skin changes resembling ichthyosis; treatment consists of restricting animal fats and milk products (foods that contain phytanic acid), and green leafy vegetables containing phytol
  3. Usher's syndrome, Types I and II: 15 to 20% of patients with retinitis pigmentosa have associated hearing loss, referred to as Usher's syndrome; type I patients have profound congenital deafness, unintelligible speech, vestibular

ataxia; type II patients have partial hearing loss, intelligible speech, and no ataxia

4. Laurence-Moon-Bardet-Biedl syndrome: associated with mental retardation, polydactyly, truncal obesity, and hypogonadism; neurologic findings are found primarily in patients with the Laurence-Moon form and polydactyly is found primarily in patients with the Bardet-Biedl form; renal disease can be a part of these syndromes and patients should have blood pressure and urine checked periodically

5. Kearns-Sayre syndrome: associated with ptosis, chronic progressive external ophthalmoplegia, respiratory distress, and heart block; ERGs usually reduced; muscle biopsy shows ragged red fibers; associated with mitochondrial DNA mutation

6. Olivo pontocerebellar atrophy: associated with tremor, ataxia, and dysarthria; autosomal dominant inheritance with variable penetrance; reduced ERG

7. Hereditary cerebroretinal degeneration including Batten's disease: neuronal ceroid lipofuscinosis: Batten's disease has multiple forms—infantile form (psychomotor deterioration, ataxia, microcephaly, granular inclusions on conjunctival biopsy); late infantile form (seizures, rapid mental deterioration, curvilinear inclusions on conjunctival biopsy); juvenile form (mental deterioration, bullseye maculopathy, fingerprint inclusions on conjunctival biopsy); adult onset form (seizures, slow dementia, abnormal inclusions on muscle biopsy)

8. Cockayne's syndrome: associated with dwarfism, deafness, mental deterioration, and premature aging; extensive loss of vision by second decade of life

9. Alström's disease: associated with diabetes, obesity, deafness, renal failure, baldness, hypogenitalism; profound loss of vision in the first decade of life, and very reduced ERG

10. Leber's congenital amaurosis
    a. epidemiology
        1) autosomal recessive inheritance
        2) some patients have associated mental retardation, neurologic deficit, seizures, deafness, renal disease
    b. clinical features

       1) severe reduction in vision during infancy
       2) biomicroscopic findings: nystagmus, hyperopia, poor pupillary reflex, may have keratoconus
       3) ophthalmoscopic findings: may be normal in some cases; usual changes include granularity, white flecks, or intraretinal bone spicule pigmentation; some cases have macular coloboma and vascular attenuation
    c. diagnosis
       1) ERG: profoundly abnormal or absent ERG in infancy
    d. treatment
       1) none
  11. Choroideremia
    a. epidemiology
       1) x-linked recessive inheritance
       2) onset young adulthood
    b. clinical features
       1) bilateral and symmetric
       2) biomicroscopic findings: normal
       3) ophthalmoscopic findings: peripheral fundus shows granularity and depigmentation in the early stages; with advanced disease, extensive choroidal atrophy and clumped pigment are visible around the periphery (carrier females may have patchy depigmentation of the retinal pigment epithelium and coarse pigment granularity or pigment clumps in the periphery)
    c. pathogenesis
       1) the gene has been localized to the long arm of the X-chromosome (Xq21 band)
    d. diagnosis
       1) ERG: reduced in amplitude with delay in b-wave implicit time; in advanced stages, ERG is undetectable (carriers usually normal)
       2) VF: constriction develops and progresses gradually (carriers usually normal)
    e. treatment
       1) none
  12. Gyrate atrophy
    a. epidemiology
       1) autosomal recessive inheritance
       2) onset first decade

b. clinical features
  1) bilateral and symmetric
  2) presenting symptoms: nyctalopya, visual field constriction, myopia, and decreased vision (20/20 to light perception)
  3) biomicroscopic findings: normal
  4) ophthalmoscopic findings: chorioretinal atrophy distributed around the peripheral fundus and sometimes near optic disc; sharply defined scalloped borders separated by normal retina; these lesions increase in size and number, gradually coalescing and involving more of the posterior pole, until there is complete chorioretinal atrophy
  5) clinical course: cataracts develop; disc pallor and attenuated vessels occur late; blindness by age 40 to 55 years
c. pathogenesis
  1) clinical findings are due to a 10 to 20 fold increase in plasma ornithine; deficiency in the enzyme ornithine aminotransferase; the gene has been localized to chromosome 10
d. diagnosis
  1) ERG: nondetectable
  2) VF: constriction develops and progresses gradually
e. treatment
  1) vitamin B_6 (300 to 500 mg/day) may result in improvement (30 to 50% decline in plasma ornithine level); low protein (15 g/day) diet; low arginine diet has been shown to delay progression of the chorioretinal dystrophy
13. Retinitis punctata albescens—a rod-cone degeneration; can be associated with signs and symptoms of retinitis pigmentosa
  a. epidemiology
    1) usually autosomal recessive inheritance; rarely autosomal dominant
  b. clinical features
    1) presenting symptoms/signs: nyctalopia, gradual loss of peripheral vision, decreased color vision, decreased acuity, photophobia
    2) biomicroscopic findings: normal
    3) ophthalmoscopic findings: multiple white punctate deposits at level of RPE

in the midperipheral fundus which fan out from posterior pole in a radial pattern and usually spare the macula; retinal arteriolar attenuation; occasional bone spicule pigmentation in midperiphery; occasional mild optic atrophy

    4) clinical course: variable; usually slowly progressive

  c. diagnosis

    1) FA: in advanced stages, RPE atrophy causes window defect and increased visualization of choroidal circulation; arteriolar attenuation; white punctate deposits may have corresponding hypofluorescence (due to blockage) or hyperfluorescence (due to leakage)

    2) ERG: nonrecordable ERG in advanced stages, even after dark adaptation; in early stages, scotopic ERG more severely affected than photopic ERG

    3) VF: constricted

    4) differential: fundus albipunctatus, fundus flavimaculatus, fundus xerophthalmicus, abetalipoproteinemia

  d. treatment

    1) none

14. Congenital stationary night blindness (CSNB)

  a. five different forms:

    1) autosomal dominant CSNB

    2) autosomal recessive CSNB

    3) x-linked CSNB

    4) Oguchi's disease (autosomal recessive)

    5) fundus albipunctatus (autosomal recessive)

  b. clinical features

    1) presenting symptoms/signs: congenital nyctalopia; visual acuity normal

    2) biomicroscopic findings: normal

    3) ophthalmoscopic findings: normal fundus in autosomal dominant, autosomal recessive, and x-linked CSNB (x-linked form may have fundus findings of myopia); Oguchi's disease patients have a golden brown fundus which changes to normal color when dark-adapted (Mizuo phenomenon); fundus albipunctatus patients have yellow-white deposits in the deep retina outside the macula (no RPE degeneration, pigment deposition, vessel attenuation, or optic atrophy)

4) clinical course: these are all stationary (i.e., nonprogressive); long-term prognosis is good

c. diagnosis
  1) ERG: normal cone ERG; may have reduced or nondetectable rod ERG, however, this normalized after 1/2 to 3 hours of dark adaptation
  2) VF: normal
  3) differential: (for fundus albipunctatus) retinitis punctata albescens, fundus flavimaculatus, fundus xerophthalmicus, abetalipoproteinemia

d. treatment
  1) none

XXVIII. TOXIC RETINOPATHY

A. Phenothiazines—Retinal Toxicity
   chlorpromazine (Thorazine)
   thioridazine (Mellaril)

1. Epidemiology
   a. chlorpromazine: doses greater than 2,000 mg/day or cumulative dose of 500 g; an antipsychotic medication

2. Clinical features
   a. bilateral, usually symmetric
   b. presenting symptoms: chlorpromazine—asymptomatic; rarely causes mild visual loss; thioridazine—blurred vision, nyctalopia, reddish/ brownish discoloration of vision
   c. biomicroscopic features: chlorpromazine—skin pigmentation, interpalpebral conjunctival pigmentation, deep corneal stromal and endothelial pigmentation, granular anterior subcapsular cataracts in a stellate configuration; thioridazine—none
   d. ophthalmoscopic features: chlorpromazine—mild stipling of the pigment epithelium; thioridazine—early changes include salt-and-pepper fundus in midperiphery; later changes include coarse pigment clumping with geographic areas of atrophy and hyperpigmentation; late stages may include diffuse pigment epithelial and choriocapillaris atrophy
   e. clinical course: thioridazine—usually, visual acuity remains stable or improves

        when the drug is stopped; however, the pigmentary changes may continue to progress even after the drug is stopped; optic atrophy may develop

    3. Pathogenesis

        a. unknown; phenothiazines bind to melanin and accumulate in uveal tissue; phenothiazines alter retinal enzyme kinetics, which may result in toxic inhibition of oxidative phosphorylation and subsequent derangements in rhodopsin synthesis

    4. Diagnosis

        a. thioridazine—color vision: abnormal

        b. VF: paracentral or ring scotomas

        c. ERG: both rod and cone function affected

        d. EOG: abnormal

    5. Treatment

        a. discontinue the medication

B. Chloroquine/Hydroxychloroquine and Quinine—Retinal Toxicity

    chloroquine (Aralen)

    hydroxychloroquine (Plaquenil)

    quinine (Quinamm)

    1. Epidemiology

        a. chloroquine: doses greater than 250 mg/day or cumulative dose of 300 g; maximum daily dose more critical than total cumulative dose; initially used as an antimalarial, now used to treat rheumatoid arthritis, discoid lupus erythematosis, and systemic lupus erythematosis

        b. hydroxychloroquine: doses greater than 400 mg/day; maximum daily dose more critical than total cumulative dose; retinal toxicity identical to chloroquine but the incidence is much lower

        c. quinine: toxicity occurs at extensive doses, greater than 4 g (accidental ingestion, suicide attempts); used for malaria and nocturnal muscle cramps

    2. Clinical features

        a. bilateral, usually symmetric

        b. presenting symptoms/signs: chloroquine/hydroxychloroquine—may be asymptomatic in early stages; may progress to blurred vision, nyctalopia, and scotomas; quinine—acute poisoning causes cinchonism (visual loss, dizziness, dysacusis, tinnitus, nausea), severe visual loss (often no light perception) which resolves over time, dilated pupils, vermiform iris movements, hippus, constricted visual fields

   c. biomicroscopic features: chloroquine/hydroxychloroquine—early stage may include subtle perifoveal pigment granularity and loss of foveal light reflex; later changes may include bullseye configuration or a prominent pigmentary disturbance which may also involve the peripheral retina; late stages may include optic atrophy and vascular attenuation; quinine—retinal edema, macular cherry red spot

   d. clinical course: chloroqine/hydroxychloroquine—the subtle macular changes of early retinopathy may be reversible; usually, the retinal changes and visual function remain stable after the drug is stopped; rarely the retinopathy and visual loss progress even after the drug is stopped; quinine—vision, pupillary function, and visual fields improve but retinal arterial constriction and optic nerve pallor develop

3. Pathology

   a. chloroquine/hydroxychloroquine: unknown; chloroquine binds to melanin and accumulates in uvea and retinal pigment epithelium

   b. histopathology: early changes occur in ganglion cells and photoreceptor outer segments; destruction of rods and cones with loss of outer nuclear layer

   c. quinine: direct toxic effect of quinine on retinal neurons and retinal pigment epithelium

4. Diagnosis

   a. chloroquine/hydroxychloroquine

      1) VF: paracentral scotomas with red test objects (may occur before symptoms and fundus changes develop)

      2) Amsler grid: may show abnormalities

      3) FA: macular pigmentary abnormalities

      4) ERG: may be abnormal in late stages

      5) EOG: may be abnormal in late stages

   b. quinine

      1) ERG: decreased a-wave and loss of oscillatory potentials which return to normal within 24 hours; b-wave decreases over time

      2) EOG: decreased

5. Treatment

     a. discontinue the medication

C. Nicotinic Acid—Retinal Toxicity

   nicotinic acid (Niacin)

  1. Epidemiology

    a. doses greater than 3 to 5 g/day; used to treat hypercholesterolemia (incidence of maculopathy is 0.7% of hyperlipidemic patients treated with nicotinic acid)

  2. Clinical features

    a. bilateral, usually symmetric

    b. presenting symptoms: systemic symptoms include cutaneous flushing, nausea, abdominal distress, rashes, and exacerbation of peptic ulcer disease; ocular symptoms include blurred vision (worse upon awakening), metamorphopsia, halos around lights

    c. biomicroscopic findings: normal

    d. ophthalmoscopic findings: cystoid macular edema associated with wrinkling of the inner retina in a starburst configuration; foveola is uninvolved by cystic changes and may appear as a bright yellow spot

    e. clinical course: visual symptoms and fundus findings resolve in 1 to 2 months after stopping the medication

  3. Pathogenesis

    a. possibly a direct toxic effect on Müller cells resulting in intracellular edema

  4. Diagnosis

    a. FA: no retinal vascular leakage; may show faint transmitted choroidal fluorescence consisting of several wedge-shaped patches of fluorescence pointing toward the fovea

  5. Treatment

    a. discontinue the medication

D. Methoxyflurane

   a nonflammable inhalational anesthetic

   see chapter on oxalosis

  1. Epidemiology

    a. may occur after prolonged administration of methoxyflurane anesthesia; associated with irreversible renal failure in a form of secondary hyperoxaluria with subsequent retinal oxalosis

  2. Clinical features

    a. bilateral and symmetric

    b. VA: 20/20 to 20/30

    c. biomicroscopic findings: normal

         d. ophthalmoscopic findings: yellow-white crystalline lesions involving the posterior pole and midperiphery; may have a predilection for retinal arteries

         e. clinical course: nonprogressive

      3. Pathogenesis

         a. methoxyflurane is metabolized to oxalic acid which combines with calcium to form an insoluble salt; this is deposited throughout the body

         b. birefringent crystals in retinal pigment epithelium, inner plexiform, and inner nuclear layers of the retina

      4. Diagnosis

         a. FA: window defects correspond with yellow-white dots

         b. VF: normal

         c. ERG: normal

         d. color: normal

      5. Treatment

         a. none

E. Tamoxifen

    tamoxifen (Nolvadex)

      1. Epidemiology

         a. patients with metastatic breast carcinoma and positive estrogen receptor tumors who are treated with tamoxifen; an antiestrogen drug

         b. may occur within normal dose range (20 to 30 mg/day; total dose 8 to 12 g) but is more significant in higher doses

      2. Clinical features

         a. bilateral and symmetric

         b. VA: usually 20/20 to 20/30 but may be worse

         c. biomicroscopic findings: rarely whorl-like corneal opacities may be present

         d. ophthalmoscopic findings: white refractile lesions of the inner retinal layers, most concentrated in perimacular area; punctate macular retinal pigment epithelial changes; cystoid macular edema

         e. clinical course: refractile lesions do not change after discontinuing the drug; visual improvement may occur after cessation of therapy

      3. Pathogenesis

         a. small intracellular spherical lesions have been noted in the perimacular area located in the nerve fiber layer and inner plexiform layer; these stained positive for glycos-aminoglycans; the refractile lesions may represent products of axonal degeneration

4. Diagnosis
    a. FA: punctate retinal pigment epithelial changes are nonfluorescent
    b. VF: normal, constricted, or paracentral scotoma
    c. ERG: normal or slightly decreased photopic and scotopic a- and b-wave amplitude
5. Treatment
    a. discontinue the medication

F. Canthaxanthine
  1. canthaxanthine (Orobronze)
      a. a naturally occurring carotenoid
      b. used as a red food coloring agent
      c. used to treat photosensitivity disorders (erthropoietic protoporphyria, polymorphous light eruption, vitiligo, photosensitive eczema, discoid lupus, malignant melanoma, dysplastic nevus syndrome, dermatomyositis, rosacea, light sensitive psoriasis, and systemic lupus erythematosus); dose 60 to 120 mg/day for 4 to 7 months of the year
      d. used as an oral skin tanning agent (orobronze; not approved for this in the United States) dose 30 to 150 mg/day
  2. Epidemiology
      a. canthaxanthine crystalline retinopathy has been seen in patients using canthaxanthine as an oral tanning agent and in patients being treated for photosensitivity disorders
      b. seen with doses ranging from 3.6 g to 178 g; related to total dose
      c. older patients with ocular hypertension or retinal pigment epithelial changes may be at higher risk for the development of retinopathy
  3. Clinical features
      a. bilateral and symmetric
      b. VA: normal; patients are asymptomatic
      c. biomicroscopic findings: normal
      d. ophthalmoscopic findings: golden-yellow crystalline deposits in the perifoveal area
      e. clinical course: reversible anatomic (number of crystalline deposits) and functional changes (static perimetry) with cessation of the drug
  4. Pathogenesis

           a. crystals in perifoveal region of the neurosensory retina (only in inner layers, most concentrated around blood vessels), retinal pigment epithelium, and choroid

    5. Diagnosis
        a. FA: normal
        b. VF: minor defects
        c. ERG: prolongation of dark adaptation

    6. Treatment
        a. discontinue the medication

G. Digitalis Glycosides
    digoxin and digitoxin

    1. Epidemiology
        a. used for congestive heart failure and cardiac arrhythmias
        b. narrow margin between therapeutic effect and drug toxicity
        c. factors relating to the development of toxicity include hypokalemia, decreased renal function, and concomitant administration of quinidine

    2. Clinical features
        a. presenting symptoms: decreased visual acuity, dyschromatopsia (yellow hue), hemeralopia (worsening of vision in bright illumination), and paracentral scotomas
        b. biomicroscopic findings: normal
        c. ophthalmoscopic findings: normal
        d. clinical course: symptoms resolve with cessation of the drug

    3. Pathogenesis
        a. digitalis glycosides have a direct effect on retinal neurons due to the inhibition of sodium potassium adenosine triphosphatase (which is an essential enzyme for the development of neuroaction potentials) of retinal photoreceptors

    4. Diagnosis
        a. ERG: decreased photopic flickering ERG amplitudes indicative of cone dysfunction

    5. Treatment
        a. decrease the dosage to normalize the drug levels

XXIX. TRAUMATIC RETINAL BREAKS, DIALYSIS, AND DETACHMENT

A. Epidemiology

      1. Occurs after penetrating and nonpenetrating trauma to the globe

B. Clinical Features

    1. Presenting symptoms/signs: floaters, photopsia; visual acuity and visual field reduced when retinal detachment involves the macula; visual field affected with extramacular retinal detachment

    2. Biomicroscopic findings: evidence of injury to the external or anterior structures of the eye; pigmented cells in anterior vitreous indicate high probability of a retinal break

    3. Ophthalmoscopic findings:

        a. retinal breaks: horseshoe-shaped retinal tears and operculated retinal holes in periphery, especially at areas of lattice degeneration or at edges of chorioretinal scars; formed vitreous is attached to the elevated flap of a horseshoe tear and to the operculum of an operculated hole

        b. retinal dialysis: a separation of the peripheral retina from the pars plana epithelium at the ora serrata; inferotemporal quadrant is most common location

        c. retinal detachment: retinal breaks and retinal dialyses may result in retinal detachment if liquified vitreous passes between the sensory retina and the retinal pigment epithelium

    4. Clinical course: retinal breaks—vitreous traction on the elevated flap of a horseshoe tear holds the tear open and therefore likely results in retinal detachment; retinal dialysis—dialyses are less likely to result in retinal detachment; if detachment is present, it is often localized and minimally elevated, especially if the dialysis is small or located inferiorly

C. Pathogenesis

    1. Trauma produces sudden deformation of the vitreous, and retinal tearing may occur in areas of strong vitreoretinal adhesion, such as the vitreous base

    2. Retinal damage at the vitreous base may result in peripheral retinal breaks and retinal dialysis

    3. Retinal breaks and dialyses result in retinal detachment when liquid vitreous enters the subretinal space

D. Diagnosis

      1. Based on clinical setting of trauma and on ophthalmoscopic findings

E. Treatment

    1. Retinal breaks treated with photocoagulation or cryopexy as prophylaxis for retinal detachment; scleral buckling surgery is indicated for retinal breaks associated with retinal detachment (success rate greater than 80%)

    2. Retinal dialysis treated with photocoagulation or cryopexy as prophylaxis for retinal detachment; scleral buckling surgery is indicated for retinal dialysis associated with retinal detachment (success rate 90%)

Essentials of Eye Care, edited by Rohit Varma.
Lippincott–Raven Publishers,
Philadelphia © 1997.

10

Intraocular Tumors

I. RETINOBLASTOMA

A. Most Common Intraocular Malignancy of Childhood

B. Epidemiology:

1. Incidence 1:14,000 to 1:20,000 live births, 200 to 300 new cases in United States per year. Average age of diagnosis 18 months, 90% diagnosed before age 3, rare after age 7. Majority of cases sporadic, minority autosomal dominant with 80% penetrance.

C. Clinical Features:

1. Asymptomatic or decreased vision
2. Leukocoria, strabismus, anisocoria, proptosis, red pain-ful eye, spontaneous hyphema, heterochromia irides
3. Calcification and vitreous seeding
4. Tumor may grow into the vitreous (endophytic) or from the retina outward (exophytic)
5. 30 to 35% are bilateral and usually present by age 1 year
6. May rarely involve pineal gland (trilateral retinoblastoma)
7. May undergo spontaneous regression
8. Metastasis may occur to skull or long bones, lymph nodes, spinal cord, or visceral organs
9. Patients with heritable (bilateral) retinoblastoma may develop other tumors later in life (e.g., osteogenic sarcoma)
10. Patients treated with ocular irradiation may develop sarcomas of the orbit

D. Pathology:

1. Tumor composed of small round cells with hyperchromatic nuclei and scant cytoplasm. Flexner-Wintersteiner rosettes or fluorettes considered pathognomonic.
2. Optic nerve invasion beyond lamina cribrosa associated with poor prognosis

E. Diagnosis:
  1. Characteristic clinical features, family history
  2. Ultrasonography may demonstrate calcium in the tumor
  3. CT may demonstrate calcium or metastasis
  4. Additional evaluation may include bone marrow biopsy, bone scans, or cerebrospinal fluid (CSF) cytology
  5. Differential diagnosis includes glial hamartoma, posterior pole granuloma from nematode infection, Coats' disease, persistent hyperplastic primary vitreous, retinopathy of prematurity, congenital cataract, Norrie's disease, retinal detachment or schisis, or large chorioretinal coloboma

F. Treatment:
  1. Appropriate genetic counseling
  2. Examination of siblings and parents
  3. Enucleation for advanced intraocular tumors is usually treatment of choice
  4. Treatment of second eye may involve external beam irradiation or brachytherapy
  5. Photocoagulation or cryotherapy may be used to treat small peripheral tumors
  6. Systemic chemotherapy for advanced cases or metastatic disease

II. CHOROIDAL METASTASIS

A. Most Common Solid Intraocular Malignant Tumor, Spread by Hematogenous Dissemination

B. Epidemiology:
  1. Incidence estimated at 4% of all patients dying of carcinoma, middle aged, and older patients
  2. Site of primary tumor; gender-dependent: breast most common overall, lung most common in males and second most common in females; other sites include gastrointestinal tract, skin melanoma, kidneys, and thyroid. Other primary carcinomas rarely metastasize to the choroid; in some patients the primary cancer remains unknown.

C. Clinical Features:
  1. May or may not have a history of previous malignancy. Varies with primary source.
  2. Choroidal metastasis has a predilection for the macula and may cause blurring of vision
  3. 25% bilateral or multifocal involvement
  4. Ophthalmoscopic findings include homogenous, creamy placoid lesions of the choroid. Typically

        develop serous retinal detachment or alterations of the retinal pigment epithelium.

D. Pathology:

    1. If well differentiated, may retain features of the primary tumor

    2. May be poorly differentiated

E. Diagnosis:

    1. Clinical features and history of malignancy

    2. Fluorescein angiography may show hypofluorescence in arterial phase and early venous phase and progressive hyperfluorescence. Useful to help differentiate tumor from nonneoplastic lesions, but not useful to differentiate from a choroidal melanoma or hemangioma.

    3. Ultrasound: A-scan—high initial spike with high to moderate internal reflectivity. B-scan—choroidal mass with moderate to high acoustic solidity.

    4. Fine needle biopsy via pars plana or subretinal approach or wedge biopsy via scleral flap may confirm diagnosis. A biopsy is not typically required.

    5. CT/MRI may be helpful to detect extraocular lesions

    6. Differential diagnosis includes amelanotic melanoma, amelanotic nevus, choroidal hemangioma, choroidal osteoma, and nonneoplastic disorders such as posterior scleritis, choroiditis, rhegmatogenous retinal detachment, central serous chorioretinopathy, and the uveal effusion syndrome.

F. Treatment:

    1. Systemic evaluation

    2. If tumor appears inactive (flat without retinal detachment) or if disc or macula is not threatened, observation is often advised

    3. Active tumors with accompanying retinal detachment usually require treatment

    4. Symptomatic patients with macular or optic nerve involvement may benefit from external beam irradiation

    5. Enucleation reserved for painful eyes with poor vision and uncontrolled tumor. It is rarely required.

III. LEUKEMIA

A. Epidemiology:

    1. Incidence of leukemic infiltration of ocular structures is about 3% of patients with leukemia. Age of onset variable.

B. Clinical Features:
  1. Asymptomatic or blurred vision
  2. Leukemic infiltration of iris with diffuse white thickening or small nodules at the pupillary margin. May develop pseudohypopyon.
  3. Leukemic infiltration of anterior chamber angle may lead to glaucoma
  4. Ophthalmoscopic findings include intraretinal hemorrhage, cotton-wool spots, white centered hemorrhages, central retinal vein occlusion, vitreous hemorrhage, and yellow infiltrates of retina, choroid, or optic nerve head

C. Pathology:
  1. Diffuse infiltration of retina, uvea, or optic nerve with leukemic cells

D. Diagnosis:
  1. Clinical features in presence of known systemic disease
  2. Cytologic diagnosis by fine needle aspiration biopsy or vitrectomy
  3. Differential diagnosis includes iritis, endophthalmitis, opportunistic infection, cytomegalovirus (CMV) retinitis

E. Treatment:
  1. Systemic evaluation by oncologist
  2. Chemotherapy or ocular irradiation
  3. Optic nerve involvement requires consideration of prompt irradiation to prevent visual loss
  4. Prognosis for vision variable depending on extent of involvement, prognosis for life guarded in most cases

IV. LARGE CELL LYMPHOMA (RETICULUM CELL SARCOMA, HISTIOCYTIC LYMPHOMA)

Infiltration by malignant lymphoid cells usually associated with systemic lymphoma

A. Epidemiology:
  1. Age of onset usually after 50, no sex predilection

B. Clinical Features:
  1. Usually presents unilaterally but becomes bilateral in about 80% of cases
  2. Vitreo-retinal form: more common and may present with blurred vision, anterior uveitis, keratic precipitates, aqueous cell, vitreous cell, retinal

infiltrates, or optic neuropathy. Commonly associated with central nervous system (CNS) lymphoma.

3. Uveal form: single or multiple well defined creamy yellow fundus lesions, may involve the iris. Often associated with visceral or nodal lymphoma.

C. Pathology.
1. Infiltration of uvea and retina with poorly differentiated mononuclear cells with large hyperchromatic nuclei
2. Pathogenesis: manifestation of systemic lymphoma, in rare instances may be an isolated primary malignancy

D. Diagnosis:
1. Clinical features, may have known systemic lymphoma
2. Histopathologic diagnosis from fine needle aspiration biopsy, iridectomy, or vitreous aspirate from pars plana vitrectomy
3. Immunohistochemical studies aid diagnosis
4. Differential diagnosis includes amelanotic melanoma, metastatic tumor, uveitis, cytomegalovirus retinitis, choroidal hemangioma, reactive lymphoid hyperplasia

E. Treatment:
1. Systemic evaluation by oncologist
2. Intrathecal chemotherapy
3. CNS and ocular irradiation
4. Visual prognosis variable, most patients die within 2 years of diagnosis

V. CHOROIDAL MELANOMA (CILIARY BODY AND CHOROID)

A. Epidemiology:
1. Incidence estimated at 4.9 to 7.6 per million per year. Mean age of diagnosis 55 to 66 years. More common in whites than in nonwhites.

B. Clinical Features:
1. Asymptomatic, blurred vision, visual field loss, floaters, or pain
2. External features include sentinel vessels (dilated episcleral vessels) and episcleral pigment from extrascleral extension
3. Lenticular astigmatism from tumor growing into or tilting the lens
4. Extension of tumor into the iris, iris neovascularization

5. Secondary glaucoma from angle closure, neovascularization, or melanomalytic process
6. Ophthalmoscopic findings include variably pigmented uveal mass (may be amelanotic), may have a collar button configuration from extension through Bruch's membrane, often an orange coloration to the surface of the tumor from lipofuscin laden macrophages, retinal pigment epithelium (RPE) atrophy and hypertrophy, choroidal neovascularization, cystic retinal degeneration, retinal detachment, invasion of retina by tumor, vitreous seeding, or vitreous hemorrhage
7. Extrascleral extension of tumor into the orbit
8. Metastasis most common to the liver, lung, skin, and others

C. Pathology:
1. Tumor may be composed of predominately one cell type or mixed
2. Spindle A cells: spindle-shaped cells with flattened nuclei, rare mitosis
3. Spindle B cells: spindle-shaped cells with oval nuclei, prominent nucleoli, and rare mitosis
4. Epithelioid cells: round to polyhedral cells with abundant cytoplasm, large nuclei, and prominent nucleoli
5. Pathogenesis: several risk factors have been postulated, including possible viral association, sunlight exposure, fair patient pigmentation, occupational exposure

D. Diagnosis:
1. Ophthalmologic findings
2. Ultrasound: A-scan—high initial spike with low to medium internal reflectivity. B-scan—identify size and extent of tumor. Lesions of more than 2.0 mm in height usually melanoma, less than 1.0 mm in height usually benign nevus.
3. Fluorescein angiography pattern variable, may help differentiate tumor from nonneoplastic lesions, but not of value to differentiate metastasis or hemangioma
4. CT and MRI may be helpful to identify extraocular disease
5. Fine needle aspiration biopsy for atypical clinical or ultrasound characteristics, or patient requests 100% certainty of diagnosis prior to therapy. Not typically performed.
6. Metastatic evaluation including liver function tests, chest X-rays, detailed physical examina-

tion, and CT or MRI of abdomen if liver function tests are abnormal

7. Differential diagnosis includes nevus, congenital hypertrophy of the RPE, RPE hyperplasia, choroidal metastasis, age-related macular degeneration, disciform scarring, melanocytoma of the optic disc, posterior scleritis, retinal detachment, choroidal detachment

E. Treatment:

1. Observation of small tumors less than 2.0 mm in height with serial photography to evaluate for growth

2. Definitive therapy should be considered for tumors showing evidence of growth or activity, or larger tumors

3. Most tumors are treated by enucleation, enucleation following preoperative external beam irradiation, or scleral plaque brachytherapy. These modalities are currently being evaluated by the Collaborative Ocular Melanoma Study.

4. Orbital exenteration may be considered for extraocular extension

5. Management of metastasis with palliative radiation therapy or chemotherapy

6. Prognosis varies with tumor cell type, tumor size, location of anterior margin of the tumor, and extrascleral extension. Twenty to 30% five year mortality for medium sized tumors, patients with metastasis usually die within 1 year.

VI. MELANOCYTOMA

Variant of nevus at the disc or anywhere in the uveal tract

A. Epidemiology:

1. Incidence unknown, age of diagnosis 14 to 79 with a mean of 50, 37% to 50% occur in African-Americans; those that occur in Caucasians tend to be in darkly pigmented individuals.

B. Clinical Features:

1. Optic disc melanocytoma:

   a. asymptomatic or blurred vision

   b. one third have an afferent pupillary defect

   c. elevated black or brown heavily pigmented lesion located over the optic disc, more common over the inferior portion of the disc, often a fibrillated margin to the tumor. About one half have a typical choroidal nevus contiguous with the disc portion of the melanocytoma.

        d. retinal vascular occlusion can occur rarely with secondary neovascular glaucoma
        e. large tumors can undergo necrosis
        f. in about 15%, enlargement can be documented by serial photos
        g. malignant degeneration very rare but can occur
    2. Extrapapillary melanocytoma:
        a. similar to a nevus but more deeply pigmented, occurs on the iris, ciliary body, or choroid

C. Pathology:
    1. Densely pigmented, uniform appearance
    2. Round to oval cells with abundant cytoplasm, small nuclei, and prominent nucleoli
    3. Pathogenesis possibly related to excess accumulation of ectopic melanocytes derived from neural crest cells during embryogenesis

D. Diagnosis:
    1. Characteristic clinical features
    2. Ultrasound may show elevation but cannot differentiate melanocytoma from other lesions
    3. Fluorescein angiography shows hypofluorescence throughout
    4. Visual fields may demonstrate progressive loss with tumor growth
    5. Serial fundus photography may demonstrate tumor growth
    6. Differential diagnosis includes choroidal melanoma, choroidal nevus, hyperplasia or hypertrophy of the retinal pigment epithelium, and combined hamartoma of the retina and retinal pigment epithelium

E. Treatment:
    1. Observation with periodic followup and serial photos
    2. If optic disc melanocytoma shows evidence of progressive growth or malignant transformation, consider consultation with ocular oncologist
    3. If iris melanocytoma shows evidence of progressive growth, consider complete excision by sector iridectomy
    4. Visual prognosis variable

VII. CHOROIDAL HEMANGIOMA

A. Classification
    1. Circumscribed: benign, well defined vascular tumor of the choroid
    2. Diffuse: benign vascular tumor of the choroid with poorly defined borders which extends over

a broad area. May be part of Sturge-Weber syndrome. Discussion below limited to circumscribed tumors only. Please see accompanying section on Sturge-Weber syndrome for discussion of diffuse choroidal hemangioma.

B. Epidemiology:
1. Incidence unknown, age of diagnosis usually 20s to 30s

C. Clinical Features:
1. May present with metamorphopsia or decreased vision
2. Usually no associated cutaneous manifestations
3. Ophthalmoscopic findings include unilateral, unifocal, red-orange mass with a predilection for the posterior pole
4. Often develop secondary, nonrhegmatogenous serous retinal detachment and cystic degeneration of the retina overlying the tumor

D. Pathology:
1. Vascular tumor composed of vascular channels, loose connective tissue, and capillary channels lined by a single layer of endothelial cell

E. Diagnosis:
1. Based on clinical features and characteristic red-orange color
2. Ultrasound: A-scan—high initial spike and high internal reflectivity. B-scan—rounded choroidal tumor with internal acoustic solidity.
3. Fluorescein angiography shows irregular hyperfluorescence of large choroidal vessels in the tumor in prearterial phase, progressive staining, and late intraretinal hyperfluorescence of cystic retinal degeneration. Pattern variable and not pathognomonic.
4. CT/MRI may help differentiate the size of the tumor
5. Differential diagnosis includes amelanotic melanoma, choroidal metastasis, choroidal osteoma, retinoblastoma, central serous choroidopathy, and posterior scleritis

F. Treatment:
1. Observation if asymptomatic
2. For serous detachment of the macula or threatening the macula, photocoagulation can be considered, using light-to-moderate evenly spread burns over the entire surface of the lesion to promote chorioretinal adhesion. Spot size: 200 to 500 μm, burn exposure 0.1 to 0.5 seconds, intense enough to cause slight whitening of the tumor surface. No

evidence from any clinical trial, however, that this approach is preferable to observation.
3. For extensive retinal detachment, consider surgical intervention
4. Low dose external beam or brachytherapy may have a role in management
5. Visual prognosis is guarded as recurrence of serous retinal detachment is common with cystic retinal degeneration in the macula
6. Prognosis for life excellent, visual prognosis guarded

VIII. JUVENILE XANTHOGRANULOMA

A. Epidemiology:
   1. Infants and young children affected. Reported rarely in adults. Incidence unknown.
B. Clinical Features:
   1. Benign, self-limited disorder
   2. Ocular:
      a. iris infiltration with focal yellow-gray poorly demarcated nodules, or diffuse thickening of iris stroma
      b. may develop heterochromic irides, spontaneous hyphema, secondary glaucoma, and buphthalmos from elevated intraocular pressure
      c. rarely the eyelid, orbit, cornea, choroid, retina, or optic nerve may be infiltrated
      d. bilateral involvement rare
   3. Systemic:
      a. multiple cutaneous orange or yellow papules that present early in infancy and usually regress spontaneously after a few years
C. Pathology:
   1. Diffuse, benign granulomatous inflammatory reaction composed of normal histiocytes, lymphocytes, eosinophils, and Touton giant cells. Pathogenesis obscure.
D. Diagnosis:
   1. Clinical diagnosis based on above findings
   2. Fine needle biopsy of anterior chamber mass to confirm diagnosis
   3. Differential diagnosis includes uveitis, retinal detachment, posterior segment tumor including retinoblastoma, intraocular foreign body, and leukemic infiltrate
E. Treatment:

1. Treatment of iris lesions advised because of the risk of hyphema, corneal blood staining, glaucoma, and amblyopia
2. Corticosteroids: topical, subconjunctival, or systemic
3. Local excision, irradiation, and irradiation combined with corticosteroids have been utilized
4. Prognosis for life excellent, visual prognosis variable

IX. NEUROFIBROMATOSIS (VON RECKLINGHAUSEN'S SYNDROME)

A. Epidemiology:
   1. Autosomal dominant, 80% penetrance. Fifty percent of cases sporadic. Frequency of new mutations 1:2500 to 1:3000.
   2. Ocular findings usually detected after age 5, most skin changes apparent at puberty
B. Clinical Features:
   1. Ocular:
      a. neurofibromatosis type 1 (NF1)
         1) neurofibromas of the eyelid, S-shaped curvature of upper eyelid from plexiform neurofibroma, pulsating proptosis
         2) diffuse or nodular conjunctival thickening, increased diameter of corneal nerves, increased incidence of congenital glaucoma, and Lisch nodules (lightly pigmented elevations of the iris)
         3) choroidal involvement includes choroidal hamartoma, diffuse thickening of the uveal tract, increased incidence of choroidal melanoma, and multifocal congenital hypertrophy of the retinal pigment epithelium
         4) retinal astrocytic hamartoma, myelinated nerve fiber layer, and optic nerve glioma or meningioma all associated
      b. neurofibromatosis type 2 (NF2): consists of above features of NF1 combined with early onset of posterior subcapsular cataract
   2. Systemic:
      a. skin manifestations include neurofibromas of the skin, "Café au lait" spots (pigmented macules), and nevi
      b. CNS findings include gliomas, pituitary tumors, and meningiomas
      c. neurofibromatosis is associated with an increased incidence of sarcomas, malignant pe-

ripheral nerve sheath tumors, breast cancer, pheochromocytoma, gastrointestinal and genito-urinary tumors, and melanomas of both the skin and choroid

  d. NF2: associated with above clinical features and bilateral acoustic neuromas, may present with tinnitus and hearing loss

C. Pathology:

  1. Lisch nodule is composed of aggregates of melanocytes and glial cells

  2. Tumors of peripheral and cranial nerves composed of Schwann cells

  3. Tumors of CNS composed of glial cells

  4. Pathogenesis of NF1 related to a defect of chromosome 17 and NF2 related to a defect of chromosome 22

D. Diagnosis:

  1. Based on general medical and systemic findings, autosomal dominant pattern of inheritance

  2. Some consider more than 6 "Café au lait" spots each larger than 1.5 cm in diameter pathognomonic

  3. Ancillary testing may include neuroimaging of the orbit and brain, EEG, audiography, and urine levels for catecholamines

E. Treatment:

  1. Supportive. Appropriate genetic counseling.

X. TUBEROUS SCLEROSIS (BOURNEVILLE'S SYNDROME)

A. Epidemiology:

  1. Autosomal dominant with incomplete penetrance, incidence unknown, usually diagnosed in infancy or childhood

B. Clinical Features:

  1. Ocular:

   a. astrocytic hamartoma of the retina or optic disc. White mulberry-like mass considered almost patho-gnomonic. If tumor is not calcified it may appear like thickening of the nerve fiber layer.

  2. Systemic:

   a. skin manifestations include adenoma sebaceum (slightly elevated papules which may resemble acne), shagreen patches (thickened redundant areas of skin), depigmented areas similar to vitiligo (ash leaf sign), and "Café au lait" spots

      b. CNS changes include seizures and mental changes from subependymal and cortical astrocytomas

      c. associated with renal angiolipoma, cardiac rhabdomyoma, irregular thickening of the bones, and hamartomas of the liver, thyroid, pancreas, and testes

C. Pathology:

    1. Astrocytic hamartoma arises from astrocytes of the nerve fiber layer. Pathogenesis uncertain.

D. Diagnosis:

    1. Based on general medical and ocular findings. Classic triad of epilepsy, mental retardation, and adenoma sebaceum may be present in about 30% of cases.

    2. Ultrasonography may help differentiate astrocytic hamartoma from other lesions

    3. Ancillary testing may include neuroimaging, EEG, echocardiogram, CXR, abdominal CT

    4. Differential diagnosis of retinal astrocytic hamartoma includes retinoblastoma, myelinated nerve fiber layer, toxocara or toxoplasma choroiditis, optic disc drusen, and Coats' disease

E. Treatment:

    1. Appropriate genetic counseling and referral to other specialists

XI. ENCEPHALOFACIAL CAVERNOUS HEMANGIOMATOSIS (STURGE-WEBER SYNDROME)

Diffuse choroidal hemangioma associated with ipsilateral facial hemangioma

A. Epidemiology:

    1. Nonhereditary, incidence unknown, usually diagnosed in childhood

B. Clinical Features:

    1. Ocular:

      a. visual impairment from hyperopia or secondary serous retinal detachment, may develop amblyopia

      b. facial hemangioma may involve the eyelid

      c. ipsilateral to the facial hemangioma findings include dilated, tortuous conjunctival and episcleral vessels, iris heterochromia

      d. glaucoma (more common when hemangioma involves the upper eyelid), may lead to buphthalmos

   e. ophthalmoscopic findings include diffuse
      choroidal hemangioma with red-orange thick-
      ening of the posterior choroid (tomato catsup
      appearance), retinal venous tortuosity and ar-
      teriovenous malformations, retinal pigment
      abnormalities, serous retinal detachment, and
      cystic retinal degeneration
   2. Systemic:
      a. skin findings include the facial hemangioma
         typically along the first and second divisions
         of the trigeminal nerve and often referred to as
         port wine stain or nevus flammeus; however,
         cutaneous pattern may be variable, rarely bilat-
         eral
      b. CNS findings include diffuse leptomeningeal
         hemangioma ipsilateral to the facial heman-
         gioma, secondary calcification, seizures, and
         mental changes
C. Pathology:
   1. Diffuse thickening of the choroid from prolifera-
      tion of small and large vessels
   2. Pathogenesis of disorder uncertain; pathogenesis
      of glaucoma may be related to high episcleral ve-
      nous pressure, incomplete cleavage of the an-
      terior chamber angle, neovascularization, often
      when retinal detachment is present, or hyper-
      secretion of aqueous
D. Diagnosis:
   1. Based on general medical and ophthalmic find-
      ings
   2. Ultrasound may show diffuse thickening of the
      choroid
   3. Fluorescein angiography similar to circumscribed
      hemangioma except for diffuse involvement
   4. Should consider obtaining MRI or CT of the
      brain, EEG
E. Treatment:
   1. Treatment of amblyopia if present
   2. Retinal detachment may be treated with scatter
      photocoagulation similar to circumscribed cho-
      roidal hemangioma. The outcome is variable.
   3. Extensive retinal detachment may require surgi-
      cal reattachment
   4. Treatment of glaucoma, including medical man-
      agement with a topical beta blocker and/or car-
      bonic anhydrase inhibitor. If ineffective consider
      trabeculectomy. Serous or hemorrhagic choroidal
      detachments may occur after trabeculectomy and
      usually resolve as intraocular pressure rises.

     5. Referral to appropriate specialists, anticonvulsants

XII. RETINOCEREBELLAR CAPILLARY HEMANGIOMATOSIS (VON HIPPEL-LINDAU SYNDROME)

Isolated capillary hemangioma of the retina can occur, known as von Hippel's disease

20% of patients with capillary hemangioma have associated cerebellar lesions known as von Hippel-Lindau syndrome, described by Lindau

A. Epidemiology:
  1. Autosomal dominant with incomplete penetrance. Sporadic cases occur frequently. Prevalence and incidence unknown. Ophthalmic manifestations usually present in second or third decade, CNS symptoms usually begin in the fourth decade of life.

B. Clinical Features:
  1. Ocular:
     a. early lesions consist of small, red to gray, capillary clusters without associated feeder vessels
     b. lesions may enlarge and develop feeder vessels and classic "pink balloon" configuration
     c. capillary hemangiomas usually in midperiphery but may involve the optic disc. Often multiple and bilateral.
     d. vision may be affected by subretinal exudate, retinal detachment, or vitreous hemorrhage
     e. eyes may go on to develop glaucoma or phthisis
  2. Systemic:
     a. skin uninvolved
     b. CNS hemangioblastoma found in cerebellum, medulla, pons, spinal cord, and cerebrum
     c. association with pheochromocytoma, renal cell carcinoma, and pancreatic cysts

C. Pathology:
  1. Tumor composed of small capillary-like or larger blood vessels lined by fenestrated endothelium which leak protein and blood constituents. Large tumors may contain vacuolated cells which show features of fibrous astrocytes that have become lipidized.

D. Diagnosis:
  1. Based on general medical and ocular findings
  2. Fluorescein angiography helpful to treat retinal capillary hemangioma

3. Ancillary testing should include brain MRI, abdominal CT, urinary catecholamine levels, and renal ultrasound
4. Differential diagnosis includes racemose hemangiomatosis and Coats' disease

E. Treatment:
1. Clinical course without treatment variable but tumors will grow and lead to retinal detachment, glaucoma, and phthisis.
2. Flat lesions effectively treated with argon photocoagulation, burn duration 0.2 to 1.0 seconds, 500 to 1000 μm spot size, intense enough to create a dense white burn over the angioma
3. Cryotherapy may be needed for larger tumors or those with subretinal fluid. Extensive cryotherapy may contribute to proliferative vitreoretinopathy or increased exudation.
4. Scleral buckle and/or vitrectomy may be necessary for vitreous traction
5. Followup examinations every 6 months
6. Examination of all family members is indicated
7. Appropriate genetic counseling and referral to specialists to detect and treat systemic complications

XIII. RACEMOSE HEMANGIOMATOSIS (WYBURN-MASON SYNDROME)

Arteriovenous malformations of the retina, optic nerve and brain

A. Epidemiology:
1. Nonhereditary, congenital, vast majority unilateral. Most symptomatic patients present in second and third decade of life.

B. Clinical Features:
1. Ocular:
a. vision may be normal or compromised if posterior pole involvement is present. Patients may present with acute loss of vision from hemorrhage or gradual loss from compression of the optic nerve or chiasm.
b. racemose hemangiomas of the orbit may cause proptosis
c. ophthalmoscopic findings include enormously dilated, tortuous retinal vessels with arteriovenous communications without intervening

capillaries. No distinct mass or subretinal exudate.

    2. Systemic:

      a. racemose hemangiomas of midbrain may cause seizures, hemiparesis, intracranial hemorrhage, and mental status changes

      b. racemose hemangiomas may be present in the mandible, maxillae, and bony palate, and cause severe hemorrhaging during dental or facial surgery

C. Pathology:

    1. Abnormal vascular communication rather than tumor. Affected vessels may become hypertrophied, causing difficulty in differentiating arteries from veins. Retinal thinning and cystic degeneration may be present.

D. Diagnosis:

    1. Based on ophthalmic and general medical findings

    2. Fluorescein angiography shows arteriovenous communications without intervening capillaries and no angiographic leakage

    3. Neuroimaging to detect CNS involvement

    4. Differential diagnosis includes retinal capillary hemangioma and congenital tortuosity of retinal vessels

E. Treatment:

    1. Treatment not indicated for retinal lesions

    2. Appropriate referral to neurologist

XIV. ATAXIA-TELANGIECTASIA (LOUIS-BAR SYNDROME)

A. Epidemiology:

    1. Autosomal recessive, incidence unknown. Carrier state may be as common as 1 in 60.

B. Clinical Features:

    1. Ocular:

      a. conjunctival telangiectasia most prominent in the exposed canthal regions

      b. neuro-ophthalmic manifestations including strabismus, nystagmus, oculomotor apraxia, impaired convergence, loss of opticokinetic nystagmus (OKN)

    2. Systemic:

      a. skin manifestations include cutaneous telangiectasias on face, ears, base of neck, and extensor surfaces; follicular keratosis, seborrheic dermatitis, and pigmentary changes

    b. progressive cerebellar ataxia presents when child learns to walk

    c. recurrent sinus and pulmonary infections from decreased IgA and impaired T cell function

    d. may develop leukemia or lymphoma

    e. associated mental retardation, dysarthric speech, testicular or ovarian atrophy, hypoplastic or atrophic thymus

C. Pathology:

    1. Diffuse cerebral degeneration with gliosis and demyelinization of white matter, atrophy of cerebellum with loss of Purkinje fibers and granular cells

D. Diagnosis:

    1. Based on general medical and ophthalmic findings, autosomal recessive pattern of inheritance

    2. Ancillary testing may show elevated alpha-fetoprotein and carcinoembryonic antigen, chromosomal instability, and immunodeficiency

    3. MRI may show cerebellar atrophy

    4. CXR may show stigmata of recurrent pulmonary infections

E. Treatment:

    1. Supportive, treatment of systemic complications as necessary; many die in childhood or early adulthood from recurrent infections, leukemia, or lymphoma

    2. Appropriate genetic counseling

XV. COMBINED HAMARTOMA OF THE RETINA AND RETINAL PIGMENT EPITHELIUM (CHR-RPE)

Idiopathic benign tumor of the retina and RPE
Hamartoma—benign overgrowth of cells that are normally present at the involved site

A. Epidemiology:

    1. Mean age is 15 years, but may occur in young children and older adults

    2. Possibly more common in males

    3. Rarely associated with neurofibromatosis type I and type II (in cases with bilateral tumors)

B. Clinical Features:

    1. Usually unilateral

    2. Presenting symptoms: painless visual loss; strabismus and leukocoria in children; degree of visual impairment varies with the location of the tumor (worse with involvement of disc or macula)

   3. Biomicroscopic findings: normal

   4. Ophthalmoscopic findings: usually located at optic disc and juxtapapillary region, and in the macula; rarely located in midperiphery; tumor appears slightly elevated with varying amounts of pigmentation, vascular tortuosity, and epiretinal membrane formation (usually one type of tissue tends to predominate)

   5. Clinical course: usually nonprogressive; rarely associated with vitreous hemorrhage and choroidal neovascular membrane; enlargement of the tumor occasionally occurs

C. Pathology:

   1. Marked disorganization of retinal architecture such that individual layers cannot be delineated; proliferation of glial tissue and retinal pigment epithelium (retinal pigment epithelium may extend into the inner retina)

D. Diagnosis:

   1. FA: degree of hypofluorescence tends to parallel the degree of hyperpigmentation; marked vascular tortuosity and telangiectasia; leakage of tortuous vessels

   2. US: minimally elevated; no characteristic sonographic pattern

   3. Differential: choroidal melanoma; melanocytoma; epiretinal membrane

E. Treatment:

   1. Amblyopia treatment in children; tractional distortion of macula has been treated by vitrectomy and epiretinal membrane peeling but visual acuity rarely improves

XVI. CHOROIDAL OSTEOMA

Idiopathic benign tumor of the choroid

A. Epidemiology:

   1. Age 10 to 30 years, but may occur in children and older adults

   2. Usually female

   3. Possibly more common in Caucasians

   4. No associated systemic disease

B. Clinical Features:

   1. Bilateral 20 to 50%

   2. Visual impairment absent or mild initially (80%—20/30 or better, 10%—20/200 or worse)

3. Ophthalmoscopic findings: yellow-white to or-ange-red choroidal lesion; 2 to 22 mm basal dimension, 0.5 to 2.5 mm elevation; well demar-cated geographic border with pseudopod projec-tions; irregular elevations and depressions; cho-roidal vascular tufts often visible on tumor surface (these do not represent choroidal neovas-cular membrane [CNVM]); may have subretinal fluid; usually juxtapapillary but may be peripap-illary or macular

4. Clinical course: slow growth in 50%; visual im-pairment may occur gradually due to degenera-tion of overlying RPE and sensory retina; visual impairment may occur suddenly due to CNVM (CNVM occurs in approximately 1/3 of patients); with followup, 50%—20/30 or better, 24%—20/200 or worse

C. Pathology:
1. Ossification occurs when blood vessels grow into a tissue and bring in osteoblasts
2. Histopathology: bony trabeculae with endothe-lial-lined cavernous spaces; osteoblasts, osteo-cytes, and osteoclasts present; thinned choriocap-illaris; overlying RPE variably depigmented

D. Diagnosis:
1. FA: early patchy hyperfluorescence and diffuse late staining; choroidal vascular tuft on tumor surface fills early but fades in later phases; if CNVM present, local area of lacy hyperfluores-cence with increasing leakage throughout the an-giogram
2. A-scan: high echo spike from surface of tumor
3. B-scan: highly reflective, mildly elevated cho-roidal mass with posterior acoustic shadowing; because of calcium content, echoes persist at de-creased sensitivity
4. CT: radiopaque plaque at level of choroid iso-dense with bone
5. MRI: hyperintense to vitreous on T1 weighted im-age; hypointense to vitreous on T2 image
6. Differential: amelanotic choroidal melanoma, amelanotic choroidal nevus, choroidal metasta-sis, cho-roidal hemangioma, age-related macular degeneration (AMD), sclerochoroidal calcifica-tion

E. Treatment:
1. No treatment for tumor unassociated with CNVM; observe closely for signs of CNVM

      2. If CNVM, argon or krypton laser has been applied when CNVM is outside foveal avascular zone (FAZ); difficulty in producing satisfactory burns because of thinned and depigmented RPE; may need repeat treatment

XVII. CAVERNOUS HEMANGIOMA

Benign retinal vascular hamartoma

A. Epidemiology:
    1. Any age, race, gender
    2. May be associated with skin hemangiomas (usually back of the neck) and CNS hemangiomas (occasional seizures, rare intracranial hemorrhage)
    3. Some pedigrees with varying manifestations; incomplete penetrance/variable expressivity; possible autosomal dominant inheritance

B. Clinical Features:
    1. Unilateral
    2. Presenting signs: usually asymptomatic, occasional mild visual dysfunction
    3. Visual impairment absent or mild (10% located in macula, 10% associated with vitreous hemorrhage)
    4. Ophthalmoscopic findings: cluster of saccular intraretinal aneurysms ("cluster of grapes"); aneurysms range in size from microaneurysms to an entire quadrant; usually gray-white fibroglial membrane on surface; layering of red blood cells (RBCs) within aneurysms results in plasma-erythrocyte separation; may cause simultaneous subretinal, intraretinal, and preretinal hemorrhage; no feeder vessels, no exudates
    5. Clinical course: usually nonprogressive; mild vitreous hemorrhage in 10%

C. Pathology:
    1. Multiple endothelium-lined (nonfenestrated) thin-walled veins separated by thin fibrous septa and surrounded by pericytes and fibrous astrocytes; located in inner retina; preretinal membrane attached to internal limiting membrane and inner retina

D. Diagnosis:
    1. FA: gray-white fibroglial tissue may autofluoresce; early hypofluorescence; aneurysms fill slowly and incompletely; late phases demonstrate plasma-erythrocyte separation with fluorescein pooling in the superior portion (fluorescein-

erythrocyte separation); no leakage A-scan: high initial spike and high internal reflectivity
   2. B-scan: surface irregularity; internal acoustic density; no choroidal excavation
E. Treatment:
   1. Periodic observation; evaluate family members; evaluate for systemic angiomas (head CT or MRI)

Essentials of Eye Care, edited by Rohit Varma.
Lippincott–Raven Publishers,
Philadelphia © 1997.

11

Neuroophthalmology

I. TOPICAL DIAGNOSIS OF LESIONS

  A. Optic Nerve

    1. Symptoms: visual loss

    2. Signs

      a. decreased visual acuity, afferent pupillary defect (APD) (may be absent if bilateral optic nerve involvement is present), impaired color vision

      b. ophthalmoscopic examination: normal appearing optic disc, optic nerve pallor, or disc swelling

    3. Visual field defects

      a. central, cecocentral and paracentral scotomas: involvement of papillomacular bundle—the fibers that enter the temporal aspect of the disc

      b. arcuate scotomas: involvement of the retinal nerve fibers temporal to the disc that enter the superior and inferior poles of the disc—respect the horizontal meridian

      c. wedge-shaped scotomas with apex at the blind spot: involvement of fibers nasal to the disc that enter the nasal aspect of the disc

      d. altitudinal defect: involvement of the retinal nerve fibers either superiorly or inferiorly to the horizontal meridian

  B. Chiasm

    1. Symptoms: ± visual loss, difficulties with side vision, diplopia, headache, endocrine dysfunction

    2. Signs

      a. ± decreased visual acuity, APD, impaired color vision

      b. ophthalmoscopic examination: normal appearing optic disc, or optic disc pallor

    3. Visual field defects

      a. junction scotoma (central scotoma accompanied by contralateral superotemporal visual field defect): compression at the junction of the intracranial optic nerve and the chiasm—the nasal crossing fibers of the fellow eye course anteriorly into the opposite nerve before running back to the optic tract

b. bitemporal hemianopia: compression of the chiasm—nasal retina fibers of each eye cross in the chiasm to the contralateral optic tract

C. Optic Tract
  1. Symptoms: vague visual complaints
  2. Signs
    a. normal visual acuity, APD on opposite side from lesion
    b. ophthalmoscopic examination: normal appearing optic discs or temporal pallor of the ipsilateral disc and pallor in a bow-tie pattern in the contralateral disc
  3. Visual field defects: incongruous homonymous hemianopia—temporal nerve fibers from the ipsilateral eye and nasal fibers from the contralateral eye

D. Lateral Geniculate Body
  1. Signs
    a. normal visual acuity, no APD
    b. ophthalmoscopic examination: normal appearing optic discs or temporal pallor of the ipsilateral disc and pallor in a bow-tie pattern in the contralateral disc
  2. Visual field defects
    a. incongruous homonymous hemianopia
    b. relatively congruous homonymous horizontal sectoranopia

E. Optic Radiations
  1. Temporal lobe
    a. signs
      1) normal visual acuity, no APD, normal appearing optic discs
      2) dominant lobe: aphasic, contralateral motor difficulties and hemianesthesia
      3) nondominant lobe: loss of body recognition, contralateral motor difficulties and hemianesthesia
      4) partial complex seizures
      5) formed visual hallucinations
      6) deja-vu phenomenon
    b. visual field defects: relatively congruous homonymous superior quadrantanopia—inferior fibers subserving superior visual field course anteriorly around the temporal horn to form

Meyer's loop; extensive temporal lobe lesions will cause field defects that extend into the inferior quadrants

F. Parietal lobe
  1. Signs
  a. normal visual acuity, no APD, normal appearing optic discs
  b. dominant lobe (left hemisphere 85% of patients): finger agnosia, agraphia, acalculia, right-left confusion
  c. nondominant lobe: neglect of contralateral visual and nonvisual environment
  d. spasticity of conjugate gaze: tonic deviation of the eyes to side opposite lesion on attempt at eye closure, producing Bell's phenomenon
  e. optokinetic nystagmus asymmetry: the evoked nystagmus is dampened when the stimuli are moved in the direction of the parietal lobe lesion
  2. Visual field defects: inferior quadrantanopia or congruous homonymous hemianopia denser inferiorly

G. Occipital Cortex
  1. Signs
  a. normal visual acuity, no APD, normal appearing optic discs
  b. cortical blindness: total blindness with normal pupillary response to light due to bilateral occipital lobe involvement; patients may deny blindness (Anton's syndrome) but OKN is absent
  c. palinopsia: persistence of a visual image after the stimulus has been removed
  d. unformed visual hallucinations
  2. Visual field defects
  a. congruous homonymous hemianopia
  b. central homonymous hemianopia: the macular representation is located on the tips of the occipital lobes and is separated from the cortical representation of the midperipheral and peripheral visual fields
  c. preservation of the temporal crescent: a portion of the nasal retina corresponds to an anterior area of visual cortex which may be spared by the lesion
  d. macular sparing: the hemianopia may preserve a small area around fixation rather than typically respecting the vertical meridian through fixation

II. OPTIC NEUROPATHIES

A. Optic Neuritis
1. Epidemiology:
    a. age of onset: second to fifth decades
    b. association with multiple sclerosis: after 15 years approximately 75% of patients with optic neuritis will develop definite multiple sclerosis
2. Clinical Features:
    a. history: acute unilateral loss of vision, progressing rapidly for hours to days, reaching its lowest level by 1 to 2 weeks, and gradually improving
    b. symptoms: usually monocular loss of vision but commonly bilateral in children; orbital pain exacerbated by eye movements; 6 Uthoff's sign—visual loss with exercise or other elevations of body temperature
    c. signs: visual acuity 20/20—no light perception (NLP); APD; impaired color vision
    d. visual fields defects: central, cecocentral, arcuate, altitudinal, general constriction
    e. ophthalmoscopic findings: swollen or normal appearing disc; pallor may develop choroidally; posterior vitreous cells can be seen in cases associated with systemic inflammatory conditions
    f. natural history: 20 to 30% have a second clinical episode
3. Diagnosis:
    a. MRI: obtain to assess for the risk of the development of multiple sclerosis
    b. laboratory tests: obtain in atypical cases; complete blood count (CBC), syphilis serologies, antinuclear antibody (ANA), erythrocyte sedimentation rate (ESR)
    c. lumbar puncture and neurologic examination: for those patients with additional neurological symptoms/signs
    d. differential: post viral optic neuritis, ischemic optic neuropathy, compressive optic neuropathy, Leber's hereditary optic neuropathy, syphilis, nutritional optic neuropathy, toxic optic neuropathy, sarcoidosis, systemic lupus erythematosus
    e. Lyme disease
4. Treatment:
    a. observation

    b. medical therapy: methylprednisolone 250 mg IV q 6 hours times 3 days followed by 11 days of oral prednisone 1 mg/kg/day

    c. followup: 1 and 2 weeks, then 1 and 3 months

    d. prognosis: 75 to 90% of patients recover vision to 20/30 or better, IV steroids accelerate recovery; however, do not affect the final visual acuity

B. Ischemic Optic Neuropathies

  1. Anterior ischemic optic neuropathy—ischemic infarction of the prelaminar portion of the optic nerve

    a. epidemiology:

      1) age of onset: 45 to 80 years

      2) associated systemic diseases: diabetes mellitus, hypertension, arteriosclerosis

      3) other associations in nonidiopathic cases: anemia, blood loss, surgical hypotension, postcataract surgery, postradiation therapy, migraine

    b. clinical features:

      1) symptoms: acute painless monocular visual loss

      2) signs: decreased visual acuity, minimal to severe 20/15—NLP; APD, impaired color vision

      3) visual field defects: altitudinal, arcuate or central defects

      4) ophthalmoscopic findings: pale disc swelling, often segmental with small flame hemorrhages, small cup-to-disc ratio in fellow eye; disc pallor develops over weeks to months

      5) natural history: visual loss usually maximal at onset, but may progress over a few weeks; recurrences in same eye are rare; second eye subsequently affected in 30 to 40% of cases

    c. pathology:

      1) pathogenesis: insufficiency in posterior ciliary artery circulation results in infarction of prelaminar retinal nerve fiber bundles

    d. diagnosis:

      1) laboratory tests

      2) question patient for history of giant cell arteritis (GCA) symptoms and consider obtaining ESR; if elevated, consider GCA

3) for atypical cases workup as follows: r/o diabetes, CBC, ANA, syphilis serology (workup by internist)

4) differential: giant cell arteritis, systemic lupus erythematosus, optic neuritis, syphilis, sarcoidosis, compressive optic neuropathy, Leber's hereditary optic neuropathy

e. treatment:
1) medical: no effective therapy
2) followup: one month
3) prognosis: improvement in visual function in 5 to 14%

2. Arteritic ischemic optic neuropathy (giant cell arteritis)—inflammatory disease of large and medium size arteries in patients over 55 years of age

a. epidemiology:
1) age of onset: greater than 55 years of age; peak 70 to 80
2) female to male ratio: 3:1
3) racial prevalence: more common in Caucasians

b. clinical features:
1) ocular symptoms: acute painless severe monocular visual loss, transient monocular visual loss
2) systemic symptoms: headache, jaw claudication, scalp tenderness, proximal muscle weakness and joint aches (polymyalgia rheumatica), anorexia, weight loss, fever
3) signs: severe decrease in visual acuity (majority of patients HM-NLP), APD, impaired color vision
4) visual field defects: altitudinal, arcuate or central defects
5) ophthalmoscopic findings: pale disc edema with small flame hemorrhages or normal appearing disc; disc pallor develops
6) other presentations: patients may also present with central retinal arterial occlusion, a cranial nerve palsy, or ocular ischemia symptoms
7) natural history: visual loss usually maximal at onset, 65 to 70% lose vision in second eye within 10 days without treatment, recurrences in same eye may occur

c. pathology:
1) pathogenesis: infarction secondary to inflammatory process of posterior ciliary arteries

        2) histopathology: granulomatous inflammation with giant cells, epithelioid cells, lymphocytes, and disruption of the internal elastic lamina

    d. diagnosis:

        1) laboratory tests: ESR is commonly elevated: top normal values are AGE/2 for males and (AGE + 10)/2 for females

        2) temporal artery biopsy

            a) is indicated even without visual symptoms, if GCA is suspected from symptoms, signs, or ESR (the ESR can be normal)

            b) should be performed within one week of starting systemic steroids

            c) a negative biopsy does not exclude GCA

        3) differential: idiopathic anterior ischemic optic neuropathy (AION), systemic lupus erythematosus, syphilis, sarcoidosis, optic neuritis, compressive optic neuropathy, Leber's hereditary optic neuropathy

    e. treatment:

        1) medical

            a) systemic steroids are given immediately, before biopsy, once GCA is suspected

            b) prednisone 1.5 mg/kg given po qd; may consider IV therapy for first 48 to 72 hours, methylprednisolone 250 mg q 6 hours

            c) continue prednisone 1.5 mg/kg for 2 weeks, then decrease dose 10% per week if symptoms and ESR normalize

        2) followup

            a) 1 month

            b) an internist should monitor symptomatic response and depression of the ESR, and adjust the steroid dosage accordingly

        3) prognosis: improvement in visual function is rare

C. Hereditary Optic Neuropathies

    1. Leber's hereditary optic neuropathy

        a. epidemiology:

            1) age at onset: 3 to 80 years, peak 20 to 30 years

            2) inheritance: maternal transmission of a mitochondrial DNA mutation—only females transmit the disease to their children, and all children inherit the mutation

            3) 70% of affected individuals are male

  b. clinical features:
    1) symptoms: acute or subacute painless loss of central vision: simultaneous involvement of both eyes or sequential involvement within 6 months
    2) signs: decreased visual acuity (20/200—NLP), ± APD, impaired color vision
    3) visual field defect: central or cecocentral scotomas
    4) ophthalmoscopic findings: normal appearing discs or pseudoedema of the disc with peripapillary telangiectatic vessels; optic atrophy develops
    5) natural history: visual loss progresses for up to 1 year then stabilizes, recurrences are rare
  c. pathology:
    1) mitochondrial DNA mutations; the four primary mutations are the 11778, 3460, 15257, and 14484; many secondary mutations have also been identified
  d. diagnosis:
    1) molecular genetic analysis: should be performed to identify the mitochondrial DNA mutation
    2) fluorescein angiography: demonstrates non-leaking peripapillary telangiectatic vessels if present
    3) differential: optic neuritis, nutritional or toxic optic neuropathies
  e. treatment:
    1) genetic counseling
    2) medical: no proven effective therapy, however may treat with Coenzyme Q 90 to 120 mg qd,
    3) vitamin C 2 gm qd, and Vitamin E 400 IU qd
    4) followup: 1 week, 1 and 3 months, 1 year
    5) prognosis: visual acuity stabilizes after a year in most patients; however, between 5 and 40% of individuals experience visual recovery to 20/40 or better a year or more after the onset of symptoms (dependent on the specific mutation)
2. Dominant optic atrophy
  a. epidemiology:
    1) age of onset: 4 to 10 years
    2) inheritance: autosomal dominant
  b. clinical features:
    1) symptoms: insidious bilateral loss of central vision

2) signs: decreased visual acuity (usually 20/30 to 20/70 but as poor as 20/200), impaired color vision

3) visual field defects: central, cecocentral or midzonal temporal defects

4) ophthalmoscopic findings: temporal pallor of discs, focal excavation of the temporal disc

    c. diagnosis:

1) differential: optic neuritis, nutritional or toxic neuropathies, other hereditary optic neuropathies, compressive optic neuropathy

    d. treatment:

1) no effective therapy
2) followup: 1, 3 and 6 months
3) prognosis: very slowly progressive with good prognosis

D. Traumatic Optic Neuropathy

    1. Epidemiology:

      a. two types: anterior and retrobulbar

    2. Clinical features:

      a. history: usually associated with closed head injury

      b. symptoms: decreased vision

      c. signs: decreased visual acuity, APD, impaired color vision

      d. visual field defects: central scotomas, arcuate defects, altitudinal defects, contralateral temporal defect

      e. ophthalmoscopic findings: anterior type—disc swelling with hemorrhages; retrobulbar type—normal appearing disc; chronically both types develop disc pallor

      f. natural history: visual loss usually remains static from the initial to the subsequent examinations; however, improvements and declines are observed

    3. Pathology:

      a. pathogenesis

1) shearing injury from blunt trauma; laceration by penetrating foreign body; compression by bone, hemorrhage, or edema

2) the nerve is most vulnerable in its intracanalicular portion where it is tightly adherent to the periosteum and lies in a nondistensible space

    4. Diagnosis:

           a) neuroimaging study: may demonstrate structural abnormalities adjacent to the intracanalicular optic nerve

           b) differential: other causes of decreased visual acuity following trauma

    5. Treatment:

      a. anterior type: consider optic nerve sheath fenestration

      b. retrobulbar type: steroids should be given within 8 hours of the trauma; methylprednisolone 30 mg/kg loading dose followed 2 hours later by 15 mg/kg every 6 hours for 48 hours; taper with oral prednisone over 7 to 10 days; consider surgical decompression of the canal if visual loss is delayed or if visual acuity decreases despite treatment with steroids

      c. followup: daily examinations initially; continue close followup during the steroid taper as visual acuity can relapse

      d. prognosis: irreversible severe visual loss is common despite treatment

E. Compressive Optic Neuropathy

  1. Clinical features:

    a. symptoms: transient visual obscurations; slowly progressive visual loss, may have acute onset; progressive proptosis

    b. signs: decreased visual acuity, APD, impaired color vision

    c. visual field defects: central scotomas, peripheral loss with sparing of central vision, bitemporal hemianopia

    d. external: proptosis

    e. ophthalmoscopic examination: normal appearing optic nerve, disc pallor or edema; optociliary shunt vessels; retinochoroidal striae

  2. Pathology:

    a. etiology: mass lesions including pituitary adenoma, craniopharyngioma, optic nerve glioma, malignant optic nerve glioma, meningioma; thyroid eye disease; paranasal mucocele; aneurysm

  3. Diagnosis:

    a. neuroimaging study: obtain immediately

    b. differential: optic neuritis, ischemic optic neuropathy, hereditary optic neuropathy

  4. Treatment:

    a. dependent on etiology

F. Toxic Optic Neuropathy

1. Clinical features:
   a. symptoms: painless progressive bilateral loss of vision
   b. signs: visual acuity 20/40—NLP, APD or bilaterally sluggish pupils, impaired color vision
   c. visual field defects: central or cecocentral
   d. ophthalmoscopic findings: temporal disc pallor; swollen or normal appearing discs
   e. natural history: optic atrophy
2. Pathology:
   a. etiology: tobacco/alcohol use, malnutrition (thiamine deficiency), pernicious anemia (B_{12} deficiency), medications/toxins including ethambutol, methanol, chloramphenicol, toluene, penicillamine, lead, streptomycin, isoniazid, quinine, thallium, halogenated hydroquinones, digitalis, placidyl, Antabuse, chlorpropamide
3. Diagnosis:
   a. neuroimaging study: obtain to rule out mass lesion
   b. laboratory tests: B_{12}, RBC folate, heavy metal screen
   c. differential: bilateral optic neuritis, hereditary optic neuropathies
4. Treatment:
   a. eliminate causative agent
   b. medications: thiamine 100 mg po bid, folate 1 mg po qd, and multivitamin tablet qd; vitamin B_{12} replacement for B_{12} deficiency
   c. referral to internist if patient is B_{12} deficient
   d. followup: 1, 3 and 6 months
   e. prognosis: the degree of reversibility on discontinuing the drug depends on both the total dose and nature of the drug
G. Infiltrative Optic Neuropathies
   1. Clinical features:
      a. symptoms: acute or subacute unilateral or bilateral visual loss (some patients with leukemia have asymptomatic disc swelling)
      b. signs
         1) decreased visual acuity, APD, impaired color vision
         2) ophthalmoscopic findings: normal appearing disc or disc swelling, may have a grayish-white appearance or a visible mass; disc pallor develops
   2. Pathology:
      a. etiology: tumors—glioma, leukemia, lymphoma, plasmacytoma, metastasis, meningeal carcino-

matosis; inflammatory conditions—pseudotumor, sarcoidosis; infections—cytomegalovirus,
toxoplas-mosis, tuberculosis, Lyme borreliosis,
syphilis, cryptococcosis, coccidiomycosis

3. Diagnosis:
  a. neuroimaging study, lumbar puncture
  b. workup by internist if indicated
4. Treatment
  a. dependent on etiology

III. OPTIC DISC ANOMALIES

A. Colobomas
  1. Epidemiology:
    a. age of onset: congenital
    b. inheritance: usually sporadic
  2. Clinical features:
    a. signs
      1) normal or decreased visual acuity
      2) external: associated hypertelorism or midfa-
        cial malformations may indicate a basal en-
        cephalocele
      3) ophthalmoscopic findings: enlarged disc
        with deep excavation, enlarged disc with re-
        tained glial tissue or vascular remnants, ex-
        cavated disc contiguous with retinocho-
        roidal coloboma located inferiorly
  3. Pathology:
    a. pathogenesis: faulty closure of the fetal fissure
      of the optic stalk and cup
  4. Diagnosis
    a. neuroimaging: indicated in patients with ac-
      companying hypertelorism or midfacial mal-
      formations
B. Pits
  1. Epidemiology:
    a. age of onset: congenital
  2. Clinical features:
    a. signs: usually normal visual acuity
    b. visual field defects: nerve fiber bundle defects
      extending from the blind spot towards fixation
      in the papillomacular zone
    c. ophthalmoscopic findings:
      1) pearly gray dimple or slit just within the
        disc margin approximately 1/3 of the disc
        diameter, usually single in an inferotempo-
        ral location
      2) may be associated with a serous detachment
        of the macula

3. Treatment:
   a. laser treatment may be indicated for large detachments
C. Hypoplasia
   1. Epidemiology:
      a. age of onset: congenital
      b. associations: young maternal age, maternal diabetes mellitus, use of anticonvulsants, alcohol, or hallucinogens during pregnancy
   2. Clinical features:
      a. ocular signs
         1) normal or decreased visual acuity, nystagmus
         2) visual field defects: arcuate, altitudinal, or sector; bitemporal if malformations of the chiasm are present
         3) ophthalmoscopic findings: unilateral or bilateral small disc, often surrounded by two pigmented rings (double ring sign)
      b. systemic signs (septo-optic dysplasia): central nervous system anomalies—agenesis of the septum pellucidum and hypothalamus; neuroendocrine abnormalities—growth hormone deficiency, deficiencies or hypersecretions of corticotropin and prolactin
   3. Diagnosis:
      a. MRI and endocrine evaluation: obtain in bilateral cases and in unilateral cases accompanied by growth or developmental delays
   4. Treatment:
      a. trial of occlusion therapy for amblyopia in unilateral cases in children
D. Optic Nerve Drusen
   1. Epidemiology:
      a. incidence: 0.3 to 1% of the population
      b. race: almost exclusively Caucasians
      c. inheritance: sporadic and autosomal dominant
   2. Clinical features:
      a. symptoms: transient visual obscurations
      b. signs
         1) normal visual acuity
         2) visual field defects: blind spot enlargement, arcuate defects or irregular peripheral contraction
         3) ophthalmoscopic findings: irregular, glistening, yellow globules on the disc surface; drusen may be buried creating pseudopapilledema; usually no optic cup is present and the vessels arise from the center of the

disc; frequently the vascular pattern is anomalous; bilateral in 66 to 73%

  c. natural history: buried drusen may become visible with advancing age

3. Pathology:

  a. histopathology: hyaline bodies located anterior to the lamina cribrosa; acellular laminated concretions which are often partially calcified

4. Diagnosis:

  a. ultrasonography: can confirm the presence of calcified drusen

  b. fluorescein angiography: drusen show autofluorescence prior to fluorescein dye injection

  c. CT scan: with bone window settings shows calcification

  d. differential: disc edema, papilledema

IV. PUPILLARY ABNORMALITIES

A. Anisocoria

   pupils of unequal size

1. Etiology

  a. if the pupils are normally reactive:
     1) physiologic
     2) Horner's syndrome
  b. if the pupils are abnormally reactive:
     1) iris damage
     2) Adie's tonic pupil
     3) third nerve palsy
     4) pharmacologic

2. Diagnosis

  a. determination of abnormal pupil:
     1) if there is more anisocoria in dim illumination or a good light reaction is present in both pupils, then the smaller pupil is abnormal
     2) if there is more anisocoria in bright illumination or a poor light reaction is present in one eye, then the larger pupil is abnormal

B. Horner's Syndrome

1. Clinical features

  a. symptoms: ptosis, asymmetric pupils
  b. ocular signs: the smaller pupil is abnormal with greater anisocoria with dim illumination, dilation lag is present in the affected pupil, mild ptosis on same side as small pupil, iris heterochromia in congenital cases (lighter color on involved side)
  c. other signs: anhidrosis ipsilateral side of body (first order neuron involvement), anhidrosis ip-

silateral face (second order neuron), no anhidrosis or involving only the forehead (third order neuron)

   2. Pathology
      a. pathogenesis: lesion involving the sympathetic pathway
      b. etiology
         1) first order neuron disorder: CNS lesions, infarction, tumor, demyelination
         2) second order neuron disorder: apical lung tumor, metastasis, trauma to the brachial plexus, thoracic aortic aneurysm, thyroid neoplasm
         3) third order neuron disorder: cluster headaches, migraine, Raeder's paratrigeminal syndrome, dissection of the carotid artery, herpes zoster
   3. Diagnosis
      a. instill cocaine 10% into both eyes; if both eyes dilate, the anisocoria is physiologic; Horner's is present if the smaller pupil fails to dilate
      b. to locate lesion wait 48 hours post cocaine instillation: instill 1% hydroxyamphetamine into involved eye; if the pupil dilates then the lesion involves a first or second order neuron (preganglionic); if the pupil fails to dilate the lesion involves a third order neuron (postganglionic)
      c. if preganglionic: obtain chest imaging (x-ray, CT, MRI), especially of apex, and neurologic examination
      d. if postganglionic: usually a benign lesion and further evaluation is usually unnecessary
C. Adie's Tonic Pupil
   1. Epidemiology:
      a. age of onset: peak 20 to 40 years
      b. female predilection: 70% female, 30% male
   2. Clinical features:
      a. symptoms: asymmetric pupils, blurred vision
      b. ocular signs: the larger pupil is abnormal with an increase in anisocoria in bright illumination; the pupil is poorly reactive to light, slowly constricts to convergence and slowly redilates; can be bilateral
      c. systemic signs: deep tendon reflexes are diminished or absent
      d. natural history: pupil may get smaller with time, opposite pupil becomes involved in 4% of patients per year

   3. Pathology:
      a. etiology: unknown; other causes of tonic pupils include herpes zoster and varicella, trauma, temporal arteritis, diabetes, syphilis, Riley-Day syndrome
   4. Diagnosis:
      a. instill pilocarpine 0.1% in both eyes; if the anisocoria is due to Adie's, the involved pupil will constrict and the normal pupil will not
      b. differential: Parinaud's syndrome
   5. Treatment:
      a. pilocarpine 0.05% for photophobia
D. Third Nerve Palsy
   1. Clinical features:
      a. signs: the larger pupil is abnormal with an increase in anisocoria in bright illumination, unreactive to light or convergence
   2. Pathology:
      a. pathogenesis: involvement of the parasympathetic pathway
      b. etiology: isolated pupillary dilation without other signs of third nerve palsy occurs with uncal herniation and basal meningitis
   3. Diagnosis:
      a. instill pilocarpine 0.1% in both eyes; if neither eye constricts, the anisocoria may be due to a third nerve palsy or pharmacologic block
      b. instill pilocarpine 1%; if the dilated pupil fails to constrict while the normal pupil constricts, the dilated pupil is secondary to pharmacologic mydriasis. If both pupils constrict, the cause is a third nerve palsy
   4. Treatment:
      a. immediate medical attention is necessary
E. Argyll Robertson Pupils
   1. Clinical features
      a. symptoms: usually asymptomatic
      b. signs
         1) small pupils, often irregular, do not react to light but do react to convergence, dilation is poor after instillation of mydriatics
         2) slit lamp: iris atrophy, portions of the iris transilluminate, interstitial keratitis may be present
         3) ophthalmoscopic findings: old chorioretinitis, optic atrophy
   2. Pathology:
      a. pathogenesis: tertiary syphilis in most cases; also seen rarely in diabetes, sarcoid, and encephalitis
   3. Diagnosis:

    a. syphilis serology: FTA-ABS or MHA-TP will be positive; VDRL or RPR may be negative

    b. lumbar puncture: greater than 5 WBC/mm^3, protein greater than 45mg/dl, or positive VDRL may indicate neurosyphilis

4. Treatment:

    a. referral to internist or neurologist for workup including

        1) HIV serology

        2) IV penicillin 2 to 4 million units q 4 hours times 10 to 14 days

V. SUPRANUCLEAR CONTROL OF EYE MOVEMENTS

A. Control of Conjugate Horizontal Eye Movements

    1. Saccadic system

        a. saccades: fast eye movements that bring objects of interest onto the fovea; may be voluntary or involuntary

        b. anatomy: horizontal saccades originate in the contralateral frontal lobe, the descending pathway decussates at the midbrain-pontine junction and terminates in the paramedian pontine reticular formation (PPRF) contralateral to the hemisphere of origin

        c. pathology:

            1) congenital oculomotor apraxia: inability to initiate normal voluntary horizontal saccades while random saccades and smooth pursuit movements are preserved; head thrusting is used to change fixation

            2) frontal gaze palsy: trauma to one frontal lobe produces a gaze preference toward the side of the lesion and a paucity of saccades contralaterally, the uninjured frontal lobe can produce ipsilateral saccades with effort

            3) opsoclonus: chaotic multidirectional saccades associated with a postviral encephalopathic syndrome, neuroblastoma, and visceral carcinomas

            4) progressive supranuclear palsy: progressive slowing and diminishing of amplitude of voluntary saccades and eventual loss of pursuit; frequently affecting downward gaze first followed by upward gaze and horizontal movements; associated with axial rigidity, dementia, dysarthria, and death over a course of 5 to 10 years

5) degenerative disorders associated with slowed or paretic conjugate saccades: multiple sclerosis, Wilson's disease, ataxia telangiectasia, Whipple's disease, Huntington's chorea, progressive multifocal leukoencephalopathy, lipid storage diseases

2. Paramedian pontine reticular formation (PPRF)

    a. brainstem center subserving conjugate ipsilateral horizontal eye movements

    b. anatomy: the PPRF sends axons to the ipsilateral sixth nerve nucleus which consists of large motor cells whose axons form the ipsilateral sixth cranial nerve and small interneurons whose axons cross immediately and ascend in the contralateral medial longitudinal fasciculus (MLF) to end in the medial rectus subnuclei of the third cranial nerve

    c. pathology: gaze paresis—injury either to the PPRF or sixth nerve nucleus produces an ipsilateral gaze paresis; the ipsilateral eye is unable to abduct and the contralateral eye is unable to adduct

3. Smooth pursuit system

    a. slow eye movements: used for tracking continuously moving targets

    b. anatomy: smooth pursuits originate in the ipsilateral parieto-occipital lobe; the projection pathways in the brainstem are unknown

    c. pathology:

        1) unilateral pursuit paresis: a lesion in the region of the parieto-occipital junction produces a loss of ipsilateral pursuit, contralateral homonymous visual field defect, and an attenuation of the optokinetic response when the stimulus is rotated toward the side of the lesion; a lesion in the cerebellar flocculus similarly produces loss of ipsilateral pursuit

        2) bilateral pursuit paresis: caused by diffuse posterior hemispheric, cerebellar, or brainstem disease; sedative drugs can cause saccadic pursuit

B. Control of Conjugate Vertical Eye Movements

    1. Anatomy: the detailed neuroanatomy is unknown; the rostral end of the PPRF probably acts as a vertical gaze center with projections to the rostral interstitial nucleus of the medial longitudinal fasciculus—the final common pathway for conjugate vertical saccades; the interstitial nucleus of Cajal in the rostral mesencephalon may also play a role

2. Pathology:
   a. paralysis of upgaze: associated with compressive lesions at the level of the posterior commissure, such as pineal region tumors, hydrocephalus, and hemorrhage
3. Parinaud's syndrome consists of paralysis of upgaze and occasionally downgaze, lid retraction (Collier's sign), light-near dissociation of the pupils, convergence retraction nystagmus, papilledema
   a. skew deviation: is a nonlocalizing vertical misalignment of the eyes, may be seen in conjunction with a unilateral internuclear ophthalmoplegia

C. Vergence System
1. Disconjugate slow eye movements that allow bifoveal fixation at all points in space from infinity to the near point of convergence; convergence is a component of the "near triad" which also includes accommodation and pupillary constriction
2. Anatomy: the detailed neuroanatomy is not known
3. Pathology: spasm of the near reflex, convergence paralysis, divergence insufficiency, and paralysis

VI. INTERNUCLEAR OPHTHALMOPLEGIA (INO)

A. Clinical features:
1. Symptoms: ± diplopia
2. Signs: ipsilateral eye adducts slowly, incompletely, or not at all, while the abducting eye exhibits horizontal nystagmus; ± skew deviation (either eye is turned up but the pattern of deviation is not isolated to a specific muscle); ± vertical upbeat nystagmus in upgaze
3. Walled-eyed bilateral INO (WEBINO) occasionally patients exhibit an exotropia "One-and-a-half" syndrome (Fisher's paralytic pontine exotropia): injury to the PPRF or sixth nerve nucleus results in an ipsilateral paralysis of gaze (the one) and simultaneous injury to the adjacent MLF results in an ipsilateral INO (the half)

B. Pathology:
1. Pathogenesis: lesion in the ipsilateral medial longitudinal fasciculus which extends from the contralateral PPRF to the ipsilateral third nerve nucleus
2. Etiology: multiple sclerosis, ischemic vascular disease of the brainstem, brainstem tumor

3. Diagnosis:
   a. special maneuvers: optokinetic testing or repetitive horizontal saccadic refixations can be used to diagnose more subtle cases where the only sign is a slowed saccadic response of the medial rectus muscle
   b. neuroimaging of the brainstem and midbrain required
   c. differential: myasthenia gravis
4. Treatment:
   a. directed at underlying cause

VII. NYSTAGMUS

A. Physiologic
   1. Endpoint nystagmus: a fine amplitude horizontal jerk nystagmus found in extreme gaze positions
   2. Optokinetic nystagmus: a jerk nystagmus elicited by moving a repetitive visual pattern within the visual field
   3. Vestibular jerk nystagmus: a jerk nystagmus which can be induced by stimulating the peripheral vestibular apparatus by either rotational or caloric testing
   4. Latent nystagmus: a jerk nystagmus induced by covering one eye
B. Congenital
   1. Epidemiology:
      a. onset: 2 to 3 months of age
   2. Clinical features:
      a. symptoms: no complaint of oscillopsia
      b. signs
         1) can exist with or without afferent visual system dysfunction
         2) can vary from an overt jerk nystagmus to what appears as purely pendular, almost always conjugate and horizontal
         3) may worsen with attempted distance fixation and dampen with convergence and near fixation
         4) usually a null point is present—a position of gaze where the oscillatory movements are minimized; patients frequently develop a head turn to place the null point in the straight ahead position
         5) a head nod may develop that may be compensatory or part of the pathologic process
   3. Pathology:
      a. etiology

        1) idiopathic
        2) associated with afferent visual system dysfunction: Leber's congenital amaurosis, aniridia, albinism, achromatopsia, bilateral optic nerve hypoplasia, etc.

   4. Treatment:
      a. Kestenbaum procedure—recession of one pair of yoke muscles with simultaneous resection of the other pair to move the null point from an eccentric position to the primary position

C. Spasmus Nutans
   1. Epidemiology:
      a. onset: 4 to 14 months or as late as 3 1/2 years
   2. Clinical features:
      a. triad of signs
         1) nystagmus: horizontal or vertical, low amplitude, pendular; appears monocular but fine conjugate shimmering motions are usually present in the other eye
         2) torticollis
         3) head nodding: rhythmic, disappearing with sleep and change in head position
      b. natural history: often lasts less than 1 month but may last months to years; usually disappears by age 5
   3. Diagnosis:
      a. MRI: exclude chiasmal gliomas and third ventricular tumors which may present similarly

D. Acquired Horizontal Nystagmus
   1. Vestibular nystagmus
      a. dysfunction of the vestibular end organ, nerve or nuclear complex
      b. symptoms: vertigo
      c. signs: primary position horizontal jerk nystagmus which may have a torsional component; the intensity increases with gaze toward the fast phase
      d. causes: peripheral—labyrinthitis, neuronitis, trauma, ischemia; CNS—tumor, trauma, ischemia
   2. Gaze-evoked nystagmus
      a. signs: a jerk nystagmus elicited by the attempt to maintain an eccentric eye position, the fast phase is in the direction of gaze
      b. causes: bilateral—sedative or anticonvulsant medications, brainstem lesion, cerebellar disease; unilateral—labyrinthine dysfunction
   3. Rebound nystagmus

        a. signs: jerk-type horizontal nystagmus with rapid phase initially directed toward the position of gaze, but which reverses direction after several seconds of eccentric gaze; it fatigues with sustained fixation

        b. causes: cerebellar or brainstem parenchymal disease or other posterior fossa lesions

    4. Periodic alternating nystagmus

        a. may be congenital in some cases

        b. signs: a periodic reversal of the direction of the horizontal jerk nystagmus

        c. causes: craniocervical junction anomalies, posterior fossa tumors, multiple sclerosis, ischemia, syphilis

        d. treatment: baclofen abolishes some acquired cases of nystagmus

E. Acquired Vertical Nystagmus

    1. Upbeat nystagmus

        a. signs: primary position nystagmus with the fast phase beating upward

        b. causes: anterior vermis or lower brainstem lesions, drug intoxication or Wernicke's encephalopathy

    2. Downbeat nystagmus

        a. symptoms: oscillopsia

        b. signs: primary position nystagmus with the fast phase beating downward

        c. causes: disorders of the craniocervical junction (especially Chiari malformations), spinocerebellar degeneration, alcohol abuse, multiple sclerosis

    3. See-saw nystagmus

        a. signs: one eye rises and intorts while the other eye falls and extorts

        b. field defects: bitemporal hemianopias (third ventricle tumors)

        c. causes: third ventricle tumors, upper brainstem vascular disease, head trauma

VIII. OCULOMOTOR PALSIES

A. General Clinical Features

    1. Symptoms: double vision which disappears when one eye is closed, droopy eyelid, ± pain

    2. Signs: ptosis; loss of adduction, elevation, and depression; pupil may be dilated, sluggish, or spared

B. Nuclear Lesions

    1. Signs

    a. third nerve palsy on same side as lesion with paresis of the contralateral superior rectus muscle: each superior rectus is innervated by the contralateral third nerve nucleus while the inferior rectus, medial rectus and inferior oblique are innervated by the ipsilateral third nerve nucleus

    b. bilateral ptosis: both levators are innervated by one structure, the central caudal nucleus

    c. pupillary involvement either bilateral or absent: parasympathetic innervation to the pupils is from a midline structure, the visceral nucleus

  2. Etiology: infarction, demyelination, tumor

C. Fascicular Lesions

  1. Signs

    a. ipsilateral third nerve paresis and contralateral cerebellar ataxia (Nothnagel's syndrome): lesion in area of the superior cerebellar peduncle

    b. ipsilateral third nerve paresis with contralateral hemitremor (Benedikt's syndrome): lesion in the region of the red nucleus

    c. ipsilateral third nerve paresis with contralateral hemiparesis (Weber's syndrome): lesion in the area of the cerebral peduncle

  2. Etiology: infarction, demyelination, tumor

D. Interpeduncular Lesions

  1. Uncal herniation

    a. signs: unilateral dilated and fixed pupil: compression of the third nerve on the tentorial edge by the uncal portion of the temporal lobe

    b. etiology: supratentorial space-occupying mass

  2. Posterior communicating artery aneurysm

    a. symptoms: ± symptoms of subarachnoid hemorrhage

    b. signs

      1) painful third nerve paresis with pupillary involvement: compression of the third nerve at the junction of the posterior communicating artery and the internal carotid artery

      2) ± signs of subarachnoid hemorrhage

    c. pathogenesis: hemorrhage suddenly enlarges the sac to which the nerve is adherent or there is actual hemorrhage into the nerve itself

    d. diagnosis: acute third nerve palsy with pupillary involvement requires emergent arteriography to exclude an aneurysm

E. Cavernous Sinus Lesions

  1. Signs

a. third nerve palsy associated with other cranial nerve involvement: fourth, fifth, sixth and sympathetic paresis
b. third nerve paresis tends to be partial and the pupillary fibers tend to be spared

2. Etiology: carotid-cavernous fistula, granulomatous inflammation (Tolosa-Hunt), aneurysm, pituitary tumor, meningioma, extension of primary paranasal sinus or nasopharyngeal carcinoma, metastatic tumor, fungus (especially mucormycosis), herpes zoster

F. Orbital Lesions
   1. Signs
      a. third nerve palsy with ± proptosis, lid edema, chemosis, conjunctival hyperemia, other cranial nerve involvement
      b. the superior or inferior division may be individually involved: superior division innervates the superior rectus and levator palpebrae; the inferior division innervates the inferior and medial rectus, the inferior oblique, the iris sphincter, and ciliary muscle
   2. Etiology: pseudotumor, trauma, tumor, mucormycosis

G. Isolated Pupil-Sparing Third Nerve Palsy
   1. Signs: ± painful third nerve paresis which tends to be complete except for sparing of the pupillary fibers
   2. Etiology: most commonly due to ischemia, however neoplasm, inflammation, and even aneurysm are possible
   3. Diagnosis
      a. if patient is over 40 years of age with a history of diabetes or hypertension observe; followup within 5 days to assess for the development of pupillary involvement, if no pupillary involvement f/u every 6 weeks until recovery; improvement should begin in 1 month and complete resolution in approximately 3 months
      b. if patient is over 40 without a history of diabetes or hypertension or is less than 40, workup as follows: blood pressure, CBC, ESR, r/o diabetes, syphilis serology, ANA, and neuroimaging study
      c. if palsy is progressive or chronic, aberrant regeneration occurs, pupil becomes involved, or other neurologic signs develop: obtain neuroimaging study

    d. if above studies are negative obtain cerebral angiogram to exclude aneurysm

    e. consider a tensilon test to rule out myasthenia

4. Differential: myasthenia gravis, thyroid eye disease, chronic progressive external ophthalmoplegia

5. Treatment:

    a. directed at underlying cause

    b. patch the involved eye to relieve diplopia

    c. strabismus surgery may be performed in symptomatic patients after the examination has been stable for at least 6 months

H. Special Syndromes of the Third Nerve

  1. Aberrant regeneration

    a. misdirected regeneration of disrupted third nerve fibers

      1) primary: no preceding acute third nerve palsy; usually a sign of intracavernous meningioma or aneurysm

      2) secondary: weeks to months after acute third nerve palsy; almost never seen in an ischemic third nerve palsy

    b. signs

      1) the upper lid may elevate on attempted adduction or depression

      2) retraction of the globe may occur with attempted vertical gaze

      3) segmental constriction of the pupil may occur with attempted vertical gaze, adduction, or both (especially down and in)

  2. Ophthalmoplegic migraine

    a. epidemiology: extremely rare, usually occurring in children before age 8, family history of migraine

    b. symptoms: pain around eye, nausea, and vomiting may accompany third nerve paresis, often with pupillary involvement

    c. natural history: usually complete resolution within 1 month

    d. diagnosis: obtain MRI to rule out other causes; however, if negative, the need to obtain angiography is controversial

  3. Cyclic oculomotor palsy

    a. epidemiology: extremely rare, onset at birth or early childhood

    b. signs: intermittent third nerve palsy alternating with normal eye movement

IX. TROCHLEAR NERVE PALSIES

A. General Clinical Features
   1. Symptoms: vertical or oblique double vision which disappears when one eye is closed, sensation that objects appear tilted, difficulty reading
   2. Signs: deficiency of movement of the eye in a down and in position, hypertropia of the involved eye unless patient fixates with involved eye, patient maintains a head tilt toward the contralateral shoulder to prevent double vision
B. Nuclear-Fascicular Lesions
   1. Signs
      a. fourth nerve palsy on the opposite side of the lesion: the fourth nerve fascicles cross in the anterior medullary vellum, prior to exiting posteriorly and coursing anteriorly to innervate the contralateral superior oblique muscle
      b. an associated Horner's syndrome in the contralateral eye may be seen in fascicular lesions: the sympathetic fibers pass through the dorsolateral tegmentum of the midbrain adjacent to the trochlear fascicles
      c. relative afferent pupillary defect (RAPD) may occur on ipsilateral or contralateral side with involvement of afferent fibers in the brachium of the superior colliculus
   2. Etiology: infarction, hemorrhage, demyelination, trauma, tumor
C. Subarachnoid Space Lesions
   1. Etiology: trauma is most common, others include meningitis or tumor
   2. Pathogenesis: contrecoup forces are transmitted to the brainstem by the free tentorial edge; the nerve is injured in the anterior medullary velum as it emerges from the dorsal brainstem
D. Cavernous Sinus Lesion
   1. Signs: fourth nerve palsy associated with other cranial nerve involvement: third, fifth, sixth, and sympathetic paresis
   2. Etiology: carotid-cavernous fistula, granulomatous inflammation (Tolosa-Hunt), aneurysm, pituitary tumor, meningioma, extension of primary paranasal sinus, or nasopharyngeal carcinoma, metastatic tumor, fungus (especially mucormycosis), herpes zoster
   3. Diagnosis: a coexisting fourth nerve palsy in the setting of a third nerve palsy can be diagnosed by assessing for the presence of intorsion as the eye

is abducted and the patient is instructed to look down

E. Orbital Lesion
  1. Signs: fourth nerve palsy with ±proptosis, lid edema, chemosis, conjunctival hyperemia, other cranial nerve involvement
  2. Etiology: pseudotumor, trauma, tumor, mucormycosis

F. Isolated Fourth Nerve Palsy
  1. Congenital
    a. epidemiology: most often seen in children and in adults greater than 40 years of age (decompensation later in life)
    b. diagnosis:
      1) examine old photographs to detect long-standing head tilt
      2) perform the Parks-Bielschowsky three-step test to confirm fourth nerve palsy:
        a) Which eye is higher in primary position?—the paretic superior oblique is present in the eye with hypertropia
        b) Is the hypertropia worse in right or left gaze?—the paretic S.O. will cause a worsening of the hypertropia in the position of gaze where the involved eye is adducted
        c) Is the hypertropia worse on head tilt to the right or left shoulder?—the paretic S.O. will cause a worsening of the hypertropia when the head is tilted to the shoulder on the same side as the involved eye
      3) large vertical fusion amplitudes are seen in congenital fourth nerve palsies (10 to 15 prism diopters)
      4) double Maddox rod test to quantitate torsional component of diplopia; greater than 10 degrees is suggestive of bilateral fourth nerve palsies
      5) no neuroimaging study is necessary for congenital palsies
    c. treatment: strabismus surgery is indicated for symptomatic patients
  2. Acquired
    a. signs: absence of both longstanding head tilt and large vertical fusion amplitudes
    b. etiology: trauma, infarction, inflammation, tumor, aneurysm
    c. diagnosis:

1) perform the Parks-Bielschowsky three-step test to confirm fourth nerve palsy
2) if patient is over 40 years of age with a history of diabetes or hypertension observe: improvement should begin in 1 month and complete resolution in approximately 3 months
3) if patient is over 40 without a history of diabetes or hypertension or is less than 40, workup as follows:
   a) blood pressure, CBC, ESR, r/o diabetes, syphilis
   b) serology, ANA and neuroimaging study
4) if palsy is progressive or chronic, or other neurologic signs develop obtain neuroimaging study
5) consider a tensilon or prostigmine test to rule out myasthenia

d. differential: myasthenia, thyroid eye disease, skew deviation
e. treatment:
   1) directed at underlying cause
   2) followup every 6 weeks until recovery
   3) patch involved eye to relieve diplopia—prisms usually not helpful
   4) strabismus surgery may be performed in symptomatic patients after the examination has been stable for at least 6 months

G. Superior Oblique Myokymia
  1. Symptoms: blurred vision from the tremor, oscillopsia, oblique diplopia
  2. Signs: arrhythmic twitching of the superior oblique muscle documented by observing a conjunctival vessel at the slit lamp or a retinal vessel on ophthalmoscopy in one eye only
  3. Pathogenesis: unknown
  4. Natural history: remission and exacerbations lasting years
  5. Diagnosis: by history and observation at slit lamp; neuroimaging to rule out intracranial mass unnecessary
  6. Treatment: reassurance, carbamazepine, surgery (superior oblique tenotomy, inferior oblique myotomy)

X. ABDUCENS NERVE PALSIES

A. General Clinical Features

       1. Symptoms: horizontal double vision which disappears when one eye is closed, worse at distance than at near, worse in right or left gaze

       2. Signs: deficiency of abduction in one eye, esotropia

B. Nuclear Lesions

       1. A lesion in the sixth nerve nucleus causes a horizontal gaze palsy and not a sixth nerve palsy: the sixth nerve nucleus consists of both motor cells whose axons form the ipsilateral sixth cranial nerve, and small interneurons whose axons ascend in the contralateral medial longitudinal fasciculus to end in the medial rectus nuclei

C. Fascicular Lesions

       1. Signs:

           a. may be isolated

           b. sixth nerve palsy associated with ipsilateral seventh nerve palsy and contralateral hemiparesis (Millard-Gubler's syndrome)

           c. sixth nerve palsy associated with contralateral hemiparesis (Raymond's syndrome)

       2. Etiology: infarction, demyelination, tumor, infection (e.g., Listeria)

D. Subarachnoid Space Lesions

       1. Etiology:

           a. increased intracranial pressure; downward displacement of the brainstem causes stretching of the sixth nerve which is tethered where it exits the pons and enters Dorello's canal

           b. pseudotumor cerebri; 30% of patients have a sixth nerve palsy secondary to increased intracranial pressure, in addition to papilledema or visual field deficits

           c. postlumbar puncture, epidural, or spinal anesthesia

           d. hemorrhage, meningitis, inflammation, infiltration, tumor

E. Petrous Bone Lesions

       1. Petrous bone abscess

           a. signs: sixth nerve palsy associated with ipsilateral seventh and eighth nerve palsy and pain in the distribution of the fifth nerve (Gradenigo's syndrome)

           b. pathogenesis: the portion of the sixth nerve in Dorello's canal is affected by an extradural abscess of the petrous apex following complicated otitis media

       2. Petrous bone fracture

           a. signs:

           1) the fifth, sixth, seventh, and eighth nerves may be involved following head trauma

           2) associated findings: hemotympanum, CSF otorrhea, Battle's sign (ecchymosis over the mastoid)

      b. pathogenesis: basal skull fracture

F. Cavernous Sinus Lesions

    1. Signs: sixth nerve palsy usually associated with other cranial nerve involvement: third, fourth, fifth, and sympathetic paresis

    2. Etiology: carotid-cavernous fistula, granulomatous inflammation (Tolosa-Hunt), aneurysm, pituitary tumor, meningioma, extension of paranasal or nasopharyngeal carcinoma, metastatic tumor, fungus (especially mucormycosis), herpes zoster

G. Orbital Lesions

    1. Signs: sixth nerve palsy with $\pm$ proptosis, lid edema, chemosis, conjunctival hyperemia, other cranial nerve involvement

    2. Etiology: inflammation, trauma, tumor, infection (e.g., bacterial, fungal, viral)

H. Isolated Sixth Nerve Palsy

    1. Etiology: postviral syndrome (children), infarction, trauma, tumor, demyelination, inflammation, infection

    2. Diagnosis:

      a. if patient is under 14 years of age observe: initially evaluate every 2 weeks to assess for progression or development of other neurologic signs; neuroimaging study at discretion of physician and parents

      b. if patient is over 40 years of age with a history of diabetes or hypertension, observe: improvement should begin in 1 month and complete resolution in approximately 3 months

      c. if patient is over 40 without a history of diabetes or hypertension or is between 15 and 40, workup as follows: blood pressure, CBC, ESR, r/o diabetes, syphilis serology, ANA, and neuroimaging

      d. if palsy is chronic or other neurologic signs develop, obtain neuroimaging study

      e. consider a tensilon test to rule out myasthenia and forced ductions to rule out a restrictive myopathy

    3. Differential: myasthenia gravis, thyroid eye disease, Duane's syndrome, spasm of the near reflex, congenital esotropia with break in fusion, restrictive myopathy secondary to orbital wall fracture

4. Treatment
   a. directed at underlying cause
   b. followup every 6 weeks until recovery
   c. patch involved eye to relieve diplopia
   d. occlusion therapy may be needed for patients less than 8 to 10 years old to prevent amblyopia (also true for third and fourth nerve palsies)
   e. strabismus surgery may be performed in symptomatic patients after the examination has been stable for at least 6 months

XI. FACIAL NERVE PALSY AND RELATED DISORDERS

A. Supranuclear Lesions
  1. Signs
     a. contralateral weakness of the lower two-thirds of the face: the precentral motor cortex of the frontal lobe controls volitional facial movement; the fibers subserving the upper face distribute to both facial nuclei, while those subserving the lower face solely supply the contralateral nucleus; thus a unilateral hemispheric lesion spares the forehead
  2. Etiology: infarction, tumor
B. Nuclear Lesions
  1. Signs:
     a. seventh nerve palsy with weakness of the ipsilateral side of the face associated with other pontine disturbances including fifth and sixth nerve involvement, horizontal gaze palsy, cerebellar ataxia, and contralateral hemiparesis
     b. a dissociation between the autonomic, sensory, and motor functions of the facial nerve may be present: lacrimation and salivation are supplied by parasympathetic fibers from the superior salivatory nucleus, and taste and other visceral and somatic sensory functions are supplied by sensory fibers from the solitary nucleus; the parasympathetic and sensory fibers join to form the nervus intermedius, which join the motor fibers to become the facial nerve
  2. Etiology: tumor, infarction, demyelination, infection
C. Infranuclear Lesions
  1. Cerebellopontine angle tumor
     a. signs: seventh nerve palsy with weakness of the ipsilateral side of the face associated with

decreased tearing, hyperacusis, decreased taste on the anterior two-thirds of tongue
   b. other associated neurologic signs: fifth, sixth, and eighth nerve palsies, Horner's syndrome, horizontal gaze palsy, cerebellar ataxia
   c. etiology: acoustic neuroma, meningioma, metastatic carcinoma
2. Geniculate ganglionitis (Ramsey-Hunt syndrome)
   a. signs:
      1) seventh nerve palsy with weakness of the ipsilateral side of the face associated with decreased tearing, hyperacusis, decreased taste on the anterior two-thirds of tongue
      2) vesicles over tympanic membrane and along the posterior aspect of the external auditory meatus (sensory distribution of the facial nerve)
   b. other associated neurologic signs: ± eighth nerve palsy: the seventh and eighth travel together in the internal auditory canal
   c. etiology: herpes zoster
3. Vidian nerve or sphenopalatine ganglion lesion
   a. signs:
      1) isolated ipsilateral tearing deficiency: the parasympathetic fibers leave the genu as the greater superficial petrosal nerve, join the deep petrosal nerve to become the vidian nerve and then synapse in the sphenopalatine ganglion before supplying the lacrimal gland via the zygomaticotemporal branch of V2 and the lacrimal branch of V1
      2) ± sixth nerve palsy if cavernous sinus is involved
   b. etiology: nasopharyngeal carcinoma
4. Bell's palsy
   a. an acute peripheral facial palsy of unknown etiology (a diagnosis of exclusion)
   b. symptoms: weakness of one side of the face, pain around the ear, facial numbness, numbness of the tongue, changes in taste, decreased tearing
   c. signs:
      1) seventh nerve palsy with weakness of the ipsilateral side of the face associated with ±decreased tearing, hyperacusis, decreased taste on the anterior two-thirds of tongue
      2) absence of other neurological deficits

    d. pathogenesis: idiopathic facial nerve palsy—secondary to edema of nerve within the fallopian canal

    e. diagnosis: if the facial nerve palsy progresses for longer than 3 weeks obtain neuroimaging study to rule out tumor

    f. treatment: the use of oral steroids is controversial, monitoring for corneal exposure is necessary in those patients with significant involvement of the orbicularis oculi

    g. prognosis: 75% of patients experience complete recovery, others have incomplete recovery and aberrant degeneration

D. Special Syndromes of the Seventh Nerve

    1. Möbius syndrome

      a. congenital bilateral seventh nerve palsies; ± bilateral sixth nerve palsies, palatal and lingual palsies, deafness, syndactyly, supernumerary, or absent digits

    2. Essential blepharospasm

      a. signs: bilateral involuntary contracture of the orbicularis oculi: may involve the lower facial musculature—Meige's syndrome

      b. etiology: unknown

      c. diagnosis: rule out causes of reflex blepharospasm (e.g., dry eye, intraocular inflammation)

      d. treatment: botulinum toxin or surgical orbicularis stripping

    3. Hemifacial spasm

      a. signs: unilateral spasm of the facial muscles; episodic, lasting several minutes

      b. pathogenesis: aberrant vascular loop causing compression of the seventh nerve as it exits the pons

      c. diagnosis: obtain MRI

      d. treatment: botulinum toxin or craniotomy with placement of sponge between vascular loop and seventh nerve

XII. CAVERNOUS SINUS LESIONS

A. Clinical Features:

    1. Symptoms: diplopia, ptosis, facial pain, or numbness

    2. Ocular signs:

      a. usually no visual acuity loss, ipsilateral pupil may be miotic (from oculo-sympathetic involvement) or dilated, ± APD

        b. external: ipsilateral ptosis, ± proptosis, decreased sensation in V1, V2, and V3 distribution

        c. motility: third, fourth, and sixth nerve palsies (see respective chapters)

        d. ophthalmoscopic findings: usually normal

B. Pathology
    1. Etiology: trauma; vascular—carotid cavernous fistula, cavernous sinus thrombosis, posterior cerebral artery aneurysm, intracavernous carotid artery aneurysm; neoplasm—carcinomatous meningitis, craniopharyngioma, pituitary adenoma, meningioma, neurofibroma, chordoma, perineural spread of squamous cell carcinoma, metastases; inflammation—sinusitis, mucocele, periostitis, herpes zoster, mucormycosis, tuberculosis, sarcoidosis, Wegener's granulomatosis, Tolosa-Hunt syndrome

C. Diagnosis
    1. Neuroimaging
    2. Differential: myasthenia, giant cell arteritis, thyroid eye disease, orbital lesions, chronic progressive external ophthalmoplegia (CPEO), brainstem disease

D. Arterial—Venous Fistula
    1. Epidemiology:
        a. associations: 25% spontaneous, 75% cerebral trauma
    2. Clinical features:
        a. history: recent or remote head trauma
        b. symptoms: red eye, pain in or around eye, subjective bruit, proptosis
        c. signs: (can be unilateral or bilateral, large spectrum of clinical findings)
            1) normal or decreased visual acuity
            2) external: lid edema, pulsating exophthalmos, ocular or cephalic bruit
            3) motility: third, fourth, and sixth nerve palsies or generalized mechanical limitation of motion
            4) slit lamp: conjunctival arterialization, chemosis, corneal edema, anterior chamber cell/flare, iris rubeosis, rapidly progressive cataract, increased intraocular pressure
        d. ophthalmoscopic findings: venous congestion, disc edema, retinal hemorrhage
        e. natural history: spontaneous closure occurs in 10 to 60%, usually the slow-flow dural variety
    3. Pathology:

      a. pathogenesis: a rent in the wall of the artery allows short circuiting of the arterial blood into the venous complex of the cavernous sinus; either a direct shunt between internal carotid artery and the cavernous sinus (direct or high-flow carotid cavernous sinus fistula) or a dural shunt between meningeal branches of the internal carotid or external carotid arteries (low flow)

   4. Diagnosis:

      a. CT scan or MRI: prominence of the superior ophthalmic vein, lateral bulging of the cavernous sinus, extraocular muscle enlargement

      b. ultrasound: shows increase in the size of the superior ophthalmic vein

      c. color doppler: shows increase in the size of the superior ophthalmic vein with reversal of blood flow

      d. angiography: definitive diagnosis—must look at both internal and external carotid arteries to determine all feeders

   5. Treatment:

      a. indication for intervention: visual deterioration, intolerable subjective bruit, head or eye pain unresponsive to medical treatment, involvement of cortical veins

      b. goal: thrombosis of fistula

      c. methods: controlled embolization or intravascular closure with detachable balloon through arterial or venous routes

E. Cavernous Sinus Thrombosis

   1. Clinical features:

      a. systemic symptoms: headache, nausea, vomiting, somnolence

      b. ocular signs (unilateral signs may become bilateral):

         1) visual loss, miotic or dilated pupil, APD

         2) external: lid edema, proptosis

         3) motility: early sixth nerve palsy evolves to complete paresis

         4) slit lamp: chemosis, corneal anesthesia, increased intraocular pressure

         5) ophthalmoscopic findings: venous congestion, disc edema

      c. natural history: 30% mortality regardless of treatment

   2. Pathology:

      a. etiology:

           1) aseptic: trauma, vasculitis, pregnancy, arteriovenous (AV) malformation, polycythemia, sickle cell anemia, intracranial surgery, dehydration, paraneoplastic hypercoagulability syndrome, obstruction by expanding intracranial mass

           2) septic: infections of the face, sinusitis, dental infections, orbital cellulitis

     3. Diagnosis:
        a. MRI
     4. Treatment:
        a. antibiotic: if septic etiology
        b. anticoagulant therapy: heparin
        c. corticosteroids: ±
        d. surgery: for sinusitis or abscess

F. Tolosa-Hunt Syndrome
     1. Clinical features:
        a. symptoms: pain in or around eye, diplopia
        b. signs: rare visual loss, pupil miotic, dilated, or APD
        c. external: hypesthesias V1 distribution
        d. motility: third, fourth, and sixth nerve paresis
        e. natural history: spontaneous remission can occur; episodes may recur at monthly or yearly intervals
     2. Pathology:
        a. pathogenesis: idiopathic inflammation
     3. Diagnosis:
        a. neuroimaging and arteriography: to rule out other etiologies (diagnosis of exclusion)
     4. Treatment:
        a. therapy: prednisone 1 to 3 mg/kg po qd, taper slowly as pain subsides
        b. prognosis: dramatic response to steroids within 48 hours but may get "rebound" if taper too rapidly (remember—noninflammatory lesions, including tumors, may respond initially to steroids)

XIII. PAPILLEDEMA

A. Clinical features:
     1. Symptoms: episodes of transient bilateral visual loss lasting a few seconds; double vision; headache; nausea; vomiting
     2. Signs:
        a. rarely a decrease in visual acuity acutely, unless exudates are present in the macula or

          cause is a tumor or other mass that affects the anterior visual system; however, can occur chronically

    b. visual field defects: enlarged blind spot acutely, peripheral defects chronically, especially inferonasally

    c. motility: unilateral or bilateral sixth nerve palsy can be present

    d. ophthalmoscopic findings: bilaterally swollen hyperemic discs with blurring of the disc margins, papillary and peripapillary hemorrhages and soft exudates, loss of venous pulsations, dilated veins; disc elevation may decrease, small refractile drusen-like bodies may appear on the disc surface, sheathing and narrowing of the peripapillary retinal vessels may develop chronically

B. Pathology:
    1. etiology: aqueductal stenosis, pseudotumor cerebri, intracranial tumors, subdural or epidural hematomas, subarachnoid hemorrhage, arteriovenous malformation, sagittal sinus thrombosis, brain abscess, meningitis, encephalitis

C. Diagnosis:
    1. neuroimaging study
    2. lumbar puncture: if CT or MRI does not reveal etiology
    3. differential: pseudopapilledema (i.e., optic disc drusen), malignant hypertensive retinopathy, diabetic papillitis, infiltration of the discs (i.e., leukemia), Leber's hereditary optic neuropathy, bilateral optic neuritis or ischemic optic neuropathy, ocular hypotony

D. Treatment:
    1. directed at underlying cause

XIV. PSEUDOTUMOR CEREBRI

A. Epidemiology:
    1. Age of onset: first to fifth decade
    2. Female to male ratio: 8:1
    3. Risk factors: obesity, pregnancy, hypertension, head trauma, middle ear disease, radical neck dissection, medications including oral contraceptives, vitamin A, nalidixic acid, tetracycline, lithium, amiodarone, danzol, steroid withdrawal

B. Clinical Features:

1. Symptoms: headache, nausea, vomiting, double vision, episodes of transient visual loss, progressive visual loss, tinnitus, dizziness
2. Ocular signs: normal visual acuity (acute cases), decreased visual acuity (chronic cases), normal pupils or APD, normal or impaired color vision, ± sixth nerve palsies
3. Systemic signs: no other neurologic signs usually present other than unilateral or bilateral sixth nerve palsy
4. Visual field defects: blind spot enlargement, generalized constriction, arcuate nerve fiber bundle defects, nasal contraction
5. Ophthalmoscopic findings: bilateral swollen, hyperemic discs with blurring of the disc margins; optic nerve pallor may develop
6. Natural history: a chronic disease but in some patients the headaches may resolve and the optic disc swelling may disappear; other patients experience progressive loss of vision with development of optic atrophy

C. Diagnosis:
   1. CT or MRI: r/o mass lesion; normal study ± small ventricles
   2. Lumbar puncture: increased intracranial pressure with normal CSF composition
   3. Differential: other causes of papilledema; diagnosis of exclusion

D. Treatment:
   1. Indications: intractable headaches or progressive visual acuity or visual field loss
   2. Medical:
      a. weight reduction
      b. diuretics: acetazolamide 500 mg, 2 g per day; lasix 40 to 120 mg per day
      c. discontinuation of causative agents
      d. serial lumbar punctures
      e. steroids (controversial)
   3. Surgical (if medical treatment fails)
      a. optic nerve sheath fenestration
      b. lumbo-peritoneal shunt
   4. Followup: initially every 2 to 3 weeks to assess for visual acuity or visual field loss, then 1 to 3 months depending on the response to treatment

XV. THYROID EYE DISEASE

A. Epidemiology

    1. Age of onset: all ages, occurring rarely under age 20

    2. Associations: hyperthyroid, hypothyroid, and euthyroid states; may appear prior to or concomitantly with systemic symptoms of dysthyroidism or after control of the dysthyroid state; often develops or worsens after radiotherapy of thyroid

    3. Most common cause of unilateral and bilateral proptosis in adults; most common cause of spontaneous double vision in middle-age and early senescence

  B. Clinical Features:

    1. History: acute or chronic presentation

    2. Symptoms: prominent eyes, double vision, eyelid swelling, decreased vision, foreign body sensation, pain

    3. Ocular signs:

      a. normal or decreased visual acuity, normal pupils or APD, normal or impaired color vision

      b. visual field defects (if optic nerve compression is present): generalized constriction, increased blind spot size, nasal step, arcuate defects, paracentral and central scotomas

      c. external: retraction of the upper eyelid, eyelid lag on downgaze, inferior scleral show, lid edema, proptosis, resistance to retropulsion

      d. motility: limitation of elevation, adduction, depression, and abduction

      e. slit lamp: conjunctival hyperemia over insertion of involved ocular muscles, chemosis, corneal superficial punctate keratitis, corneal ulceration, elevation of intraocular pressure on attempted upward gaze

      f. ophthalmoscopic findings: normal appearing disc, optic nerve swelling, or disc pallor

    4. Systemic signs: hyperthyroidism—tachycardia, goiter, weight loss, muscle wasting, proximal muscle weakness, hand tremor; hypothyroidism—lethargy, fatigue, dry skin, weight gain, bradycardia, myxedema

    5. Natural history: Graves' orbitopathy usually occurs within 2 years of diagnosis of hyperthyroidism—usually "burns out" over 5 to 20 years

  C. Pathology:

    1. Pathogenesis: unknown, probably immune-mediated

    2. Histopathology: enlargement of extraocular muscles due to endomysial fibrosis, mucopolysaccharide deposition, and perivascular lymphocyte and plasmacyte infiltration

D. Diagnosis:

1. Forced duction testing: identify mechanical resistance
2. Neuroimaging: rule out orbital mass; reveals enlargement of multiple muscles in both orbits (enlargement of the muscle with sparing of the tendon)
3. A-scan ultrasonography: reveals enlarged extraocular muscles
4. Thyroid function tests: T3, T4, thyroid stimulating hormone (TSH), T3 resin uptake
5. Tensilon test: for suspected coexisting myasthenia gravis
6. Differential: third nerve palsy with aberrant regeneration, Parinaud's syndrome, myasthenia, orbital mass

E. Treatment:

1. Control of systemic thyroid disease by internist to obtain euthyroid state
2. Lid edema: elevate head of bed at night
3. Exposure keratopathy: artificial tears and ointment, taping lids closed, or applying saran wrap or goggles at night
4. Diplopia: patch one eye, muscle surgery once disease is quiescent for 6 months; some patients benefit from steroids or botulinum toxin injections
5. Worsening exposure despite treatment: prednisone 100 mg po q day for 1 to 2 days followed by orbital decompression
6. Severe acute inflammation: prednisone 100 mg po q day; if improvement, taper slowly; if no improvement taper quickly and treat with radiation therapy
7. Visual loss from optic neuropathy: prednisone 100 mg q day is started immediately in anticipation of radiation therapy or orbital decompression
8. Followup: those patients with an optic neuropathy or severe exposure keratopathy need immediate attention and frequent followup until stable; those patients with only mild to moderate proptosis or lid retraction, and minimal exposure keratopathy may be followed every 3 to 6 months

XVI. MYASTHENIA GRAVIS (MG)

A. Epidemiology:

      1. Age of onset: any age

      2. Associations: 5% of patients with myasthenia will also have thyroid dysfunction; increased incidence of thymoma and immune disorders, especially in older persons

B. Clinical Features:

      1. Symptoms: ptosis and/or diplopia which is variable; often worse at the end of the day

      2. Signs:

          a. normal visual acuity, normal pupillary exam

          b. external: ptosis, lid fatigue—ptosis becomes more pronounced with sustained upward gaze; lid-twitch sign (Cogan)—when the patient looks down and then quickly refixes in primary position, the lid will display an upward overshoot before falling to the ptotic position, weakness of obicularis oculi

          c. motility: any of the extraocular muscles may be involved, so any ocular movement pattern may develop; may mimic ocular motor cranial nerve palsies or central gaze disturbances; phoria and tropia measurements may be variable during the same examination

      3. Natural history: remissions and exacerbations often triggered by infection or trauma

C. Pathology:

      1. Pathogenesis: antibodies to acetylcholine receptors block the receptors, leading to a reduction of the available acetylcholine receptors in the motor endplate of striated muscles

D. Diagnosis:

      1. Tensilon test: 1 cc of tensilon (10 mg/1 ml) is drawn up in a TB syringe and IV access is established. 0.2 cc is injected and the patient is observed for one minute. If no response is observed 0.8 cc is injected. The patient's ptosis or tropia is measured prior, immediately after, and three to four minutes following the injection, or red-green glasses and a light are used to chart change in diplopia. An improvement or major change in the measurements is usually diagnostic of MG. A negative test does not rule out myasthenia. A worsening or reversal are consistent with MG but not diagnostic. Atropine must be on hand for bradycardia, bronchospasm, etc.

      2. Neostigmine test: an alternative test for children or uncooperative adults. 0.4 mg of atropine is given IM 15 minutes prior to the injection of neostigmine. Dose = [weight (kg)/70 kg] × 1.5 mg.

Resolution of signs should occur within 30 to 45 minutes

3. Sleep test: photograph lids, sleep 45 minutes, then photograph again
4. Ice test: photograph lids, place ice on lids, photograph again
5. Laboratory tests: acetylcholine receptor antibody level (diagnostic, however only present in two-thirds of patients with ocular MG), thyroid function tests—T3, T4, TSH; ANA, ESR
6. Electromyography (EMG): a decremental muscular response is seen with repetitive supramaximal motor nerve stimulation (helpful if present; however, may see normal response if extremity musculature is uninvolved)
7. Chest CT or MRI scan: must obtain to investigate thymoma
8. Neurologic evaluation: referral to neurologist
9. Differential: partial third or sixth nerve palsy, internuclear ophthalmoplegia, Eaton-Lambert syndrome, CPEO, thyroid eye disease, myotonic dystrophy—uniocular signs should be assessed with neuroimaging, even if pharmacological tests are positive

E. Treatment:
1. Local ocular therapy: occlusion or prism for diplopia, tape or spectacle crutches for ptosis: surgery occasionally helpful for stable, chronic ptosis or strabismus
2. Referral to a neurologist
3. Mestinon: 30 mg tid to start, may increase to 90 to 120 mg every 3 hours
4. Systemic steroids: admit patient to hospital, begin prednisone 100 mg qd, follow pulmonary function tests for several days, then discharge; taper to prednisone 60 mg qid and once remission is achieved taper by 5 mg increments each month
5. Thymectomy, other immunosuppressives, and plasmaphoresis: reserved for patients who are refractory to steroids or who cannot tolerate them
6. Followup: if systemic symptoms are present (breathing or swallowing difficulties) patient needs immediate medical attention by neurologist; if ocular symptoms are acute, initially follow the patient every week until stable and advise patient to seek immediate medical care if systemic symptoms should develop, otherwise patients can be followed every 3 to 6 months

7. Prognosis: if symptoms remain isolated to the eyes after 2 years, development of systemic MG is unlikely; eye symptoms are frequently unresponsive to mestinon, but may respond to alternate day steroids or thymectomy

XVII. MYOTONIC DYSTROPHY

A. Epidemiology
1. Age at onset: late childhood, adolescence or early adult life
2. Inheritance: autosomal dominant
B. Clinical Features:
1. Symptoms/signs: myotonia
a. persistent activity of muscle fibers after a strong contraction
b. accompanied by dystrophic changes in other tissues and organs
2. Ocular findings: ptosis, symmetric external ophthalmoplegia, myotonia of lid closure and gaze holding, orbicularis weakness, sluggish miotic pupils, polychromatic lenticular deposits, iris neovascular tufts, ocular hypotony, pigmentary retinopathy
3. Systemic findings: frontal balding, testicular atrophy, cardiac abnormalities, face, neck and limb myopathy with atrophy
4. Natural history: progressive
C. Pathology:
1. Histopathology: muscle biopsy reveals an increased number of nuclei which are located centrally and arranged in long rows (pathognomonic), variation in caliber of fibers, ringed fibers, and sarcoplasmic masses
D. Diagnosis:
1. Electromyography: reveals a typical incremental response
2. Differential: CPEO
E. Treatment:
1. No effective treatment

XVIII. CHRONIC PROGRESSIVE EXTERNAL OPHTHALMOPLEGIA (CPEO)

A. General
1. Clinical features:
a. symptoms: diplopia usually is not present
b. ocular signs
1) normal acuity, normal pupillary exam

            2) external: ptosis, weak orbicularis oculi

            3) motility: symmetric limitation of ocular motility (eye movements remain limited with doll's head and caloric stimulation)

            4) slit lamp: exposure keratopathy

    2. Pathology:

        a. histopathology: ragged-red muscle fibers are seen admixed with relatively normal muscle fibers

        b. electron microscopy: ragged-red muscle fibers demonstrate strikingly abnormal mitochondria

    3. Diagnosis:

        a. tensilon test: to rule out myasthenia

        b. differential: myasthenia gravis, thyroid disease, progressive supranuclear palsy

    4. Treatment:

        a. lubricants for exposure problems, prism in spectacles for reading, lid crutches or surgical repair of ptosis

B. Kearns-Sayre Syndrome

    1. Epidemiology:

        a. age of onset: before age 20 years

        b. inheritance: usually sporadic

    2. Clinical features:

        a. ocular signs: CPEO with retinal pigmentary degeneration

        b. systemic signs: cardiac conduction defects, neurosensory hearing loss, cerebellar signs, vestibular system dysfunction, mental retardation, delayed puberty, short stature

    3. Pathology:

        a. histopathology: ragged-red muscle fibers in skeletal muscle and vacuolization of the cerebrum and brain stem

    4. Diagnosis:

        a. lumbar puncture: elevated cerebrospinal fluid protein

    5. Treatment:

        a. referral to cardiologist for yearly electrocardiograms, ± cardiac pacemaker

C. Oculopharyngeal Dystrophy

    1. Epidemiology:

        a. age of onset: fifth and sixth decades

        b. inheritance: usually autosomal dominant, French Canadians; can be sporadic

    2. Clinical features:

        a. signs: ptosis, CPEO, temporalis wasting

    3. Pathology:

      a. histopathology: marked reduction in the number of muscle fibers; and significant degenerative changes and characteristic nuclear inclusions in remaining fibers

   4. Treatment:

      a. cricopharyngeal surgery to prevent aspiration

XIX. MIGRAINE

A. Epidemiology:

   1. Age of onset: 50% begin before age 20

   2. Incidence: affects 15 to 19% of males and 25 to 29% of females

   3. Inheritance: familial incidence in 65 to 90% of cases

   4. Associations: history of car sickness

B. Clinical Features:

   1. Symptoms:

      a. severe unilateral throbbing or boring headache, 30% generalized; anorexia, nausea, vomiting, desire to avoid light and noise

      b. ± typical aura: present in 20% of migraine patients; a sharply defined aura precedes the headache phase, lasting 5 to 40 minutes; usually visual, characterized by a scintillating scotoma—a central scotoma slowly expands peripherally, outlined by shimmering lights; the aura may also be neurologic, sensory or motor; patients over 40 may lose the headache phase and still experience the aura (acephalgic migraine, ocular migraine or migraine equivalent)

      c. prolonged aura: neurologic deficits may persist into and after the headache phase; may persist for hours or weeks; hemiparesis, dysarthria, hemianesthesia

      d. without aura: may be triggered by food substances containing tyramine or phenylalanine such as cheeses, chocolate, yogurt, red wine, or containing aspartame such as diet soda; attacks may be related to hormonal changes in women

      e. ophthalmoplegic: paralysis of the third or sixth nerve occurring during or following the headache, lasting for days or weeks; starting during childhood

   2. Signs: normal ocular examination (except for a third and sixth nerve paresis in the ophthalmoplegic variety)

    C. Diagnosis:
- **1.** CT or MRI: obtain in any cases with atypical features—headache always on same side; onset during middle age without a family history or history of car sickness; when neurologic signs outlast the headache; headache that awakens patient from sleep, worsening or increased frequency of headaches
- **2.** Differential: muscle contraction (tension) headache, cluster headache, giant-cell arteritis, increased intracranial pressure, malignant hypertension, meningitis, vascular malformation of the brain, subarachnoid bleed

    D. Treatment:
- **1.** Referral to internist or neurologist
- **2.** Abortive therapy:
  - **a.** analgesics: trial of aspirin or acetaminophen; Fiorinal or Fioricet are extremely effective; however, contain a barbiturate
  - **b.** ergotamine compounds: most effective when administered in the prodromal phase
  - **c.** sumatriptan: new drug, very effective, administered SQ
- **3.** Prophylactic therapy:
  - **a.** avoidance of triggering factors
  - **b.** tricyclic antidepressants: amitriptyline
  - **c.** beta blockers: propranolol (should not be used for patients with visual aura)
  - **d.** calcium channel blockers: diltiazem, verapamil, nifedipine (best for patients with visual aura with or without headache)
  - **e.** serotonin antagonists: methysergide
  - **f.** MAO inhibitors: Parnate, Nardil

XX. FUNCTIONAL (NONORGANIC) VISUAL LOSS

    A. Subjective visual loss not attributable to an organic cause

    B. Clinical Features:
- **1.** Symptoms: loss of vision in a malingerer or hysteric, or a patient with Munchausen's
- **2.** Signs: no ocular signs are present to account for the decreased vision

    C. Diagnosis:
- **1.** Document better visual acuity than that to which the patient will admit
- **2.** For patients claiming hand motion to no light perception:

      a. pupillary exam: an APD should be present if one eye has visual loss to this degree

      b. optokinetic test: if nystagmus can be evoked by rotating the optokinetic tape in front of the eye, then vision is better than hand motions

      c. mirror test: slowly move a large mirror in front of the patient's face beyond the range of hand-motion vision; if the eyes move, following the image, the vision is better than hand motions

3. For patients claiming 20/40 to 20/400

      a. visual acuity checking: start with the 20/10 line; if patient cannot read this, inform him or her that you will put up an easier line to read, the 20/15 line; continue in this fashion; the patient may read a line or two before reaching the 20/40 line

      b. test near vision: this should correlate with the distance vision; if better patient has nonphysiologic visual loss or myopia

      c. retest distance visual acuity 10 feet from the chart: patient's vision should be twice as good; if better or worse then nonphysiologic

      d. stereoscopic visual testing: identification of the smaller stereoscopic circles on the Titmus test requires good vision in both eyes

      e. red-green glasses: one can test monocular acuity with both eyes opened; the letters in the red zone are seen with the eye behind the red lens, and those in the green zone with the eye behind the green lens

      f. visual field testing: may demonstrate a nonphysiologic response such as a tunnel visual field

4. Differential: amblyopia, cone-rod dystrophy, cortical blindness

D. Treatment:

  1. If nonphysiologic visual loss is suspected but cannot be documented, reevaluate in 1 week; if still unable to document better visual acuity, obtain ancillary tests; ERG, VER, CT or MRI, fluorescein angiogram

  2. Reassure patient that no ocular abnormality can be found that accounts for their visual loss (helpful for malingering children, less useful for malingering adults, particularly those attempting monetary gains)

XXI. TRANSIENT MONOCULAR VISUAL LOSS

A. Clinical Features:

1. Ocular symptoms: acute onset of monocular visual loss usually lasting several minutes although can last hours; all or a portion of field of vision is affected, recovery of vision is rapid
2. Systemic symptoms: ±neurologic, motor, or sensory
3. Signs: usually a normal examination, however an embolus may be seen within a retinal arteriole; cholesterol emboli—orange or yellow, refractile, globular usually at bifurcation; platelet emboli—gray-white, long smooth shape, mobile, can lodge anywhere; calcium emboli—chalk white, large at first or second bifurcations (other emboli include tumor, fat, air, organisms, foreign body)

B. Pathology:
1. Etiology:
   a. embolic sources: diseased blood vessels, cardiac wall or valve, injection of particulate matter
   b. thrombosis: lipohyalinosis associated with systemic hypertension; vasculitis including giant cell arteritis, lupus erythematosis, polyarteritis nodosa; hypercoagulable states including sickle cell anemia, multiple myeloma, polycythemia, macroglobulinemia
   c. vasospasm: migraine

C. Diagnosis:
1. Patients 40 years or over
   a. if cholesterol emboli are present: origin is common or internal carotid artery, need carotid duplex scanning and possibly arteriography (patients also need a physical examination and cardiac workup for associated heart disease)
   b. if either platelet or calcific emboli are seen: origin may be arteries, heart wall, or valves; need carotid duplex scanning and possibly arteriography, transthoracic echocardiography, holter monitor; a CBC should also be drawn for platelet emboli to rule out a hematologic disorder
   c. if no emboli are seen: need to first obtain CBC and ESR (must rule out giant cell arteritis); next carotid duplex scanning and possibly arteriography; if carotids are negative, obtain transthoracic echocardiography (only occasionally is transesophageal echocardiography necessary), then holter monitor
2. Patients under 40 years of age

    a. if cholesterol, platelet, or calcific emboli are seen: workup is similar to that of patients over 40 years of age

    b. if no emboli are seen: obtain CBC, ESR, ANA, PTT, anticardiolipin and antiphospholipid antibodies, antithrombin III, protein S and C, consider transesophageal echocardiography for patent foramen ovale, consider carotid duplex for atherosclerosis or carotid dissection (possibly followed by MRI, MRA, arteriography), consider transthoracic echo-cardiography for cardiac wall or valve abnormalities, atrial myxoma

   3. Differential: must be distinguished from visual obscurations which are briefer, seconds; causes include papilledema, disc drusen, compressive orbital tumors (may or may not be gaze-evoked); also distinguish from Uhthoff's phenomenon, transient visual loss induced by exercise or heat associated with optic neuritis or vasospasm

D. Treatment:

    a. Therapy: individualized depending on etiology

    b. Prognosis: depends on etiology

      1) patients over 40: approximately 1%/year risk of some visual loss; 2%/year risk of stroke; 2%/year risk of mortality secondary to cardiac disease, increasing to 4 to 8%/year risk of mortality if embolus seen

      2) patients under 40: usually benign condition secondary to vasospasm

XXII. TRANSIENT BINOCULAR VISUAL LOSS

A. If episodes of transient binocular visual loss are preceded by scintillating scotomata lasting 15 to 20 minutes, then etiology is most likely migraine (see Migraine for details).

B. Vertebrobasilar Insufficiency

   1. Clinical features:

    a. ocular symptoms: transient bilateral blurring of vision usually lasting at least 30 seconds, occasionally minutes, rarely hours

    b. systemic symptoms: transient ataxia, vertigo, dysarthria, dysphagia, drop attacks, hemiparesis, hemisensory loss

    c. signs: normal examination

   2. Pathology:

    a. pathogenesis: decreased blood flow in the vertebral, basilar, and posterior cerebral arteries

      b. etiology: atheromatous occlusion, hypertensive vascular disease, embolization, decrease in cardiac output, subclavian steal, cervical spondylosis, anemia, polycythemia, congenital hypoplasia; vasospasm common in young

   3. Diagnosis:

      a. blood pressure reading: assess for subclavian steal

      b. EKG and holter monitor

      c. CBC, ±ESR, antiphospholipid antibodies

      d. ±cervical spine films

      e. differential: migraine, papilledema, giant cell arteritis

   4. Treatment:

      a. referral to neurologist, may consider admission for anticoagulation in certain cases

      b. directed at underlying cause

C. Seizures Within the Visual Cortex

   1. Symptoms: typically the transient visual loss is preceded by unformed hallucinations, usually flickering lights that do not move across the visual field

   2. Etiology: neoplasms, arteriovenous malformations, ischemia, meningoencephalitis, trauma

   3. Diagnosis: electroencephalography and MRI

   4. Therapy: supervised by neurologist

Essentials of Eye Care, edited by Rohit Varma.
Lippincott–Raven Publishers,
Philadelphia © 1997.

12

Ocular Genetics*

I. CRITERIA FOR GENETIC DISORDERS

A. Autosomal Dominant Traits

1. The trait appears in every generation (vertical transmission).
2. The gene defect is expressed in the heterozygote.
3. The affected person transmits the trait to the offspring on the average of 50% of the time. A homozygous patient would have virtually a 100% chance of passing the trait to each of his or her children.
4. Unaffected persons do not transmit the trait to their children except in nonpenetrance.
5. Affected children have affected parents except in isolated cases caused by new germinal mutations.
6. Usually there is equal sex incidence of affected persons.
7. The trait is transmitted to either sex from either sex. Male-to-male transmission is only seen in autosomal dominant disorders.

B. Autosomal Recessive Traits

1. The trait does not cause clinical disease in the heterozygote.

Notes On This Chapter

*1. Genetic disorders described elsewhere in this handbook include corneal dystrophies, retinoblastoma, phacomatoses, hereditary neuroophthalmic conditions, and oculoplastic conditions.
2. The *Mendelian Inheritance in Man* number is provided for most disorders. (McKusick, V.A., *Mendelian Inheritance in Man*, 9th Edition, Johns Hopkins Press. Baltimore, 1990.)
3. Question marks within text refer to a likely, but not definite, mode of inheritance.
4. Some especially rare or controversial conditions are not included.

      2. Individuals with two mutant alleles (homozygote) express the disorder.

      3. The trait appears only in siblings, not in parents, or offspring (horizontal distribution of cases in a pedigree).

      4. Parents of affected patients may be consanguinous.

      5. There is equal sex incidence among affected persons.

      6. One fourth of siblings of the proband are affected on the average.

C. X-Linked Dominant Traits

      1. The trait is always expressed in a heterozygous individual.

      2. Heterozygous females transmit the trait to both sexes with equal frequency.

      3. Affected males transmit the trait to all their daughters but none of their sons.

      4. There are about twice as many affected women as men (because women have 2/3 of all X chromosomes).

      5. May be lethal in males.

D. X-Linked Recessive Traits

      1. The carrier female ordinarily does not manifest the disease.

      2. The trait is much more common in males.

      3. The trait is passed from males, through all the daughters and to one half of those daughters' sons.

      4. The trait never is transmitted from an affected father to his children of either sex.

      5. The affected males in the family are either brothers or related to one another through carrier females, for example, maternal uncles (oblique pedigree).

E. Mitochondrially (Cytoplasmically) Inherited Traits

      1. Females transmit the trait to both male and female offspring.

      2. The trait is never transmitted from an affected father to his children of either sex.

      3. Heterogeneity in expression between individuals can be due to a difference in the percentage of affected mitochondria.

      4. Heterogeneity in expression can vary within the cells of a single individual due to a difference in the percentage of affected mitochondria.

II. CHROMOSOMAL SYNDROMES

A. Trisomy 21 Syndrome (Down Syndrome)

      1. Epidemiology: the most common chromosomal syndrome in humans with an incidence of 1 in 672 to 1 in 1,000 live births; frequency increases with age of the mother, with about 1 in 2,300 live births for mothers between the ages of 15 and 19 to about 1 in 40 live births to those 44 years and older

2. Ocular clinical features:
   a. almond-shaped palpebral fissures
   b. upslanting (mongoloid) palpebral fissures
   c. prominent epicanthal folds
   d. blepharitis, usually chronic
   e. cicatricial ectropion
   f. strabismus, usually esotropia
   g. aberrant retinal vessels ("crowded disc")
   h. iris stromal hypoplasia
   i. Brushfield's spots
   j. keratoconus
   k. cataract
   l. myopia and astigmatism
   m. nystagmus
   n. glaucoma
   o. infantile retinal detachment

B. Turner Syndrome
   1. Epidemiology: occurs in about 1 of every 2,500 to 3,500 women
   2. Ocular clinical features:
      a. pigmented areas on eyelids
      b. prominent epicanthal folds
      c. accentuated downslanting of palpebral fissures
      d. ptosis
      e. strabismus
      f. nystagmus
      g. bruised sclera
      h. pupillary heterotopia
      i. anterior axial embryonic cataract
      j. color deficiency in Turner's syndrome is the same as that in the normal male population
      k. anticipate complete expression of other X-linked disorders

C. Trisomy 18 Syndrome (Edwards' Syndrome)
   1. Epidemiology: incidence of 1 in 5,000 to 1 in 8,000 newborns: 50% die before four months of age and 90% die before one year; a few have lived as long as 15 years; preponderance of females 3:1
   2. Ocular clinical features:
      a. epicanthal folds
      b. ptosis
      c. blepharophimosis with unusually small or oblique fissures
      d. unusually thick lower lid
      e. hypertelorism (sometimes hypotelorism)

      f. hypoplastic supraorbital ridges
      g. congenital glaucoma
      h. corneal opacities
      i. micophthalmia
      j. optic disc anomalies
      k. iris and uveal colobomata

D. Trisomy 13, Patau's Syndrome, Bartholin Syndrome

  1. Epidemiology: frequency of 1 in 4,000 to 1 in 14,500 live births; 50% of infants die within the first month, 70% die by the sixth month, and fewer than 5% survive for more than three years

  2. Ocular clinical features:
      a. hypotelorism (sometimes hypertelorism)
      b. shallow supraorbital ridges
      c. absent eyebrows
      d. epicanthal folds
      e. cyclopia
      f. microphthalmia, sometimes clinical anophthalmia
      g. corneal clouding
      h. cataracts
      i. uveal colobomata
      j. iridoschisis
      k. intraocular connective tissue, including cartilage
      l. persistent hyperplastic primary vitreous
      m. retinal dysplasia
      n. optic nerve hypoplasia, atrophy, or occasionally colobomata
      o. anterior segment dysgenesis

E. Short Arm 5 Deletion ("Cat's Cry" Syndrome)

  1. Ocular clinical features:
      a. hypertelorism
      b. mongolian slant
      c. epicanthal folds
      d. myopia
      e. exotropia
      f. iris colobomata
      g. optic atrophy

F. Long Arm 13 Deletion (13q14) Syndrome
    Short Arm 11 Deletion (11p13) Syndrome

III. DISORDERS OF THE LENS

A. Congenital Cataracts

  1. Congenital cataracts as an isolated ocular finding #115650-116700,123660
      a. inheritance: autosomal dominant (most common) X-linked, or recessive (least common); be-

tween 8.3 and 25% of all congenital cataracts are familial. Anterior polar, crystalline, lamellar, nuclear, posterior polar, and total cataracts have been described.

2. Congenital cataract as part of a syndrome of systemic disease

   a. Alport syndrome #301050
      1) inheritance: X-linked dominant
      2) clinical features: hereditary hemorrhagic nephritis, sensorineural hearing loss, and ocular findings, which may include congenital cataract or postnatally developed posterior cortical cataract, subretinal flecks, and anterior lenticonus

   b. cataract-dental syndrome (Nance-Horan syndrome) #302350
      1) inheritance: X-linked recessive
      2) clinical features: dense nuclear cataracts, microcornea, abnormal ears and teeth
      3) diagnosis: carrier females may show Y-sutural cataracts and dental anomalies

   c. chondrodysplasia punctata
      1) inheritance: autosomal recessive (#215100), autosomal dominant (Conradi-Hunermann disease #118650), X-linked dominant (#302950)
      2) clinical features: irregular calcification of the cartilage of epiphyses and congenital cataracts (72% recessive form, 17% dominant form), children often die within first two years from recurrent infection in recessive form; sectoral cataract in X-linked dominant form

   d. galactokinase deficiency #230200
      1) inheritance: autosomal recessive
      2) clinical features: congenital cataract is the only clinical manifestation of the disease
      3) treatment: cataract can probably be prevented by dietary restriction of galactose

   e. galactosemia #230400
      1) inheritance: autosomal recessive
      2) clinical features: failure to thrive, hepatosplenomegaly, cirrhosis, mental retardation, galactosemia, galactosuria, and infantile cataracts that appear during the first year of life
      3) diagnosis: oil-drop cataract, progression to nuclear or total cataract
      4) treatment: cataracts are preventable and can regress completely by withholding galactose

    f. Hallermann-Streiff syndrome (Francois Dyscephalic syndrome)

        1) inheritance: autosomal dominant vs. all new mutations

        2) clinical features: dyscephaly with bird-like head, dental anomalies, proportional dwarfism, hypotrichosis, skin atrophy, bilateral microphthalmos and, in most cases, bilateral congenital cataract

    g. incontinentia pigmenti (Bloch-Sulzberger) syndrome

    (See section IVD. Pigmentary Retinopathy Associated with Systemic Disease)

    h. Lowe's Oculocerebrorenal syndrome #309000

        1) inheritance: X-linked recessive

        2) clinical features: mental retardation, amino aciduria, hyperammonemia, tubular acidosis, dwarfism with ricketts, congenital cataract, and congenital glaucoma

        3) pathology: lens is small and thin

        4) diagnosis: female carriers may show spoke-like or flake-like opacities in the peripheral cortex

    i. Marinesco-Sjögren syndrome #248800

        1) inheritance: autosomal recessive

        2) clinical features: congenital spinocerebellar ataxia, mental retardation, and congenital cataract

    j. myotonic dystrophy #160900

        1) inheritance: autosomal dominant

        2) clinical features: "Christmas tree cataracts" (multicolor flecks within lens), macular degenerative changes, myotonia, muscle wasting, premature frontal balding

    k. Smith-Lemli-Opitz syndrome #270400

        1) inheritance: autosomal recessive

        2) clinical features: microcephaly and mental retardation associated with congenital cataracts in 15% of patients

    l. Down, Edwards' and Patau's syndromes

    (See Chromosomal Syndromes)

  3. Treatment of congenital cataracts: if cataracts are suspected to interfere with vision, several approaches can be taken. Optical iridectomy and mydriatics provide temporary treatment in cases of incomplete congenital cataracts. For complete or central cataracts, surgical extraction is the necessary approach with irrigation and aspiration of the lens material, posterior capsulotomy, anterior vitrectomy and consideration of intraocular lens (IOL) insertion. Early fitting of aphakic contact lens and antiamblyopic treatment is critically important (add at least 1.50 diopters to provide optical correction for near objects).

B. Ectopia Lentis
  1. Ectopia lentis et pupillae #225200
     a. inheritance: usually autosomal recessive
     b. clinical features: usually bilateral, commonly not symmetrical with lenses and pupils displaced in opposite directions from each other; cataract formation, glaucoma, and retinal detachment can occur
     c. treatment: same as for simple ectopia lentis
  2. Homocystinuria #236200, 236250
     a. inheritance: autosomal recessive
     b. clinical features:
        1) skeletal manifestations, excessive height, and low ratio of upper segment to lower segment; generalized osteoporosis with vertebral collapse, scoliosis, deformities of the anterior chest
        2) cardiovascular manifestations: thrombotic vascular occlusion, main threat to survival (coronary artery occlusion can occur in children)
        3) ocular manifestations: ectopia lentis is ocular hallmark and detected in 90% of patients. Dislocation is bilateral and symmetrical with lens usually migrating inferiorly or inferonasally; myopia; retinal degeneration; pupillary block glaucoma can occur.
     c. treatment: dietary manipulation can treat the metabolic defect (about 1/2 of cases respond to pyridoxine) and prevent lens dislocation and progression of myopia if instituted shortly after birth
  3. Hyperlysinemia #238700
     a. inheritance: autosomal recessive
     b. clinical features: mental retardation, hypotonic muscles; ectopia lentis has been described
  4. Marfan syndrome #120160
     a. inheritance: autosomal dominant with variable expressivity, 15% have no family history; all patients presumably have mutations in fibrillin gene on chromosome (chr.) 15
     b. clinical features:

1) skeletal manifestations: excessive height, loose jointedness, scoliosis, and anterior chest deformity
2) cardiovascular manifestations include: aortic root dilatation, dissecting aortic aneurysm, and mitral valve prolapse
3) ocular manifestations: enophthalmos in severely affected children caused by reduced retrobulbar fat, moderate to high myopia is most frequent; ectopia lentis appears in 50 to 80% of patients, almost always bilateral and symmetrical, most commonly superotemporal; retinal detachment and glaucoma may occur
   c. treatment: includes management of systemic disease and ectopia lentis if present
5. Simple ectopia lentis #129600
   a. inheritance: autosomal dominant more common than autosomal recessive
   b. clinical features: usually bilateral symmetric upward and temporal displacement of the lens; one variant with spontaneous late subluxation occurs between ages 20 to 65 years; glaucoma can occur
   c. treatment of ectopia lentis: early diagnosis and prompt optical correction through the phakic or aphakic zone may decrease incidence of amblyopia. Mydriatic instillation may improve vision. Laser iridoplasty can be used to enlarge pupillary opening. Lens extraction can be considered if optical correction is impossible
6. Sulfocysteinuria (sulfite oxidase deficiency) #272300
   a. inheritance: autosomal recessive
   b. clinical features: mental retardation, seizures, ectopia lentis has been described
7. Weill-Marchesani syndrome #277600
   a. inheritance: autosomal recessive with partial expression in heterozygote
   b. clinical manifestations:
      1) skeletal manifestations, large thorax and stubby spade-like hands, increased subcutaneous tissue, head often brachycephalic with depressed nasal bridge
      2) ocular manifestations: microspherophakia, ectopia lentis in over 80% of patients with diagnosis at mean age of 18 years, glaucoma
   c. treatment: includes the management of ectopia lentis

IV. DISORDERS OF THE RETINA AND CHOROID

A. Retinal Detachment and Vitreoretinal Degenerations
1. Arthroophthalmopathy, hereditary progressive (Stickler syndrome) #108300
   a. inheritance: autosomal dominant
   b. clinical features: optical findings are identical to Wagner's syndrome except, in addition, there are frequently retinal detachments caused by large circumferential tears. Systemic findings include joint disease, characteristic facial bone hypoplasia (flat midface, depressed nasal bridge, maxillary hypoplasia, micrognathia), cleft palate, and hearing loss; mutations in collagen type 2A1 gene have been reported
   c. treatment: follow for and treat retinal detachment
2. Autosomal dominant vitreoretinochoroidopathy (ADVIRC) #193220
   a. inheritance: autosomal dominant
   b. clinical features: chorioretinal hyper- and hypopigmentation, choroidal atrophy, cystoid macular edema, cataracts
3. Familial exudative vitreoretinopathy (FEVR) #133780
   a. inheritance: autosomal dominant
   b. clinical features: first stage manifested by white with and without pressure; second stage has abnormal vessels in the temporal periphery (tortuous vessels, multiple arteriolar-venular shunts and subretinal exudates); third stage has retinal vascular changes, vitreoretinal proliferation develops with subsequent retinal detachment
   c. treatment: may require laser photocoagulation or retinal detachment repair
4. Goldmann-Favre's syndrome (macrofibrillar vitreoretinal degeneration)
   a. inheritance: autosomal recessive
   b. clinical features: extensive vitreous degeneration associated with peripheral pigmentary retinal degeneration. Pockets of liquified vitreous scattered among fibrillar vitreous membranes; peripheral retinoschisis; night blindness
5. Norrie disease (congenital progressive oculo-acoustico-cerebral degeneration) #31600
   a. inheritance: X-linked recessive
   b. clinical features: males; bilateral retinal malformation, retinal detachment, vitreous hemorrhage, deafness, mental retardation

6. Sickle cell hemoglobin retinopathy
(See Retina Chapter 9)
7. Wagner syndrome
   a. inheritance: autosomal dominant
   b. clinical features: moderate myopia but may be severe, strabismus, cataract, usually beginning around puberty, mainly posterior cortical punctate opacities, nuclear sclerosis, complicated cataract, vitreous degeneration with syneresis, and liquefaction which produces an optically empty vitreous except for some vitreous membranes; fundus changes include choroidal atrophy, peripheral retinal pigmentation which may be perivascular, vascular sheathing, sclerosis, and caliber changes; retinal detachment can uncommonly occur; subnormal electroretinogram (ERG)

B. Macular Dystrophies
   1. Choroidal sclerosis (central areolar dystrophy) #215500
      a. inheritance: autosomal dominant
      b. clinical features: age of onset in third to fifth decades; slowly progressive decreased central vision; ophthalmoscopy reveals nonspecific foveal granularity, early and geographic RPE atrophy with loss of choriocapillaris. Progressive central scotoma
      c. pathology: well-demarcated area of retinal pigment epithelial (RPE) and choriocapillaris atrophy with no evidence of choroidal sclerosis
      d. treatment: low vision aids
   2. Cystoid macular dystrophy
      a. inheritance: autosomal dominant
      b. clinical features: age of onset first to second decade; decreased central vision from 20/25 to 20/80, progressive to 20/200 to counting fingers late in disease; ophthalmoscopy and fluorescein angiography reveal cystoid macular edema early, and RPE derangement and atrophy late; some cases may have RPE changes in "bull's-eye" pattern
   3. Degenerative myopia #160700
      a. inheritance: majority autosomal recessive
      b. clinical features: age of onset in first decade; increased axial length with gradual decrease in central vision which may worsen with development of lacquer cracks through the fovea and/or choroidal neovascularization
      c. diagnosis: characteristic peripapillary atrophy and/or posterior staphyloma and other charac-

teristic fundus changes; A-scan for axial length measurement

    d. treatment: laser treatment for choroidal neovascularization; retinal detachment (RD) repair

4. Familial drusen #126700

    a. inheritance: autosomal dominant with variable penetrance

    b. clinical features: age of onset second to fourth decade; asymptomatic in most, however, patients may develop choroidal neovascular and disciform scarring which results in decreased vision, round yellow-white depositions in the posterior pole in midperiphery turning to colorless with time

    c. pathology: RPE and Bruch's membrane change similar to that seen in age-related macular degeneration

    d. treatment: laser treatment for choroidal neovascularization; low vision aids

5. Familial foveal retinoschisis

    a. inheritance: autosomal recessive

    b. clinical features: onset in first decade; decreased central vision from 20/30 to 20/50, possibly progressive; foveal retinoschisis identical to the X-linked form, but no peripheral retinoschisis

6. Fenestrated sheen macular dystrophy

    a. inheritance: autosomal dominant

    b. clinical features: onset in the first decade; progressive paracentral scotomas with preservation of normal central vision; ophthalmoscopy reveals refractile sheen of fovea with red, cyst-like lesions; RPE atrophy in "bull's-eye" pattern may be seen late; fluorescein angiography reveals RPE transmission defects in advanced cases; normal to subnormal photopic ERG; normal scotopic ERG; normal to subnormal electro-oculogram (EOG)

7. Fovea macular vitelliform dystrophy, adult type (adult-onset foveomacular pigment epithelial dystrophy) #153700

    a. inheritance: likely autosomal dominant

    b. clinical features: age of onset in fourth to sixth decades; decreased vision in the 20/30 to 20/40 range. Ophthalmoscopy reveals symmetrical round or oval slightly elevated, yellow subretinal lesions in the macular area with or without small drusen in the paracentral region

    c. diagnosis: fluorescein angiography reveals irregular ring of hyperfluorescence surrounding a central hypofluorescent spot; no evidence of perifoveal leakage

8. Fundus flavimaculatus #230100
   a. inheritance: autosomal recessive more than autosomal dominant
   b. clinical features: age of onset in first to second decade; may be asymptomatic without macular findings; ophthalmoscopy reveals yellow-white flecks in the posterior pole in midperiphery; majority of patients show macular change as only finding: Stargardt's disease (both may be the same disorder)
   c. pathology: yellow flecks shown to be enlarged RPE cells packed with lipofuscin
   d. diagnosis: normal to subnormal photopic ERG and subnormal electro-oculogram (EOG); silent choroid on fluorescein angiography
   e. treatment: low vision aids

9. Juvenile retinoschisis #312700
   a. inheritance: X-linked recessive
   b. clinical features: age of onset in first decade; slowly progressive decreased central vision; ophthalmoscopy reveals foveal retinoschisis in 100% and peripheral (vitreous veils) retinoschisis in 50%
   c. pathology: splitting of retina in the nerve fiber layer
   d. diagnosis: selective decrease in B-wave amplitude on ERG
   e. treatment: follow for retinal detachment

10. Macular degeneration, juvenile (Stargardt's disease) #248200
    a. inheritance: autosomal recessive with an autosomal dominant variety (#153900)
    b. clinical features: age of onset in first to second decades decreased central vision in patient with previous normal vision, defective color vision. Ophthalmoscopy reveals "beaten bronze" macular changes with or without flecks in the posterior pole and midperiphery similar to fundus flavimaculatus
    c. diagnosis: ERG and EOG may be normal to subnormal
    d. treatment: low vision aids

11. Macular degeneration, polymorphic vitelline, Best disease, vitelliform macular dystrophy #153700
    a. inheritance: autosomal dominant with variable penetrance

b. clinical features: age of onset in first decade; minimal decreased vision early with worsening later in life; ophthalmoscopy reveals "egg yolk" lesion in the fovea which may rupture to give a "scrambled egg" appearance; choroidal neovascularization can occur; lesions may be multifocal

c. diagnosis: EOG characteristically abnormal and ERG normal with characteristic fundus appearance

d. treatment: low vision aids; laser treatment for choroidal neovascularization

12. North Carolina macular dystrophy #136550

    a. inheritance: autosomal dominant

    b. clinical features: drusen usually present; severity from mild to severe, evacuated macular appearance; vision from normal to 20/200 with median near 20/40; believed congenital and typically nonprogressive; ERG is normal

13. Patterned dystrophy of the retinal pigment epithelium, butterfly-shaped pigment dystrophy of the fovea #169150

    a. inheritance: autosomal dominant

    b. clinical features: age of onset in second to fifth decades; asymptomatic or mild decrease in vision. Ophthalmoscopy reveals symmetrical reticular pattern of pigmentary change in the macula; choroidal neovascularization may occur

    c. diagnosis: subnormal EOG, normal ERG

    d. treatment: laser treatment for choroidal neovascularization

14. Pericentral pigmentary retinopathy (inverse retinitis pigmentosa) #268060

    a. inheritance: autosomal recessive

    b. clinical features: age of onset in second to third decade; gradual decrease in central vision; perimacular RPE derangement and atrophy; may have pigment change to midperiphery; progressive color defect

    c. diagnosis: normal to subnormal ERG

15. Progressive cone rod dystrophy #120970

    a. inheritance: autosomal dominant, more common than autosomal recessive

    b. clinical features: age of onset in first to third decade; decreased central vision, severe photophobia, severe defective color vision; ophthalmoscopy reveals bull's-eye maculopathy and temporal optic disc pallor

      c. diagnosis: abnormal to nonrecordable photopic ERG and normal to near normal scotopic ERG; color vision testing reveals severe deutan-tritan defect or achromatopsia; peripheral visual field is normal

      d. treatment: red lenses can help photophobia; low vision aids

  16. Pseudoinflammatory fundus dystrophy of Sorsby #136900

      a. inheritance: autosomal dominant

      b. clinical features: onset within fourth to fifth decades; bilateral progressive hemorrhagic maculopathy secondary to choroidal neovascularization

C. Primary Pigmentary Retinopathies

  1. Autosomal Dominant Retinitis Pigmentosa

      a. typical autosomal dominant retinitis pigmentosa #180380

          1) clinical features: progressive visual field loss, night blindness; classic triad is attenuated arterioles, bone spicule pigmentation and waxy pallor of the optic disc; may see cystoid macular edema, vitreous cells and condensates; optic nerve drusen and late choroidal atrophy; gene mutations identified include:

              a) chr. 3, rhodospin gene mutations

              b) chr. 6p, rds gene for peripherin

              c) chr. 8, pericentric variety

              d) chr. 11g rom-1 gene (subunit peripherin complex)

              e) chr. 7p and 7q

          2) diagnosis: ERG is abnormal or nonrecordable

      b. pigmented paravenous chorioretinal atrophy #172870

          1) inheritance: autosomal dominant, may be X-linked recessive

          2) clinical features: bone spicule pigmentation in a paravenous distribution; minimal if any progression; patients are usually asymptomatic; may have associated hyperopia, esotropia and vitreoretinal degeneration

      c. progressive cone rod dystrophy
         (See section IVB. Macular Dystrophies)

      d. Leber congenital amaurosis
         (rare; see under recessive type below)

  2. Autosomal recessive retinitis pigmentosa

      a. Goldmann-Favre disease
         (See section IVA. Retinal Detachment and Vitreoretinal Degenerations)

    b. Leber congenital amaurosis #20400, #204100

        1) inheritance: autosomal recessive, rarely autosomal dominant

        2) clinical features: four general types;

            a) nonseeing infant with nonrecordable ERG, fundus examination initially appears normal but pigmentary deposits usually develop

            b) infantile night blindness—symptoms of visual field loss frequently are noted by four years of age with severely reduced ERG; child maintain central field with visual acuity in the 20/70 to 20/200 range

            c) pigmentary retinal degeneration and macular coloboma, occasional keratoconus and mild skeletal abnormalities also found

            d) rare autosomal dominant type, behaves like early onset cone rod dystrophy

        3) diagnosis: for all ERG severely affected

    c. progressive cone rod dystrophy
       (See section IVB. Macular Dystrophies)

    d. retinitis pigmentosa with preserved para-arteriolar retinal pigment epithelium (PPRPE) #268030

        1) clinical features: findings of RP with relative preservation of para-arteriolar RPE, hyperopia

    e. retinitis punctata albescens (progressive form)

        1) clinical features: discrete white to yellow spots throughout fundus which may become pigmented with time; night blindness, progressive field loss and retinal vessel attenuation

  3. X-linked recessive pigmentary retinopathies

    a. X-linked retinitis pigmentosa #312600, #312610

        1) clinical features: RP findings; two chromosomal loci known on Xp

    b. choroideremia
       (See section IVG. Choroidal Dystrophies)

    c. juvenile retinoschisis
       (advanced stage may mimic RP; see IVB. Macular Dystrophies)

D. Pigmentary Retinopathies Associated with Systemic Disease

  1. Autosomal dominant pigmentary retinopathies

    a. arthroophthalmopathy, hereditary, progressive (Stickler syndrome)
       (See section IVA. Retinal Detachment and Vitreoretinal Degenerations)

      b. Charcot-Marie-Tooth disease #118200
- **1)** clinical features: pigmentary retinopathy, degeneration lateral horn spinal cord, optic atrophy

      c. cholestasis with peripheral pulmonary stenosis (Alagille syndrome) #118450
- **1)** clinical features: intrahepatic cholestatic syndrome, posterior embryotoxon, Axenfeld anomaly, congenital heart disease, flattened facies and bridge of nose, bony abnormalities, myopia, pigmentary retinopathy

      d. Flynn-Aird syndrome #136300
- **1)** clinical features: atypical pigmentary retinopathy, cataract, myopia, nerve deafness, ataxia, skin atrophy, baldness, cystic bone changes

      e. myotonic dystrophy #160900
(See section III. Disorders of the Lens)

      f. olivopontocerebellar atrophy III (OPCA with retinal degeneration) #164500
- **1)** clinical features: retinal degeneration (peripheral and/or macular), cerebellar ataxia, external ophthalmoplegia may occur

      g. Paget disease of bone (PDB) #167250
- **1)** clinical features: occasionally angioid streaks, one pedigree of pigmentary retinopathy

      h. Wagner syndrome
(See section IVA. Retinal Detachment and Vitreoretinal Degenerations)

  2. Autosomal recessive pigmentary retinopathies

      a. abetalipoproteinemia (Bassen-Kornzweig disease) #200100
- **1)** clinical features: secondary vitamin A and E deficiency, acanthocytosis, anemia, celiac syndrome
- **2)** treatment: night blindness and retinopathy respond to supplementation with vitamin A and E

      b. Alströms disease #203800
- **1)** clinical features: pigmentary retinopathy, diabetes, obesity, normal mental capacity, and neurosensory deafness

      c. asphyxiating thoracic dystrophy of the newborn (Jeune syndrome) #208500
- **1)** clinical features: dwarfing skeletal dysplasia leading to respiratory insufficiency, retinal disease, liver fibrosis, pigmentary retinopathy

      d. Bardet-Biedl syndrome #209900

      1) clinical features: pigmentary retinopathy, mild mental retardation, polydactyly, obesity, hypogenitalism, barely to nonrecordable ERG, progressive visual field loss

e. carotenemia, familial #115300

      1) clinical features: retinal degeneration from vitamin A deficiency; failure of absorption or cleavage of betacarotene

f. cerebrohepatorenal syndrome (Zellweger syndrome)

(See section VID. Other Disorders of Metabolism)

g. Cockayne syndrome #216400

      1) clinical features: pigmentary retinal degeneration, optic atrophy, deafness, cachectic dwarfism, precociously senile appearance, mental retardation

h. cystinosis, late onset juvenile or adolescent nephropathic type

(See section VID. Other Disorders of Metabolism)

i. homocystinuria

(See section III. Disorders of the Lens)

j. hyperostosis corticalis deformans juvenilis (juvenile Paget disease) #239000

      1) clinical features: large head, expanded and bowed extremities, chronic idiopathic hyperphosphatemia, occasional retinal degeneration, and angioid streaks seen

k. Joubert syndrome with bilateral chorioretinal coloboma #243910

      1) clinical features: Joubert syndrome (aplasia of the cerebellar vermis with episodic hyperpnea, abnormal eye movements, rhythmic protrusion of the tongue, ataxia, retardation) associated with bilateral chorioretinal coloboma; subtype with Leber congenital amaurosis-type of retinal dystrophy

l. Laurence-Moon syndrome #245800

      1) clinical features: similar to Bardet-Biedl with paraplegia and without polydactyly and obesity

m. mannosidosis

(See section VIC. Disorders of Combined Carbohydrate and Lipid Metabolism)

n. Marinesco-Sjögren syndrome

(See section III. Disorders of the Lens)

o. microphthalmia with hypermetropia, retinal degeneration, macrophakia and dental anomalies #251700

      1) clinical features: as titled

p. mucopolysaccharidosis I-H, I-S and III
(See section VIB. Disorders of Carbohydrate Metabolism)

q. neuronal ceroid lipofuscinosis
   1) clinical features and pathology:
      a) Haltia-Santavuori, occurs in infancy with rapid deterioration, fine granular inclusions on EM
      b) Jansky-Bielschowsky, onset 2 to 4 years, rapid CNS deterioration, curvilinear inclusions on EM (#204500)
      c) Vogt-Spielmeyer, onset 6 to 8 years, slowly progressive, CNS disease, visual loss precedes dementia, "finger-print" inclusions on EM (#204200)

r. osteopetrosis (Albers-Schönberg disease) #259700
   1) clinical features: defective resorption of immature bone, macrocephaly, progressive deafness, hepatosplenomegaly, anemia, retinal degeneration with abnormal or extinguished ERG

s. pallidal degeneration, progressive with retinitis pigmentosa #260200
   1) clinical features: progressive pigmentary retinopathy, extrapyramidal rigidity, dysarthria, destruction of pallida and substantia nigra

t. pseudoxanthoma elasticum (PXE) #264800
   1) clinical features: angioid streaks, some patients with focal fine exudates mainly in equator of retina, characteristic plaque-like skin lesions on skin of neck, axilla, and areas of flexion of limbs; GI bleeds

u. Refsum disease
(See section VIA. Disorders of Lipid Metabolism)

v. retinal dysplasia and retinal aplasia #266900
   1) clinical features: congenital blindness, kidney developmental abnormalities

w. sickle cell hemoglobin retinopathy
(See Chapter 9)

x. Sjögren-Larsson syndrome #270200
   1) clinical features: Swedish family, mental deficiency, spasticity, pigmentary retinal degeneration (characteristic glistening white dots), may have cataracts

y. Usher syndrome #276900, #276910
   1) inheritance: two forms, both autosomal recessive

2) epidemiology: 6 to 10% of RP patients are profoundly deaf and 3 to 6% of severely deaf patients have RP; overall prevalence 3 per 10,000
3) clinical features:
   a) type 1—RP plus profound neurosensory deafness and no vestibular function (#267900)
   b) type 2—RP and congenital partial deafness with intact vestibular function (#276910)
4) treatment: low vision aids; important to teach tactile forms of communication before blindness occurs

  3. X-linked recessive pigmentary retinopathies
    a. incontinentia pigmenti (Bloch-Sulzberger syndrome) #308310 (familial), #308300 (sporadic)
     1) clinical features: females; skin pigmentation in lines and whorls, alopecia, dental anomalies, optic atrophy, falciform folds, cataract, nystagmus, strabismus, patchy mottling of fundi, conjunctival pigmentation
    b. mucopolysaccharidosis II (Hunter syndrome) (See section VIB. Disorders of Carbohydrate Metabolism)
    c. Pelizaeus-Merzbacher Disease #312080
     1) clinical features: infantile progressive leukodystrophy, cerebellar ataxia, limb spasticity, mental retardation, may have pigmentary retinopathy with absent foveal reflex
  4. Mitochondrially inherited pigmentary retinopathies
    a. progressive external ophthalmoplegia (Kearns-Sayre syndrome)
     1) clinical features: ptosis, pigmentary retinopathy, heart block; normal to abnormal ERG
     2) treatment: check EKG for heartblock

E. Stationary Night Blindness
  1. Congenital stationary night blindness
    a. inheritance: autosomal dominant (#163500) or X-linked forms (#310500)
    b. clinical features: history of nonprogressive night blindness since childhood, normal appearing fundus, myopia in X-linked form, abnormal scotopic ERG
  2. Fleck retina of Kandori #228990
    a. inheritance: autosomal recessive
    b. clinical features: irregular fundus flecks with macular sparing
  3. Fundus albipunctatus #136880

       a. inheritance: autosomal recessive
       b. clinical features: discrete uniform white dots over the entire fundus with greatest density in the midperiphery and no macular involvement; night blindness
    4. Oguchi disease #258100
       a. inheritance: autosomal recessive
       b. clinical features: night blindness; higher incidence in Japanese; fundus has a yellowish metallic sheen which reverts to a normal appearance after prolonged dark adaptation (Mizuo phenomenon)

F. Cone Dystrophies
    1. Achromatopsia (total color blindness) #216900
       a. inheritance: autosomal recessive
       b. clinical features: poor vision (20/200 range) and nystagmus since birth, day blindness, photophobia, absent color discrimination
    2. Color blindness
       a. inheritance: X-linked or autosomal dominant (tritan)
       b. clinical features:
         1) deutan (#303800): about 6% of western European male population; green cone pigment affected; luminosity loss throughout color spectrum
         2) protan (#303900): about 2% of western European male population; red cone pigment affected; luminosity loss at red end of spectrum
         3) blue-monochromatic (incomplete achromatopsia; #303700): poor central and color discrimination, infantile nystagmus, nearly normal fundus appearance; intact blue photopic and scotopic ERGs; red and green cone pigment affected
         4) tritan (#190900): lack of blue-yellow discrimination but intact red-green discrimination (chr. 7q22)
    3. Progressive cone dystrophy
       a. inheritance: X-linked (#304020, #304030) or autosomal dominant (#304030)
       b. clinical features: progressive loss of central vision and color discrimination beginning in second to fourth decades; day blindness and photophobia; there may be a bull's-eye maculopathy, normal macula or a golden tapetal sheen; abnormal photopic and normal scotopic ERG

G. Choroidal Dystrophies

1. Aicardi syndrome #304050
   a. inheritance: X-linked dominant
   b. clinical features: females; round, widespread depigmented chorioretinal lesions; microphthalmos and coloboma occur; agenesis of the corpus collosum; infantile spasms, and severe mental retardation
2. Choroideremia #303100
   a. inheritance: X-linked recessive
   b. clinical features: affected males develop peripheral vision loss and night blindness from age 4 to 20 years. Ophthalmoscopic examination reveals loss of RPE and choriocapillaris which begins at the equator and progresses anteriorly and posteriorly
   c. diagnosis: ERG shows rod cone degenerations, EOG is abnormal, wide angle fluorescein angiogram shows choriocapillaris and RPE dropout with preservation of larger choroidal vessels
   d. treatment: low vision aids and genetic counseling
3. Gyrate atrophy #258870
   a. inheritance: autosomal recessive
   b. clinical features: manifest by 6 to 8 years of age or later with progressive visual field loss and night blindness; patients develop loss of RPE and choriocapillaris, and intact RPE has more pigmentation than normal. Myopia and cataracts commonly found
   c. diagnosis: deficiency of ornithine aminotransferase leads to ornithine plasma elevations 6 to 10 times normal range. ERG is abnormal.
   d. treatment: low vision aids; dietary arginine restriction and vitamin B6 supplementation appears to halt progression of the disease

V. ALBINISM

A. Albinism with Hemorrhagic Diathesis and Pigmented Reticuloendothelial Cells (Hermansky-Pudlak Syndrome) #203300
   1. Inheritance: autosomal recessive
   2. Clinical features: there may be freckles, easy sunburning with or without petechiae and ecchymoses, the hair is white to brown, the iris is blue to brown with transillumination defects; there is a bleeding diathesis; pulmonary fibrosis can be fatal

3. Diagnosis: clinical appearance, tyrosinase activity in hair bulbs is normal, skin shows incomplete melanization, platelet defect and catechol-like material in urine. Common in Puerto Rico
4. Treatment: low vision aids, patient should be advised to avoid platelet-inhibiting medicines, such as aspirin and other nonsteroidal anti-inflammatory agents. Patients may require cryoprecipitate infusion to lower bleeding time. Use of vitamin E as a membrane stabilizer may decrease epistaxis. Patients often have pulmonary symptoms in the third to fifth decades, secondary to ceroid-like deposits in the lung, requiring cough suppressants and oxygen supplementation

B. Autosomal Recessive Ocular Albinism #203200
   1. Inheritance: autosomal recessive, represents a form of oculocutaneous albinism with predominant ocular involvement
   2. Clinical features: very rare, patients may have easy sunburning and may tan, hair is normal, iris is normal with transillumination defects
   3. Diagnosis: clinical appearance, tyrosinase activity in hair bulbs is normal, skin melanosomes are normal; carriers have normal ocular examination. Represents mild form of oculocutaneous albinism with predominant ocular manifestations. Mutations in tyrosinase gene demonstrated
   4. Treatment: low vision aids, genetic counseling

C. Chediak-Higashi Syndrome #214500
   1. Inheritance: autosomal recessive
   2. Clinical features: skin may vary from no pigmentation to normal, hair may have a silvery sheen, iris is light blue to brown with or without transillumination defects. These patients are predisposed to infections and have a reduced survival
   3. Diagnosis: tyrosinase activity in hair bulbs is normal, macromelanosomes may be seen in skin biopsy, giant azurophilic staining granules are seen inside the cytoplasm of neutrophils (thought to be of normal lysosome), and clinical appearance; there may be enlarged leukocyte granules in carriers
   4. Treatment: various treatments have been described for the accelerated phase of this syndrome, including iron and folic acid supplementation to treat anemia, ascorbate to improve leukocyte function and chemotherapy for treatment of pancytopenia (most promising has been combination of vincristine and corticosteroids), genetic counseling

D. Nettleship-Falls Ocular Albinism #300500

1. Inheritance: X-linked recessive
2. Clinical features: only type of pure ocular albinism; there may be congenital hypopigmented skin macules, and these patients may show some tanning; hair is normal, iris is normal color with transillumination defects
3. Diagnosis: clinical appearance and macromelanosomes are seen on skin biopsy; partial transillumination defects, areas of RPE hypopigmentation, and macromelanosomes may be seen in carrier females
4. Treatment: low vision aids and genetic counseling

E. Tyrosinase Negative—Oculocutaneous Albinism (OCA 1) #203100
   1. Inheritance: autosomal recessive
   2. Clinical features: no skin pigmentation, easy sunburning, no tanning, hair is white, iris is light blue with transillumination defects
   3. Diagnosis: clinical features, no tyrosinase activity in hair bulbs, no melanin
   4. Treatment: low vision aids and genetic counseling

F. Tyrosinase Positive—Oculocutaneous Albinism (OCA 2) #203200
   1. Inheritance: autosomal recessive
   2. Clinical features: skin pigmentation present in nevi, easy sunburning, some tanning, hair is white to light yellow, iris is light blue to hazel with transillumination defects
   3. Diagnosis: clinical appearance, there is normal or increased tyrosinase activity in hair bulbs and trace melanin in skin
   4. Treatment: low vision aids and genetic counseling

G. Yellow Mutant—Oculocutaneous Albinism #203100
   1. Inheritance: autosomal recessive
   2. Clinical features: skin is creamy colored, there is easy sunburning and no tanning, hair is yellow, iris is blue with transillumination defects, Amish population
   3. Diagnosis: clinical appearance, there is trace tyrosinase activity in hair bulbs, hair bulb incubation in L-cysteine increases pigment
   4. Treatment: low vision aids and genetic counseling

VI. DISORDERS OF METABOLISM

A. Disorders of Lipid Metabolism
   1. Apolipoprotein A-1 deficiency #107680.0012
      a. inheritance: autosomal dominant
      b. clinical features: low high density lipoproteins (HDL), diffuse corneal clouding

2. Cerebral cholesterinosis (cerebrotendinous xanthomatosis) #213700
   a. inheritance: autosomal recessive
   b. clinical features: progressive neurologic dysfunction, premature atherosclerosis, cholesterol deposition in most tissues and cataracts
3. Fabry's disease (angiokeratoma corporis diffusum) #301500
   a. inheritance: X-linked recessive
   b. clinical features: telangiectatic skin lesions, hypohidrosis, febrile episodes, peripheral neuropathy, renal failure, cardiovascular disease, gastrointestinal symptoms, and central nervous system disturbances
      1) ocular findings: corneal opacification by fine superficial white, yellow or brown dots distributed in a vortex pattern (90% female carriers), opacities do not affect vision, dilation and tortuosity of conjunctival vessels, sometimes with aneurysm formation (50% of patients), posterior spoke-like sutural cataracts (50% of patients), periorbital edema (25% of patients), papilledema, retinal edema, optic atrophy, and dilation and tortuosity of retinal vessels
      2) dermatologic findings: small round red to blue-black spots
   c. pathology: intracytoplasmic lamellar inclusions, especially in basal epithelial cells. Similar inclusions also seen in conjunctival epithelium
4. Farber lipogranulomatosis #228000
   a. inheritance: autosomal recessive
   b. clinical features: increased tissue ceramide, corneal clouding and conjunctiva granulomas
5. Fish eye disease #136120
   a. inheritance: probably autosomal dominant
   b. clinical features: increased LDL triglyceride, VLDL low HDL white-yellow corneal, dot-like opacities
6. Gaucher disease #230800
   a. inheritance: autosomal recessive
   b. clinical features: hematologic abnormalities with hypersplenism, bone lesions, skin pigmentation, and pingueculae; cherry red spot can occur
   c. pathology: pingueculae contained foamy epithelial cells (Gaucher cells)
7. GM1 gangliosidosis #230500

     a. inheritance: autosomal recessive

     b. clinical features: infantile form characterized by coarse facies, macula cherry red spot (50% of cases), infants survive only 1 to 2 years, mild diffuse corneal clouding can occur

8. Hyperlipoproteinemia

     a. inheritance: autosomal recessive, autosomal dominant, or multiple genetic factors involved

     b. clinical features:

       1) type I

          a) elevated chylomicron and triglyceride (#238600)

          b) eruptive xanthomata in lids

          c) lipemia retinalis

       2) type IIA

          a) elevated low density lipoproteins (LDL) and cholesterol (#143890)

          b) premature corneal arcus

          c) xanthelasma

          d) lid and conjunctival xanthomata

       3) type IIB

          a) elevated LDL and very low density lipoproteins (VLDL) (#144010)

          b) elevated cholesterol and triglycerides

          c) premature corneal arcus

       4) type III

          a) elevated VLDL remnants (#107741)

          b) triglycerides and cholesterol

          c) premature corneal arcus

          d) xanthelasma

          e) lipemia retinalis

       5) type IV

          a) elevated VLDL and triglycerides (#144600)

          b) lipemia retinalis

       6) type V

          a) elevated VLDL and chylomicrons (#144650)

          b) elevated triglycerides and cholesterol

          c) rarely eruptive xanthomata

          d) lipemia retinalis

9. Lecithin—cholesterol acyltransferase insufficiency (LCAT) #245900

     a. inheritance: autosomal recessive

     b. clinical features: high VLDL, unasterified cholesterol, diffuse arcus-like, dot-like corneal opacities

10. Metachromatic leukodystrophy #250100

     a. inheritance: autosomal recessive

     b. clinical features: congenital and infantile forms can show corneal clouding, optic atrophy, ab-

normal extraocular movements, pupillary abnormalities, and graying of the macula

11. Niemann-Pick disease #257200
   a. inheritance: autosomal recessive
   b. clinical features: may rarely be associated with
      clouding of corneas; cherry red spot can occur
12. Refsum disease #266500
   a. inheritance: autosomal recessive
   b. clinical features: phytanic acid storage, thick-
      ened corneal epithelium, pannus, increased
      visibility of corneal nerves, corneal guttate,
      corneal edema; pigmentary retinopathy
13. Tangier disease #205400
   a. inheritance: autosomal recessive
   b. clinical features: absent HDL, stromal corneal
      clouding with normal vision, yellow-orange
      conjunctival tinge
B. Disorders of Carbohydrate Metabolism

Mucopolysaccharidosis (MPS)

	Genetics	Corneal Clouding	Retinal Pigmentary Degeneration	Optic Atrophy
I-H: Hurler #252800	AR	+++	R	R
I-S: Scheie (formerly (MPS V)	AR	+++	R	R
II: Hunter #309900				
A. Severe pheno-type	XR	–	R	R
B. Mild phenotype	XR	+	R	R
III: Sanfilippo				
A. Sulfatase-deficient #252900	AR	–	R	R
B. Glucosamini-dase-deficient #252920	AR	–	R	R
C. Acetyl-CoA-a glucosaminidase N acetyl transfer-ase deficient #252930	AR	–	R	R
D. N-acetylglucos-aminidase-6 sulfate sulfatase deficient #252940	AR	–	R	R
IV: Morquio #253000	AR	++	NR	R
V: Vacant; now MPS I-S				

VI: Maroteaux-Lamy #253200				
A. Severe phenotype	AR	++	NR	R
B. Mild phenotype	AR	++	NR	NR
VII: Sly #253220	AR	++	NR	NR

R - Reported

NR - Not Reported

    a. pathology: corneal findings similar in all mucopolysaccharidosis (MPS) disorders; vacuolization of the conjunctiva and corneal epithelium, endothelium, and keratocytes; ultrastructurally vacuoles are single membrane-bound structures containing fibrillogranular material or membranous lamellar inclusions, less marked changes in MPS II, MPS III

    b. treatment: corneal transplantation can result in at least short-term clear corneas; vision may still be limited by optic nerve or retinal disease; corneal clouding and retinal function can stabilize or even improve with bone marrow transplantation to correct enzymatic insufficiency

C. Disorders of Combined Carbohydrate and Lipid Metabolism

  1. Fucosidosis #230000

    a. inheritance: autosomal recessive

    b. clinical features: superficial corneal clouding, retinopathy, dilated tortuous conjunctival vessels, cytoplasmic membrane-bound inclusions containing fibrogranular and multilaminated material are found in corneal conjunctival and vascular endothelium on EM

  2. Mannosidosis #248500

    a. inheritance: autosomal recessive

    b. clinical features: superficial corneal clouding

  3. Mucolipidosis type II—(I cell disease) #252500

    a. inheritance: autosomal recessive

    b. clinical features: corneal clouding occurs commonly, retinopathy can occur

  4. Mucolipidosis type III (pseudohurler polydystrophy) #252600

    a. inheritance: autosomal recessive

    b. clinical features: mild corneal clouding, retinopathy

  5. Mucolipidosis type IV (Berman syndrome)

    a. inheritance: autosomal recessive

    b. clinical features: severe corneal clouding in infancy; retinal dystrophy

      6. Neuraminidase deficiency (sialidosis) #256550
- **a.** inheritance: autosomal recessive
- **b.** clinical features: corneal clouding, cherry red spot

D. Other Disorders of Metabolism

  1. Alkaptonuria #203500
- **a.** inheritance: autosomal recessive
- **b.** clinical features: ochre-colored deposits in limbal area, interpalpebral pigmentation of conjunctiva and episclera, sclera, and rectus tendons
- **c.** pathology: pigment is extracellular, attached to collagen fibers and fibrocytes (conjunctiva and sclera)

  2. Amyloidosis #204850
- **a.** inheritance: autosomal dominant or autosomal recessive
- **b.** clinical features: primary localized amyloidosis can affect bulbar or palpebral conjunctiva, Tenon's capsule, tarsus, limbus, lacrimal gland, or orbit; dominantly inherited, primary systemic amyloidosis, familial amyloid polyneuropathy type IV or Meretoja's syndrome, associated with lattice dystrophy of the cornea

  3. Bietti crystalline retinopathy #210270
- **a.** inheritance: autosomal recessive
- **b.** clinical features: onset in second decade; tapetoretinal degeneration with small glittering crystals in posterior pole; atrophy of RPE; sparkling yellow crystals in superficial paralimbal cornea in some patients
- **c.** pathology: cholesterol-like crystals in corneal or conjunctival fibroblasts and in circulating lymphocytes

  4. Cerebrohepatorenal syndrome (Zellweger syndrome) #214100
- **a.** inheritance: autosomal recessive
- **b.** clinical features: disorder of peroxisome biogenesis; cloudy corneas and cataracts present in most cases, glaucoma, Brushfield spots, persistent pupillary membrane, epicanthus, rapidly progressive retinal degeneration, and optic disc pallor can be present; muscular hypotonia, high forehead, and hypertelorism, hepatomegaly, deficient cerebral myelination, nonrecordable ERG

  5. Congenital erythropoietic porphyria #263700
- **a.** inheritance: autosomal recessive, manifested shortly after birth, recognized by excretion of pink or red urine

    b. clinical features: optic nerve atrophy and retinal hemorrhages occur; scarring and depigmentation of the eyelid, entropion, keratoconjunctivitis, conjunctival necrosis, scleromalacia, and corneal melting and scarring can occur

6. Cystinosis, late onset juvenile or adolescent nephropathic type #219750, #219800, #219900
    a. inheritance: autosomal recessive
    b. clinical features: three forms, infantile, adolescent and adult, diffuse corneal stromal crystals, recurrent erosions can occur and crystals can cause intense photophobia; crystal deposits also seen in conjunctiva, bulbar and fornicial areas; retinal pigmentary changes with extensive depigmentation in the periphery seen consistently in #219900
    c. pathology: corneal crystals are intracellular within an epithelium and keratocytes and are membrane bound; crystal deposition results in thinning and focal breaks in Bowman's membrane; crystals also in subepithelial conjunctiva, sclera, iris, ciliary body, choroid, extraocular muscles, and RPE
    d. diagnosis: conjunctival biopsy can confirm diagnosis; should be fixed in absolute phenol and examined with polarized light, can also use leukocyte cystine assay
    e. treatment: cysteamine can reduce corneal crystal content; given as 10 millimolar drop hourly; crystals can recur in corneal transplants; renal transplantation for renal failure

7. Hemochromatosis #235200
    a. inheritance: can be autosomal recessive
    b. clinical features: rusty brown pigmentation of the perilimbal bulbar conjunctiva has been described

8. Hyperuricemia
    a. inheritance: combination of genetic and environmental factors
    b. clinical features: monosodium urate deposition in cornea, conjunctiva and sclera; acute conjunctival inflammation can occur with complaints of photophobia, burning and pain; conjunctival tophi can also occur; foreign punctate or needle-like refractile crystals can appear in the anterior corneal stroma and epithelium, and are most dense in the palpebral fissure
    c. treatment: corneal epithelial deposits can be removed by scraping or superficial keratectomy

9. Multiple carboxylase deficiency, late onset (biotinidase deficiency) #253260
   a. clinical features: conjunctivitis in 50% of patients, one of initial findings in 10% of patients, optic atrophy may be seen
10. Phenylketonuria (PKU) #261600
    a. inheritance: classically autosomal recessive
    b. clinical features: cataracts, partial albinism and photophobia can be seen
11. Porphyria cutanea tarda (PCT) #176100
    a. inheritance: probably autosomal dominant
    b. clinical features: recurrent vesiculation of lid skin with secondary scarring and cicatricial entropion and punctal stenosis; conjunctiva can be hyperemic with vesicle formation leading to necrosis scarring and symblepharon formation; corneal scarring can occur
12. Tyrosine transaminase deficiency (tyrosinemia type II) #276600
    a. inheritance: autosomal recessive
    b. clinical features: dust-like corneal opacities randomly distributed in lower aspect of cornea; these do not stain with fluorescein nor are they associated with vascularization; dendritic lesions may simulate herpes simplex keratitis
    c. pathology: hypoplastic stratified epithelium with intracellular edema, thickening of basement membrane, conjunctiva plaques reveal membrane-bound inclusions in superficial epithelial cells and blood vessel endothelium
    d. treatment: diet low in tyrosine and phenylalanine can lead to resolution of eye and skin lesions; disease recurs in corneal transplants
13. Wilson's disease #277900
    a. inheritance: autosomal recessive
    b. clinical features: Kayser-Fleischer ring (95% of patients), sunflower cataract (15 to 20% of patients); Kayser-Fleischer ring seen best with gonioscopy
    c. pathology: corneal pigmentation caused by granular copper deposition in peripheral Descemet's membrane
    d. treatment: removal of deposits with D-penicillamin which prevents and reverses clinical manifestations

Essentials of Eye Care, edited by Rohit Varma.
Lippincott–Raven Publishers,
Philadelphia © 1997.

13

Trauma

I. ORBITAL AND ADNEXAL TRAUMA

A. General Principles

1. Always perform a careful and complete eye evaluation prior to an orbital and adnexal exam; the first priority in periorbital trauma is to rule out a globe injury

2. Carefully document the circumstances of injury in the patient's own words for clues as to the presence of a foreign body or penetrating injury as well as for medicolegal purposes; photographs are helpful to document the patient's exam

3. CT scans are preferred over roentgenograms; any injury suspicious enough for fracture, foreign body, or hemorrhage based on clinical exam should be evaluated by CT imaging whether or not plain X-ray yields information; thin (2 mm) sections should be obtained with axial and direct coronal sections if possible; reformatted coronal sections are usually adequate, however, if the patient cannot lie prone

4. Most orbital fracture repairs may be delayed for several days unless bony fragments impinge on vital orbital structures or complications such as orbital hemorrhage or intraorbital foreign body are present

5. Orbital fractures involving the paranasal sinuses should be treated with oral antibiotics; subcutaneous emphysema suggests sinus fracture and air in the orbit; the patient should avoid noseblowing and the Valsalva maneuver until repair is performed

6. Medial wall fractures are suggested by epistaxis, acquired telecanthus, or flattening of the nasal bridge

7. Exquisite care should be given to repair of the eyelid because of its great functional and cosmetic im-

portance; use fine, nonabsorbable suture for periorbital skin repair and evert skin edges to reduce scarring; lids require continuous tarsal margin for proper conformation with meticulous layered closure

B. Eyelid and Canalicular Lacerations

    1. Epidemiology

        a. several studies have shown that young males in the second and third decades have the highest incidence of periorbital trauma including lid lacerations

        b. canalicular lacerations often seen after penetrating injury with a sharp object or avulsion (forcible separation) of medial canthal tendon by blunt trauma; they are seen particularly with fist injury (often a glancing blow) or animal bite (see below)

    2. Clinical features:

        a. a careful history of injury circumstances is important; a lid laceration and accompanying lid and conjunctival edema may mask a globe perforation or an intraorbital foreign body

    3. Pathology

        a. a rich blood supply is present in the eyelids, which are supplied by branches of the internal and external carotid arteries; infection is uncommon unless the wound is contaminated by foreign material

    4. Diagnosis

        a. primary attention should be paid to integrity of the globe and absence of an intraorbital foreign body; lacerations should be gently and carefully explored to determine their extent and depth

        b. suspect canalicular laceration if medial canthal tendon laxity is present; probe and irrigate through punctum; patient should feel saline in throat if the lacrimal excretory system is patent

        c. often see rounding of medial canthus and acquired telecanthus (increased distance between medial canthus and midline)

    5. Treatment

        a. infiltrative anesthesia (2% lidocaine with 1:100,000 epinephrine) may be used locally for lid anesthesia and akinesia

        b. it is sometimes best to wait to allow lid hemorrhage and edema to abate; repair may be safely delayed up to 48 hours if necessary due to excellent vascular supply of the lids

c. wound edges may be trimmed with minimal tissue sacrifice if ragged tissue edges are present

d. wound should be copiously irrigated with sterile saline to remove foreign material prior to repair

e. oral antibiotics may be given for 5 to 7 days as follows: dicloxacillin 250 mg qid (pediatric dose, 25 mg/kg/day in four divided doses) or Ceclor 250 mg tid (pediatric dose, 25 mg/kg/day in three divided doses)

f. wait 6 to 12 months for correction of any residual deformities; scar remodeling may occur for up to a year

g. wounds to the lacrimal gland are uncommon; be careful not to sever lacrimal ductules when exploring and repairing in the superolateral quadrant, or severe dry eye may result

h. where extensive tissue loss exists and major eyelid reconstruction is required, copious lubrication, including fashioning of a moisture chamber if necessary, is indicated; a textbook of oculoplastic surgery should be consulted for advanced techniques of lid repair

6. Extracanalicular marginal lacerations

a. may be repaired under local anesthesia in most adults; general anesthesia is preferred in children

b. horizontal lid defects with tissue loss of up to 25% in young patients, 33% in older patients, may be repaired primarily if lateral canthotomy/cantholysis is performed

c. repair technique

1) place 6-0 silk sutures at the gray line first in a vertical mattress fashion to reapproximate tarsus and check alignment and conformation, then place 6-0 silk sutures at lash line and posterior tarsus

2) extramarginal tarsus should then be closed with a series of interrupted 6-0 Vicryl sutures; tie knots on anterior surface of tarsus

d. close muscle separately with interrupted 5-0 or 6-0 chromic suture; the skin may be closed with 6-0 silk or nylon

1) margin sutures should be left in place for 10 to 14 days; skin suture may be removed after 5 to 7 days

2) excessive medial mobility of the eyelid may be a sign of transection of the lateral

canthal tendon; may reattach tendon (if visible) or lateral aspect of tarsus to periosteum of lateral orbital tubercle with 4-0 Mersilene or nylon

7. Canalicular marginal lacerations
    a. there is controversy whether to repair isolated canalicular lacerations; experimental evidence suggests that only one functional canaliculus is required for lacrimal drainage; one study suggests a 50% risk of intermittent epiphora in those with unrepaired monocanalicular injury
    b. bicanalicular silicone intubation through the lacrimal sac and nasolacrimal duct is the preferred method of repair
    c. general anesthesia is preferred for canalicular lacerations requiring silicone intubation and any pediatric eyelid laceration; a magnifying loupe or the operative microscope gives the best visualization of the canaliculus
    d. repair technique
        1) a punctal dilator may be used prior to insertion of a Bowman probe into punctum to identify distal end of canaliculus; use operating scope to identify proximal end; look for shiny pinkish-white mucosa with rolled edges; if still occult may try saline, air, or Healon irrigation through other punctum; if unable to identify proximal canaliculus after several attempts simply close the laceration with attention to alignment
        2) once identified the canaliculus should be irrigated to assure patency of the proximal system, particularly in blunt trauma where a medial wall fracture may coexist; the silicone tube is introduced into the punctum and is passed through the distal and proximal canaliculus until meeting the bony medial wall of the orbit; it is then directed inferiorly and its tip is retrieved from the nose with a grooved director; the ends are then tied off in the nose; leave tube in place 6 to 12 months before removal

8. Traumatic ptosis
    a. many periorbital injuries will exhibit traumatic ptosis due to mechanical ptosis of swollen lid as well as protective reflex present when eye is injured; injury to the oculomotor nerve is also a possible mechanism of ptosis

      b. may have direct transection of levator complex by sharp instrument; blunt trauma may cause dehiscence or otherwise impair levator function by edema or hemorrhage; absence of lid fold on injured side may indicate levator dehiscence

      c. the presence of orbital fat indicates penetration beyond the orbital septum and possible levator transection; orbital fat should be gently repositioned and any freely prolapsing fat may be excised; the orbital septum should not be sutured together

      d. lacerations to the levator complex should be repaired within the first 24 hours; most adults can be repaired under local anesthetic; patient cooperation under local anesthesia may be used to allow easy identification of the levator by voluntary movement of the eyelid

      e. irrigate thoroughly with sterile saline to remove any foreign material; identify ends of aponeurosis and suture to other end or to tarsal plate with 5-0 or 6-0 Vicryl or Dexon

      f. repair of ptosis due to blunt trauma should be delayed at least 6 months to prevent overcorrection and to allow for any spontaneous recovery of levator function; an exception is made for children in the critical period for amblyopia; in these children a temporary brow suspension may be used

   9. Periorbital lacerations

      a. follow lines of skin tension (Langer's lines) in repair; this will help to conceal and limit the extent of scarring

      b. close in layers, first repositioning orbital fat; 5-0 or 6-0 Vicryl suture is appropriate for orbicularis closure, and 6-0 nylon for skin

      c. undermine skin locally if a small defect is present and then close directly with interrupted nonabsorbable sutures (e.g., 6-0 nylon); may be removed after 5 to 7 days

      d. use a skin graft if a larger defect is present; preferred donor sites are ipsilateral or contralateral lid skin, retroauricular skin, supraclavicular skin

      e. can "freshen up" ragged edges but generally don't remove tissue unless obviously devitalized

C. Intraorbital Foreign Bodies

   1. Epidemiology

    a. a penetrating orbital injury should be considered to harbor an intraorbital foreign body until proven otherwise by imaging tests; any penetrating orbital injury should be evaluated thoroughly to rule out intraorbital foreign body or occult ruptured globe; these injuries may occur despite normal visual acuity

    b. the most common site of foreign body entry is the medial canthus, followed by the upper and lower lids; entry in the lateral canthus is least common

    c. intraorbital foreign body may present with delay in diagnosis, months to years after seemingly minor trauma; be sure to elicit history of trauma in any case of inflammatory orbitopathy

2. Clinical features

    a. visual acuity may range from 20/20 to no light perception (NLP); excellent acuity may be present despite an intraorbital foreign body

    b. history of penetrating trauma, particularly wooden sticks, branches, or pencils; metal objects such as knives, pens, BBs, etc.

    c. may have impaired motility due to mass effect of foreign body or direct muscle or nerve injury; defer forced duction testing

    d. suspect intraorbital foreign body particularly if orbital fat is present in wound

3. Pathology

    a. direct damage to orbital structures may be caused by the foreign body, secondary edema, or hemorrhage; copper and copper alloys may cause an acute purulent inflammation; wood and vegetable matter may cause fungal or anaerobic bacterial infection and lead to meningitis and brain abscess, osteomyelitis or chronic draining fistula

4. Diagnosis

    a. it is important to suspect an orbital foreign body based on history and clinical exam; many patients will be intoxicated or unconscious and may not recall the circumstances of injury

    b. CT scan (preferred) or ultrasound; MRI should not be used if there is a chance that a metallic foreign body is present; the radiologist should be alerted to the suspicions of an intraorbital foreign body, particularly one with radiodensity between bone and soft tissue such as glass or wood; scan should include sinus and cranial imaging if any clinical suspicion exists

c. penetrating orbitocranial injuries are rare but may be catastrophic; neurologic status should be monitored and the presence of cerebrospinal fluid (CSF) should be noted; all such cases should receive prompt neuroimaging

5. Treatment

a. the entry wound and any removed foreign material should be cultured

b. the location and composition of an intraorbital foreign body (or bodies) dictate its management; copper, wood, vegetable, or other organic matter should as a rule be removed; other metals, glass and stone may be left in place unless easy surgical access exists or if sharp edges are apparent on imaging and the risk of injury due to foreign body migration is high

c. intravenous antibiotics should be given (e.g., a second generation cephalosporin such as cefoxitin or cefotetan) (third generation cephalosporins have weaker anaerobic coverage); an alternative is penicillin G 10 million units IV qd divided into 3 to 4 doses

d. an anterior foreign body may be removed through original wound; more posterior material may require formal orbitotomy

e. careful dissection along tissue planes, wide exposure, and gentle retraction of intraorbital contents are essential for surgical success; a fiber optic headlight may be helpful in more posterior dissections; choose surgical route to always keep foreign body between the surgeon and optic nerve; use magnet if magnetic foreign body is suspected

f. obtain ear, nose, and throat (ENT) and neurosurgical consultations if indicated by exam and imaging studies

D. Blowout Fractures

1. Epidemiology

a. as in most facial trauma, young adult males are likeliest to sustain a blowout fracture

b. blowout fractures are the second most common facial fracture after nasal fracture

2. Clinical features

a. typically see limited upgaze, diplopia on upgaze, pain on attempted upgaze, enophthalmos, hypophthalmos, cheek hypesthesia in distribution of infraorbital nerve; may see proptosis acutely due to orbital and periorbital edema; restricted downgaze may be present if there is entrapment of the inferior rectus muscle; globe ptosis with herniation of the eye or its inferior muscles into the maxillary sinus

b. a positive forced duction test (i.e., resistance to traction) will be present when there is attempted rotation into upgaze

c. enophthalmos may produce a pseudoptosis with a pronounced superior lid sulcus

d. a ring of periorbital ecchymosis may be associated with a basilar skull fracture; appropriate imaging tests should rule out this condition

3. Pathology

    a. two theories advanced to account for fracture:

        1) "hydraulic" theory with compression of orbital contents, increased intraorbital pressure, and fracture of the thin orbital floor

        2) "buckling" theory with stress transmitted directly from the orbital rim to the orbital floor; may be a combination of forces

    b. fractures may range from thin "hairline" fracture with minimal or no entrapment to extensive disruption of the orbital floor with globe ptosis and widespread herniation of orbital contents

4. Diagnosis

    a. history, clinical exam, and CT scan, particularly coronal sections; palpation of the periorbital area may reveal an associated zygoma fracture with inferior displacement of the lateral canthus and flattening of the cheek

5. Treatment

    a. controversial—most surgeons would operate after a period of 7 to 14 days if there is disabling primary or upgaze diplopia or enophthalmos of 2 mm or more when compared to unaffected eye

    b. blowout fractures are not to be repaired acutely; delayed repair (4 to 6 weeks) is indicated in cases of concurrent ruptured globe or hyphema, because repeated forced duction testing and other globe manipulation is necessary at the time of surgery

    c. exposure of the orbital contents to sinus flora should be covered with oral antibiotics (e.g., amoxicillin 250 mg tid or cefuroxime 250 mg bid) for 5 to 7 days

E. Periorbital Animal and Human Bites
  1. Epidemiology
    a. vast majority are dog bites, most occur in young children; face-biting behavior of dogs thought to establish dominance of animal over similar-sized children
    b. annual incidence of 44,000 facial dog bites in U.S.A. with 8% of these sustaining periorbital bites; one study found that greater than half of periorbital dog bites occurred in children less than 5 years old
  2. Clinical features
    a. avulsed medial canthal tendon (see separate section on canalicular laceration) is very common in dog bites; fortunately, direct injury to globe is uncommon
    b. immunocompromised are at risk for systemic infection with DF-2, a common species of the flora of the dog oral cavity; may lead to fulminant infection with sepsis, disseminated intravascular coagulation, and shock
  3. Pathology
    a. most common cause of infection after dog bite is *Pasteurella multocida,* a gram-negative coccobacillus; treat with penicillin G, 8 to 12 million units per day in four divided doses; tetracycline (250 to 500 mg qid), oxacillin or cefuroxime may be used in the penicillin-allergic
    b. DF-2 bacteria is a gram-negative rod; treat with prompt intravenous penicillin G or chloramphenicol if penicillin-allergic (50 to 100 mg/kg/day divided into four doses)
  4. Diagnosis
    a. history, evidence of bite or puncture wounds; lacrimal probing may be performed if the patient is cooperative
    b. it is important to document the circumstances of the bite injury for reporting to public health authorities and for medicolegal purposes
  5. Treatment
    a. tetanus prophylaxis required if greater than 5 years elapsed since last booster
    b. repair of lacrimal canaliculus laceration (see separate section); the role of antibiotics is controversial in clean wounds; a broad spectrum intravenous late-generation cephalosporin for 24 hours followed by outpatient oral antibiotic therapy may be appropriate; copious saline ir-

      rigation and removal of any foreign material are mandatory

  c. healing by secondary intention should be allowed only when a wound infection is present

  d. human bites are treated similarly to dog bites, i.e., with irrigation, conservative debridement of devitalized tissue, meticulous primary repair, and antibiotic coverage; avulsion injuries are uncommon in human bites; feral animals such as raccoon, skunk, or bat are known to carry rabies with a high prevalence; consult with local public health authorities in these cases

  e. in most jurisdictions offending animal must be quarantined and tested for rabies; consult with ER physician or public health authorities for guidance as to local laws

F. Periocular Burns

  1. Epidemiology

    a. periocular burns present in 14% of burns, 67% of facial burns in one study; 50% of these were partial-thickness that healed within one week; only 12% of patients required skin grafts

  2. Clinical features

    a. may have thermal burns, explosive injury, chemical burns

  3. Pathology

    a. first-degree burns are confined to the epidermis; second-degree burns affect the epidermis and part of the dermis; third-degree burns of the eyelid extend through the epidermis and dermis into the underlying orbicularis

  4. Diagnosis

    a. usually obvious from history and clinical exam; see edema and tissue necrosis; rule out foreign bodies on skin or eye surface, especially in blast injuries; careful inspection for corneal surface injury

    b. a thorough general eye exam is always indicated, although fortunately the ocular surface is often spared due to the Bell's reflex; always check ability to close eyes and integrity of Bell's reflex

  5. Treatment

    a. examine for foreign bodies and check pH to prevent further injury from chemical burn

    b. primary goal is to protect the ocular surface and prevent secondary corneal infection; burn patients may be unconscious or sedated and will have a decreased protective reflex; aggressive lubrication with artificial tears and bland ointment with daily exam of the corneal surface is indicated initially; topical antibiotics should be used in presence of corneal epithelial defect or infectious conjunctivitis (e.g., bacitracin-polymyxin ointment bid-qid); any discharge should be cultured and Gram-stained

c. avoid early debridement unless tissue clearly devitalized; the excellent vascular supply of the eyelids will often allow retention of tissue that looks compromised in the early postburn period

d. tarsorrhaphies are generally to be avoided in burn patients unless they are comatose or have severe exposure; they are always a temporizing measure and cannot resist the contracture and separation forces from a severe burn

e. early split-thickness skin grafting (preferred donor sites include the anterolateral neck or medial upper arm) after conservative debridement is suggested in second- and third-degree burn patients after the burn eschar sloughs in the first 1 to 2 weeks; contracture is minimized but not eliminated by split-thickness grafts, and contracture may continue for 6 to 12 months

f. avoid symblepharon if conjunctiva burned by sweeping fornices with antibiotic ointment and early buccal mucous membrane grafting

g. late deformities include ectropion, distorted lid margin, epicanthal folds, lid retraction and symblepharon

II. CORNEAL ABRASION

A. Epidemiology
1. Occurs after blunt or penetrating injury to the globe; common agents include fingers, fingernails, edges of paper, foreign bodies, and contact lenses

B. Clinical Features
1. Presenting symptoms/signs: severe pain, redness, photophobia, tearing, decreased vision
2. Biomicroscopic findings: irregularly shaped area of absent corneal epithelium; irregular corneal light reflex; topical fluorescein stains areas of absent epithelium green when viewed under cobalt blue light; in the absence of infection, the corneal

stroma remains clear; evidence of injury to other anterior segment structures may be present

3. Ophthalmoscopic findings: evidence of posterior segment injury may be present
4. Clinical course: most small abrasions will heal spontaneously overnight; occasionally, corneal infection may result; spontaneous recurrent corneal erosion may occur weeks to months later

C. Pathogenesis
1. In patients with recurrent corneal erosion, the corneal epithelium fails to bind adequately to the basement membrane during the healing process

D. Diagnosis
1. Slit lamp examination using fluorescein is essential to determine the extent and depth of the corneal defect

E. Treatment
1. It is important to evert the lids and examine the palpebral conjunctiva and cul-de-sac to rule out the presence of retained foreign body
2. For small abrasions, only antibiotic ointment or drops may be necessary
3. For larger abrasions, antibiotic ointment, cycloplegics, and pressure patching usually are necessary

III. CHEMICAL INJURIES

A. Epidemiology
1. Most commonly occurs in industrial and agricultural settings; may occur in domestic environment; may be assault-related
2. Alkali burns are much more serious than acid burns; ammonium hydroxide is the worst offender, followed by sodium hydroxide (lye), potassium and magnesium hydroxide, and calcium hydroxide (lime); ammonium hydroxide is present in household ammonia, window cleaner, and fertilizer
3. Acid burns commonly include sulfuric and nitric acids; automobile battery explosions are the usual cause

B. Clinical Features
1. Presenting symptoms/signs: pain, redness, tearing, photophobia, decreased vision; eye may be painless and appear white (a poor prognostic sign due to severe anterior segment ischemia)
2. Biomicroscopic findings: partial or total loss of the corneal epithelium; corneal stroma may appear

clear, mildly hazy, or opaque; limbal blanching (may indicate loss of anterior segment vascular supply); elevated intraocular pressure (IOP)

3. Ophthalmoscopic findings: may appear normal but view often limited by anterior segment damage

4. Clinical course: healing of conjunctival and corneal epithelium usually occurs; corneal stroma may clear, become vascularized, or ulcerate, and can ultimately develop a descemetocele and perforate; symblepharon, dry eye, entropion, and trichiasis may develop; IOP may remain elevated, or hypotony may develop with resultant phthisis

C. Pathogenesis

1. Strong alkalis cause saponification of fatty acids in cell membranes and subsequent disruption of cells; the cation determines the penetrability and the hydroxyl concentration determines the extent and severity of the injury; ammonia is highly lipid-soluble and rapidly penetrates the eye; calcium hydroxide penetrates poorly because it reacts to form calcium soaps which precipitate and hinder further penetration; with very high pH, collagen fibers swell, thus elevating IOP

2. For corneal healing, there is a balance between collagen synthesis and degradation (proteolysis); degradation occurs via collagenase (synthesized in polymorphonuclear leucocytes (PMNs), epithelial cells, and fibroblasts); if the rate of proteolysis exceeds the rate of collagen synthesis, stromal ulceration results (usually 2 to 3 weeks after injury)

3. Acid burns produce denaturation and coagulation of protein, which precipitate and prevent further penetration; damage is usually limited to surface of eye

D. Diagnosis

1. Based on clinical history and on biomicroscopic findings

E. Treatment

1. Immediate treatment for any chemical injury, whether documented or suspected, is copious irrigation with the nearest available water or bland fluid; irrigation should be continued during transport to the nearest hospital; upon presentation, irrigation should be continued with sterile saline; topical anesthetics and lid speculum may be necessary; conjunctival fornices should be swept for potential particulate chemical matter; monitor pH with a dipstick

2. For mild injuries, use topical antibiotics, cyclo-plegics, and pressure patch
3. For severe injuries, topical steroids may be also used for approximately 5 to 7 days; steroids enhance collagenase activity, and if steroids are used they should be rapidly tapered and discontinued beyond the first week; topical collagenase inhibitors (L-cysteine, acetyl-cysteine, or ethylenediamine tetraacetic acid [EDTA]) may be used; ascorbic acid promotes collagen synthesis and may be used topically (10% solution) and systemically (2 to 4 gm po qd)
4. Glaucoma therapy may be necessary, especially during the initial management
5. Lysis of symblepharon with an ointment-coated glass rod may be useful
6. Late treatment includes surgical correction of cicatricial entropion, conjunctival or mucous membrane autografts, and penetrating keratopathy

IV. TRAUMATIC HYPHEMA

A. Epidemiology
   1. Occurs after blunt or penetrating trauma to the globe
B. Clinical Features
   1. Presenting symptoms/signs: asymptomatic or pain, photophobia, decreased vision
   2. Biomicroscopic findings: circulating and/or layered red blood cells in anterior chamber; iris sphincter tear; may have evidence of injury to orbit (e.g., blowout fracture) or to other interior structures of the eye (e.g., phacodonesis)
   3. Ophthalmoscopic findings: may have evidence of injury to posterior segment (e.g., retinal dialysis)
   4. Clinical course: gradual resolution of hyphema usually occurs; rebleeding occurs in 5 to 10% or more, usually within 5 to 7 days (if rebleed occurs, the size of the hyphema is usually larger than the primary hyphema); medications (aminocaproic acid, prednisone) may reduce the incidence of rebleeding; elevated intraocular pressure may develop and produce corneal blood staining, retinal arteriolar occlusion, and glaucomatous optic atrophy
C. Pathogenesis
   1. Trauma induces compressive forces that rupture iris and ciliary body vessels

2. Rebleeding may be related to normal clot retraction and lysis
D. Diagnosis
    1. Based on clinical setting of trauma and on biomicroscopic findings; gonioscopy and scleral depression should be deferred until well after the risk of rebleed (highest risk at 5 to 7 days)
E. Treatment
    1. Eye shield, topical steroids (pred forte), cycloplegics (homatropine)
    2. Follow IOP closely; if IOP is elevated, aqueous suppressants and hyperosmotic agents are useful
    3. Systemic steroids (prednisone 40 mg/d) may reduce the incidence of rebleeding
    4. Systemic aminocaproic acid (Amicar 50 mg/kg q 4°) may reduce the incidence of rebleeding; associated with potential complications (syncope, orthostatic hypotension, nausea, vomiting); antiemetics and orthostatic precautions may minimize the complications; do not use in pregnancy
    5. Consider surgery for persistent elevated IOP (>60 for 2 days, >50 for 5 days, >35 for 7 days); anterior chamber washout via paracentesis site(s) may be beneficial
    6. Obtain sickle cell test (sickle prep, hemoglobin electrophoresis) in all African-American and Hispanic patients; hyphema in sickle cell disease or sickle trait patients is a much more serious condition; there is a higher incidence of glaucoma because red blood cells tend to sickle in aqueous humor (because of low oxygen and low pH) and have difficulty passing through the trabecular meshwork; in addition, the optic disc is much more sensitive to elevated IOP due to potentially compromised microvascular perfusion; avoid repetitive carbonic anhydrase inhibitors (acetazolamide) since these lower aqueous pH and may increase sickling; avoid adrenergic agents (epinephrine) since these lower aqueous oxygen and may increase sickling; avoid repetitive hyperosmotic agents since these cause hemoconcentration and may increase sludging; consider surgery to prevent corneal blood staining and optic atrophy

V. TRAUMATIC GLAUCOMA (ANGLE RECESSION)

A. Trauma May Produce Glaucoma by a Variety of Mechanisms: secondary open angle glaucomas include obstruction of the trabecular meshwork by white blood cells and inflamed tissues (traumatic uveitis), red blood cells (hyphema), hemoglobin-laden macrophages (hemolytic glaucoma), degenerated red blood cells (ghost cell glaucoma), lens cortex (lens particle glaucoma), and granulomatous inflammation (phacoanaphylaxis); management depends on controlling or eliminating the specific causative agent(s); angle recession glaucoma is a specific type of traumatic glaucoma that is discussed below

B. Epidemiology

　　1. Occurs after blunt or penetrating trauma to the globe

C. Clinical Features

　　1. Usually unilateral

　　2. Presenting symptoms/signs: asymptomatic or pain, redness, photophobia, loss of visual field, decreased visual acuity

　　3. Biomicroscopic findings: gonioscopy is necessary for diagnosis; an irregular widening of the ciliary body band indicates angle recession; the number of clock hours involved should be documented

　　4. Ophthalmoscopic findings: evidence of injury to the posterior segment may be present

　　5. Clinical course: all eyes with angle recession must be followed indefinitely; the greater the extent (clock hours) and severity of angle recession, the greater the risk of glaucoma; glaucoma may develop soon after trauma or up to years later

D. Pathogenesis

　　1. Histopathology: a tear through the ciliary body between the longitudinal and circular muscle layers

　　2. The cause of the diminished outflow may either be direct damage to the trabecular meshwork or extension of an endothelial layer (and subsequent Descemet's membrane) from the cornea over the iridocorneal angle

　　3. Since up to 50% of fellow eyes develop elevated IOP, those eyes with angle recession glaucoma may have been predisposed to develop open angle glaucoma

E. Diagnosis

　　1. Based on history of trauma and on gonioscopic findings

F. Treatment

　　1. Aqueous suppressants useful

　　2. May get paradoxical response with miotics

　　3. Laser trabeculoplasty has limited success

　　4. Trabeculectomy may be necessary

VI. COMMOTIO RETINAE

A. Epidemiology
  1. Occurs after blunt trauma to the front of the eye
B. Clinical Features
  1. Visual acuity reduced in cases with macular involvement
  2. Biomicroscopic features: evidence of injury to the external and anterior structures of the eyes
  3. Ophthalmoscopic findings: whitening or opacification of the deep sensory retina opposite to the site of impact (contrecoup injury); may involve fovea and/or extensive areas of the retinal periphery; other features of posterior segment trauma (choroidal rupture, macular hole) may also be present
  4. Clinical course: typically, there is complete resolution in several days and visual acuity returns to normal; with more severe blunt trauma, visual loss may persist and the retinal opacification may be replaced by pigment epithelial mottling or even by heavy intraretinal pigment deposition
C. Pathogenesis
  1. Blood-retinal barrier is often intact as assessed by fluorescein angiography and vitreous fluorophotometry
  2. Retinal opacification is probably due to photoreceptor outer segment disruption; outer segments are particularly susceptible to damage due to absence of the Müller cell skeletal system (Müller cells occupy the retina from the internal limiting membrane to the photoreceptor inner segment and support all cellular layers except the photoreceptor outer segments)
D. Diagnosis
  1. Based on clinical setting of acute blunt trauma and ophthalmoscopic features
E. Treatment
  1. None

VII. CHOROIDAL RUPTURE

A. Epidemiology
  1. Occurs after penetrating and nonpenetrating trauma to the globe
  2. Patients with pseudoxanthoma elasticum have a relatively brittle Bruch's membrane and are particularly susceptible to choroidal rupture following minor ocular trauma
B. Clinical Features

1. Visual acuity affected with macular involvement of choroidal rupture or subretinal hemorrhage (usually 20/200 or worse)
2. Biomicroscopic features: evidence of injury to the external or anterior structures of the eye
3. Ophthalmoscopic features: *direct choroidal ruptures*—located anteriorly at the site of impact; oriented parallel to the ora; rare. *Indirect choroidal ruptures*—occur opposite to the site of impact (contrecoup injury); crescent-shaped lesion of the posterior pole oriented concentric with the disc margin; the initial injury often involves subretinal hemorrhage; the choroidal rupture may not be apparent acutely due to the hemorrhage
4. Clinical course: choroidal rupture develops a gliotic scar within a few weeks; hyperpigmentation develops at the margins of the healed lesions; choroidal neovascularization from the margins of the lesion may develop at any time and may result in retinal pigment epithelial and/or retinal hemorrhagic or serous detachment; some cases develop chorioretinal vascular anastomosis

C. Pathogenesis
1. Trauma induces compressive forces that rupture the relatively inelastic Bruch's membrane and its adjacent choriocapillaris (resulting in acute subretinal hemorrhage) and retinal pigment epithelium (resulting in late pigment changes); the retina and sclera do not rupture as the retina is relatively elastic and the sclera is strong
2. Choroidal ruptures are tears of the choroid, Bruch's membrane, and retinal pigment epithelium

D. Diagnosis
1. Fluorescein angiography (FA): may be useful acutely in detecting and localizing small choroidal ruptures and suspected ruptures beneath subretinal hemorrhage; healed ruptures typically demonstrate early hypofluorescence within the rupture (due to the damaged choriocapillaris) and late hyperfluorescence (due to diffusion from the surrounding intact choriocapillaris); in cases with choroidal neovascularization, fluorescein angiography demonstrates early lacy subretinal vessels with late leakage

E. Treatment
1. Argon laser photocoagulation of choroidal neovascular membrane may result in resolution of serous macular detachment

VIII. SCLOPETARIA/TRAUMATIC CHORIORETINAL RUPTURE

A. Epidemiology
   1. Occurs after nonpenetrating trauma to the globe involving a high velocity projectile that directly strikes or passes tangential to the globe
   2. Usually caused by shotgun or BB pellets
   3. A rare manifestation of nonpenetrating trauma
B. Clinical Features
   1. Visual acuity affected with macular involvement
   2. Biomicroscopic findings: evidence of injury to the external or anterior structures of the eye
   3. Ophthalmoscopic findings: full thickness defect in retina, retinal pigment epithelium, Bruch's membrane, and choroid in the same quadrant as the projectile injury; bare sclera visible, although this may not be apparent acutely as there is often overlying vitreous hemorrhage and adjacent intraretinal and subretinal hemorrhage
   4. Clinical course: the lesion ultimately develops irregular, scarred, and pigmented borders; retinal detachment does not develop acutely but rarely may develop as a late complication; vitreous hemorrhage may also develop later
C. Pathogenesis
   1. High velocity projectiles cause rapid deformation of the globe and a sudden increase in the tensile stresses in the ocular tissues; these stresses may exceed the tensile strength of the retina and choroid, but not the relatively elastic posterior hyaloid and the relatively strong sclera; rupture of the choroid is followed by retraction of these tissues to expose the bare sclera
D. Diagnosis
   1. Based on clinical setting of acute nonpenetrating trauma with a high velocity projectile and on ophthalmoscopic findings of bare sclera
E. Treatment
   1. No immediate surgical intervention is needed; scleral buckling surgery and/or vitrectomy may be needed if late retinal detachment or vitreous hemorrhage develops

IX. TRAUMATIC RETINAL BREAKS, DIALYSIS, AND DETACHMENT

A. Epidemiology

1. Occurs after penetrating and nonpenetrating trauma to the globe
B. Clinical Features
   1. Presenting symptoms/signs: floaters; photopsia; visual acuity and visual field reduced when retinal detachment involves the macula; visual field affected with extramacular retinal detachment
   2. Biomicroscopic findings: evidence of injury to the external or anterior structures of the eye; pigmented cells in anterior vitreous indicate high probability of a retinal break
   3. Ophthalmoscopic findings: *retinal breaks*—horseshoe-shaped retinal tears and operculated retinal holes in periphery, especially at areas of lattice degeneration or at edges of chorioretinal scars; formed vitreous is attached to the elevated flap of a horseshoe tear and to the operculum of an operculated hole; *retinal dialysis*—a separation of the peripheral retina from the pars plana epithelium at the ora serrata; inferotemporal quadrant is most common location; *retinal detachment*—retinal breaks and retinal dialyses may result in retinal detachment if liquified vitreous passes between the sensory retina and the retinal pigment epithelium
   4. Clinical course: *retinal breaks*—vitreous traction on the elevated flap of a horseshoe tear holds the tear open and therefore likely results in retinal detachment; *retinal dialysis*—dialyses are less likely to result in retinal detachment; if detachment is present, it is often localized and minimally elevated, especially if the dialysis is small or located inferiorly
C. Pathogenesis
   1. Trauma produces sudden deformation of the vitreous, and retinal tearing may occur in areas of strong vitreoretinal adhesion, such as the vitreous base
   2. Retinal damage at the vitreous base may result in peripheral retinal breaks and retinal dialysis
   3. Retinal breaks and dialyses result in retinal detachment when liquid vitreous enters the subretinal space
D. Diagnosis
   1. Based on clinical setting of trauma and on ophthalmoscopic findings
E. Treatment
   1. Retinal breaks treated with photocoagulation or cryopexy as prophylaxis for retinal detachment; scleral buckling surgery is indicated for retinal

breaks associated with retinal detachment (success rate substantially greater than 80%)
2. Retinal dialysis treated with photocoagulation or cryopexy as prophylaxis for retinal detachment; scleral buckling surgery is indicated for retinal dialysis associated with retinal detachment (success rate 90%)

X. PURTSCHER'S RETINOPATHY

A. Epidemiology
   1. A similar fundus appearance may be seen in a variety of traumatic injuries and diseases: severe head trauma without direct trauma to the globe; acute pancreatitis; long bone fracture; chest compression injuries; air embolization; amniotic fluid embolization; childbirth; hydrostatic pressure syndrome; connective tissue diseases such as lupus, scleroderma, and dermatomyositis
B. Clinical Features
   1. Typically bilateral; unilateral cases have been described; however, in apparent unilateral cases the fellow eye may demonstrate very subtle findings
   2. Presenting symptoms/signs: asymptomatic, central or paracentral scotomas, decreased vision (visual acuity ranges from 20/20 to count fingers)
   3. Biomicroscopic findings: normal
   4. Ophthalmoscopic findings: multiple patches of superficial retinal whitening; may have intraretinal hemorrhages; may have papillitis
   5. Clinical course: unpredictable; some patients experience resolution of visual loss and fundus changes over several weeks to months; some patients develop permanent visual loss associated with macular pigmentary disturbance, nerve fiber layer loss, and optic atrophy
C. Pathogenesis
   1. Uncertain; severe trauma and acute pancreatitis have been shown to activate complement; complement activation results in intravascular granulocyte aggregates or "leukoemboli" measuring 60 to 80μ; retinal arteriolar embolization by granulocyte aggregates may produce the fundus findings
D. Diagnosis
   1. Based on clinical setting of the conditions listed above and on ophthalmoscopic findings
   2. FA: variable findings which may include normal choroidal filling, focal areas of retinal arteriolar

obstruction, patches of capillary nonperfusion, venous staining, and disc leakage

E. Treatment
   1. None

XI. TERSON'S SYNDROME

A. Intraocular hemorrhage (usually vitreous hemorrhage) in association with any form of intracranial hemorrhage
B. Epidemiology
   1. Occurs in patients with any form of intracranial hemorrhage; most common setting is subarachnoid hemorrhage
   2. The majority result from spontaneous rupture of an intracranial aneurysm (20% of patients with subarachnoid hemorrhage develop intraocular hemorrhage); may also occur after subdural hemorrhage
C. Clinical Features
   1. Unilateral or bilateral
   2. Presenting symptoms/signs: asymptomatic, decreased vision (visual acuity ranges from 20/20 to light perception)
   3. Biomicroscopic findings: may have red blood cells in anterior vitreous
   4. Ophthalmoscopic findings: vitreous hemorrhage; multiple preretinal, intraretinal, and subretinal hemorrhages may be present in peripapillary region
   5. Clinical course: two-thirds develop a clinically apparent epiretinal membrane which may result in significant visual loss; many eyes with nonclearing hemorrhage undergo vitrectomy; 83% achieve 20/50 or better at 4-year followup (whether managed with observation or vitrectomy)
D. Pathogenesis
   1. Uncertain; intracranial hemorrhage produces an acute elevation of intracranial pressure that is transmitted within the optic nerve sheath to obstruct the venous drainage from the eye; the acute rise in venous pressure causes distention and rupture of fine papillary and retinal capillaries; the hemorrhage may spread to the subretinal space, within the retina, the subinternal limiting membrane space, the subhyaloid space, or the vitreous cavity
E. Diagnosis
   1. Based on clinical setting of intracranial hemorrhage and on ophthalmoscopic findings

F. Treatment
   1. Indications for conservative management include rapidly clearing vitreous hemorrhage, unilateral involvement with a normal fellow eye, associated ocular damage that precludes good vision, and poor health
   2. Indications for vitrectomy include visually immature eyes in which early rehabilitation may prevent amblyopia, and bilateral involvement
   3. No difference in final visual acuity between eyes managed conservatively and eyes that undergo vitrectomy
   4. Visual recovery faster in eyes managed with vitrectomy

XII. VALSALVA RETINOPATHY

A. Epidemiology
   1. Occurs during Valsalva maneuver; activities include heavy lifting, coughing, vomiting, sexual activity, and straining during bowel movement
B. Clinical Features
   1. Usually unilateral
   2. Presenting symptoms/signs: asymptomatic, decreased vision
   3. Biomicroscopic findings: normal
   4. Ophthalmoscopic findings: dumbbell-shaped hemorrhage beneath the internal limiting membrane at or near the central macula; may have large or oval hemorrhage; subinternal limiting membrane hemorrhage may break through to the subhyaloid space or vitreous cavity
   5. Clinical course: usually gradual resolution of hemorrhage and visual acuity
C. Pathogenesis
   1. Sudden elevation of intrathoracic or intraabdominal pressure is transmitted to the eye because of incompetent or absent valves in the venous system of the head and neck; superficial retinal capillaries rupture from the sudden elevation of ocular venous pressure
D. Diagnosis
   1. Based on clinical setting of Valsalva maneuver and on ophthalmoscopic findings
E. Treatment
   1. Continued observation while the hemorrhage gradually resorbs; occasionally vitrectomy may be considered

XIII. MANAGEMENT OF CORNEOSCLERAL LACERATIONS

A. Patient Evaluation
1. General considerations
   a. with simultaneous chemical injury, sterile irrigation should be completed immediately; otherwise completely assess the nature of the injury by careful history and directed physical examination
2. History
   a. should include (for medical as well as legal purposes):
      1) complete circumstances of injury
      2) exact time of injury; location (job, home, etc.)
      3) mechanism of injury; objects involved (metal, vegetative material)
      4) wearing safety glasses?
      5) preexisting state of eyes—injured and fellow
         a) history of amblyopia
         b) history of prior ocular trauma
         c) history of refractive error
         d) family history of ocular diseases
      6) tetanus immunization status
      7) past medical history
      8) past surgical history
      9) current medications
      10) allergic or adverse reaction to medications
      11) most recent food intake:
         a) last solid food
         b) last oral intake
3. Ocular examination—caution: be cognizant of possible coexistent injuries, especially intracranial injury; assure medical stability prior to completing ocular assessment
4. Visual acuity:
   a. perform initial measurement as accurately as possible; push patient to achieve best recorded acuity
   b. perform quick refraction if situation warrants
   c. utilize near card (Rosenbaum pocket screener or equivalent) in emergency room. Carry +2.00 or +2.50 spherical add and record reading distance.
   d. use pinhole as necessary (if glasses broken)
5. Pupillary examination:

    a. assess configuration; if pupil contour not round, consider occult rupture or laceration with peaking toward wound

    b. assess reactivity to light

    c. assess possible relative afferent pupillary defect (swinging flashlight test)

    d. if pupil size unequal, consider:

        1) ciliary ganglion injury or sympathetic chain injury (Horner's syndrome); preganglionic versus postganglionic

6. Visual fields—subjective testing to confrontation via counting fingers and red test object if able

7. Extraocular motility:

    a. steady fixation at distance and near?

    b. full ductions and versions?

    c. limitations or deviations (simultaneous orbital blowout fracture)?

8. External examination (perform external drawings or preferably obtain external and slit lamp photographs for documentation of injury at presentation)

    a. possible eyelid margin trauma?

    b. possible nasolacrimal system trauma?

    c. levator injury?

    d. wound contamination or purulence?

9. Slit lamp biomicroscopic examination—important to visualize globe completely

    a. utilize Desmarres retractor if there is severe facial and lid swelling

    b. a +20 prism diopter lens or direct ophthalmoscope may be used in ER if portable slit lamp not available

    c. perform Seidel test using sterile fluorescein sodium 2% solution or sterile fluorescein-impregnated filter paper

    d. perform gonioscopy when possible, but not if eye is perforated or ruptured. Look for:

        1) angle recession

        2) cyclodialysis cleft

        3) intraocular foreign body

10. Intraocular pressure measurement

    a. perform measurement using applanation, pneumotonometry, Tonopen, carefully, as indicated

    b. if patient cooperation suboptimal, do not pursue measurement aggressively

    c. do not perform if central corneal scleral laceration present or if anterior chamber obviously flat and eye soft

    d. in occult ruptured globes, IOP may be normal

B. Ophthalmoscopic examination
   1. Perform dilated direct/indirect ophthalmoscopy early, before lens opacity develops or hemorrhage obscures media
   2. Inform neurosurgery colleagues and nurses of pupillary dilation in advance if intracranial or spinal injuries coexist or are suspected; place note on forehead of unconscious or obtunded patients
   3. Use sterile tropicamide 0.5% (defer phenylephrine usage if possible with open globe)
      Perform dilation of both eyes
C. Ancillary diagnostic studies:
   1. Roentgenography (use plastic rather than metallic eye shield)
   2. Bone-free dental films
   3. B-scan ultrasonography—perform with extreme caution if suspected ruptured or lacerated/perforated globe; helpful with hyphema or vitreous hemorrhage
   4. Computed tomography—axial/coronal, sagittal planes (directly or reconstructed)
      a. cut thinnest possible slices (less than 1.5 mm if possible) through the orbits with overlapping cuts if a small foreign body is suspected
      b. caution with one or more foreign bodies having a sufficient attenuation coefficient and volume to cause streak and artifacts
   5. Magnetic resonance imaging—provides superior tissue definition; CAUTION: be careful of ferromagnetic retained foreign bodies in ocular trauma
      a. T1-weighted sequence provides most contrast and detail for ocular and orbital imaging
      b. normal T2-weighted image of the eye and orbit; the vitreous and aqueous have highest signal intensity
D. Fundamental Principles in Anterior Segment Trauma
   1. Suspect that trivial injury may mask actual ocular penetration, if:
      a. conjunctival hemorrhage is associated with:
         1) ocular hypotony
         2) shallowing of the anterior chamber
         3) hyphema or vitreous hemorrhage
      b. perform complete ocular exam, ultrasonography, computed tomography, or MRI as indicated
   2. Topical anesthetic allows more thorough evaluation; NEVER prescribe or allow patient to confiscate topical anesthesia, as it may lead to:
      a. severe epithelial toxicity

    b. an anesthetic cornea that may result in ulcerative keratitis

3. Systemic narcotic medications are rarely necessary for pure ocular trauma
4. Use sterile diagnostic drops if ruptured globe suspected
5. Do not use ophthalmic ointment preparations as they may:
   - **a.** obscure further visualization
   - **b.** penetrate intraocularly
6. Protect globe from further trauma with rigid eye shield (plastic or metallic)
7. Ensure adequate tetanus prophylaxis
   - **a.** clostridia contamination usually follows severe crushing injury
   - **b.** may follow extensive eyelid injury. Tetanus can theoretically occur following any wound or puncture.
     1) primary immunization for tetanus consists of a series of three injections at timed intervals
     2) adults with an uncertain history of a completed primary series should receive the primary series
     3) significant proportion of persons over 60 years of age lack the protective antibody against tetanus toxoid
     4) when prophylaxis is indicated in children under the age of 7, use DPT
     5) after age 7, use tetanus toxoid (Td) 0.5 ml intramuscularly
     6) patients with an unknown or negative history of tetanus vaccination should be considered nonimmunized and for prophylaxis may require passive immunization with tetanus immunoglobulin (TIG) 250 units intramuscularly
     7) Td and TIG administered at the same session are given in different syringes at separate sites
     8) infection prophylaxis—posttraumatic endophthalmitis is a devastating complication, which may occur in 2 to 7% of severe ocular injuries
8. Guidelines for antiobiotic prophylaxis—consider:
   - **a.** most common and suspected pathogens
   - **b.** antibiotic susceptibilities of locally prevalent strains

    c. potential antibiotic toxicities (ocular and systemic)

    d. current standards of care (medical, legal)

    e. posttraumatic endophthalmitis—most frequent organisms isolated are:

        1) *Staphylococcus*

        2) bacillus, especially *B. cereus*

        3) Streptococcus

        4) gram-negative rods, including Pseudomonas

        5) various fungi

    f. broad spectrum antibiotic coverage—always begin systemic antibiotics as soon as the diagnosis of ruptured or perforated/lacerated globe is confirmed. Immediate delivery is essential. A recommended combination is:

        1) vancomycin 1 gm IV q12h or cefazolin 1 gm IV q6h

        2) gentamicin (100 mg loading dose, then 80 mg IV q8h)

        3) clindamycin 600 mg IV q8h if soil contamination or intraocular foreign body is present

    g. alternative systemic antibiotic selections:

        1) ceftriaxone or cefotaxime 1 gm IV q12h

        2) ciprofloxacin or ofloxacin if gram-negative organism suspected

    h. use topical antibiotic drops only in the absence of uveal prolapse

        1) cefazolin 50 mg/ml q30min until surgery

        2) gentamicin 14 mg/ml q30min until surgery

        3) ciprofloxacin or ofloxacin 3 mg/ml q30min until surgery

    i. subconjunctival antibiotic injection should be avoided initially until after surgery, so as to avoid further prolapse of ocular contents and/or inadvertent intraocular administration of toxic doses

    j. intravitreal antibiotics should be considered if penetrating injury violates lens capsule or involves vitreous cavity with contaminated foreign body. A recommended combination is:

        1) vancomycin 1 mg/0.1 ml and amikacin 4 mg/0.1 ml (but see below)

        2) clindamycin may also be given if very high suspicion for bacillus cereus infection

        3) ceftazidime 2 mg/0.1 ml if gram-negative organism suspected, to avoid potential aminoglycoside toxicity

E. Preoperative Checklist for Lacerations of the Globe

1. From the moment it is ascertained that an injured eye will require surgical repair, the plan should be formulated in logical sequential steps.
   a. Determine that surgery is definitely needed
   b. Organize the ocular surgical team, including corneal, vitreoretinal, and oculoplastic specialists, if required
   c. Follow specific preoperative checklist. This includes:
      1) detailed ocular history
      2) directed physical examination
      3) ancillary/radiologic tests
      4) microbial cultures
      5) begin systemic (parenteral) and topical antibiotics if indicated
      6) apply rigid protective eye shield
      7) check nothing by mouth status (NPO)
      8) obtain informed consent for surgical repair (including possible primary enucleation) and general anesthesia
      9) administer antiemetics as needed
      10) administer pain medications and sedatives as needed
      11) notify anesthesiology and operating room
      12) administer tetanus prophylaxis
      13) perform preoperative lab tests
      14) obtain anesthesia clearance and get other consultants if necessary
      15) arrange for special equipment, as required in operating room:
         a) Jaffe-style speculum to avoid further mechanical pressure on globe
         b) canalicular involvement: silicone intubation set
         c) stellate corneal laceration: tissue adhesive, donor tissue, therapeutic soft contact lens
         d) traumatic lens involvement: irrigation-aspiration equipment, specialized cannulas, vitrectomy instrument, phacoemulsification unit
         e) intraocular foreign body: specialized magnets, intraocular forceps
F. Repair of Corneal and Scleral Lacerations
   1. Repair versus enucleation
      a. primary repair should almost always be attempted, regardless of severity
      b. enucleation can be performed as a secondary procedure in the early postoperative period to avoid sympathetic ophthalmia

      c. delayed enucleation, with demonstration to patient of lack of useful visual function, is beneficial psychologically

      d. delayed secondary enucleation is desirable for allowing complete written informed consent (especially if patient's level of consciousness is reduced from trauma or inebriation)

      e. primary enucleation is justified only when total disorganization of the globe has resulted from trauma

2. Closure of corneal and scleral lacerations

    a. goals of surgical repair:

        1) to close all lacerations

        2) to restore normal intraocular pressure

        3) to avoid incarceration of ocular tissue in wounds

        4) to restore and protect visual axis

    b. principles of surgical repair: the four "Rs"

        1) REMOVE disorganized tissue and hemorrhage

        2) REPOSIT viable tissue, including uvea

        3) REPAIR the wound accurately

        4) RESTORE normal anatomical relationships

    c. general surgical considerations

        1) reassess damage extent under general anesthesia

        2) if eyelid and facial lacerations are present, address injury to the globe first

        3) do not cut cilia when an open wound of the globe is present (may cover using sterile adhesive drape)

        4) adequate exposure of wound is essential for accurate repair

          a) Jaffe-type speculum to avoid mechanical pressure

          b) do not use traction sutures under rectus muscles in hypotonous globes to avoid needle perforation

          c) limbal sutures may be placed using 6-0 silk/vicryl

3. Close all lacerations

    a. conjunctiva

        1) a conjunctival laceration raises suspicion for possible underlying, occult scleral laceration or rupture

        2) conjunctival chemosis and hemorrhage may obscure vitreous, uveal, or retinal prolapse

3) conjunctival lacerations require careful exploration under topical or general anesthesia in uncooperative patients

   a) dissection of conjunctiva and Tenon's fascia off the sclera is required to definitively observe and delineate the extent of the laceration, puncture, or rupture

   b) possible occult foreign body may be buried under torn/hemorrhagic conjunctiva

4) surgical repair of conjunctival laceration is rarely necessary for less than 1 cm due to rapid healing. Prophylactic antibiotic drops or ointment is suggested:

   a) erythromycin

   b) bacitracin

   c) polymixin-B/trimethoprim

   d) gentamicin or tobramycin

   e) ciprofloxacin or ofloxacin

5) if surgical repair of the conjunctiva is required, reapproximate laceration edges carefully with interrupted or continuous 7-0 or 8-0 vicryl or collagen sutures. Carefully reapproximate conjunctival edges to prevent:

   a) implantation of conjunctival epithelium in the subconjunctival space—inclusion cyst

   b) inclusion of Tenon's fascia in the wound—white herniation

   c) plica semilunaris or caruncular manipulation

4. Nonperforating corneal laceration

  a. rule out occult perforation of Descemet's membrane by:

    1) Seidel's test with sterile 2% fluorescein sodium solution or fluorescein-impregnated filter paper

    2) apply gentle pressure against upper lid during testing to uncover otherwise self-sealing wounds

    3) careful slit lamp biomicroscopy of Descemet's membrane to search for breaks

  b. if Descemet's break is present, hospitalization and antibiotic therapy required

  c. if partial thickness, patient treatment may consist of medical therapy alone in ambulatory setting

  d. treatment goals:

1) prevention of infection
2) promote epithelial and stromal healing
3) minimize scarring and surface irregularity
4) promote epithelial adhesion
5) prevent irregular astigmatism

e. treatment options
1) pressure patching with antibiotic ointment if no wound gape
2) therapeutic soft contact lens (TSCL) to shield deeper nonperforating injury from eyelid movement
3) antibiotic prophylaxis—ofloxacin 0.3% bid to qid or gentamicin 0.3% bid to qid
4) cycloplegic agent (homatropine 5% or cyclopentolate 1 to 2% tid to qid)
5) keep TSCL in place for 2 to 4 weeks until healing complete

f. long, partial thickness corneal wounds:
1) may require suturing if there is significant wound gape or override
2) if flap of tissue avulsed, secure with sutures oriented toward apex of the triangular avulsion to improve tissue apposition

g. simple full thickness corneal lacerations—laceration does not violate the limbus or have uveal or vitreous incarceration

h. treatment options for self-sealed small lacerations:
1) therapeutic soft contact lens—may be used for small self-sealing corneal perforation to support the wound as it heals. Best for lacerations less than 3 mm in length that are self-sealing. Assess anterior chamber depth stability.
   a) consider adjunctive aqueous humor suppressants (e.g., acetazolamide, methazolamide, topical beta blockers)
   b) topical antibiotic prophylaxis (ofloxacin 0.3%/ ciprofloxacin 0.3% or gentamicin/tobramycin 0.3%)
   c) topical cycloplegia (homatropine 5% or cyclopentolate 1 or 2%)
   d) protective metallic shield; avoid rubbing
2) tissue adhesive. Cyanoacrylate tissue adhesive useful for puncture wounds or small (less than 2 mm) lacerations that do not self-seal or would require excessive suture placement in the central visual axis. Preferred method of application:

a) patient lying down under operating microscope
b) topical anesthesia
c) lid speculum
d) remove epithelium around perforation site with blade or forceps
e) carefully dry area with cellulose sponges
f) apply small amount of tissue adhesive (less than a drop) using a fine gauge (30) disposable needle. Apply additional small amounts sequentially as required for sealing
g) maintain lid speculum in place to allow polymerization of the adhesive for 3 to 5 minutes postapplication
h) apply therapeutic soft contact lens over dried tissue adhesive
i) NOTE: cyanoacrylate tissue adhesive is not currently approved for clinical ophthalmic use by the U.S. FDA

  i. simple full thickness corneal lacerations requiring corneal suture placement

1) surgical preparation and draping in usual sterile fashion
2) place lid speculum with caution to avoid pressure application to open globe
  a) lid retraction sutures may be used if necessary
  b) limbal traction sutures through cornea (6-0 silk) may also be used as necessary
3) if anterior chamber is formed, self-sealed wound may be sutured directly
4) if anterior chamber is shallowed or flattened, reformation with viscoelastic through the wound or through a separate limbal stab incision may be required to protect the lens, iris, and corneal endothelium (air may alternatively be used for chamber reformation if viscoelastic unavailable)
  a) limbal stab incision may be preferable to avoid manipulation of wound edges with instrument
  b) place limbal incision with a 15 degree sharp microsurgical knife approximately 90 degrees from the wound (in phakic patients, avoid injury to iris or lens)

  j. definitive corneal suturing placement

1) initial shallow temporary sutures may be used to approximate wound for deeper definitive suture placement
2) monofilament 10-0 nylon on fine spatula design microsurgical needle optimal
3) simple interrupted sutures easiest with progressive halving of the wound
   a) make definitive corneal sutures 1.5 mm long
   b) place definitive sutures at approximately 90% depth in the corneal stroma
   c) place definitive corneal sutures of equal depth on both sides of the wound to avoid malapposition (shallow sutures will cause internal wound gape; asymmetric sutures will result in wound override; full thickness suture bite may provide a potential route of entry for microbial invasion or harm the corneal endothelium)
4) for shelved lacerations, place sutures at equal distance with respect to the internal aspect of the wound and tie with minimal tension to optimize tissue apposition
5) if edges of wound are macerated or edematous, place longer suture bites for security
6) avoid suture bites through visual axis
   a) if sutures are required near center of visual axis, make bites progressively shorter, more proximal to center of the cornea
   b) straddle visual axis by placing sutures at each side of the visual axis
   c) utilize "no touch" technique (i.e., no forceps) placing the tip of the suturing needle perpendicular to the corneal surface and following the path of the needle through the tissue
7) complicated laceration
   a) suture perpendicular rather than beveled areas of the wound first
   b) place long-deep sutures at the wound's periphery
   c) place shorter, shallower appositional sutures toward the visual axis
8) use 1-1-1 slip knot or locked 2-1-1 knot for easier suture burial and subsequent removal

      a) trim knot short and rotate beneath surface with smooth forceps

      b) reverse orientation of the knot and direct ends away from surface to facilitate subsequent suture removal

      c) bury knots superficially on the side of the wound away from the visual axis

        i. reform/deepen anterior chamber through the separate limbal paracentesis

      d) use fluorescein 2% solution to verify watertightness

k. stellate corneal lacerations—watertight closure may be particularly challenging

    1) use multiple interrupted sutures

    2) utilize bridging sutures as necessary

    3) use of purse-string sutures may be helpful

    4) use therapeutic soft contact lens, tissue adhesive, or patch grafting if persistent central leak

l. corneal laceration with iris incarceration

    1) reform/deepen a flat or shallow anterior chamber with viscoelastic through a separate limbal paracentesis site

    2) properly reposit incarcerated iris tissue or excise exposed iris tissue if repair delayed more than 24 hours or devitalized

    3) place preliminary, temporary corneal sutures to stabilize the wound to allow chamber deepening in select cases

    4) consider instillation of acetylcholine for pharmacologic repositing of peripherally incarcerated iris

    5) with central corneal iris incarceration, mydriasis with intraocular epinephrine 1:10,000 may atraumatically reposit iris

    6) viscoelastic dissection may assist in mechanical repositioning of iris

    7) direct sweeping with a cyclodialysis spatula may drag iris from the wound

      a) caution: avoid iatrogenic iridodialysis

      b) avoid damage to corneal endothelium

      c) avoid damage to crystalline lens

    8) corneal laceration should be completely sutured for watertight closure

      a) wound inspected for any iris or vitreous incarceration

      b) intracameral acetylcholine or air may assist in identifying vitreous strands

      9) repeat sweeping through the paracentesis, if necessary

     10) anterior chamber should be reformed through the paracentesis site with balanced salt solution

     11) wound tested for residual leakage

m. corneal laceration with lens involvement

     1) small penetrating injuries caused by small projectiles or puncture wounds may cause significant lens damage

     2) lens removal at the time of surgical repair of laceration usually not an emergency

     3) fibrinous anterior chamber reaction or pupillary membrane may masquerade as a flocculent traumatic cataract

     4) significant lens injury with obviously disrupted capsule and liberated cortical material should be removed to prevent phacoantigenic postoperative inflammation

     5) lens surgery should be performed under controlled circumstances with adequate visualization and appropriate equipment

     6) if any doubt regarding lens injury, delay lens surgery for a second procedure

     7) with capsular rupture and vitreous involvement, lensectomy combined with vitrectomy is advisable. Surgical approach from:
        a) limbus
        b) pars plana

     8) with young trauma patients, aspiration and cutting of the lens alone usually sufficient

     9) sonication with harder nuclei may be required

     10) posterior chamber intraocular lens placement depends on:
        a) patient age and growth state of eye
        b) zonular and capsular support integrity
        c) presence of residual vitreous or posterior segment trauma

     11) secondary posterior chamber intraocular lens can be performed under controlled circumstances following primary repair of trauma

n. corneal laceration with vitreous involvement

     1) frequently accompanies corneal laceration with lens involvement

     2) principal goal to relieve vitreous incarceration from traumatic wound

3) removal of vitreous incarceration reduces risk of:
   a) chronic intraocular inflammation
   b) cystoid macular edema
   c) vitreous fibrosis
   d) retinal detachment
   e) intraocular infection from vitreous wick
4) automated vitrectomy instruments are helpful as are bimanual techniques. A separate infusion port apart from the cutting instrument is preferred for optimal control. Options include:
   a) irrigating bulb syringe
   b) 23-gauge butterfly infusion canula
   c) sutured infusion canula
5) corneal wound first closed to allow reformation of anterior chamber
   a) dry cellulose sponges may gently withdraw vitreous strands. Cut vitreous strands flush with wound using sharp scissors.
6) following wound closure, use sharp keratome to enter limbus and place vitrectomy probe to remove vitreous strands to cortical remnant and to perform anterior vitrectomy
   a) use high cutting rates (approximately 400 cps)
   b) use low suction (approximately 100 mmHg)
7) resweep wound with sweep instrument through paracentesis
8) observe pupil contour
9) reinstill acetylcholine solution to constrict pupil
10) place air bubble to visualize and tamponade vitreous

o. scleral-corneal laceration (corneoscleral lacerations)
   1) key steps in repair of corneoscleral lacerations are:
      a) make stab incision into anterior chamber
      b) place traction sutures
      c) perform extensive conjunctival peritomy as indicated
      d) first approximate the limbus
      e) repair scleral laceration
      f) remove extraocular muscles if necessary

g) consider cryotherapy or diathermy if scleral wound extends beyond the ora serrata, or if indirect ophthalmoscopy shows retinal tears. Delayed retinopexy may be safer when visualization has improved or at time of subsequent vitrectomy.

h) repair corneal lacerations

i) sweep iris from corneal wound

2) approximate limbus using nonabsorbable 8-0 nylon or silk suture

3) reposit prolapsed iris

4) close corneal wound completely

5) assess extent of scleral laceration using conjunctival peritomy as needed

6) close sclera with nonabsorbable 8-0 nylon or silk or 7-0 vicryl. Use retractors to expose sclera.

7) lacerations extending underneath extraocular muscles may be repaired with the assistance of a muscle hook or bridle suture to retract muscle

8) if the complete extent of the laceration cannot be determined, the muscle may be first secured with a double armed 6-0 vicryl suture, then disinserted to provide adequate exposure

9) in cases with extremely posterior scleral extensions toward the optic nerve, the posterior extent of the wound may be left unsutured, rather than distorting the globe with improperly placed sutures

p. corneoscleral lacerations with uveal and vitreous prolapse

1) prolapsed vitreous through a scleral laceration is gently withdrawn with a dry cellulose sponge and cut flush with the sclera

2) mechanical vitrectomy may also be completed if visualization is adequate

3) principal goal of initial surgery is to secure watertight closure of the globe

4) secondary procedures to repair posterior segment injuries may be required

5) reposit uveal tissue through gape in scleral laceration if possible, or shrink with light cautery diathermy. Send any excised tissue for histopathologic examination.

a) excised retina indicates poor prognosis

6) close sclera from anterior to posterior with successive interrupted sutures spaced closely, in order to over-sew prolapsed uveal tissue with the sclera

7) assistant may reposit uvea while surgeon places sutures

q. corneoscleral lacerations with tissue loss

    1) tight suturing of small puncture wounds and avulsive injuries may result in tissue distortion and excessive postoperative astigmatism and scarring

    2) with larger corneal tissue loss, full thickness and lamellar patch grafting are preferred

      a) fresh donor tissue is ideal

      b) glycerin-preserved or frozen corneal/scleral tissue may be used for patch graft

      c) partial thickness lamellar bed carefully fashioned with blade

      d) donor tissue prepared as with lamellar keratoplasty

      e) nonviable donor epithelium removed by scraping

      f) limbal incision created and lamellar dissection carried from limbus to limbus

      g) cut donor button 0.5 mm larger than the recipient bed diameter (may require hand-fashioned graft if recipient bed is irregular)

      h) secure on-lay graft with interrupted 10-0 nylon sutures

      i) full-thickness patch grafting:

        i. debride wound margins to form a rim of healthy tissue

        ii. remove donor epithelium if nonviable tissue is used

        iii. use corneal trephine or hand-fashioned graft to be slightly larger than the defect

        iv. secure graft with interrupted 10-0 nylon sutures

        v. penetrating keratoplasty—rarely indicated in primary repair after trauma. Keratoplasty usually delayed until eye has healed from trauma and inflammation subsided to optimize graft survival and prevent rejection.

G. Postoperative Management of Ocular Trauma Patient
  1. Control infection
  2. Suppress inflammation
  3. Stabilize ocular surface
  4. Promote wound healing
     a. prevention of infection
        1) subconjunctival antibiotics:
           a) cefazolin 100 mg
           b) gentamicin 40 mg (administer with caution well away from wound)
        2) parenteral antibiotics for 4 to 7 days:
           a) cefazolin 1 gm IV q6h or vancomycin 1 gm IV q12h
           b) gentamicin 100 mg IV loading dose; then 80 mg IV q12h
           c) clindamycin 600 mg IV q8h (if soil contamination and bacillus likely)
           d) cefotaxime or ceftriaxone 1 gm IV q12h as alternatives
        3) topical antibiotics
           a) fortified cefazolin 50 mg/ml
           b) gentamicin 14 mg/ml
           c) ciprofloxacin 3 mg/ml or ofloxacin 3 mg/ml (dosage q1h for 24 hours, then q2h for 48 hours, then taper according to clinical response)

Essentials of Eye Care, edited by Rohit Varma.
Lippincott–Raven Publishers,
Philadelphia © 1997.

14

Ophthalmic Histopathology

I. THE EYELIDS

A. Cysts
1. Dermoid cyst
   a. gross: smooth, oval mass, does not transilluminate
   b. microscopic: lined by stratified squamous epithelium, skin appendages within cyst walls. Contains keratin. Rupture results in foreign body granulomatous inflammation.
2. Epidermal inclusion cyst
   a. gross: elevated, whitish, dome-shaped lesion, does not transilluminate
   b. microscopic: lined by stratified squamous epithelium, no skin appendages, contains desquamated keratin. Rupture results in foreign body granulomatous inflammation.
3. Apocrine hidrocystoma
   a. gross: dome-shaped mass, usually solitary, contains clear fluid. Transilluminates.
   b. microscopic: cyst lined by convoluted epithelial walls with inner cuboidal (single or multiple) and outer myoepithelial layer. Intracytoplasmic vacuoles and surface secretory projections of inner cuboidal layer.
4. Eccrine hidrocystoma
   a. gross: solitary or multiple, tense bluish vesicle(s)
   b. microscopic: variably-sized intradermal cyst(s) lined by several layers of flattened epithelial cells. No secretory projections of inner cell layer.
B. Inflammations
1. Blepharitis
   a. gross: thickened, erythematous, ulcerated lid margin with grayish polymorphic scales along eyelashes

    b. microscopic: acanthosis, hyperkeratosis, chronic nongranulomatous inflammatory infiltrate
  2. Hordeolum
    a. gross: external type—erythematous, discrete, elevated, superficial pustule or papule near or on lid margin; internal type—diffuse, erythematous, deep lesion involving most of eyelid
    b. microscopic: polymorphonuclear leukocytes (PMNs), edema, vascular congestion, and cellular debris centered around hair follicles (external) or around meibomian glands within tarsal plate (internal)
  3. Chalazion
    a. gross: hard, variably-sized nodule within eyelid
    b. microscopic: lipogranulomatous inflammation, including multinucleated giant cells, lymphocytes, and plasma cells with scattered clear spaces (preparation artifact due to dissolved lipid). Oil red O stains fat on frozen tissue sections not exposed to processing solvents.
  4. Pyogenic granuloma
    a. gross: rapidly enlarging, painless, polypoid mass
    b. microscopic: granulation tissue with fibroblasts, endothelial cells of budding capillaries, and an inflammatory cell infiltrate including lymphocytes and plasma cells
C. Infections
  1. Molluscum contagiosum
    a. gross: dome-shaped, small, waxy nodule(s) with unbilicated center on lid or lid margin. May have associated follicular tarsal reaction.
    b. microscopic: thickened epithelium arranged in a cup-shaped configuration with keratin and large, degenerated cells with large eosinophilic inclusions filling the cup. Epithelial cells with large, round, eosinophilic intracytoplasmic inclusion bodies progressively increase in size toward the surface.
  2. Preseptal cellulitis
    a. gross: erythema, edema of involved lid tissues anterior to orbital septum
    b. microscopic: diffuse infiltration of PMNs within tissue planes of lid with associated vascular congestion and edema. Bacteria (special stains).
D. Systemic
  1. Amyloid
    a. gross: variably-sized brownish red nodules, systemic process if only lid skin involved, local process if only palpebral conjunctival involved

    b. microscopic: amorphous, eosinophilic hyaline deposits in connective tissue or associated with blood vessel walls. Variable inflammatory reaction. Green birefringence in unstained, hematoxylin and eosin (H&E), and Congo red sections. Metachromasia with crystal violet stain, fluorescence with thioflavine-T, dichroism with polarized light.

  2. Juvenile xanthogranuloma
    a. gross: elevated, yellow-orange nodules on lids, single or multiple
    b. microscopic: diffuse granulomatous inflammatory reaction with dermal foam cells (lipid-containing macrophages), Touton giant cells (central eosinophilic cytoplasm separated from peripheral clear cytoplasm by ring of nuclei), and numerous blood vessels

  3. Xanthelasma
    a. gross: multiple, yellowish, soft plaques on medial portion of lids
    b. microscopic: clusters of foam cells in superficial dermis around venules. Can involve vessel wall.

E. Benign Tumors
  1. Inverted follicular keratosis
    a. gross: small reddish papule, usually solitary, rarely with central umbilication or pigmentation
    b. microscopic: keratinized central area surrounded by squamous cells that are surrounded by acantholytic squamous cells that are surrounded by basaloid cells (squamous eddy). Hyperkeratosis, acanthosis.

  2. Pseudoepitheliomatous hyperplasia
    a. gross: elevated, irregular surface at edge of an area of chronic inflammation or carcinoma
    b. microscopic: acanthosis with protrusion (not infiltration) into dermis by squamous cells in the overlying epidermis. Many mitotic figures but no atypia or dyskeratosis. PMNs in squamous proliferations.

  3. Seborrheic keratosis
    a. gross: discrete, brownish lobulated plaques with overlying scales
    b. microscopic: variable. Acanthosis, hyperkeratosis, dyskeratosis, papillomatosis, and benign proliferation of basaloid cells.

  4. Keratoacanthoma
    a. gross: solitary, firm, dome-shaped lesion with crusted, umbilicated center

        b. microscopic: noninvasive, keratin-filled crater with irregular proliferation of underlying epithelium and extension of adjacent epidermis over crater, low nuclear-to-cytoplasmic ratio, acanthosis, well-demarcated from adjacent normal epithelium

    5. Pyogenic granuloma

        a. gross: fleshy-red, pedunculated lesion

        b. microscopic: loose fibrous stroma with numerous capillaries (granulation tissue) and an acute and chronic nongranulomatous inflammatory cell infiltrate

    6. Actinic keratosis

        a. gross: elevated, erythematous lesion with scaly, whitish surface

        b. microscopic: hyperkeratosis, parakeratosis, papillomatosis, nuclear atypia in basal layer, dermal chronic inflammatory cell infiltrate

F. Nevi

    1. Junctional nevus

        a. gross: well-circumscribed, flat, homogenous brownish lesion

        b. microscopic: clusters of melanocytes with basophilic, polyhedral nuclei (nevus cells) at epidermal-dermal junction

    2. Intradermal nevus

        a. gross: elevated, papillomatous, fleshy to brown or black lesion

        b. microscopic: nevus cells in dermis without associated inflammatory cells. Nuclei become smaller, thinner, or spindle-shaped deeper in dermis (normal polarity of nevus).

    3. Compound nevus

        a. gross: flat or elevated, fleshy to brown or black lesion

        b. microscopic: nevus cells at epidermal-dermal junction and in dermis, dermal portion with normal polarity

    4. Blue nevus

        a. gross: flat, bluish-gray lesion

        b. microscopic: intertwining cords of elongated, spindle-shaped nevus cells in deep dermis. Occasionally very cellular.

    5. Congenital oculodermal melanocytosis (nevus of Ota)

        a. gross: bluish-gray discoloration of lids, brow, sclera, uvea

        b. microscopic: fusiform, bipolar, dendritic, pigmented melanocytes in upper and mid-dermis, parallel to skin surface

G. Malignant Tumors
1. Malignant melanoma
   a. gross: flat or elevated, variably pigmented lesion with associated erythematous base
   b. microscopic: large, atypical cells with increased nuclear-to-cytoplasmic ratio, epithelial and/or dermal invasion, mitoses, lymphocytic inflammatory infiltrate. Different classification than uveal melanomas; further discussion is beyond the scope of this text.
2. Squamous cell carcinoma
   a. gross: indurated, poorly demarcated nodule, or plaque with ulceration
   b. microscopic: pleomorphic cells with hyperchromatic nuclei, scant cytoplasm, atypical mitotic figures, invasion of tumor cells into dermis, abnormal keratinization. If no invasion into dermis and intact epithelial basement membrane—carcinoma-in-situ (Bowen's disease).
3. Basal cell carcinoma: nodular variant
   a. gross: painless, firm, indurated, pearly nodule usually on lower lid with overlying telangiectasia. May have a central crater (rodent ulcer).
   b. microscopic: lobules of small, regularly-shaped cells with scant cytoplasm, hyperchromatic nuclei, palisading of peripheral row of nuclei around outer rim of tumor with retraction artifact from surrounding stroma. Mitoses. Overlying epidermis thinned, atrophied without prominent hyperkeratosis. Central crater with raised epithelial borders.
4. Basal cell carcinoma: sclerosing variant (morphea form)
   a. gross: indurated, pale plaque
   b. microscopic: small cords of cells scattered within dense hyalinized stroma in dermis
5. Sebaceous adenoma
   a. gross: solitary, firm, yellowish, smooth, round nodule
   b. microscopic: irregularly shaped and sized lobules of differentiated sebaceous gland, rows of benign basaloid cells between sebaceous proliferations
6. Sebaceous gland adenocarcinoma
   a. gross: well-circumscribed, firm, yellowish growth. Encapsulated, ulcerated, or infiltrative. May masquerade as chalazion or chronic blepharitis.
   b. microscopic: basophilic cells ranging from undifferentiated to mature sebaceous cells with

hyperchromatic nuclei, central nucleoli, intracytoplasmic lipid, abundant mitoses forming ir-
regularly-shaped lobules along the epithelium
(pagetoid spread). Four patterns: lobular, come-
docarcinoma, papillary, mixed.

II. THE LACRIMAL GLAND

A. Cysts
  1. Lacrimal duct cyst
     a. gross: bluish, dome-shaped cystic structure
     b. microscopic: lined by outer flattened basal ep-
        ithelial cell layer and inner cuboidal to colum-
        nar layer with goblet cells. Wall may contain
        lacrimal gland acini, inflammation, fibrosis.
B. Inflammations
  1. Acute dacryoadenitis
     a. gross: focal or diffuse thickening of normal lac-
        rimal gland tissue
     b. microscopic: acute inflammatory cell infiltrate
        (PMNs), edema with preservation of acini archi-
        tecture
  2. Chronic dacryoadenitis
     a. gross: focal or diffuse thickening of lacrimal
        gland tissue
     b. microscopic: chronic inflammatory infiltrate
        (lymphocytes, plasma cells), loss of acini, pres-
        ervation of ductules, variable fibrosis
  3. Sarcoidosis
     a. gross: diffuse enlargement of lacrimal gland
     b. microscopic: many noncaseating granulomas,
        usually near vessels, with minimal to no lym-
        phocytic cuffing, multinucleated giant cells
        with acidophilic (asteroid) or calcified ba-
        sophilic (Schaumann's) bodies
  4. Lymphoepithelial lesion of Sjögren's syndrome
     a. gross: diffuse enlargement of lacrimal gland
     b. microscopic: marked chronic inflammatory cell
        infiltrate with prominent germinal centers, lack
        of gland acini. Scattered epithelial cell islands
        without lumina and surrounded by inflamma-
        tory cells.
C. Lacrimal Gland Tumors
  1. Pleomorphic adenoma (benign mixed tumor)
     a. gross: bosselated mass with tumor nodule(s)
        protruding through fibrous capsule
     b. microscopic: scattered small ductules, lined by
        inner low columnar and outer spindle-shaped
        layer, that blends into surrounding mesenchy-

      mal tissue matrix with cartilaginous, adipose, bony, or myxoid characteristics. May have stellate collagen deposition and tyrosinase crystals.

2. Adenoid cystic carcinoma
   a. gross: variably sized lacrimal gland mass
   b. microscopic: different patterns: basaloid (solid), cribriform (Swiss cheese), comedocarcinomatous, tubular, or sclerosing. In all patterns: small cells with small nucleoli, sparse cytoplasm. Alcian blue-positive material (probable multilaminated basal lamina) in scattered spaces. Perineural invasion, eosinophilic osteoblastic change on bony trabeculae.
3. Malignant mixed tumor
   a. gross: lacrimal gland mass
   b. microscopic: features of pleomorphic adenoma and adenoid cystic carcinoma or poorly differentiated adenocarcinoma

III. THE CONJUNCTIVA

A. Congenital
   1. Limbal dermoid
      a. gross: well-circumscribed, firm, solitary mass. Usually inferotemporal. Varies from small (2 to 3 mm), slightly elevated, whitish nodule to large (12 to 15 mm), round, tan mass. May protrude through interpalpebral fissure. Adjacent corneal stromal lipid deposition.
      b. microscopic: connective tissue matrix with pilosebaceous material and lipid drop-out spaces
B. Conjunctivitis: Infectious and Noninfectious
   1. True (inflammatory) membrane
      a. gross: whitish, mucoid material on conjunctival surface adherent to underlying epithelium. Conjunctiva bleeds when membrane is removed.
      b. microscopic: fibrin-cellular debris
   2. Pseudomembrane
      a. gross: whitish, mucoid material on conjunctiva. Removed without bleeding.
      b. microscopic: fibrin-cellular debris
   3. Papillary conjunctivitis
      a. gross: raised, polygonal hyperemic areas less than 1 mm in size, with central vessel, in mosaic pattern separated by pale channels. On palpebral conjunctiva or bulbar limbus.
      b. microscopic: marked foldings of hyperplastic conjunctival epithelium with central fibrovascu-

lar core, inflammatory cell infiltrate in substantia propria, edema between connective tissue septa anchoring overlying epithelium to deeper collagenous tissues.

4. Giant papillary and vernal conjunctivitis
   a. gross: large papillae greater than 1 mm in size in upper palpebral conjunctiva
   b. microscopic: disruption of connective tissue septa in upper palpebral conjunctiva, inflammatory cells (eosinophils, mast cells) in substantia propria, clumps of eosinophils along bulbar limbus (Horner-Trantas' dots)

5. Follicular conjunctivitis
   a. gross: smooth elevation of palpebral conjunctiva without central vascular core
   b. microscopic: chronic lymphocytic infiltrate with active germinal centers in substantia propria

6. Trachoma
   a. gross: MacCallan stage I—immature follicles on superior tarsal conjunctiva, no scarring; stage II—mature follicles, no scarring; stage III—mature follicles, with scarring, round to ovoid relatively lucent areas within superior limbal pannus (Herbert's pits); stage IV—no follicles, marked scarring
   b. microscopic: intracellular parasites resembling gram-negative basophilic cocci; stage I—lymphocytic infiltrate in superior tarsal substantia propria, perinuclear inclusions (of Halberstaedter and Prowazeck) in epithelial cells; stage II—collections of lymphocytes with germinal centers, macrophages with phagocytosed debris; stage III—lymphoid follicles, round areas of scattered fibrocellular scarring within superior limbal neovascularization (Herbert's pits), stage IV—marked fibrocellular scarring, disruption of normal architecture

7. Sarcoidosis
   a. gross: round translucent cysts in conjunctival fornix
   b. microscopic: discrete granuloma—multinucleated giant cells with asteroid and/or Schaumann's bodies and rim of lymphocytes and plasma cells

C. Degenerations
   1. Pingueculum
      a. gross: localized, yellowish-gray, elevated lesion close to nasal or temporal limbus on interpalpebral portion of bulbar conjunctiva

      b. microscopic: mild thinning and degeneration or acanthosis of epithelium without cellular atypia, parakeratosis or hyperkeratosis; basophilic degeneration of collagen (elastotic: stains with elastic tissue stains but no elastolysis)

    2. Pterygium

      a. gross: similar to pingueculum, except usually nasal and involves adjacent peripheral cornea

      b. microscopic: subepithelial accumulations of amorphous, eosinophilic, hyalinized or granular-appearing material similar to degenerated collagen interspersed with fragmented or coiled fibers similar to abnormal elastic tissue. Increased number of stromal fibrocytes. Elastotic degeneration. Invades corneal epithelium with breakdown of Bowman's layer.

D. Systemic

    1. Amyloidosis

      a. gross: nodular or diffuse conjunctival thickening

      b. microscopic: nodular or diffuse eosinophilic homogeneous material interspersed among islands of entrapped atrophic epithelium. Orange-red appearance, dichroism, birefringence with polarized light (Congo red stain). Metachromatic (crystal violet stain), yellowish-green fluorescence (fluorochrome thioflavine T).

    2. Lymphoid lesions

      a. gross: salmon-pink, relatively flat, smooth lesion(s) with soft consistency, usually in fornices

      b. microscopic: lymphocytes comprising irregularly-shaped germinal centers in substantia propria

    3. Bitot's spot

      a. gross: thickened, rough, bubbly appearance near limbus

      b. microscopic: thickened, keratinized epithelium, occasional with rete pegs. Loss of goblet cells. Corynebacterium xerosis.

E. Cysts

    1. Epithelial inclusion cyst

      a. gross: elevated, mobile, opaque, localized conjunctival lesion

      b. microscopic: dislodged epithelium within stroma with central cavitation. Lined by nonkeratinized, stratified squamous epithelium with goblet cells. Contains mucin.

F. Benign Tumors

    1. Congenital melanosis oculi (ocular melanocytosis)

      a. gross: slate-gray or blue areas within episclera and not conjunctival epithelium (does not move with conjunctiva)

      b. microscopic: elongated, spindle-shaped cells with branching processes in substantia propria

  2. Congenital oculodermal melanocytosis (nevus of Ota)

      a. gross: bluish-gray discoloration of lids, brow, conjunctiva, uvea

      b. microscopic: elongated, spindle-shaped pigmented cells in substantia propria

  3. Primary acquired melanosis (PAM)

      a. gross: unilateral flat area with speckled brown pigmentation and irregular margins. Moves with conjunctiva if no associated malignancy.

      b. microscopic:

        1) without atypia: variable number of nevus cells in epithelium at epidermal-substantia propria junction, without hyperplasia of melanocytes or atypical features

        2) with atypia: variable number of nevus cells with cellular atypia in epithelium at epidermal-substantia propria junction. No basilar hyperplasia or epithelioid melanocytes.

  4. Squamous papilloma

      a. gross: sessile or pedunculated exophytic tumor. Usually in inferior fornix or at limbus. Multiple, often bilateral.

      b. microscopic: vascular cores covered by acanthotic, nonkeratinized stratified squamous epithelium

  5. Inverted papilloma

      a. gross: endophytic mass

      b. microscopic: benign epithelial and goblet cells extending into substantia propria

G. Malignant

  1. Carcinoma in situ

      a. gross: lesion, usually in interpalpebral fissure, with keratin scale

      b. microscopic: thickening of epithelium, cytologic atypia (spindle-shaped cells with hyperchromatic nuclei or epidermoid cells with large vesicular nuclei, loss of polarity, mitoses above basilar [germinal] layer). Demarcation line between atypical and normal cells.

  2. Squamous cell carcinoma

      a. gross: sessile or papillary growth in interpalpebral area near limbus

      b. microscopic: malignant squamous cells with hyperchromatic nuclei beyond basement membrane into substantia propria

   3. Kaposi's sarcoma

      a. gross: patch of elevated "hemorrhage" that does not resolve over time

      b. microscopic: spindle-shaped cells, vascular channels with poorly defined endothelial cell lining

IV. THE SCLERA

  A. Congenital

    1. Blue sclera

      a. gross: translucent sclera (brown uvea shows through as blue)

      b. microscopic: thinning of sclera—may also be thicker and more cellular. Abnormal collagen fibers (25% reduction in corneal thickness, >50% scleral).

  B. Inflammations

    1. Episcleritis

      a. gross: hyperemia, edema of episcleral tissue. May have associated mobile intraepiscleral nodule.

      b. microscopic: chronic, nongranulomatous inflammatory infiltrate in episcleral tissue with lymphocytes, plasma cells, edema. Chronic granulomatous inflammation (rare).

    2. Scleritis, diffuse anterior

      a. gross: diffuse vascular hyperemia

      b. microscopic: zonal granulomatous inflammation with central necrotic sclera surrounded by inner zone of polymorphonuclear leukocytes and histiocytes and outer zone of lymphocytes and plasma cells. Fibroblastic transformation of scleral stromal cells.

V. THE CORNEA

  A. Congenital

    1. Microcornea

      a. gross: greatest diameter less than 11 mm

      b. microscopic: normal histologically except for overall small size

    2. Megalocornea

      a. gross: smallest diameter greater than 13 mm

      b. microscopic: normal histologically except for overall large size

   3. Corneal opacity: facet
   a. gross: small, superficial spot; distorted corneal light reflex
   b. microscopic: abraded area of epithelium replaced with thickened epithelial layer, Bowman's, and sometimes anterior corneal stroma; no scar tissue
   4. Corneal opacity: nebula
   a. gross: mild, diffuse, cloudlike opacity with indistinct borders
   b. microscopic: superficial stromal scarring
   5. Corneal opacity: macula
   a. gross: moderately dense opacity with distinct border
   b. microscopic: dense scar in corneal stroma
   6. Corneal opacity: leukoma
   a. gross: white, opaque scar
   b. microscopic: stromal scarring, iris adherent to posterior corneal surface
   7. Anterior embryotoxon
   a. gross: whitish ring around full or partial circumference of corneal periphery separated from limbus by clear cornea
   b. microscopic: lipid in anterior and posterior stroma as two triangles apex to apex. Bases of triangles are Bowman's and Descemet's.
   8. Posterior embryotoxon
   a. gross: ring- or bow-shaped opacity in peripheral cornea
   b. microscopic: anterior displacement of Schwalbe's ring
   9. Sclerocornea
   a. gross: whitening of affected cornea, usually superiorly, difficult to distinguish from sclera
   b. microscopic: increased numbers of collagen fibrils of variable diameters, thin Descemet's
   10. Central corneal dysgenesis: Peter's anomaly
   a. gross: central corneal opacity
   b. microscopic: absence of Bowman's, Descemet's, and endothelium from central cornea
B. Inflammations
   1. Punctate epithelial erosions
   a. gross: punctate epithelial defects
   b. microscopic: basal cell edema of epithelium, epithelial cell separation and absence from Bowman's
C. Infections
   1. Bacterial keratitis

    a. gross: variably-sized whitish corneal infiltrate with epithelial defect

    b. microscopic: acute inflammatory cell infiltrate (PMNs), necrotic debris, edema, destruction of affected corneal tissue. Organisms (special stains).

  2. Fungal keratitis

    a. gross: opacification of stroma, overlying ulceration, satellite lesions

    b. microscopic: necrotic centrally with variable inflammatory cell infiltrate (granulomatous, nongranulomatous, or rarely, acute), fungi (Gomori methenamine silver, periodic acid Schiff [PAS], Giemsa) or Candida and those causing mucormycosis (H&E)

  3. Herpes simplex keratitis

    a. gross: corneal epithelial dendrite, arborizing pattern of opacification

    b. microscopic: epithelial stage: viral inclusions, multinucleated giant cells (coalescence of infected corneal epithelial cells, corneal scrapings, Giemsa). Stromal involvement: granulomatous reaction to Descemet's, herpes simplex virus (HSV) antigen in stroma.

  4. Interstitial keratitis (congenital syphilis)

    a. gross: nonulcerating inflammation of stroma, vascularization, scarring

    b. microscopic: stromal vascularization anterior to Descemet's, irregularly-shaped, almost confluent posterior nodularity

  5. Acanthamoeba keratitis

    a. gross: ring infiltrate

    b. microscopic: numerous acanthamoebic cysts in corneal stroma, PMNs

D. Degenerations

  1. Band keratopathy

    a. gross: whitish stippled opacification with irregular borders on surface

    b. microscopic: basophilic granules (calcium) in interpalpebral epithelial basement membrane, Bowman's layer, anterior stroma

  2. Arcus, adult

    a. gross: whitish line around corneal circumference parallel to limbus with intervening clear zone

    b. microscopic: noncrystalline cholesterol and phospholipid (frozen section, fat stains), present as inverted triangle at Bowman's and upright triangle with base anterior to Descemet's

3. Pannus
   a. gross: whitish, vascularized tissue extending onto cornea from limbus
   b. microscopic: degenerative pannus: fibrous connective tissue interposed between epithelium and Bowman's. Basophilic stippling superficially (calcification). Inflammatory pannus: fibrous connective tissue, inflammatory cell infiltrate with destruction of Bowman's.
E. Dystrophies
   1. Map-dot-fingerprint (Cogan's microcystic) dystrophy
      a. gross: gray patches, microcysts, and/or fine lines in central epithelium
      b. microscopic: map and fingerprint pattern: thickened or multilaminar strips of epithelial basement membrane extending into epithelium. Dot pattern: intraepithelial spaces with desquamating epithelial cells.
   2. Meesman's dystrophy
      a. gross: tiny epithelial vesicles extend to limbus in interpalpebral fissure
      b. microscopic: thickened epithelium, multilaminar thickened basement membrane with projections into basal epithelium. "Peculiar substance" (PAS-positive material) within epithelium.
   3. Reis-Bückler's dystrophy
      a. gross: superficial, geographic, grayish reticular opacification centrally
      b. microscopic: focal areas of disruption, replacement of Bowman's with fibrocellular tissue
   4. Granular dystrophy
      a. gross: discrete, focal, white, granular deposits in anterior stroma, clear intervening areas. Does not extend to limbus.
      b. microscopic: hyaline stromal deposits, most prominent anteriorly, stain red with Masson's trichrome
   5. Lattice dystrophy
      a. gross: refractile lines, central subepithelial white dots, ground-glass appearance of stroma. Clear peripherally.
      b. microscopic: amyloid deposits (orange-red with Congo red stain, metachromatic with crystal violet, birefringence, dichroism) in anterior stroma and subepithelial area
   6. Macular dystrophy
      a. gross: focal, grayish superficial stromal opacities at various depths, extend to corneal periphery. Cloudy intervening stroma.

        b. microscopic: keratocytes and vacuolated cells filled with glycosaminoglycans (acid mucopolysaccharides) within stroma (PAS, colloidal iron, alcian blue)

  7. Guttata

        a. gross: round, dark defects at Descemet's and endothelium

        b. microscopic: diffuse thickening of Descemet's with localized nodularity

  8. Fuchs' endothelial dystrophy

        a. gross: variable. Round defects of Descemet's and endothelium to decompensated cornea with epithelial bullae, subepithelial fibrosis, stromal edema, and Descemet's folds.

        b. microscopic: large, polymorphic endothelial cells, thickened Descemet's with localized excrescences. Subepithelial fibrosis.

  9. Posterior polymorphous dystrophy

        a. gross: variable. Grouped vesicles, geographic-shaped discrete gray lesions, broad bands with scalloped edges, stromal edema, iridocorneal adhesions.

        b. microscopic: abnormal endothelial cells with epithelialization: multilayered, microvilli, keratin, intercellular desmosomes.

 10. Congenital hereditary endothelial dystrophy (CHED)

        a. gross: diffuse, blue-gray, ground-glass appearance

        b. microscopic: uniform thickening of Descemet's, increased corneal thickness, nonbullous epithelial edema

 11. Keratoconus

        a. gross: conical deformation, central or paracentral thinning, Fleischer's iron ring, Vogt's stromal striae, Descemet's tear

        b. microscopic: fragmentation of Bowman's, thinning of stroma and overlying epithelium, folds or breaks in Descemet's, variable diffuse scarring. Iron deposition (Perls' stain) in basal epithelial cells.

 12. Keratoglobus

        a. gross: globular deformation of cornea, midperipheral thinning

        b. microscopic: areas of thickening of Descemet's

F. Pigmentations

  1. Krukenberg spindle

        a. gross: melanin on endothelium as vertical ellipse

       b. microscopic: melanin within endothelial cells, free on posterior corneal surface and within macrophages

    2. Iron lines (see table)

Iron Lines

Barraquer-Green	scar
Baum	Salzmann's nodular degeneration
Ferry	filtering bleb
Fleischer	keratoconus
Forstot-Mannis	penetrating keratoplasty—donor side, corneal suture
Hudson-Stahli	aging
Koneig	epikeratophakia, keratomileusis
Mason	penetrating keratoplasty at wound site margin
Steinberg	refractive keratectomy
Stocker	pterygium

       a. gross: iron line within epithelium

       b. microscopic: iron within basal epithelial cells (Perls' stain)

    3. Kayser-Fleischer ring

       a. gross: complete or incomplete yellowish-green ring in posterior cornea along its circumference

       b. microscopic: copper deposition in inner portion of Descemet's

    4. Blood staining

       a. gross: yellowish, granular appearance to posterior corneal surface

       b. microscopic: acute—orange particles (hemoglobin) within stroma; chronic—iron in keratocytes

VI. THE UVEAL TRACT

  A. Congenital

    1. Persistent pupillary membrane

       a. gross: pigmented or nonpigmented strand(s) of tissue attached to iris collarette, extends into anterior chamber, to posterior corneal surface, or to anterior lens surface

       b. microscopic: strands of mesodermal tissue without neovascularization

    2. Hematopoiesis

       a. gross: none

       b. microscopic: hematopoietic tissue with blood cell precursors in uveal tissue, usually choroid

    3. Hypoplasia

  a. gross: rudimentary iris connected to ciliary body. Varies in different quadrants.
  b. microscopic: rudimentary iris rim along periphery. Underdeveloped or absent iris musculature.
4. Coloboma
  a. gross: localized absence or defect of iris, ciliary body, or choroid. May be complete, incomplete, or cystic (choroid). Usually inferonasal.
  b. microscopic: iris—complete absence of all tissue in involved area, from pupil to periphery or only portions of iris; ciliary body—defect filled with mesodermal and vascular tissue with hyperplastic ciliary processes along edges; choroid—absence or atrophy of choroid and retinal pigment epithelium (RPE) with atrophic and gliotic retina, some with rosettes. Hyperplastic RPE along edges. Thinned, cystic overlying sclera, filled with proliferated glial tissue.
5. Primary iris cysts
  a. gross: at pupillary border, midiris or peripheral iris
  b. microscopic: lined by multilayered cornea-like epithelium with goblet cells or neuroepithelium from iris posterior pigmented epithelium
6. Pars plana cysts
  a. gross: radially oriented cyst-like structures on pars plana (translucent when unfixed; milky after 60 minutes of fixation with formaldehyde)
  b. microscopic: large intraepithelial cysts within nonpigmented ciliary epithelium. Contain hyaluronic acid, but appear empty on routine sections.
B. Systemic Disorders
1. Lisch nodules
  a. gross: multiple, small spider-like melanocytic nevi on anterior iris surface
  b. microscopic: collections of nevus cells in anterior iris stroma
2. Juvenile xanthogranuloma
  a. gross: diffuse or discrete iris, ciliary body, or anterior choroidal lesions
  b. microscopic: diffuse granulomatous inflammatory cell infiltrate with histiocytes and multinucleated giant cells with homogenous eosinophilic cytoplasm centrally, a rim of nuclei, and a peripheral rim of foamy cytoplasm (Touton giant cells), blood vessels
3. Lacy vacuolation of iris pigment epithelium

      a. gross: multiple punctate iris transillumination defects

      b. microscopic: intraepithelial vacuoles, contain glycogen (PAS)

    4. Angioid streaks

      a. gross: bilateral, irregular, jagged lines radiating from peripapillary area toward periphery, deep to retinal vessels

      b. microscopic: break in elastic layer of Bruch's membrane, RPE basement membrane thickening, RPE thinning. Hyperplasia of surrounding RPE.

C. Vascular

    1. Iris neovascularization

      a. gross: nonradial blood vessels on iris surface, ectropion uvea

      b. microscopic: new iris vessels with thin walls at pupillary border and/or midperiphery arising from iris stromal or ciliary body (near iris root) vessels, fibrovascular tissue on anterior iris surface. Loss of normal convoluted anterior iris surface making anterior and posterior iris surfaces parallel, pulling of posterior pigmented epithelium to iris surface, bending of sphincter muscle into J-shaped configuration, loss of dilator muscle, layer of myofibroblasts covering new vessels.

    2. Choroidal neovascularization (see "age-related macular degeneration" below)

    3. Cavernous hemangioma of choroid: Sturge-Weber syndrome

      a. gross: round or oval, slightly elevated, orangish mass, indistinct borders

      b. microscopic: dilated endothelial-lined spaces in affected area of choroid, indistinct margins

D. Uveitis

    1. Nongranulomatous inflammation

      a. microscopic: lymphocytic cellular infiltrate, mostly T-lymphocyte subtypes, but also B-lymphocytes and plasma cells

    2. Granulomatous inflammation

      a. gross: mutton-fat keratic precipitates, iris nodules on pupillary rim (Koeppe) or midiris (Busacca)

      b. microscopic: multinucleated giant cells (transformed macrophages) with eosinophilic (vimentin filaments) cytoplasm, lymphocytes, plasma cells. Granulomas (clusters of multinucleated giant cells surrounded by rim of lymphocytes).

3. Sarcoid uveitis
   a. gross: ciliary flush, Busacca or Koeppe nodules. Iris, ciliary, choroidal, perivascular, or optic nerve granulomas
   b. microscopic: granulomatous noncaseating inflammatory infiltrates, multinucleated giant cells with asteroid and/or Schaumann's bodies
4. Fuchs' heterochromic iridocyclitis
   a. gross: iris hypochromia, no anterior or posterior synechiae
   b. microscopic: stromal iris atrophy, loss of stromal pigment, lymphocytic and plasma cell infiltration of iris and ciliary body with necrosis, arteriolar hyalinization
5. Serpiginous choroiditis
   a. gross: well-demarcated gray lesions initially at level of RPE. Eventual degeneration of RPE, choroidal geographic atrophy, and disciform scarring.
   b. microscopic: diffuse lymphocytic infiltration throughout choroid, prominent focal infiltrates along RPE margins. Choriocapillaris, RPE, and photoreceptor atrophy, choroidal neovascularization.
6. Sympathetic ophthalmia
   a. gross: choroidal thickening, small depigmented, yellowish clusters of seed-shaped lesions
   b. microscopic: diffuse choroidal thickening due to nonnecrotizing granulomatous uveal inflammation (lymphocytes, epithelioid cells, occasional eosinophils), sparing of choriocapillaris, relative lack of retinal involvement, phagocytosis of uveal pigment by epithelioid cells, epithelioid cells between RPE and Bruch's membrane (Dalen-Fuchs' nodules), extension of granulomatous process into scleral canals and optic disc
E. Choroidal Dystrophies
   1. Central areolar choroidal sclerosis
      a. gross: exudative, edematous macular area leads to well-demarcated area of atrophy
      b. microscopic: incomplete or complete loss or degeneration of choriocapillaris, RPE, and outer retinal layers
   2. Peripapillary choroidal sclerosis
      a. gross: well-demarcated atrophic area around optic nerve head. Increased visibility of large choroidal vessels.
      b. microscopic: absence of choriocapillaris, RPE and photoreceptors with decreased number of

choroidal vessels in affected area. Breaks in juxtapapillary Bruch's membrane.

3. Choroideremia
   a. gross: extensive degeneration of retina and choroid, sparing the macula
   b. microscopic: marked atrophy or absence of choroid with atrophy of overlying outer retina

4. Gyrate atrophy
   a. gross: islands of chorioretinal atrophy in mid-periphery
   b. microscopic: focal photoreceptor atrophy and RPE hypoplasia in posterior pole. In midperiphery, distinct transition between normal tissue with marked retinal, RPE, and choroidal atrophy.

F. Tumors
   1. Ephelis (freckle)
      a. gross: localized area (no nodule) of darker pigmentation on iris surface
      b. microscopic: increased pigmentation of anterior border melanocyte layer. Normal number of melanocytes.

   2. Iris nevus
      a. gross: discrete nodule or mass on anterior iris surface
      b. microscopic: increased number of atypical, benign-appearing melanocytes with variable pigmentation.

   3. Choroidal nevus
      a. gross: flat, discoid, usually pigmented lesion, less than 2 disc diameters (DD) in size
      b. microscopic: four cell types: polyhedral—plump, markedly pigmented; fusiform—plump, dendritic, moderately pigmented; spindle—slender, little to no pigment; balloon—large with abundant foamy cytoplasm

   4. Malignant melanoma of iris
      a. gross: usually at inferior pupillary zone, a discrete or diffuse mass with variable pigmentation and increased vascularity. Pupillary distortion.
      b. microscopic: (see below)

   5. Malignant melanoma of choroid or ciliary body
      a. gross: elevated, mound- or mushroom-shaped, or bilobed variably pigmented mass
      b. microscopic: six types: epithelioid—noncohesive cells with round large nuclei, prominent nucleoli, abundant cytoplasm, distinct cell borders; increased pleomorphism and nuclear area

compared to spindle cells, frequent mitoses. Intermediate epithelioid—noncohesive cells with round nuclei, prominent nucleoli, abundant cytoplasm, indistinct cell borders. Spindle A—cohesive cells with small spindle-shaped nuclei, low nuclear-to-cytoplasmic ratio, central dark strip (nuclear fold) without distinct nucleoli, indistinct cell borders, rare mitoses. Spindle B—cohesive spindle-shaped cells, spindle-shaped nuclei, higher nuclear-to-cytoplasmic ratio, prominent nucleoli, indistinct cell borders, decreased pleomorphism and nuclear area. Mixed—spindle cells (mostly spindle B) and epithelioid cells. Necrotic—no identifiable cell type. When examining melanomas, look for invasion of Bruch's membrane, scleral canals, sclera, optic nerve, vortex veins, localized retinal detachment, extrabulbar extension.

VII. THE LENS

A. Congenital
1. Zonular, axial, sutural, filiform, and membranous cataracts: nonspecific histologic findings
2. Anterior polar cataract
   a. gross: small, bilateral, symmetric, nonprogressive opacity involving anterior subcapsular cortex and lens capsule
   b. microscopic: metaplasia and proliferation of subcapsular epithelial cells, superficial cortical fiber loss
3. Lenticonus and lentiglobus
   a. gross: localized cone shape (conus) or spherical (globus) protrusion of axial portions of anterior or posterior lens
   b. microscopic: capsule normal at cone periphery, almost absent at apex. Normal subcapsular epithelium and cortex over anterior lens surface.
4. Mittendorf's dot
   a. gross: small, white opacity just inferonasal to posterior pole of lens at lenticular attachment site of hyaloid artery
   b. microscopic: fibrous tissue, residual vascular basement membrane if attached hyaloid vessel tail near posterior capsule
5. Posterior polar cataract
   a. gross: larger opacity involving posterior subcapsular cortex and lens capsule

        b. microscopic: posterior migration of lens epithelial cells in posterior subcapsular region, with epithelial cell swelling and enlargement (Wedl or bladder cells). Minimal posterior subcapsular cortical degeneration.

    6. Rubella cataract

        a. gross: uniform dense nuclear opacity or total cataract

        b. microscopic: retention of cell nuclei, variable degrees of nuclear pyknosis and karyorrhexis in fibers of embryonic-early fetal lens

B. Lens Capsule Abnormalities

    1. True exfoliation of lens capsule

        a. gross: anterior layer of anterior lens capsule splits off into sheets that curl into anterior chamber

        b. microscopic: cleavage plane lies within anterior half of lens capsule, having filamentous anterior and homogeneous posterior portions

C. Adult Cataracts

    1. Anterior subcapsular cataract

        a. gross: whitish opacities in anterior subcapsular area

        b. microscopic: necrosis of lens epithelium and subcapsular fibers, proliferation and fibrous metaplasia (to spindle cells) of adjacent cuboidal lens epithelium to form multilayered hypercellular plaque and then fibrous scar

    2. Posterior subcapsular cataract (PSC)

        a. gross: granular, vacuolar plaque in axial posterior subcapsular cortex

        b. microscopic: disorganization and metaplasia (to spindle cells) of meridional rows of lens epithelial cell nuclei at equator (absence of nuclear bow) with migration to posterior subcapsular area. Layers of round, nucleated migratory cells (Wedl or bladder cells) aggregate around PSC.

    3. Cortical cataract

        a. gross: spoke-like whitish opacities in lens cortex

        b. microscopic: water clefts—areas of cortical lamellae disrupted by swollen, degenerated lens fiber debris seen as nuclear, eosinophilic globular aggregates (Morgagnian globules) surrounded by lighter granular material; rounding off of ends of cortical cells; calcium oxalate or cholesterol in chronic cataracts; cortical material in equatorial region—Soemmerring's ring.

    4. Nuclear sclerosis
      a. gross: variable nuclear color from clear to yellow to brown (cataracta brunescens) to black (cataracta nigra). Anteroposterior thickening.
      b. microscopic: amorphous and homogenous nucleus with compaction of cells, increased eosinophilia and loss of artifactitious nuclear clefts

VIII. THE VITREOUS

A. Congenital
    1. Persistent hyperplastic primary vitreous
      a. gross: opaque plaque on posterior lens, attaching to elongated, centrally displaced ciliary processes
      b. microscopic: fibrovascular connective tissue in the retrolental vitreous, extending laterally to elongated, centrally displaced ciliary processes. Anterior aspect of plaque may extend through lens capsule into cortex. Posterior aspect may have attached hyaloid vessel.
    2. Bergmeister papillae
      a. gross: glial tissue (posterior remnants of hyaloid system) over nasal portion of optic nerve head
      b. microscopic: occluded remnants of posterior portion of hyaloid artery surrounded by glia
B. Inflammations
    1. Pars planitis (nongranulomatous peripheral uveitis)
      a. gross: whitish snow-like material accumulated along inferior vitreous base
      b. microscopic: condensed vitreous with mononuclear cells ("snowballs"), fibroglial tissue, vessels, nonpigmented ciliary epithelium, and fibrocyte-like cells
C. Infections
    1. Bacterial
      a. gross: variable debris, liquefaction, and opacification of vitreous gel with variable amount of purulent exudate
      b. microscopic: acute inflammatory cells (PMNs) along collagenous fibrils. Organisms (special stains).
    2. Fungal
      a. gross: fluffy, opaque microabscesses, satellite lesions. Associated areas of retinitis.
      b. microscopic: chronic inflammatory cell infiltrate (lymphocytes, plasma cells). Hyphae (special stains).

D. Vitreous Opacities
   1. Posterior vitreous detachment
      a. gross: previous attachment site of vitreous at optic nerve head freely mobile within central vitreous as round fibrous band (Weiss ring)
      b. microscopic: vitreous filaments collapsed anteriorly, forming condensed posterior vitreous layer. Watery fluid without collagenous filaments in posterior subvitreal space.
   2. Asteroid hyalosis (Benson's disease)
      a. gross: multiple glistening spherical opacities (calcium-containing lipid) of 0.01 to 0.1 mm diameter suspended within vitreous. No gravitational aggregation.
      b. microscopic: weakly basophilic (H&E) spherules with an outer dense ring and central homogenous zone (PAS, Von Kossa stains). Birefringent spicules in polarized light. Attached to collagenous vitreous framework.
   3. Synchysis scintillans
      a. gross: freely mobile golden opacities comprising variably-sized crystals (cholesterol) in fluid vitreous. Settles inferiorly when eye is immobile.
      b. microscopic: clefts of dissolved-out cholesterol crystals (in paraffin-embedded sections) within vitreous. Birefringent retained cholesterol esters in polarized light (frozen sections).
   4. Systemic primary amyloidosis
      a. gross: extracellular, granular opacities in sheet-like vitreous veils. Larger opacities give vitreous a glass-wool appearance.
      b. microscopic: eosinophilic pale substance with filamentous ultrastructure in vitreous. Stains with Congo red, metachromatic with crystal violet, birefringent, dichroism, fluorescent with thioflavin-T.
   5. Vitreous hemorrhage
      a. gross: blood within vitreous cavity
      b. microscopic: red blood cells and pigment-containing macrophages within vitreous or in space between retina and posterior face of detached vitreous
E. Epiretinal Membrane
   1. gross: translucent fragment of tissue
   2. microscopic: RPE cells, macrophages, fibrocytes, fibrous astrocytes, myofibroblast-like cells, hyalocytes. May or may not be vascularized. Collagen.
F. Tumors

1. Reticulum cell sarcoma (histiocytic lymphoma)
    a. gross: cells and fluffy, nondiscrete opacities in posterior cortical vitreous. May extend into central vitreous.
    b. microscopic: pleomorphic cells with oval-to-round nuclei with small, finger-like protrusions and irregular multiple nucleoli. Scanty delicate cytoplasm poorly preserved in vitreous aspirates.

IX. THE RETINA

A. Congenital
    1. Lange's fold: fixation artifact in infant eyes due to variable shrinkage of retina and sclera
        a. gross: no clinical correlate
        b. microscopic: elevated and anteriorly displaced peripheral retina at ora serrata with adhesion to vitreous base
    2. Retinopathy of prematurity
        a. stage 1
            1) gross: white demarcation line separating vascularized and nonvascularized retina
            2) microscopic: thickening of normal angiogenesis wave with two zones: anterior vanguard zone—spindle cells with gap junctions, rear guard zone (not seen clinically)—differentiating endothelial cells with new, dilated capillaries
        b. stage 2
            1) gross: elevated pink ridge
            2) microscopic: posterior extension of demarcation line, further hyperplasia to surface, vanguard tissue. Posterior proliferation of endothelial cells or rear guard tissue.
        c. stage 3
            1) gross: extraretinal fibrovascular proliferation
            2) microscopic: anterior and posterior growth of fibrovascular proliferative tissue into vitreous, placoid in ridge region, vitreous synchysis, and condensation
        d. stage 4
            1) gross: subtotal retinal detachment
            2) microscopic: traction due to proliferative vitreoretinopathy—glial proliferation, sheets of myofibroblasts proliferating in intravitreal strands along collapsed and condensed vitreous scaffold
        e. stage 5

        1) gross: total funnel-shaped retinal detachment
        2) microscopic: fibrous traction, anterior retinal folding

B. Infectious Retinitis

   1. Cytomegalovirus retinitis

      a. gross: area of coagulative, necrotizing retinitis, sharply demarcated from normal retina, with multiple variably-sized pale yellow retinal infiltrates with ill-defined margins and interspersed retinal hemorrhages ("pizza pie"), perivascular infiltration

      b. microscopic: retinal thickening with disruption of architecture by enlarged cells with prominent Cowdry type A intranuclear eosinophil inclusions with surrounding clear zones and small, multiple, basophilic intracytoplasmic inclusions (numerous virions associated with dense masses of PAS-positive matter), disruption of underlying RPE with a secondary diffuse granulomatous infiltrate in underlying choroid, intranuclear inclusions in RPE, and vascular endothelium

   2. Histoplasmosis

      a. gross: small, punched-out, atrophic chorioretinal scars in midperiphery and posterior pole, peripapillary and/or macular chorioretinal scarring. No vitreous inflammation.

      b. microscopic: chronic granulomatous inflammatory infiltrate in choroid with RPE hyperplasia, breaks in Bruch's, organizing subretinal hemorrhage, chorioretinal adhesions, choroidal neovascularization, disciform scar

   3. Toxoplasmosis

      a. gross: multifocal necrotizing retinochoroiditis, focal periarterial exudates

      b. microscopic: areas of coagulative retinal necrosis, sharply demarcated from normal retina. Underlying choroid and sclera with secondary diffuse granulomatous inflammatory infiltrate with choroid occasionally becoming necrotic with obliteration of choriocapillaris. Organism multiplying in retinal cell (pseudocyst). Intracellular protozoan (multiple tiny nuclei) multiplying within self-made membrane (true cyst), may be free in tissue (eccentrically placed tiny nuclei with tapering of opposite end of cytoplasm).

C. Retinal Vascular Occlusive Disease

1. Central or branch retinal artery occlusion
   a. gross: whitening of affected retina, particularly in posterior pole (if affected). Orange reflex from intact choroidal vasculature beneath intact foveola contrasts surrounding opaque neural retina (cherry red spot).
   b. microscopic: arteriosclerosis-related thrombosis, embolus (cholesterol, calcific, platelet-fibrin), or arteritis at level of lamina cribrosa. Acutely, edema within inner retinal layers with pyknosis and death of affected nuclei. As retinal edema clears, inner ischemic atrophy (including inner aspect of inner nuclear layer) remains in distribution of retina supplied by occluded vessel, progresses to diffuse homogeneous acellular scar.
2. Central retinal vein occlusion
   a. gross: extensive retinal edema and hemorrhage involving most of retinal layers, dilated tortuous retinal veins, cotton-wool spots
   b. microscopic: thrombosis in central retinal vein at level of lamina cribrosa, marked retinal edema, focal retinal necroses, subretinal, intraretinal and preretinal hemorrhage. With time, hemosiderin staining of retina, hemosiderin-laden macrophages, disorganization of retinal architecture, gliosis, fibrovascular preretinal membranes, and neovascularization.
3. Branch retinal vein occlusion
   a. gross: retinal hemorrhages, cotton-wool spots in affected distribution, usually superotemporal quadrant beginning at arteriovenous crossing
   b. microscopic: retinal edema, focal necrosis, subretinal, intraretinal, and preretinal hemorrhages. With time, hemosiderosis, disorganization of retinal architecture, gliosis, fibrovascular preretinal membranes.
4. Hypertensive retinopathy
   a. gross: flame-shaped and dot-blot hemorrhages, cotton-wool spots, hard exudates, Elschnig's spots (black, isolated spot of pigment with surrounding yellowish-red halo), Siegrist's streaks (pigment along choroidal vessel)
   b. microscopic: complete obstruction of terminal choroidal arterioles and choriocapillaris by fibrin thrombi (Elschnig's spot), linear chains of pigment deposition along sclerosed choroidal vessel (Siegrist's streaks), semiopaque wall of arteriolosclerotic arteriole obscures underlying

venule due to common adventitia (AV nicking), cystoid spaces in outer plexiform layers filled with eosinophilic material (hard exudate), eventual outer retinal ischemic atrophy

5. Retinal capillary hemangioma: Von Hippel-Lindau
    a. gross: arteriole and venule enter and exit a well-circumscribed, midperipheral yellow to pink retinal vascular lesion. Associated intraretinal and subretinal lipid.
    b. microscopic: small, capillary-like or slightly larger blood vessels, lined by endothelium and delicate reticulum. Many vacuolated cells in stromal interstitium between blood vessels of larger lesions. Fusiform thickening of entire retinal thickness. Scattered lipid foam cells and glial tissue throughout lesion.

D. Diabetic Retinopathy
    1. histopathologic changes at various stages of diabetic retinopathy include: capillary microaneurysms, basement membrane thickening, loss of pericytes, intraretinal microvascular abnormalities (IRMA), venous dilation, duplications, beadings, intraretinal hemorrhages, lipid exudate in outer plexiform layer, cotton-wool spots, macular edema, macular ischemia, vitreous hemorrhage, rhegmatogenous or traction retinal detachments, neovascularization and fibrous tissue proliferation (intraretinal, on retinal surface, on disc surface), and elevation of vessels into vitreous
    2. Capillary nonperfusion
        a. microscopic: mural deposition of PAS-positive plasma derivatives passing through a defective endothelium (plasmatic vasculosis)
    3. Microaneurysms
        a. gross: dot-like outpouchings adjacent to areas of capillary nonperfusion
        b. microscopic: fusiform or saccular outpouchings of capillaries (PAS or trypsin digestion) in inner nuclear layer. May hyalinize and become occluded due to thrombosis or deposition of PAS-positive material.
    4. Capillary basement membrane thickening
        a. microscopic: increased thickness of capillary basement membranes
    5. Loss of capillary pericytes
        a. microscopic: loss of pericytes that normally surround vessel's outer circumference, decrease in normal pericyte-endothelial cell ratio in retinal capillaries of a normal (1:1) young person.

Detected by balloon-like spaces (pericyte ghosts) in digest preparations.

6. Intraretinal hemorrhages
   a. gross: boat-shaped, flame-shaped, dot-blot hemorrhages, dark subretinal, and even darker, more discretely defined subRPE blood
   b. microscopic: subinternal limiting membrane or subhyaloid blood cells (boat-shaped), hemorrhage in horizontal orientation between axons of nerve fibers in the inner retina (flame-shaped), hemorrhage among outer plexiform nerve fibers (dot-blot) that restrict lateral displacement of blood, subretinal hemorrhage, hemorrhage between RPE and Bruch's membrane limited by attachments of RPE to Bruch's (subRPE blood)

7. Cotton-wool spots
   a. gross: gray, semiopaque lesions with feathery edges in superficial retina, associated with blood vessels. Variable in size, less than one-half disc diameter.
   b. microscopic: disciform, sharply circumscribed lesion, in thickened ganglion cell and nerve fiber layer, composed of cell-like cytoid bodies due to swollen nerve fiber layer (NFL) axons containing pooled mitochondria. Localized inner ischemic atrophy. Bloodless capillary lumens, loss of endothelial cells and pericytes.

8. Cystoid macular edema
   a. gross: retinal thickening with honeycomb-like cystoid spaces
   b. microscopic: intraretinal edema with fluid accumulation within Müller's cells and within spaces in outer plexiform layer (Henle's layer) and inner nuclear layer

9. Neovascularization
   a. gross: fibrovascular and glial tissue on vitreous side of internal limiting membrane
   b. microscopic: intraretinal proliferation of vessels from venous circulation, may proliferate through internal limiting membrane, along inner retinal and posterior hyaloid surfaces. Fenestrations present, tight junctions absent. Fibroglial component forming preretinal membranes.

10. Sickle Cell Retinopathy
    a. gross: midperipheral and peripheral lesions, including arteriolar occlusions, neovascularization, proliferative retinopathy, and preretinal hemorrhage

11. Salmon patch
   a. gross: well-circumscribed, slightly elevated, red-orange midperipheral retinal lesion with interspersed iridescent spots
   b. microscopic: hemorrhage within inner retinal layers beneath internal limiting membrane (ILM). Schisis cavity between ILM and remaining retina after blood resorbs. Reflection of light from hemosiderin-laden macrophages in inner retinal layers (iridescent spots) after degradation of blood cells
12. Black sunburst
   a. gross: round, well-circumscribed, hyperpigmented, peripheral chorioretinal scar
   b. microscopic: hemorrhage in deeper retinal layers, hemosiderin-laden macrophages, increased density of pigment epithelial melanin. Reactive RPE hyperplasia.
E. Retinal Detachment (RD)
   1. Distinguish an artifactitious, fixation-related RD from a true RD. An artifactitious RD lacks subretinal fluid (fluid may disappear during tissue processing of true RD), has photoreceptor destruction, attachment of pigment granules to photoreceptor outer segments, and loss of RPE apical villi.
      a. gross: retinal separation from RPE, usually with subretinal fluid
      b. microscopic: degeneration and loss of rod and cone outer segments. Cystoid degeneration in outer plexiform layer with coalescence of cystoid spaces into large cysts (orange-peel effect). Glial and connective tissue proliferation. Fibroglial membranes on external retinal surface. Serous (homogenous, eosinophilic material) or serosanguinous (red blood cells) subretinal fluid. Thickened Bruch's membrane, drusen, hyalinization of choriocapillaris. RPE proliferation with fibrous metaplasia (clinically visible demarcation line). Chronic detachments—loss of photoreceptors, retinal disorganization, gliosis, marked cystic degeneration, preretinal membranes, RPE proliferation at ora serrata (Ringschwiele).
F. Age-Related Macular Degeneration
   1. gross: pigmentary changes, geographic atrophy, drusen, hemorrhage, lipid, areas of retinal elevation
   2. microscopic: partial or complete obliteration of choriocapillaris. Thickening of Bruch's membrane

with calcification and basophilic changes. Atrophy of RPE with depigmentation, hypertrophy, or hyperplasia.

3. Drusen—located between RPE basement membrane and inner collagenous layer of Bruch's membrane, except for basal laminar deposits (see below)

4. Nodular, hard drusen
    a. gross: yellowish small discrete subretinal lesions
    b. microscopic: PAS-positive, hyaline membranous debris with lipid from one or more RPE cells. May have dystrophic calcification. Electron microscopy—finely granular or amorphous material with vesicles, tube-like structures, abnormal collagen. Hypertrophic RPE at margins.

5. Soft, granular drusen
    a. gross: larger, yellowish, small subretinal lesions with indistinct margins
    b. microscopic: pale-staining amorphous material within dome-shaped area between thickened inner aspect of Bruch's and remainder of Bruch's. Hypertrophy, attenuation, and/or loss of overlying RPE. May have dystrophic calcification. Electron microscopy—thickened area with vesicles, membranous debris, abnormal basement membrane.

6. Diffuse, confluent drusen
    a. gross: yellowish, subretinal lesions with indistinct margins; confluent
    b. microscopic: diffuse thickening of inner collagenous zone of Bruch's membrane. May have dystrophic calcification. Electron microscopy—thickening due to electron-dense material, filaments, clusters of widely-spaced collagen.

7. Basal laminar drusen (deposit)
    a. gross: multiple, small, round yellowish subretinal lesions
    b. microscopic: diffuse thickening of inner aspect of Bruch's membrane with superimposed, highly uniform, numerous, small, internal nodules. Electron microscopy—granular deposits between RPE plasma membrane and RPE basement membrane; wide-spaced collagen.

8. Basal linear deposit
    a. gross: multiple, small yellowish subretinal lesions
    b. microscopic (electron): vesicles external to RPE basement membrane, phospholipid, filamentous

9. Choroidal neovascularization
   a. gross: small, translucent fragment of tissue, usually with pigment or hemorrhage on its surface
   b. microscopic: endothelial-lined vascular channels between RPE and Bruch's membrane. Spindle-shaped cells (fibrocytes) and round cells (lymphocytes). Retina, RPE and its basement membrane, Bruch's membrane, choroid, and basal laminar deposits assist in orienting a surgically excised membrane. Associated fluid, hemorrhage, and lipid.
10. Disciform scar
    a. gross: whitish, subretinal, and intraretinal scarring within macula
    b. microscopic: fibrous tissue, proliferated RPE cells, degeneration of photoreceptor cells

G. Disease of Retinal Periphery
   1. Lattice degeneration
      a. gross: lesion usually parallel to ora serrata. Criss-crossing white lines of fibrosed retinal vessels in locally thinned retina with irregular, mottled subjacent RPE. Overlying vitreous liquefication.
      b. microscopic: discontinuity of internal limiting membrane, various degrees of inner retinal thinning and atrophy, overlying pocket of liquefied vitreous, thickened, hyalinized retinal vessels, RPE changes, condensation and adherence of vitreous at lesion margins. Decreased number of retinal capillaries with fibrotic degeneration of larger vessels in affected area (trypsin digested flat retinal preps).
   2. Cobblestone degeneration
      a. gross: well-demarcated, flat, pale lesions anterior to ora serrata with frequent prominent vessels at base of lesion. Usually in inferotemporal quadrant.
      b. microscopic: circumscribed area of outer retinal and RPE atrophy. Remaining inner nuclear layer adherent to Bruch's membrane. Usually normal choroid except for absent or partially obliterated choriocapillaris. Sharp boundary between normal and atrophic retina with RPE hypertrophy and hyperplasia along margins.
   3. Typical peripheral cystoid degeneration
      a. gross: grayish, transparent cysts with rounded margins just posterior to ora serrata, usually in temporal quadrant

      b. microscopic: rows of cystoid spaces in outer plexiform layer that enlarge to involve adjacent nuclear layers and form tunnels separated by Müller fibers that further coalesce to form intraretinal schisis cavities (inner wall composed of internal limiting membrane and inner portion of Müller cells, outer wall composed of photoreceptor nuclei)

   4. Reticular peripheral cystoid degeneration

      a. gross: fine, stippled surface with arborizing superficial vascular pattern just posterior to typical cystoid degeneration

      b. microscopic: cystic spaces of hyaluronic acid within nerve fiber layer, extending from internal limiting membrane to inner plexiform layer. Thinned inner retinal layers (almost only inner limiting membrane and vessels present).

   5. Typical degenerative retinoschisis

      a. gross: retinal elevation in inferotemporal quadrant with beaten metal appearance of inner layer. Occasional small, glistening yellowish dots.

      b. microscopic: splitting in outer plexiform layers and adjacent nuclear layers. Inner wall consists of internal limiting membrane, inner portions of Müller cells, nerve fiber layer remnants, and blood vessels. Outer wall consists of outer plexiform layer, outer nuclear layer, and photoreceptors. Cyst filled with hyaluronic acid.

H. Generalized Chorioretinal Degeneration

   1. Retinitis pigmentosa

      a. gross: pigment in bone-spicule configuration. Narrowed arterioles.

      b. microscopic: disorganization and loss of photoreceptors (usually rods), RPE degeneration and proliferation, intraretinal migration of pigment-filled macrophages and RPE around retinal vessels. Intact Bruch's membrane. Usually no chorioretinal scars. Thickening and hyalinization of vessel walls. Diffuse or sectoral optic nerve atrophy with gliosis.

   2. Macular hole (full-thickness)

      a. gross: round hole in fovea, may have associated epiretinal membrane

      b. microscopic: retinal defect in foveal area surrounded by rounded, detached edges. Subretinal fluid, intraretinal edema, variable photoreceptor atrophy collection of RPE, macrophages, fibrocytes, fibrous astrocytes, myofibroblast-like cells, hyalocytes, and collagen (epiretinal membrane).

I. Tumors

1. Astrocytic hamartoma: tuberous sclerosis
   a. gross: multiple yellowish-white or gray lesions, large and protuberant or small and flat
   b. microscopic: elongated fibrous astrocytes with small oval nuclei and interlacing cytoplasmic processes. Foci of calcification. Large, pleomorphic, round astrocytes in larger lesions, especially of optic nerve head.

2. Retinoblastoma
   a. gross: single or multiple whitish mass(es): exophytic (into subretinal space, retinal vessels on tumor surface) or endophytic (into vitreous cavity, no retinal vessels visible) growth
   b. microscopic: cells with round, oval, or spindle-shaped hyperchromatic nuclei, sparse cytoplasm, frequent mitoses, areas of necrosis with scattered cuffs of viable tumor cells around remaining blood vessels with intra- and extracellular calcification. Monolayer of columnar cells with eosinophilic cytoplasm and peripheral nuclei around a central lumen lined by external limiting membrane (Flexner-Wintersteiner rosettes), cells surrounding a lumen filled with eosinophilic cytoplasmic processes (Homer Wright rosette), aggregates of well-differentiated rod and cone photoreceptors with outer segments centrally (fleurette). Tumor cells may spread into optic nerve, leptomeninges, or choroid.
   c. spontaneous regression of retinoblastoma: islands of calcified cells in fibroconnective tissue mass with contours of tumor cells along its periphery filling the vitreous. RPE and ciliary epithelial cell proliferation.

3. Retinocytoma
   a. gross: may be similar to retinoblastoma
   b. microscopic: fleurettes intermixed with benign individual cells at various stages of photoreceptor differentiation. No mitoses or necrosis. Cells have more cytoplasm than retinoblastoma cells.

4. Medulloepithelioma
   a. gross: whitish mass with rough surface, areas of pigmentation, and fibrous tissue
   b. microscopic: ribbon-like structures of undifferentiated, round-to-oval shaped cells with cellular polarity and little cytoplasm. Stratified cells

(up to five layers), lined on one side by a thin basement membrane. Mucinous cysts. Flexner-Wintersteiner and Homer Wright rosettes. Cartilage or smooth muscle.

X. THE OPTIC NERVE

A. Congenital
   1. Optic nerve hypoplasia
      a. gross: decreased optic disc diameter with centrally located vessels
      b. microscopic: partial or complete atrophy and absence of neurons
   2. Congenital crescent
      a. gross: white, semilunar area along disc margin, usually inferiorly or inferotemporally, often associated with oval disc (long axis is parallel)
      b. microscopic: absence of RPE and choroid in crescent area
   3. Coloboma
      a. gross: varies from deep physiologic cup to large hole with associated retrobulbar cyst
      b. microscopic: absence of optic nerve tissue in affected area, fibrous tissue lining surrounding hypoplastic or gliotic retina. Smooth muscle fibers and adipose tissue within wall of defect.
   4. Optic nerve pit
      a. gross: triangular or circular, small depression about one-quarter of disc diameter, located inferotemporally
      b. microscopic: connective tissue capsule surrounding defect in lamina cribrosa with retinal tissue looping into optic nerve or subarachnoid space
   5. Morning glory syndrome
      a. gross: enlarged, deeply excavated optic disc with surrounding elevated tissue, indistinct margins
      b. microscopic: deeply displaced optic disc within enlarged scleral foramen, RPE and retina extend into excavation
   6. Optic disc edema
      a. gross: elevated hyperemic disc with loss of physiological cup, blurring of disc margins, hemorrhage, soft exudates
      b. microscopic: swollen axonal fibers anterior to lamina cribrosa, tissue edema, vascular congestion, characteristic S-shaped configuration, and concentric folds (Paton's lines) of outer retinal

layers with lateral displacement of peripapillary photoreceptors. Degeneration of nerve fibers with gliosis and optic atrophy due to chronic edema.

7. Optic disc drusen
   a. gross: varies from subtle disc elevation to glistening, globular bodies protruding from optic nerve head and obscuring disc margins
   b. microscopic: calcareous, basophilic, laminated acellular bodies of varying shapes and sizes within prelaminar or nonmyelinated areas of optic disc. Stain for amino acids, acid mucopolysaccharides, calcium, and hemosiderin.

8. Optic atrophy/neuropathy from a variety of etiologies
   a. gross: disc pallor, decreased nerve diameter, loss of normal spongy nerve texture
   b. microscopic: nonspecific atrophic changes: axonal degeneration with loss of myelin (removed by macrophages) and oligodendrocytes, widened subarachnoid space with redundancy of dura, pial septa widening, astrocytic proliferation with optic nerve gliosis, retinal ganglion cell loss. Histologic distribution of atrophy may be diagnostic and correlates with clinical visual field deficits.

B. Arteritic Ischemic Optic Neuropathy
   1. Temporal arteritis
      a. gross: tortuous temporal artery
      b. microscopic: intimal thickening with granulomatous reaction adjacent to a fragmented internal elastic lamina, extending into an occasionally necrotic media and adventitia. Multinucleated giant cells.

C. Tumors
   1. Glioma (juvenile pilocytic astrocytoma)
      a. gross: tubular or fusiform-shaped retrobulbar optic nerve
      b. microscopic: spindle-shaped cells with elongated nuclei, intracytoplasmic eosinophilic hyalinization of fibers (Rosenthal fibers), foci of microcystic degeneration and calcification, enlarged neural bundles between thickened pial septa, extension of spindle-shaped tumor cells into meninges with reactive hyperplasia
   2. Meningioma
      a. gross: optic nerve mass, frequently extending through dura

  b. microscopic: concentrically packed masses of cells arranged in whorls with round or ellipsoid nuclei and abundant basophilic cytoplasm with rare laminated, calcium concretions (psammoma bodies)

 3. Melanocytoma (magnocellular nevi)

  a. gross: darkly pigmented, endophytic mass on optic nerve head

  b. microscopic: large, heavily pigmented, uniform cells

XI. THE GLAUCOMAS

 A. Open-Angle Glaucoma

  1. Primary open-angle glaucoma (early changes have not been well categorized)

   a. gross: normal depth and width of anterior chamber, normal configuration of chamber angle

   b. microscopic: lower cellularity of trabecular meshwork (TM) than age-matched nonglaucomatous eyes. Thickening of basement membrane where there is loss of endothelial lining with formation of lattice collagen inclusions. Thickening and fusion of trabecular beams, composed of endothelial cells surrounding collagen cores, with narrowing and loss of intertrabecular spaces. Collapse of Schlemm's canal with glycosaminoglycans filling intertrabecular spaces. End-stage—marked hyalinization, sclerosis, compaction, and obliteration of TM.

  2. Pigment dispersion syndrome with glaucoma

   a. gross: increased trabecular meshwork pigmentation, pigment line anterior to Schwalbe's line (Sampolesi's line), iris transillumination defects, vertical line of pigment on corneal endothelium (Krukenberg spindle [KS])

   b. microscopic: variable accumulation of pigment granules, pigment-laden macrophages, and cellular debris between trabecular beams, on the anterior surface of lens (Scheie stripe), on corneal endothelium (KS). Phagocytosed pigment in trabecular and corneal endothelial cells (KS), focal loss of iris pigment epithelium (transillumination defects).

  3. Pseudoexfoliation syndrome with glaucoma

   a. gross: central disc of fibrillary protein-like material surrounded by peripheral granular area on anterior lens capsule with intervening clear area

    b. microscopic: fine fibrils embedded in homogenous matrix, open angle with unevenly distributed pigment granules. Pseudoexfoliative material in intertrabecular spaces, juxtacanalicular tissue, beneath endothelium in Schlemm's canal. Parallel, small slivers perpendicular to lens capsule centrally and thick dendritic-appearing material at right angles to capsule peripherally. Small elastic fibers (special stains) in conjunctiva.

4. Iridocorneal endothelial syndrome (ICE) with glaucoma

    a. microscopic: monolayer of endothelial cells with basement membrane covering anterior chamber structures and trabecular meshwork

5. Angle-recession glaucoma

    a. gross: increased anterior chamber depth in affected area

    b. microscopic: tear in face of ciliary body between external longitudinal muscle fibers and internal circular and oblique muscles. Concurrent injury to trabecular meshwork includes tears in iris root (iridodialysis) and longitudinal muscle detachment from scleral spur (cyclodialysis).

6. Hemolytic glaucoma

    a. gross: blood may be present in anterior chamber

    b. microscopic: degenerating red blood cells and macrophages with phagocytosed erythrocytes in trabecular channels

7. Ghost cell glaucoma

    a. gross: khaki-colored pseudohypopyon, resolving vitreous hemorrhage

    b. microscopic: thin-walled, denatured erythrocytes in anterior chamber (phase-contrast microscopy) and trabecular meshwork. Defect in anterior hyaloid.

8. Phacolytic glaucoma

    a. gross: hypermature cataract, anterior chamber debris

    b. microscopic: denatured lens protein in anterior chamber, macrophages filled with degenerated lens cortical material in angle

9. Phacoanaphylactic glaucoma

    a. microscopic: granulomatous inflammatory reaction around damaged lens. Lens particles in trabecular meshwork.

B. Closed-Angle Glaucoma
  1. Primary closed angle glaucoma
    a. gross: shallow anterior chamber, abnormal configuration of angle
    b. microscopic: oblique approach of iris to insertion. Adhesions between peripheral iris and trabecular meshwork in later stages.
  2. Neovascular glaucoma
    a. gross: blood vessels on anterior iris surface and angle structures
    b. microscopic: fibrovascular membranes on iris stromal surface, and on open angle. Peripheral anterior synechiae, endothelial cell-lined vascular channels within angle structures.

C. Primary Congenital Glaucoma
    a. gross: enlarged axial length (buphthalmos) and corneal diameter (megalocornea)
    b. microscopic: anterior attachment of iris root to meshwork, anterior attachment of ciliary muscle longitudinal fibers to trabecular bands, trabecular beam thickening, incomplete separation of angle structures with retained fetal tissue

D. Sequelae of Glaucoma
  1. Buphthalmos
    a. gross: enlargement of globe
    b. microscopic: stretched and thinned cornea and sclera, rupture of suspensory ligaments of lens
  2. Haab's striae
    a. gross: vertical, horizontal, or oblique lines in the posterior cornea
    b. microscopic: discontinuous areas in Descemet's membrane
  3. Iris
    a. gross: areas of iris atrophy
    b. microscopic: hyalinization of iris stroma, atrophy of iris pigment epithelium, formation of pigment clumps near pupillary margin
  4. Ciliary body
    a. microscopic: atrophy, blunting, and hyalinization of stroma of ciliary processes (distinguish from thickening of ciliary body basement membrane in diabetes). Decreased cellularity and vascularity of ciliary stroma.
  5. Glaucomflecken
    a. gross: multiple, grayish-white punctate anterior subcapsular opacities. Follows lines of sutures.
    b. microscopic: focal areas of necrotic lens epithelial cells, degeneration of subepithelial cortex

6. Retina
   a. gross: loss of nerve fiber layer
   b. microscopic: degeneration and disappearance of ganglion cells and their axons (nerve fiber layer), vessel attenuation. Loss of inner nuclear layer cells due to transsynaptic atrophy.
7. Optic nerve
   a. gross: variable enlargement and deepening of optic nerve cup
   b. microscopic: prominent overhanging ridges at disc margins, vessels situated under lips of ridge, backward bowing of lamina cribrosa, enlarged, excavated cup, thinning to absence of ganglion nerve fibers around edge of disc, loss of retinal ganglion cells, decrease in nerve diameter, gliosis, demyelination, numerous large spaces (containing hyaluronic acid) within optic nerve parenchyma (cavernous spaces of Schnabel)

XII. THE ORBIT

A. Congenital
   1. Microphthalmos with cyst
      a. gross: small globe with large cyst
      b. microscopic: evidence of ocular structures with defect in sclera, cyst lined by glial, retinal, and undifferentiated tissue and disorganized RPE
B. Infections
   1. Bacterial orbital cellulitis
      a. microscopic: acute inflammatory infiltrate (neutrophils) with some chronic inflammatory cells and necrotic tissue. Organisms (special stains).
   2. Mucormycosis
      a. microscopic: variable inflammatory infiltrate from many to few neutrophils, broad, irregularly shaped, nonseptate hyphae branching at right angles, necrotic tissue, invasion of vessels by organism
C. Inflammations
   1. Histiocytosis X
      a. microscopic: mono- and binucleated histiocytes with bean-shaped nuclei, prominent nucleoli, and eosinophilic cytoplasm containing the Langerhans or Birbeck granule. Eosinophils, lymphocytes, plasma cells, multinucleated histiocytes, sparse stroma.
   2. Inflammatory orbital pseudotumor

        a. microscopic: polymorphous inflammatory response (eosinophils, neutrophils, plasma cells, lymphocytes, macrophages), varying amounts of collagen deposition, vasculitis, inflammatory infiltrate within muscle tendons, diffuse fibrosis in later stages

D. Systemic

    1. Graves' ophthalmopathy

        a. gross: thickened extraocular muscles

        b. microscopic: increased water content and cellular infiltrate of mononuclear cells, lymphocytes, plasma cells, mast cells, fibroblasts within interstitial tissues of extraocular muscles, most commonly inferior and medial recti; sparing of tendons. End-stage—fibrosis, destruction of muscles with fatty infiltration.

    2. Progressive external ophthalmoplegia

        a. gross: thinned muscle(s)

        b. microscopic: atrophic muscles with variation in diameter, granular and vacuolar degeneration. Fibrous and fatty infiltration. Abnormal mitochondria in fibers.

E. Tumors

    1. Capillary hemangioma

        a. gross: solitary, red, smooth lesion

        b. microscopic: proliferating plump endothelial cells lining and crowding out capillary-sized vascular spaces containing red blood cells

    2. Cavernous hemangioma

        a. gross: purplish, encapsulated mass, spongy appearance on cut edge

        b. microscopic: large blood-filled vascular channels lined by inner layer of endothelial cells and outer smooth muscle cells, thick fibrous tissue stroma and capsule

    3. Lymphangioma

        a. gross: blood-filled, lobulated cystic mass

        b. microscopic: nonencapsulated networks of endothelially-lined channels separated by thin, loose connective tissue septa and filled with a faintly pink staining matrix. No pericytes or smooth muscle in walls of vascular structures. Scattered follicles of lymphoid tissue in interstitium.

    4. Rhabdomyosarcoma

        a. gross: well-circumscribed or irregular firm orbital mass

        b. microscopic: embryonal subtype: hypercellular areas of small, round, oval, elongate, or stellate cells with frequent mitoses separated by hypocellular myxoid areas. Occasional cross-striations. Alveolar subtype: rhabdomyoblastic cell processes comprise walls of alveolae, cells lie free in alveolae lumen, rare cross-striations.

Tissue Stains

Stain	Use
Alcian blue	mucopolysaccharide—blue
Alizarin red	calcium—red
Bodian, Cajal, Golgi	axons—black
Brown-Brenn	bacteria in tissue:
	gram-positive—blue
	gram-negative—red
	Moraxella, Acinetobacter,
	Neisseria—variable
Brown and Hopps	same as Brown-Brenn
colloidal iron	acid mucopolysaccharides—blue
Congo red	amyloid—orange/red
cresyl violet	nerve cells, glia—blue
crystal violet	birefringence in polarized light
eosin	cytoplasmic organelles—pinkish
Fite-faraco acid fast	*M tuberculosis & leprae,* atypical mycobacteria—red with blue background
Fontana Masson	melanin—black
Giemsa	chlamydia intracytoplasmic inclusion bodies
Gomori's methenamine silver	fungi, yeast—black with green background
	reticulum fibers—black
Gram	gram-positive bacteria—deep red
	gram-negative bacteria—pale pink
Grocott's modification of Gomori's	fungi—black
hematoxylin	nucleic acids—blue
Kinyoun's acid fast	acid fast bacilli—red
luxol fast blue	myelin—blue
	fungi—dark blue
Masson's trichrome	collagen fibers—blue
	ciliary muscle—red
Mayer's mucicarmine	mucin, *Cryptococcus* capsule— deep red
rhodanine	copper—bright red
melanin bleach	bleaches melanin
oil red O	lipid—red
periodic acid Schiff	glycogen, mucin (not specific), basement membranes, fungi—purplish-red
Perls' Prussian blue	iron—blue
phosphotungstic acid hematoxylin	muscle fibers, fibrin, glial fibers—blue
rhodamine B	keratinoid—red

Sudan black B	lipid (meibomian gland)—black
Van de Grief	collagen fibers—green
Verhoeff's van Gieson	collagen fibers—red elastic fibers—blue nuclei—black
Von Kossa	calcium salts—black
Warthin-Starry	spirochetes—black with yellowish background
Weigert	myelin—black
wet mount	surface parasites *(Demodes, P. pubis)*
Wilder's reticulin	reticulin—black collagen—reddish
Wright's	inflammatory cells

Essentials of Eye Care, edited by Rohit Varma.
Lippincott–Raven Publishers,
Philadelphia © 1997.

15

Anterior and Posterior Segment Surgical Procedures

I. EXTRACAPSULAR CATARACT EXTRACTION

A. Introduction

   1. Nonsurgical management

      a. patient education

      b. reassurance about cause of visual disability and prognosis

      c. changing spectacle lens correction for lenticular myopia and nuclear cataract

      d. instruction regarding appropriate lighting

      e. trial of mydriatic therapy to allow patient to view around a central lenticular opacity (e.g., axial PSC plaque)

   2. Surgical management

      a. no single test adequately describes the effect of cataract on an individual patient's visual or functional ability

      b. surgical decision should not be made on results of Snellen visual acuity measurement alone

      c. weigh likelihood of visual improvement and impact on quality of life against risk and cost of surgery

      d. indications for surgery: the purpose of cataract surgery is to reduce or eliminate functional impairment caused by the lenticular opacity

   3. Surgical considerations. Each step of the cataract surgical procedure builds upon the next step. If preliminary steps are not carefully followed, the later steps will be increasingly difficult and the overall success of surgery reduced.

      a. strive for consistency and reproducibility

      b. procedure should be as simple as possible to promote success

      c. each step should be followed carefully with minimal variation

        d. be a craftsman, not a journeyman

        e. prevent intraoperative complications

B. ECCE Surgical Objectives

    1. Safely remove nucleus with minimal stress applied to zonules

    2. Securely place an intraocular lens (IOL) within an intact capsular bag

    3. Secure wound with a watertight closure of an incision that results in minimal astigmatism

C. Preoperative Preparation

    1. Premedication

        a. no preoperative sedation usually required prior to operating room for routine patient preparation

    2. Pupillary dilation

        a. larger pupil makes ECCE easier to perform

        b. combination of long- and short-acting mydriatics preferred

            1) homatropine 5% or cyclopentolate 2%

            2) tropicamide 1%

            3) phenylephrine 2.5% or 10% (be wary with labile hypertension)

            4) flurbiprofen 0.03%

            5) apply one of each every ten minutes for at least three doses, beginning at least one hour preoperatively

            6) flurbiprofen may have a local anticoagulant effect

    3. Anesthesia

        a. sedation

            1) continuous monitoring with pulse oximetry

            2) oxygen via nasal canula

            3) intravenous short-acting hypnotic agents administered per anesthesiologist or anesthetist

        b. anesthetic techniques

            1) monitored local administration preferred over general anesthesia

            2) the use of sedation drugs that are reversible and with minimal side effects is appropriate

            3) local anesthesia may be induced by either the retrobulbar or peribulbar technique

            4) utilize a 50-50 mixture of:

                2% lidocaine hydrochloride

                0.75% bupivacaine hydrochloride

                hyaluronidase (Wydase) to promote more efficient diffusion through periocular tissues

            5) use 1.5-inch-long, blunt, modified Atkinson-type retrobulbar needle to minimize potential for retrobulbar hemorrhage or globe injury

6) do not use epinephrine, which may cause pain due to acidity (pH with plain lidocaine is about 3.5)

7) a 10-cc syringe is filled with the local anesthetic mixture

8) a two-site peribulbar-retrobulbar injection method may be preferred

9) administer 3 ml of anesthetic mixture inferior temporally

10) administer 2 ml of anesthetic mixture superior nasally. Apply povidone-iodine 10% solution around the skin and eyelashes of the operative eye to allow sufficient contact time for drying and microbicidal effect ("prepprep").

4. Ocular hypotony
   a. after the local anesthetic injections have been administered, apply the Honan balloon over the operative eye. First, apply paper tape to ensure that eyelid is closed. Apply a folded 4×4 gauze sponge; then place the Honan balloon at a pressure of 30 mm Hg for approximately 10 to 15 minutes. Alternative technique is digital ocular massage.

5. Surgical prophylaxis against ocular infection
   a. careful preoperative examination for significant external diseases
      1) anterior (staphylococcal) blepharitis
      2) lacrimal sac infection
      3) purulent conjunctival discharge
   b. treat external diseases preoperatively with appropriate local and/or systemic antibiotic therapy as indicated well in advance of the planned surgery
   c. apply topical antibiotics and antiseptics in the immediate preoperative period
      1) fluoroquinolone (ciprofloxacin 0.3% or ofloxacin 0.3%) 1 drop to operative eye every 10 minutes for six doses beginning 1 to 2 hours preoperative
      2) povidone-iodine 10% solution preprep, as well as application to periocular skin and lid margins just prior to surgery
      3) povidone-iodine 5% solution placed directly onto ocular surface of operative eye
      4) utilize occlusive adhesive surgical drape, being careful to retract cilia away from operative field

6. Exposure of operative site
  a. cut occlusive dressing carefully and keep cilia from protruding into operative field
  b. place wire or other lid speculum, carefully avoiding direct pressure to the globe
  c. adjust the tilt of the microscope in the position of the patient's head
  d. avoid placement of rectus stay sutures if exposure is adequate
  e. if inadequate superior exposure, place a 4-0 black silk superior rectus stay suture by depressing the globe with a muscle hook and grasping the superior rectus muscle with a fixation forceps. Use caution when passing the needle beneath the muscle belly to avoid direct injury to the muscle or penetration into the globe.
  f. if the superior lid speculum is in the way, remove it and use a superior rectus suture to retract the upper lid

D. Surgical Incisions
  1. Conjunctiva
    a. for ECCE technique, expose the superior surgical limbus by creating an 11-mm fornix-based conjunctival peritomy. Begin the incision at 10 o'clock and extend towards 2 o'clock. Attempt to remove Tenon's fascia in a single motion.
    b. apply wet-field electrocautery to the limbus behind the intended area of limbal or scleral incision. Avoid excessive cautery, which may result in scleral shrinkage and induction of astigmatism.
    c. dry the superior limbal zone using a Wek-Cel or equivalent sponge
    d. obtain a solid purchase on the globe using a 0.12 or 0.3 forceps to grasp the sclera behind the limbus

  2. Limbal incision
    a. clean any excess Tenon's fascia from the limbus using a crescent blade
    b. grasp the globe behind the limbus using a 0.12 or 0.3 forceps
    c. set the caliper to the distance of 10.0 mm and mark the limbal zone
    d. create a three-planed incision using a crescent blade or equivalent
      1) hold the crescent blade perpendicular to the sclera to create a 10-mm partial thickness (50 to 75%) posterior limbal incision
      2) using an angled crescent blade or equivalent, dissect tangentially from the base of

the initial incision toward the anterior limbus into the beginning of clear cornea

   3) the third plane starts by entering the anterior chamber at the anterior limbus at 12 o'clock. Plane three is further completed with extension of the wound after the anterior capsulectomy.

3. Anterior capsulectomy
   a. the anterior chamber is first reformed using a viscoelastic agent
   b. for ECCE, a large circular anterior capsulectomy measuring 6.5 to 7 mm is preferred (caution—widely dilated pupil and extending beyond the zonular insertion zone will weaken zonules)
   c. continuous curvilinear capsulorhexis provides a smooth, clean edge for easier and more confident insertion of IOL within capsular bag
   d. if visualization is inadequate, a traditional "can-opener" capsulotomy can be carefully performed with caution to avoid radial tears

4. Completion of limbal incision, plane three
   a. use the angled crescent or other disposable microsurgical blade to extend the wound to an overall 10-mm cord length at the anterior limbus
   b. place two interrupted 9-0 black nylon sutures equally spaced with the distance of the chosen IOL optic diameter between the two sutures centrally. Placement of sutures in this fashion allows passage of an irrigation/aspiration device through any of the three segments while preventing iris prolapse in most cases.

5. Problem avoidance
   a. detachment of Descemet's membrane
      1) use a sharp instrument for initial penetration into the anterior chamber
      2) exercise caution with passage of instruments into and out of the anterior chamber. Gently elevate the anterior lip of the wound with forceps when passing an instrument in and out of the eye while simultaneously depressing the posterior lip of the wound with the intraocular instrument.
   b. shallow anterior chamber
      1) search for causes of possible elevated intraocular pressure (e.g., rectus sutures, lid speculum, etc.)
   c. iris prolapse
      1) maximal pupil dilatation

        2) careful entry into the anterior chamber at the anterior limbus

        3) use 9-0 nylon safety sutures. Add additional 9-0 nylon sutures as needed if iris is prolapsing from wound.

        4) use viscoelastic to reposit iris as necessary

E. Removal of the Nucleus

  1. Hydrodissection

    a. use an anterior chamber canula attached to a syringe with balanced salt solution (BSS). Pass the tip of the canula beneath the smooth edge of the anterior capsulotomy and direct a fluid wave posteriorly in the 3 o'clock meridian. Similarly, place the tip of the canula at the 9 o'clock meridian and direct a fluid wave of BSS posteriorly for hydrodissection. Hydrodissection should be completed with injection of BSS under the anterior capsule flap until the fluid dissects around the equator, flows underneath the nucleus and separates the nucleus from its cortical attachment.

  2. Expression of the nucleus

    a. the temporary 9-0 nylon safety sutures are looped out of the wound

    b. the wound has been extended to the left and to the right for the internal distance of approximately 10 mm with the angled crescent blade

    c. gentle expression can be achieved by steady downward superior pressure over the pars plana using a lens loop. Simultaneous gentle inferior pressure on the globe with a muscle hook is applied at the inferior limbus.

    d. the assistant may gently elevate the wound by grasping at 12 o'clock and pulling upward to facilitate expression

    e. alternatively, an irrigating lens loop may be passed gently beneath the nucleus, allowing time for fluid to dissect between the nucleus and the posterior capsule. Once irrigating fluid has built up beneath it, the nucleus begins to float upwards towards the wound. The irrigating loop is then withdrawn while applying slight posterior pressure on the sclera next to the wound using the forceps held in the free hand.

  3. Facilitating extraction of lens nucleus

    a. ensure adequate pupil dilation; add epinephrine or additional viscoelastic for mechanical dilation

    b. make certain nucleus is loosened with hydrodis-section maneuver

    c. bring the superior equator of the nucleus anterior to the plane of the iris by harpooning the nucleus

    d. use the irrigating lens loop

    e. extend the incision to 11 mm or greater if the nucleus is particularly large

F. Removal of Residual Cortical Material

  1. Cortex removal

    a. following nuclear expression, irrigate loose cortex from the anterior chamber with BSS

    b. secure the two preplaced 9-0 nylon sutures

    c. remove cortex using an automated irrigation/aspiration device. Place I/A device deep beneath the anterior capsulotomy to gently and sequentially withdraw cortical material (caution—do not exert pressure on capsule during cortical cleanup).

    d. following removal of cortical material, the posterior capsule may be gently and carefully polished clean using the minimum aspiration setting or the capsular-vacuum function on the automated I/A device

    e. for difficult opacities, use a Kratz scratcher to polish the posterior capsule

  2. Potential problems

    a. rupture of posterior capsule

      1) if the vitreous humor does not present, use viscoelastic to fill the anterior chamber and support the area of break; residual cortical material may be removed through gentle aspiration with a nonirrigating instrument

      2) if vitreous presents, place a separate BSS infusion line on a 23-gauge butterfly canula and lower the infusion bottle height. Insert the anterior vitrectomy device and perform a careful anterior vitrectomy to remove the prolapsed vitreous.

      3) with the infusion bottle height lowered, the irrigation/aspiration device may be reinserted to carefully remove as much cortical material as safely possible (caution—avoid aspiration of vitreous strands)

      4) if the vitreous is adequately removed and there appears to be sufficient capsular support, a posterior chamber intraocular lens (PC IOL) may be implanted. If there is inadequate capsular support, consider a flexible anterior chamber (AC) IOL or alternatively a scleral fixated posterior chamber (PC) IOL.

G. Implantation of IOL

1. Reformation of anterior chamber and capsular bag

  a. instill viscoelastic into the anterior chamber until the normal phakic depth is achieved. The canula should be directed into the capsular bag to adequately inflate the capsular bag.

2. PC IOL insertion

  a. in general, a single-piece, all-polymethylmethacrylate (PMMA) lens of 6.5 to 7 mm diameter is preferred

  b. avoid opening the PC IOL from the sterile container and exposing to operating room air or the operative field until immediately prior to insertion

  c. grasp the PC IOL with a straight or angled McPherson or intraocular lens forceps

  d. a small amount of viscoelastic material may be placed on the anterior surface of the PC IOL for additional endothelial protection

  e. the PC IOL is advanced through the wound into the anterior chamber, directed through the pupil and into the capsular bag at the 6 to 7 o'clock position. Release the superior haptic outside of the wound. Using the free hand, a Sinsky hook may be inserted through the wound and placed on the superior central surface of the optic.

  f. while depressing the center of the optic posteriorly, the superior haptic is simultaneously grasped with the straight or angled McPherson forceps in the central part of the haptic. The haptic is then pushed straight downward towards the 5 o'clock position and gently released, such that the optic and haptic pass deep beneath the iris and the anterior capsule and into the capsular bag.

  g. the PC IOL may then be centered within the capsular bag using the Sinsky hook. The IOL may be fully rotated into a horizontal position within the capsular bag.

3. Preventing decentered IOL

  a. place both haptics within the capsular bag or, alternatively, both haptics within the ciliary sulcus

  b. abort placement of IOL in the capsular bag if a capsular rent is observed

  c. orient the haptics away from a known break in the capsule or zonule

       d. rotate the IOL to bring both haptics outside or inside the bag as indicated

H. Wound Closure

    1. Limbal closure

       a. place a cover over the central cornea to avoid possible operating microscope light-induced retinal damage

       b. close with interrupted 10-0 nylon sutures placed in a radial orientation

       c. prior to closing the final segment of the wound, reintroduce the I/A device and aspirate the residual viscoelastic agent

       d. a miotic agent such as acetylcholine or carbachol may be instilled to achieve pupillary miosis

       e. continue suturing until wound is completely closed in a watertight fashion

       f. the sutures are cut and the knots buried on the scleral side of the wound

    2. Conjunctival closure

       a. the conjunctiva may be closed using a temporary looped 10-0 nylon suture or a buried, interrupted 8- or 9-0 vicryl suture

       b. alternatively, the conjunctiva may be closed using the wet field coaptation cautery forceps

I. Postoperative Prophylaxis Against Infection

    1. Subconjunctival injection

       a. cefazolin 100 mg (or vancomycin in penicillin-allergic patient) administered inferiorly away from wound

       b. avoid aminoglycoside injection

       c. subconjunctival dexamethasone may be administered

       d. topical fluoroquinolone antibiotics (ciprofloxacin or ofloxacin 0.3%) may be instilled prior to placing an eye patch

       e. the operative eye may be dressed with antibiotic and corticosteroid ophthalmic ointment

       f. a sterile eye patch should be securely placed over the operative eye

       g. a protective metallic shield should be placed over the operative eye before moving or transporting the patient

II. EXTRACAPSULAR CATARACT EXTRACTION VIA PHACOEMULSIFICATION

    A. Introduction

      1. Cataract surgery is safe and effective in restoring vision

          a. complication rates of cataract surgery are low

              1) when complications do occur, however, they are often serious and vision-threatening

          b. method of cataract extraction via standard ECCE or phacoemulsification does not result in statistically significant differences in final visual outcome

          c. phacoemulsification and ECCE surgery appear to be equally effective in restoring vision

      2. Motivation for phacoemulsification method

          a. enhanced safety

          b. more rapid visual rehabilitation following the procedure

              1) smaller incision promotes more rapid healing, reduced postoperative astigmatism, less likelihood of wound dehiscence

      3. It is not possible to determine from current published literature whether phacoemulsification enhances the outcome compared with standard extracapsular procedure when measured by reduction or elimination of functional impairment due to cataract

   B. Preoperative Preparation

      1. Premedication

          a. preoperative oral sedation not routinely used

          b. intravenous sedation administered in operating room just prior to procedure

      2. Pupillary dilation

          a. large pupil desirable to facilitate phacoemulsification technique

          b. short-acting mydriatic agents combined with longer-acting agents

          c. tropicamide 1% 1 drop q10min 2–3 doses beginning 1 hour prior to surgery

          d. cyclopentolate 2% or homatropine 5% 1 drop to operative eye q10min 2–3 doses beginning 1 hour preop

          e. phenylephrine 2.5% 1 drop operative eye q10min 2–3 doses beginning 1 hour preop

          f. flurbiprofen 1 drop operative eye q10min ×6 doses beginning 1 hour preop (caution—local anticoagulant effect)

      3. Anesthesia and akinesia

          a. possible options:

              1) retrobulbar injection

              2) peribulbar injection

   3) combined retrobulbar and peribulbar injection
   4) sub-Tenon's infusion
   5) topical administration
   b. for beginning phacoemulsification, preferred method is probably a two-site peribulbar-retrobulbar injection
      1) use a 1.5-inch blunt-tip modified Atkinson-type retrobulbar needle on a 10-cc syringe to inject 3 ml inferior temporally
      2) use same needle to inject 2 ml superior nasally
   c. anesthetic mixture is a 50-50 solution of 2% lidocaine and 0.75% bupivacaine and with hyaluronidase
   d. do not use epinephrine, which is potentially painful due to its acid pH
   e. consider omitting bupivacaine to avoid delay in return of useful vision in the immediate postoperative period
4. Ocular hypotony
   a. following local anesthetic injections, apply a Honan balloon at 30 mm Hg for approximately 10 minutes
   b. alternatively, ocular digital massage may be applied
5. Antimicrobial prophylaxis
   a. conjunctival flushing with sterile saline actually increases species in colony counts
   b. scrubbing of lashes and lid margins increases species in colony counts
   c. topical antibiotics administered in a brief preoperative regimen immediately prior to the incision reduce the amount of lid and conjunctival bacteria compared with untreated controls
   d. topical antiseptic just prior to incision has added to effect
      1) povidone-iodine 10% solution to periocular skin and eyelashes
      2) povidone-iodine 5% solution directly on ocular surface immediately before incision
      3) do not flush ocular surface with saline
      4) occlusive draping of eyelids
C. Incisions
   1. Two components: external component, internal component
      a. surgical incision options
         1) basic incision

    a) the external incision consists of a linear groove in the sclera placed just posterior to the limbus

    b) the basic incision is completed with a stab entry into the anterior chamber

  2. Scleral pocket technique

   a. a perpendicular linear external incision is created more posteriorly from the limbus

    1) the discission is then dissected anteriorly from the groove towards the anterior chamber

  3. Corneal valve incision for sutureless surgery

   a. a scleral tunnel dissection is carried up further anteriorly into the corneal stroma prior to entry into the anterior chamber

   b. the valve incision is occluded by normal intraocular pressure against the flexible corneal tissue

  4. Clear corneal valve incision (temporal or nasal)

   a. perpendicular partial thickness incision using a diamond blade at the limbus just anterior to the conjunctival vascular arcade

   b. perform tangential dissection with diamond keratome or a crescent blade into clear cornea

   c. redirect keratome perpendicular to the plane of the cornea to enter the anterior chamber with a self-sealing valve incision

  5. Side port stab incision for two-handed technique

   a. placed 90 degrees away in peripheral clear cornea

   b. sharp pointed blade used to make incision

  6. Anterior capsulotomy

   a. reform the anterior chamber using viscoelastic

   b. insert an angled 27- or 30-gauge needle to create a small nick in the anterior capsule and to raise a capsular flap

   c. advance capsular flap by elevating the needle to create a smooth rounded edge

   d. guide the smooth rounded edge with a 27-gauge needle in a continuous curvilinear fashion (either clockwise or counterclockwise directions)

   e. change vectors to facilitate curvilinear progression

   f. if difficulty advancing with needle, grasp with a utrata-like forceps for better control

   g. regrasp frequently to complete circular tear

   h. optimal diameter approximately 5.5 to 6.0 mm to avoid anterior capsular fibrosis and to facilitate nuclear removal

         i. if radial extension of tear, stop, create new nick, and reverse direction to include zone of radial extension

  D. Removal of the Nucleus

    1. Hydrodissection

      a. principal goal of hydrodissection is to enable safe rotation of the nucleus by breaking cortical adhesions.

        1) use a 25- to 27-gauge angled canula on a 3-cc syringe filled with BSS

        2) pass tip of canula beneath the edge of the circular capsulotomy

        3) direct a fluid wave of BSS posteriorly for hydrodissection

        4) the fluid should dissect around the equator, flow underneath the nucleus, and separate the nucleus from its cortical attachments

        5) the second hydrodelineation step begins with the canula being pushed into the body of the nucleus

        6) upon injecting fluid, the "Golden Ring" will signal the true separation of nuclear layers

    2. Nucleus removal

      a. transition to phaco

      b. staged progression

      c. begin by trying central sculpting of nucleus during conventional ECCE (add additional viscoelastic to avoid cumulative endothelial damage)

      d. practice maneuvering instruments through a small incision

    3. Phacoemulsification technique

      a. judge the relative density of the nuclear cataract to initial optimal techniques

      b. central sculpting

      c. select initial machine settings with moderately high phaco power, low aspiration flow rate, and low vacuum

      d. for soft to moderately dense nuclear cataract, perform deep central sculpting of the nuclear core

      e. relaxing nucleotomy can be performed along the inferior nucleus engaging with the probe facing downward and using pulsed phaco power to create a hole in the edge of the residual bowl created from sculpting

      f. the peripheral hole in the bowl can then be extended

      g. through a side port incision, a cyclodialysis spatula or equivalent instrument can be used to rotate the nucleus 180 degrees to bring the relaxing nucleotomy to the superior position

h. in similar fashion, a relaxing nucleotomy can be created at the 12 o'clock position with symmetric enlargement

i. the posterior plate of nuclear material is then shaved thinner until the red reflex is observed (caution—avoid posterior capsule engagement)

j. the remaining lens material on each side can be eliminated using a peripheral aspiration and removal maneuver. The nuclear material is engaged with the phacoemulsification port using aspiration and lifted into the safety zone where it is emulsified and eliminated.

k. in similar fashion, the other nuclear half is engaged with the phaco port and lifted into the safety zone, where it is emulsified and eliminated

l. the outer nuclear shell is then engaged at 6 o'clock and gently separated from the capsular bag

m. a second-hand instrument can then assist with flipping the soft shell over ("chip and flip" technique)

n. for moderate to hard nuclear cataract, a nuclear cracking technique is recommended

o. first, create a long deep central trench using phacoemulsification on high power settings with low or zero vacuum

p. a spatula can then be introduced to separate one half of the nucleus from the other by applying force in the direction opposite to that applied with the phacoemulsification probe (cross-instrument technique)

q. the crack should split the nucleus down through the center of the lens. Each half of the nuclear plate can then be engaged with higher vacuum power and emulsified sequentially.

r. alternatively, a four-quadrant cracking technique can be used by similar sculpting, trench digging, clockwise rotation for 90 degrees, trench digging, repeat clockwise rotation for 90 degrees, trench digging, and rotation until a cross trench is completed

s. the posterior plate can then be cracked in similar fashion with the two-cross instrument technique to split the nucleus down through the center of the lens

t. each nuclear quadrant can then be emulsified within the capsular bag using the second-hand spatula instrument to stabilize the nuclear quadrant

    u. after each quarter is emulsified, most of the outer nucleus is removed

E. Removal of Residual Cortical Material

    1. Cortical aspiration

        a. with phacoemulsification, there is usually much less cortex to remove

            1) continuous curvilinear capsulorrhexis eliminates capsular flaps which can interfere with cortical aspiration

            2) with phacoemulsification, however, the subincisional cortex may be difficult to remove if the anterior capsulotomy is small enough in diameter

            3) if the subincisional cortex does not come out easily, then it should be left to avoid zonular weakening or capsular discission

            4) following removal of cortical material, the posterior capsule may be gently and carefully polished clean using minimum aspiration or capsular vacuum function on the automated irrigation/aspiration device

            5) for difficult subincisional cortex, a two-port system may be used to facilitate removal by accessing 90 degrees away for a more optimal approach to the retained cortex

            6) for difficult axial opacities, a Kratz scratcher may be used to polish the posterior capsule

    2. Potential problems

        a. inadvertent posterior capsular discission

            1) with phacoemulsification, there rarely may be a violation of the posterior capsule with the phaco port

            2) surgeons should immediately stop phacoemulsification and lower the infusion bottle height

            3) care should be taken to remove as much nucleus as safely possible

            4) if vitreous prolapse is present and being engaged by the phaco port, anterior vitrectomy must be carefully performed to free vitreous from around the residual nucleus

            5) the phacoemulsification unit can then be reintroduced to gently remove remaining nuclear material

            6) with the infusion bottle height at a low setting, the irrigation/aspiration device may be reinserted to carefully remove as much cor-

tical material as safely possible (caution—
avoid aspiration of vitreous strands)

3. Repeat vitrectomy if any residual vitreous strands
remain

4. If the vitreous is adequately removed and there remains sufficient capsular support away from the
rent in the posterior capsule, a PC IOL may be implanted. Care should be taken to avoid placing the
haptic through the capsular rent.

5. If there is inadequate capsular support, or a large
rent in the posterior capsule, a flexible AC IOL, or
alternatively, a scleral-fixated PC IOL should be
considered

F. Implantation of IOL

1. Small incision

a. with phacoemulsification technique, the small
incision offers the opportunity to insert a small
diameter, single-piece rigid material PC IOL, or
alternatively, a flexible foldable PC IOL

2. The anterior chamber and capsular bag are reformed

a. instill viscoelastic to the anterior chamber until
the normal phakic depth is achieved by directing the viscoelastic into the capsular bag

b. with single-piece rigid PC IOLs, the internal
wound will require extension using the angled
crescent or diamond keratome

c. with silicone plate haptic PC IOLs, the lens
should be loaded into the injection cartridge
system

d. the cartridge injector device should then be
carefully inserted into the corneal valve or scleral tunnel with the bevel directed downward

e. the plate haptic PC IOL can then be carefully injected slowly into the capsular bag

f. if the trailing portion of the silicone plate PC
IOL fails to enter the capsular bag, use Sinsky
hook to push straight forward and downward to
allow plate haptic IOL to enter the capsular bag

g. with acrylic or other foldable IOLs, the lens
should be carefully folded using the recommended lens holder

h. the trailing haptic should be folded to fit
through the small incision

i. the lens should be slowly and carefully released
into the capsular bag

j. the Sinsky hook may then be used to center the
PC IOL within the capsular bag

G. Wound Closure

1. Clear corneal valve incisions
   a. closure may be achieved using a 10-0 vicryl absorbable suture to place an interrupted radial closure
   b. a slipknot can be used to tie the 10-0 vicryl suture and adjust tension. The suture should be cut close to the knot.
   c. the surgical knot may then be rotated into the wound
   d. although many corneal valve incisions are self-sealing, an absorbable suture provides additional safety and stability
   e. stromal hydration only partially and temporarily apposes the wound edges
   f. for scleral tunnel incisions, radial sutures may increase corneal astigmatism if closed too tight
   g. horizontal sutures do not attempt to approximate the edges of an incision
   h. horizontal sutures are used simply to flatten the scleral tunnel and to make the incision watertight
   i. the sutures are cut and the knots buried in the wound
   j. for conjunctival closure, the conjunctiva may be closed using a temporary loop 10-0 nylon suture or a buried interrupted 8- or 9-0 vicryl suture
   k. alternatively, the conjunctiva may be closed using the wet field coaptation cautery forceps
H. Postoperative Prophylaxis Against Infection
   1. Subconjunctival injection
      a. cefazolin 100 mg (or vancomycin in the penicillin-allergic patient) may be administered inferiorly with a 30-gauge needle away from the wound
      b. avoid aminoglycoside injection
      c. subconjunctival dexamethasone may be administered
      d. topical fluoroquinolone antibiotics (ciprofloxacin or ofloxacin 0.3%) may be instilled prior to placing a sterile eye patch
      e. the operative eye may then be dressed with antibiotic and corticosteroid ophthalmic ointment
      f. a sterile eye patch should be securely placed over the operative eye
      g. a metallic eye shield should be placed over the sterile eye patch for safety
      h. with clear corneal phacoemulsification using topical anesthesia, no eye patch or shield may be necessary

III. PENETRATING KERATOPLASTY

A. Introduction
   1. With penetrating keratoplasty, the most important considerations involve preoperative decisions with respect to patient selection and postoperative care, including management of complications
B. Preoperative Evaluation
   1. Complete ophthalmic history and clinical examination
      a. patient history
         1) potential vision—the following factors must be considered:
            a) prior history of "normal" eyes
            b) any history of amblyopia, strabismus, "lazy eye," childhood patching, etc.
            c) results from previous eye examinations prior to current problem
            d) the best vision obtained postoperatively if the patient has had prior surgery or ocular trauma
            e) family history of eye disease, such as glaucoma, retinal detachments, or retinal degenerations
            f) the nature of the vision loss—gradual or sudden
            g) the medical history of systemic diseases, such as diabetes or inflammatory disease, that might decrease retinal potential
      b. recipient environment
         1) both local and systemic factors are important to long-term graft survival and with the preoperative history one should assess:
            a) history of increased intraocular pressure control
            b) history of ocular inflammation and how long inflammation quiescent
            c) history of associated dermatologic disease and current state of control
            d) systemic factors that preclude surgery
            e) social factors that might mitigate against successful keratoplasty, including compliance with followup
            f) history of corneal anesthesia or ocular surface disease should be specifically considered
            g) history of neurosurgery
            h) history of herpes zoster ophthalmicus

        i) history of ocular cicatricial pemphigoid
        j) prior history of radiation exposure
        k) prior history of chemical injury
        l) history of Stevens-Johnson syndrome
        m) history of severe atopic keratoconjunctivitis
        n) ocular rosacea
        o) graft-versus-host disease (GVHD)
        p) keratoconjunctivitis sicca

2. Potential vision-clinical examination
    a. standard tests
    b. afferent pupillary defect
    c. two light discrimination
    d. Maddox rod and red/green discrimination
    e. Purkinje vascular image
    f. blue field entoptic test
    g. potential acuity meter (PAM)
    h. laser interferometry
    i. electroretinogram (ERG)
    j. pattern evoked visual potential
    k. visual evoked potential (VEP)
    l. ultrasonography
    m. B-scan ultrasonography is essential to establish the presence or absence of coexistent posterior segment disease when the cornea is cloudy

C. Preoperative Preparation
  1. Systemic factors—as for any surgical procedure, success is maximized by establishment of optimal health
    a. diabetes, hypertension, endocrine disorders, and other systemic conditions should be controlled
    b. if there is a recent history of unstable cardiopulmonary disease within 6 months, keratoplasty should be deferred until the patient can be medically cleared
    c. a general medical evaluation to assess anesthesia risk is useful, especially if general anesthesia is considered
  2. Social factors
    a. patients with anticipated self-care problems or lack of compliance with followup should have family members present for counseling and arrangements with a visiting nurse associate
  3. Donor material
    a. optimal donor material should:
      1) carry minimal risk of transmission of disease from donor to recipient
      2) have ample donor endothelial reserve

            3) have minimal chance of inducing graft rejection

4. Criteria for donor material

    a. tissue from donors with the following conditions is considered potentially hazardous and requires special handling:

        1) active viral hepatitis

        2) AIDS or HIV seropositivity

        3) active viral encephalitis or encephalitis of unknown origin

        4) Creutzfeldt-Jakob disease

        5) rabies

5. Donor contraindications for keratoplasty—tissue from donors with the following conditions is considered potentially health-threatening for the recipients and is not offered for surgical purposes.

    a. death of unknown cause

    b. death from CNS diseases of unknown etiology

    c. Creutzfeldt-Jakob disease

    d. subacute sclerosing panencephalitis

    e. progressive multifocal leukoencephalopathy

    f. congenital rubella

    g. Reye's syndrome

    h. active viral encephalitis or encephalitis of unknown origin

    i. active septicemia (bacteremia, fungemia, viremia)

    j. active bacterial or fungal endocarditis

    k. active viral hepatitis, hepatitis-B surface antigen-positive donors, hepatitis-C seropositive donors

    l. rabies

    m. intrinsic ocular disease

    n. retinoblastoma

    o. malignant tumors of the anterior ocular segment

    p. active ocular or intraocular inflammation, conjunctivitis, scleritis, iritis, uveitis, vitritis, choroiditis, retinitis

    q. congenital or acquired disorders of the eye that would preclude a successful outcome (e.g., keratoconus, keratoglobus, central donor corneal scar)

    r. pterygia or other ocular surface disorders involving the central optical area of the corneal button

    s. prior intraocular or anterior segment surgery

    t. refractive corneal procedures (e.g., radial keratotomy, lamellar keratoplasty)

    u. anterior segment surgery, including cataract and IOL implantation, trabeculectomy

        v. active leukemias

        w. active lymphomas

        x. recipients of human pituitary-derived growth hormone between 1963 and 1985

        y. HIV-seropositive donors, AIDS, children and infants of mothers with AIDS

        z. active syphilis

6. Optimization of endothelial reserve

    a. donor age. Full-term birth or older. Most surgeons use an upper age limit of around 65 years and attempt to use young corneas for young patients. Caution with fetal tissue due to elasticity and potential for induced high myopia.

    b. examination of donor material. Eye Bank provides grade of tissue.

    c. surgeons should check material with slit lamp biomicroscopic examination prior to use

    d. special holders of donor material allow ease of examination at slit lamp

    e. time interval between death and surgery

    f. intervals between death, whole body refrigeration, enucleation, and preservation should be as brief as possible

    g. eyes properly preserved with modern tissue culture media can be used with satisfactory results for up to 5 to 7 days after death

7. Intraocular pressure (IOP)

    a. IOP must be adequately controlled prior to consideration for keratoplasty

    b. if topical and systemic medications are unsuccessful, consideration of prekeratoplasty trabeculectomy, transscleral YAG cyclophotocoagulation, or filtering tube implantation is advisable

8. Inflammation

    a. all efforts should be made to defer elective keratoplasty until ocular inflammation is controlled for an extended period of time

    b. if keratoplasty must be performed in the presence of active inflammation, intensive topical and systemic corticosteroids should be administered in the perioperative period

    c. for grafting in herpes simplex keratitis, consideration of prophylaxis with systemic acyclovir to prevent recurrence or rejection is strongly suggested

D. Patient Preparation and Anesthesia

  1. Pupil

    a. miosis—pupillary miosis is desirable in phakic patients. Topical pilocarpine 1 or 2% should be applied two to three times immediately prior to surgery

    b. mydriasis—if keratoplasty is to be combined with cataract extraction, the pupil should be dilated using the same eyedrop protocol as for ECCE

  2. Retrobulbar anesthesia

    a. use blunt modified Atkinson-type retrobulbar needle to administer 2% xylocaine and 0.75% marcaine mixture with hyaluronidase (Wydase) in a 50-50 mixture

    b. facial nerve block may be administered (O'Brien approach preferred to Van Lint or Nadbath approaches)

  3. General anesthesia should be used if there is a frank corneal perforation or limited patient cooperation

    a. intraocular pressure should be lowered following retrobulbar anesthesia with a pressure-reducing device, such as the Honan balloon (30 mm Hg for 10 to 15 minutes) or by digital massage

    b. acetazolamide or IV mannitol may be used in select cases unless there are systemic contraindications

  4. Antimicrobial prophylaxis

    a. make certain any external ocular infectious diseases are adequately treated prior to surgery

    b. preoperative antibiotic may be administered in the period just prior to incision

    c. a fluoroquinolone (ofloxacin 0.3% or ciprofloxacin 0.3%) is administered topically with 1 drop every 10 minutes for six doses in the hour preceding surgery

    d. povidone-iodine 10% solution is placed on the periocular skin and allowed to dry

    e. povidone-iodine 5% solution is placed directly on the eye just prior to the surgical incision

    f. do not flush or irrigate, as this may increase bacterial colony counts

    g. occlusive draping to the eyelids prevents exposure of the operative field to cilia and the surrounding skin

E. Keratoplasty Technique

  1. Lid speculum—a speculum is placed between the eyelids to provide adequate exposure; care should be taken to avoid any pressure exerted on the globe. If there is an impending or a completed perforation, use a special speculum (Jaffe or equivalent) to avoid pressure on the globe.

2. Preparation of the donor button
   a. determination of graft size—in general, the size of the graft is usually determined at the time of surgery. Grafts used to treat endothelial dysfunction should be as large as possible (8.0 to 8.5 mm in diameter).
   b. grafts larger than 8.5 mm should be avoided since they can lead to extensive synechiae and subsequent glaucoma
   c. grafts much smaller than 6.5 mm may be inadequate due to central optical distortion or insufficient area of endothelial transplantation
   d. the donor button is cut before the recipient cornea is cut
   e. important to cut around donor corneal button to prevent significant astigmatism
   f. cut the donor on a Teflon block using a trephine guide (Weck system)
   g. be certain to check the trephine size prior to cutting
   h. typically good to check sizes by first placing a disposable sterile trephine blade on the recipient cornea to gently mark the epithelium. Once an appropriate size has been chosen for the recipient bed, then 0.25 or 0.5 mm is added to determine the size of the donor.
   i. as a general rule, the donor button is cut 0.5 mm larger than the recipient in aphakic eyes. For pseudophakic and phakic eyes, the same size or 0.25 mm larger size is used (there is evidence that using a donor button 0.5 mm larger than the recipient bed in aphakic eyes reduces the chance for glaucoma. Also, the larger donor cornea material does not require tight sutures and there is less postoperative hyperopia and astigmatism).
   j. care must be taken to be certain that the Teflon block is not hot as a result of sterilization immediately prior to use
   k. after cutting the donor cornea, the button can be left in the depression of the plastic block. Use a small amount of tissue medium or BSS to moisten the endothelium, and be careful to avoid bringing the donor button onto the field prior to the time that it is needed.
   l. when cutting the recipient cornea in aphakic eyes or eyes in which cataract surgery is planned, a single or double scleral support ring

(Flieringa or equivalent) can be placed to maintain the shape of the eye during the keratoplasty
m. suture the ring with interrupted or running 7-0 vicryl or silk sutures
n. make certain the scleral support ring is centered and pass sutures so as not to destroy the globe and induce astigmatism
o. use at least six suture bites to make sure the ring is secure. Caution—avoid needle penetration of globe.
p. keep 12 and 6 o'clock sutures long as traction sutures
q. if the patient is phakic or pseudophakic, a ring may not be necessary, and inferior and superior rectus stay sutures may stabilize the globe
r. a paracentesis wound can be created near the temporal limbus. This may be used to inject viscoelastic to firm up a soft eye just prior to trephine.
s. postkeratoplasty astigmatism is a major problem, which can result from improper technique in cutting the recipient cornea
t. it is essential that the trephine be perpendicular to the cornea and centered for the optical zone
u. if the trephine is not perpendicular and centered, a decentered graft with irregular edges and high astigmatism will result
3. Free-hand technique
a. if the cornea is cut using a hand-held trephine, the corneal epithelium is first marked with a trephine to ensure centering about the optical zone
b. in the opposite hand, a forceps may be used to grasp either the scleral support ring or the globe itself to ensure three-point fixation
c. the cutting is started with a gentle downward pressure and a twisting movement alternating clockwise and counterclockwise
d. care should be taken to ensure that the cut is made perpendicular to the cornea, at equal depths in all quadrants
e. one can set the trephine up to 80% of corneal thickness and then enter the anterior chamber with a sharp blade
f. alternatively, with experience, the anterior chamber can be safely entered with the trephine
g. when aqueous humor is observed, one should stop cutting with the trephine because the col-

lapsed anterior chamber might result in cutting the iris or lens capsule

  h. a vacuum trephine (Hessburg-Barron) may be used to aid in cutting around recipient bed

  i. the center of the cornea is marked

  j. the syringe is depressed and the trephine is centered in position on the cornea

  k. after gentle pressure is applied, the syringe is released and suction is obtained after about ten seconds

  l. the trephine is gently lifted and the surgeon spins down the blade by turning the finger post until the anterior chamber has been entered

  m. suction is then released by pressing the plunger of the suction syringe fully

  n. one can also use this method to cut 80% depth and then complete the incision with a sharp blade

  o. newer trephine designs (Tampa Trephine) may result in less postoperative astigmatism

  p. once the anterior chamber is entered using whichever trephine one chooses, curved corneal scissors are used to complete the incision

  q. care is taken to introduce the lower blade of the corneal scissors into the anterior chamber under the central cornea to be removed to prevent damage to the peripheral corneal endothelium. The upper blade is placed down into the trephine cut after the lower blade is through the incision and in position. Cutting is then performed by lifting upward with the lower blade, which prevents a double cut to the wound.

  r. one always pulls up on the lower blade to avoid cutting the iris or lens capsule

  s. first, the cornea is cut in one direction and then the other to excise the corneal button and remove it from the eye

  t. if one suspects an infectious etiology that is undetermined or persistent in the tissue, a small portion of the recipient button can be excised and sent for microbial culture

  u. the remainder of the corneal button should be sent for histopathologic examination following proper fixation procedures

4. Anterior vitrectomy

  a. if vitreous is present in the anterior chamber, an anterior vitrectomy should be performed prior to placing the donor button

  b. a mechanical vitrectomy using instrumentation is preferred to a cellulosponge vitrectomy

    c. an "open sky" approach may be used with a second infusion canula with BSS

    d. care must be taken to avoid exerting traction on the vitreous face during the procedure

5. Cataract extraction

    a. if significant lenticular opacification exists, consideration towards combined cataract extraction with IOL insertion at the time of keratoplasty is undertaken

    b. if there are any posterior synechiae present, they can be swept either with a Barraquer sweep or the viscoelastic canula

    c. a circular tear continuous curvilinear capsulorrhexis of 6 to 6.5 mm in diameter is carried out with a cystotome or a utrata forceps

    d. balanced salt solution is injected beneath the anterior capsule to assist in developing a cleavage plane

    e. the lens nucleus can then usually be easily expressed with a lens loop or alternatively by harpooning the nucleus with a 25-gauge needle. The lens can be rotated in a counterclockwise fashion out of the capsular bag.

    f. once the nucleus has been removed, cortical cleanup may be carried out using a mechanical nonautomated irrigation/aspiration device (Simcoe I/A system) for better control

    g. an automated irrigation/aspiration device can be used, though there may occasionally be significant bowing of the anterior capsule forward

    h. the PC IOL (6.5 to 7.0 mm diameter, all PMMA single-piece lens preferred) can then be easily placed within the capsular bag

    i. if there is any loss of zonular or capsular bag support, the lens can then be placed intentionally in the ciliary sulcus

    j. if there is questionable support for ciliary sulcus placement, the lens may be sutured to the iris. A PC IOL containing two positioning holes on the optic is preferred and a 10-0 polypropylene suture secured to each positioning hole. The double-armed 10-0 polypropylene suture can then be placed up and out through the iris. The sutures are then tied to secure the lens.

6. Suturing the graft

    a. once any other intraocular procedures, such as vitrectomy, IOL removal, or exchange are completed, the donor graft is then sutured in position

   b. fill the anterior chamber with sodium hyaluronidase or other viscoelastic

   c. transfer the donor cornea from the Teflon block
   using a cornea spatula (Paton) or fine forceps by
   grasping the epithelial edge of the donor button
   and flipping it over onto the recipient bed

   d. after the donor button has been placed in position, epithelial side up, cardinal sutures of 10-0
   nylon should be placed in to secure the graft
   into position

   e. four cardinal sutures of 10-0 nylon are placed at
   90-degree intervals (12, 3, 6, and 9 o'clock)

   f. the needle tip should be placed about 1.5 mm
   from the edge of the donor graft and passed deep
   to a level just above Descemet's membrane
   (about 90% thickness)

   g. the needle is then passed into the recipient
   cornea at the same level and out about 1.5 to 2
   mm from the edge

   h. use 0.12 mm forceps to grasp the corneal tissue
   during suturing; the needle should always be
   passed directly under and behind the tip of the
   forceps

   i. after the four cardinal sutures have been placed,
   additional interrupted sutures or a continuous
   running suture are placed to secure the graft

   j. interrupted sutures are preferred if the recipient
   bed is highly vascularized or there is significant
   inflammation. This allows selective removal
   without disturbance of other sutures.

   k. a second set of four interrupted sutures may be
   placed by simply bisecting the initial four sutures and placing them in a radial fashion. Once
   eight sutures have been placed, an additional
   eight sutures are placed, each halfway between
   the first eight for a total of 16 sutures.

   l. the first four cardinal sutures may need to be replaced

   m. as the sutures are being placed, it is critically
   important to maintain a formed anterior chamber (use BSS, viscoelastic, or air)

   n. if viscoelastic is used to maintain the anterior
   chamber, an attempt to exchange the viscoelastic with BSS should be performed prior to placing all of the interrupted sutures

   o. after all the sutures have been placed, the excess
   sutures should be cut very close to the knots and
   the knots buried into the recipient cornea

    p. a surgical keratometer can be useful to assess intraoperative astigmatism

    q. a continuous running suture may be placed if the recipient corneal bed is not vascularized or thin

    r. a 10-0 monofilament nylon suture is used

    s. the continuous running suture is started after four or eight cardinal interrupted sutures have been placed

    t. the needle is always passed through the graft first and then through the recipient bed

    u. usually 16 to 20 passes of the needle are required

    v. the microscope may be moved to allow ease of placement

    w. avoid grasping the needle near the tip or touching the tip of the needle so as not to dull the needle

    x. after the running suture has been placed for the full 360 degrees, the suture should be secured with a triple-through surgeon's knot

        1) then using tying forceps, the slack must be pulled up to adequately tighten the running suture

        2) once the running suture has been adequately tightened, the triple-through is taken out and the sutures retied with a single-through locking knot

        3) after the single-through, a square knot is placed and the sutures cut flush with the knot

        4) the knot is then carefully buried into the stroma, being very careful not to break the suture

        5) if the running suture is broken at any time during placement, it can be spliced to allow continued passage of the suture

        6) after completing the running or interrupted suturing of the graft, the anterior chamber is deepened

        7) the wound should then be carefully tested for any leakage

        8) two percent sterile fluorescein can be placed on the eye to check for significant wound leaks

        9) if a significant wound leak is found, a single interrupted or multiple interrupted sutures are placed to close the leakage

    10) subconjunctival antibiotics (cefazolin and gentamicin) can be administered. Subconjunctival corticosteroids (dexamethasone 4 mg/ml) may also be administered.

    11) the operative eye is then dressed with topical antibiotic ointment and corticosteroid ointment

    12) a sterile eye patch and metallic shield are placed over the operative eye

F. Postoperative Care

    1. The most important consideration in keratoplasty

      a. must be tailored individually to the particular circumstances for grafting

      b. in the immediate postoperative period, the wound should be tested carefully for any microscopic leakage

      c. frequent topical corticosteroids (prednisolone 1%) should be applied in the early period and tapered according to the clinical circumstances

      d. adjunctive topical antimicrobial therapy should be applied frequently and tapered early

      e. topical lubricating ointment with or without antibiotic may be continued longer

      f. generally, patients are seen every day for several days after surgery, then once a week for 3 to 4 weeks, then once a month for 3 months, then every 2 to 3 months until a year after surgery. This schedule is obviously tailored pending clinical improvement.

    2. Suture removal

      a. suture removal is again tailored for the individual circumstances of grafting

      b. for interrupted sutures, suture removal can be started early selectively, depending on tightness or looseness

      c. usually every other interrupted suture is removed at 4 to 6 months and the remaining at 9 to 12 months

      d. a single continuous running suture should be left in place for at least 9 to 12 months and longer

      e. if a patient has little astigmatism and the sutures are causing no problems, it can be left in place for a longer period

      f. suture adjustment at the slit lamp has been proposed, but risks the possibility of breaking the suture and the need for returning the patient to the operating room

      g. corneal topography can be used as a guide to assist in selective suture removal

IV. ARGON LASER TRABECULOPLASTY (ALT)

A. Indicated When IOP Is Not Controlled by Medications at Level Necessary to Prevent Further Damage to Optic Nerve

B. Technique:

pretreat with apraclonidine 1%, argon green laser, 50-micron spot size, laser beam of 0.1 second duration aimed at anterior half of trabecular meshwork through gonioprism; place spots at least one spot in diameter apart, laser power initiated at 600 to 800 mW and then modified to achieve mild blanching/small bubble formation; approximately 80 to 100 spots should be applied to 360° of the angle; treatment may be done in two separate sessions with application of 40 to 50 spots to 180° of the angle at each session; IOP should be checked one hour after laser, the following day and at 4 to 12 weeks postoperatively; postoperatively topical steroids can be used for the first 3 to 4 days, the IOP-lowering medications should be continued postoperatively unless the IOP lowering effect is obtained; if IOP is lowered by trabeculoplasty, medications can be discontinued sequentially.

C. Complications:

prior to use of apraclonidine transient elevated IOP in up to 50% of eyes; the incidence of this compliction can be decreased by preoperative treatment with apraclonidine; iritis, peripheral anterior synechiae, pain

D. Contraindications:

uncooperative patient, hazy view of angle, closed iridocorneal angle, glaucomas associated with intraocular inflammation or trauma, patients less than 35 years of age

E. Prognostic Factors:

ALT is more effective in lowering IOP in eyes with higher preoperative IOPs, in phakic eyes, in patients aged 40 and older, in patients with pseudoexfoliation and pigmentary glaucoma; the mechanism of action of ALT is hypothesized to be either due to increased separation of the trabecular beams by shrinkage of the laser-treated trabeculum or due to increased or altered production of glycosaminoglycans by the laser activated trabecular cells.

F. The Glaucoma Laser Trial:

patients were randomized to initial treatment of glaucoma with laser or topical medications has shown that initial treatment with argon laser trabeculoplasty is at least as efficacious as initial treatment with topical medications in terms of lowering intraocular pressure, and visual field and optic disc changes over a 7-year period.

G. 80% Patients Experience Drop in IOP for 6 to 12 months, 50% patients maintain significantly lower IOP for 3 to 5 years after treatment:

H. Retreatment May be Effective if the entire angle has not been fully treated previously; if the entire angle has been treated previously, the chance of success is small

V. TRABECULECTOMY

A. Indications:
   when medical and laser treatment fail to control intraocular pressure in open-angle glaucoma. Currently, the National Eye Institute has a trial (the Collaborative Initial Glaucoma Treatment Study) under way to determine if initial treatment with trabeculectomy is more beneficial than conventional medical therapy.

B. Trabeculectomy:
   a partial thickness-filtering procedure performed by removing blocks of limbal tissue beneath a scleral flap; which reduces incidence of hypotony as compared to full thickness drainage procedures; less successful in patients with secondary glaucoma or previously failed filter; higher failure rate in African-Americans; 80 to 95% successful in lowering IOP at 1 year.

C. Technique:
   bridle suture of 4-0 silk placed around superior rectus muscle or a peripheral corneal suture with 6-0 polyglactin; limbal or fornix-based conjunctival flap created with Wescott scissors—for limbal-based flap, buttonhole through conjunctiva made with sharp dissection between Tenon's capsule and episclera, and extended superiorly 12 to 15 mm posterior to and parallel to limbus; the conjunctival flap is dissected anteriorly to the limbus by sharp dissection; bleeding is controlled with cautery; the scleral flap is created with a Beaver knife or Superblade; 2 to 4 mm circumferentially and 3 to 4 mm radially, being careful to keep the incision partial thickness and to maintain consistent depth; the flap is elevated with a forceps and dissected from the underlying sclera; if the eye is at high risk for failure, a sponge soaked in 5-fluorouracil (50 mg/ml) or mitomycin C (0.2–0.5 mg/ml) may be placed either above or below the scleral flap for approximately 5 minutes; the sponge is then removed and the area irrigated with balanced salt solution; a corneal paracentesis tract is made; the sclerostomy is then fashioned by entering the anterior chamber with a superblade paral-

lel to the most anterior edge of clear cornea; a Kelly Descemet punch is used to complete the sclerostomy; a broad peripheral iridectomy is performed; any bleeding from the iris root/ciliary processes is controlled using a taper tip cautery; the scleral flap is reapproximated by two to four 10-0 nylon sutures at the edges of the flap, tying the sutures with slip-knots to allow for adjustment of tension; the anterior chamber is reformed with a blunt 30G cannula, and adequacy of filtration at sides of flap is assessed with cellulose sponges; the nylon slip knots may be loosened or tightened depending on the adequacy of flow; the conjunctival and Tenon's flap is closed with 8-0 chromic or vicryl sutures in a running, locked manner; balanced salt solution is injected through the paracentesis tract to reform the anterior chamber while watching for elevation of the bleb and deepening of the anterior chamber; the bleb, incision, and limbus can be painted with fluorescein to identify any leaks through the conjunctiva; subconjunctival injections of cefazolin and decadron are injected in the inferior forniceal region; the eye is patched after instilling a drop of atropine sulfate 1%; postoperatively, patient is treated with a cycloplegic agent, topical steroids, and a topical antibiotic; the patient is seen on the first postoperative day to assess the depth of the anterior chamber, IOP, integrity of the wound, and signs of infection, then at day 3, 1 week, 2 weeks, 1 month, and 2 months postoperatively; the patient may need to be seen more frequently if the clinical course suggests it; postoperatively, subconjunctival injections of 5-fluorouracil may need to be given if the bleb appeasrs to be scarring down and vascularized.

D. Complications:

include early and late bleb infection, endophthalmitis, persistent hypotony, flat anterior chamber, wound leaks, hyphema, early cataract formation, dellen formation near a high bleb, transient IOP elevation, serous choroidal detachments, suprachoroidal hemorrhage, persistent uveitis, cystoid macular edema, and loss of vision; a toxic corneal epitheliopathy may develop from use of 5-fluorouracil; this can be treated by stopping the 5-fluorouracil injections and using lacrilube eye ointment.

VI. CILIODESTRUCTIVE PROCEDURES

Treatment of ciliary body with cryotherapy, diathermy, argon endolaser, Nd:YAG laser; and diode laser; complications include prolonged hypotony, pain, inflammation, cystoid macular edema, hemorrhage, and phthisis bulbi.

VII. DRAINAGE DEVICES

Tube placed in the anterior chamber to shunt aqueous to a bleb over a plate that is placed at a site posterior to the limbus; examples are the Ahmed, Baerveldt, Krupin, Molteno, and Schocket implants; generally reserved for patients in whom conventional glaucoma filtration surgery with antimetabolites has failed.

VIII. LASER SUTURE LYSIS OF THE TRABECULECTOMY FLAP SUTURES OR RELEASABLE SUTURES:

Used to increase outflow from the trabeculectomy site by loosening the adhesion between the scleral flap and the scleral bed; it may be performed in the first ten postoperative days following trabeculectomy without an antimetabolite or trabeculectomy with 5-fluorouracil or in the first month following a trabeculectomy with mitomycin C. For laser suture lysis, the corner of a Zeiss goniolens or the Hoskins lens is placed on the conjunctiva over the suture to allow a view of the suture, pretreatment with topical anesthetic and phenylephrine to blanch conjunctival vessels; the argon green or krypton red laser 500 mwatts to 1 watt power, 50 microns spot size, 0.1 second, aiming beam focused on the nylon suture; postsuture lysis digital massage or focal pressure on the flap edge with a Q-tip may be needed to achieve immediate IOP reduction and an elevation of the bleb.

IX. LASER PHOTOCOAGULATION OF THE RETINA

A. A variety of multicenter, randomized, prospective, controlled clinical trials provide a wealth of knowledge about the natural history of, as well as the beneficial effect of, laser photocoagulation upon several retinal diseases. This chapter will briefly summarize the indications and techniques set forth by these studies, as well as extrapolations from these studies which are in common use.

B. Wavelength
1. A variety of lasers and wavelengths are currently available. Although there are numerous theoretic advantages of one wavelength over another, in clin-

ical practice most of these are subtle and unproven. Xenon photocoagulation has been largely replaced because fewer side effects were demonstrated with argon laser in the diabetic retinopathy study (DRS).

2. The argon laser is currently the most widely used laser for treatment of retinal conditions. It has been proven useful in the DRS, macular photocoagulation study (MPS), branch vein occlusion study (BVOS), and an early treatment of diabetic retinopathy study (ETDRS) trials. Argon blue (488 nm) has been largely abandoned for argon green (514 nm), due to less inner retinal absorption by xanthophyll and less intraocular scattering. Furthermore, tritan color contrast sensitivity defects have been detected in ophthalmologists who used the blue-green argon laser extensively, possibly secondary to reflection of the aiming beam.

3. Dye lasers can emit yellow (577 nm) light, which penetrates nuclear sclerotic cataracts better than green and is better absorbed by hemoglobin. Although it is untested in major clinical trials, it is useful for focal treatment of microaneurysms and choroidal neovascularization (CNV) due to its good hemoglobin absorption. The krypton red (647 nm) laser is useful in treating through vitreous hemorrhage and adjacent to intraretinal hemorrhage due to its poor absorption by hemoglobin. It penetrates deeper into the choroid and can be more painful than green.

4. The diode laser emits in the infrared (805 nm) range, which accentuates the advantages and disadvantages of krypton red. Its penetration is excellent, but it is more painful than argon lasers. One major advantage is its solid-state design, which makes it much smaller and more portable than other lasers. Indocyanine green (ICG) dye absorbs infrared light, and in the future, ICG-enhanced diode treatment of CNV may prove useful.

5. The recently released frequency-doubled YAG laser produces light in the green spectrum and uses solid-state technology. This combination may prove very popular in the future.

C. Treatment Techniques

1. Specific parameters for treatment will be listed by condition in subsequent sections

2. More important than the wavelength of laser energy is the placement and intensity of the photocoagulation. For macular photocoagulation, the fluorescein

or ICG angiogram is projected on a viewer adjacent to the patient.

3. As the power density is inversely proportional to the square of the spot diameter, the energy should theoretically be cut by a factor of four when the spot diameter is cut in half

4. Certain lenses alter the retinal spot size (e.g., a 200 m spot setting is enlarged to almost 500 m on the retina by a Rodenstock lens)

5. Intensity of photocoagulation burns:
   a. grade I (light): faint retinal blanching
   b. grade II (mild): hazy, translucent retinal burn
   c. grade III (moderate): opaque, gray/dirty-white retinal burn
   d. grade IV (heavy): dense, chalky-white retinal burn

D. Laser Systems
   1. Slit lamp delivery is usually the safest way to apply macular photocoagulation
   2. The laser indirect ophthalmoscope (LIO) offers advantages in patients with very peripheral pathology (tears), media opacity, intraocular gas, or those recently having undergone eye surgery. When applying extensive PRP with the LIO, the repeat mode is useful to minimize body motion. As the size of the laser burn is very dependent upon the positioning of the handheld lens, it is easy to inadvertently decrease the spot size and increase power density while using the repeat mode. Therefore, it is recommended to set the energy level using the smallest achievable spot size in order to prevent inadvertent rupture of Bruch's membrane in the repeat mode. Duration of 0.2 seconds is often used.
   3. Endophotocoagulation is extensively used in vitreous surgery
   4. A contact transscleral delivery system is currently being evaluated for diode photocoagulation of the retinal periphery

E. Complications
   1. Although retinal photocoagulation has become a very safe procedure, numerous important potential side effects should be discussed with the patient in the form of informed consent prior to treatment
      a. pain:
         1) more common with treatment along the horizontal meridian
         2) more common with diode and krypton
      b. retrobulbar hemorrhage or central retinal artery occlusion if retrobulbar anesthesia used

    c. foveal burn or macular edema
    d. vitreous, retinal, or subretinal hemorrhage
    e. choroidal effusion or serous retinal detachment
    f. angle closure glaucoma
    g. decreased visual field and night blindness
    h. CNV due to rupture of Bruch's membrane
    i. epiretinal membrane formation
    j. cataract, iris atrophy, corneal burn
    k. RPE rip

X. SPECIFIC RETINAL CONDITIONS

A. Diabetic Macular Edema (DME)
  1. The ETDRS found that treatment of clinically significant diabetic macular edema (CSDME) lowers the chance of severe visual loss by 50 percent
  2. CSDME is defined as one of the following:
    a. retinal thickening at or within 500 microns of the macular center
    b. hard exudates at or within 500 microns of the macular center if associated with retinal thickening of the adjacent retina
    c. Retinal thickening at least one disc area in extent, any part of which is within one disc diameter of the macular center
  3. This diagnosis is not made with fluorescein angiography; however, angiography is recommended to direct treatment. A combination of two treatment modalities is recommended:
    a. focal treatment:
      1) used for microaneurysms 500 to 3,000 microns from the foveal center, which are felt to be causing CSDME
      2) microaneurysms between 300 to 500 microns from the foveal center are often left for a second treatment session
      3) treatment parameters:
        a) wavelength: yellow (better hemoglobin absorption) or green (ETDRS-proven)
        b) spot size: 50 to 100 microns (50 near foveal center)
        c) duration: 0.05 to 0.1 seconds (0.05 near foveal center)
        d) intensity: blanching of microaneurysms (if possible)
    b. grid treatment:
      1) used to treat diffuse retinal thickening or nonperfused zones felt to be causing CSDME

  2) can be used to treat clusters of microaneurysms treatment parameters:
   a) wavelength: green
   b) spot size: 100 to 200 microns
   c) duration: 0.1 second
   d) intensity: light (Grade 1)
   e) pattern: spots should be one burn width apart
 c. followup:
  1) 3 to 4 months
  2) fluorescein angiography repeated if retreatment is needed
B. Proliferative Diabetic Retinopathy (PDR)
 1. The DRS identified four risk factors for severe visual loss:
  a. presence of neovascularization (NV)
  b. NV within one disc diameter of disc (NVD)
  c. NV size: NVD $\geq$ 1/4 disc area (standard photo 10A). NVE $\geq$ 1/2 disc area.
  d. vitreous or preretinal hemorrhage
 2. Retinal photocoagulation (PRP) is strongly recommended for three or four of the above risk factors
 3. PRP can be considered for one to two risk factors based upon clinical setting (can be deferred while macular edema treatment given)
 4. Although PRP is not recommended for most nonproliferative diabetic retinopathy, when PDR is extremely severe, treatment may be given prophylactically to prevent progression to high-risk PDR
 5. Rubeosis is usually treated with urgent PRP
 6. When safe, DME is treated before PRP is administered to minimize exacerbation of the edema; however, when high-risk PDR is present with CSDME, both are usually treated concurrently
  a. treatment parameters (PRP):
   1) wavelength: green (krypton red or diode infrared if cataract or VH)
   2) spot size: 500 microns
   3) duration: 0.05 to 0.2 seconds
   4) intensity: moderate (Grade III)
   5) pattern:
    a) PRP scatter one burn width apart from arcades (or at least 300 microns from foveal center) to far periphery
    b) flat NVE is treated with almost confluent burns without directly attempting closure of NV

      c) treatment over major vessels is avoided
    6) treatment is often split into two to three sessions of approximately 800 spots each over several weeks
    7) followup is dependent upon severity of PDR and clinical response to laser
    8) additional fill-in laser is recommended if NV does not initially respond. The laser and direct ophthalmoscope may facilitate anterior treatment.
    9) vitrectomy may be considered if very severe, active NV persists despite full laser or if vitreous hemorrhage prevents PRP, especially in Type I diabetics

C. Branch Retinal Vein Occlusion (BRVO)
  1. The BRVO examined patients with macular edema secondary to BRVO and found 65% of treated patients had two or more lines of improvement vs. 37% of untreated patients. In patients with NV, scatter PRP of nonperfused areas was found to decrease the incidence of vitreous hemorrhage from 61% to 29%. Treatment is recommended after development of neovascularization.
  2. Fluorescein angiograms obtained after sufficient clearance of intraretinal hemorrhage
    a. indications for treatment:
      1) persistent macular edema with visual acuity less than 20/40
      2) neovascularization with or without vitreous hemorrhage
    b. treatment parameters: macular edema
      1) wavelength: green preferred; red or infrared if cataract, vitreous hemorrhage, or intraretinal hemorrhage present
      2) spot size: 100 μ
      3) duration: 0.1 second
      4) intensity: mild to moderate (Grade II to Grade III)
      5) pattern: grid one burn width apart in areas of capillary leakage from arcade to edge of foveal avascular zone
    c. treatment parameters: neovascularization
      1) wavelength: green preferred; red or infrared if cataract, vitreous hemorrhage, or intraretinal hemorrhage present
      2) spot size: 200 to 500 μ
      3) duration: 0.1 second
      4) intensity: moderate (Grade III)

       5) pattern: grid one burn width apart in area of nonperfusion to within 3,000 μ of foveal center
  3. Treatment is not recommended over intraretinal blood, and treatment adjacent to blood may be safer with red or infrared wavelengths
    a. followup: 3 to 4 months

D. Central Retinal Vein Occlusion (CRVO)
  1. The CVOS is evaluating the efficacy of treatment for macular edema and severe nonperfusion in CRVO. Extensive nonperfusion more than 10 disc areas, ERG abnormalities (such as decreased B-wave to A-wave ratio), and the presence of an afferent pupillary defect correlate with ischemic CRVOs and the development of rubeosis.
  2. These cases should be followed closely (every 3 weeks) for the development of rubeosis
  3. PRP may help induce regression of NV secondary to ischemic CRVO
    a. treatment parameters: CRVO
       1) wavelength: green-preferred; red or infrared if cataract, vitreous hemorrhage, or intraretinal hemorrhage present
       2) size: 500 μ
       3) duration: 0.05 to 0.2 seconds
       4) intensity: moderate (Grade III)
       5) pattern: grid one burn width apart from arcades to far periphery

E. Choroidal Neovascularization (CNV)
  1. Multicenter trials have demonstrated a beneficial treatment effect for well-demarcated CNV, which is extrafoveal (greater than 200 microns from foveal center) or juxtafoveal (1 to 200 μ from foveal center) in age-related macular degeneration (AMD), presumed ocular histoplasmosis syndrome (POHS), and idiopathic CNV. These findings have been extrapolated to CNV from other conditions, such as angioid streaks, choroidal rupture, optic nerve head drusen, and choroidal nevi and tumors. Treatment of CNV in other conditions, such as high myopia, remains controversial.
  2. Recently, treatment for certain cases of subfoveal CNV secondary to AMD has been found to be beneficial. However, subgroup analysis of subfoveal group demonstrates best treatment effect for small (less than one disc area) new CNV with poor initial visual acuity (less than 20/200). Large CNV with good initial visual acuity has a poor treatment effect.

3. The subfoveal studies define several types of presumed choroidal neovascularization based on stereoscopic fluorescein angiographic appearance:
    a. classic CNV:
        1) well demarcated boundaries
        2) discerned during transit
        3) late leakage often obscures boundaries
    b. fibrovascular pigment epithelial detachment (PED):
        1) a type of occult CNV
        2) irregular, stippled hyperfluorescent elevation of RPE
        3) boundaries may be well or poorly demarcated
        4) persistent staining or leakage of fluorescein at 10 minutes
    c. late leakage of undetermined source:
        1) a form of occult CNV
        2) boundaries always poorly demarcated
        3) source of leakage not discernible in early phase of angiogram
    d. elevated blocked fluorescence:
        1) elevated above normal RPE
        2) when adjacent to CNV, considered to harbor fibrovascular tissue
4. Eligibility criteria for extrafoveal, juxtafoveal CNV treatment
    a. evidence of classic CNV
    b. entire neovascularization (CNV plus PED, blood, or elevated blocked fluorescence) has well demarcated borders
    c. recurrent CNV that is extrafoveal, juxtafoveal and meets above criteria
    d. PED: (i) classic CNV is major component, (ii) has well demarcated boundaries
5. Eligibility criteria for subfoveal CNV treatment
    a. well-demarcated subfoveal CNV
    b. vision 20/40 to 20/320
    c. age 50 years or more
    d. size of CNV and all lesion components
        1) new CNV (never treated): up to 3 1/2 disc areas
        2) recurrent CNV:
            a) recurrent CNV + laser scar: up to 6 disc areas
            b) some untreated retina must remain within 1500 microns of foveal center
6. Pretreatment protocol:
    a. angiogram should be less than 96 hours old; reduces possibility that lesion has grown

    b. pretreatment composite drawing can be made from angiogram

        1) use microfilm reader to project the angiogram onto white notebook paper

        2) use early venous frame of angiogram to trace vessels and locate foveal avascular zone center, and include larger landmark vessels and disc

        3) trace out boundaries of the choroidal neovascularization, again use early venous phase

        4) trace blocked fluorescence and blood with separate colors

    c. informed consent of procedure, discuss natural history, 50% of risk of persistence or recurrence. Goal of treatment is to stabilize visual acuity.

    d. use retrobulbar anesthesia as needed

7. Treatment parameters for CNV:

    a. wavelength: the precise placement and intensity of treatment is more important than the wavelength. Argon blue, green, and krypton red laser all produce light energy which is converted to heat primarily at the level of the RPE. Argon green can be used for all CNVs; however, yellow and red have theoretic advantages. Krypton red produces deeper burn with less spread into the inner retina and less absorption by xanthophyll; has been used in MPS trials for juxtafoveal CNV or subfoveal. Argon blue/green photocoagulation has been used for extrafoveal CNV and argon green has been used for extrafoveal, juxtafoveal, or subfoveal lesions

    b. spot size: a 200-micron spot can be used to straddle the edge of the membrane, producing treatment 100 microns beyond the edge; 500-micron spots are used to fill in the central lesion

    c. duration: 0.2 to 1 second

    d. intensity: heavy (Grade IV lesions)

    e. pattern: treat foveal side of CNV first, then the boundaries, and finally, the remaining area is filled in with overlapping burns

    f. specific considerations: 50% risk of persistence or recurrence

        1) extrafoveal lesions—extend treatment an additional 100 microns beyond the adjacent blood, pigment, or other blocked fluorescence surrounding the lesion

      2) juxtafoveal lesions—extend treatment an additional 100 microns beyond CME or on border away from fovea. Extend treatment an additional 100 microns into any blood on foveal side if CNV is 100 microns or further from the foveal center.

      3) subfoveal lesions—the subfoveal study includes fibrovascular PED, elevated blocked fluorescence, and hemorrhage adjacent to CNV (in most cases) as lesion components to be included in the total lesion to be treated. Extend treatment an additional 100 microns beyond peripheral boundaries of all lesion components except blood. Treatment is not required 100 microns beyond blood.

      4) subfoveal recurrence—extend treatment 100 microns beyond peripheral boundaries of all lesion components except blood. Extend 300 microns into previous treatment/previous laser scar as well as beyond base of feeder vessel.

   8. Followup

     a. immediate

      1) posttreatment photographs are recommended

      2) composite drawings are then made to document the extent of laser treatment and landmark vessels

      3) the dense white photocoagulation treatment is outlined with a colored pencil

      4) the adequacy of the photocoagulation treatment, extent, and intensity is then judged by placing the posttreatment drawing over the pretreatment CNV drawing

      5) re-treat if necessary

      6) aspirin use and heavy lifting should be discouraged

     b. long-term

      1) followup examination and fluorescein angiography at 1, 3, and 6 weeks posttreatment

      2) examination is then performed 3 to 6 months and then biyearly

      3) patient should be encouraged to continue with daily Amsler grid examination

F. Central Serous Chorioretinopathy (CSR)

   1. Although focal photocoagulation can quicken the resolution of serous macular detachment secondary to central serous chorioretinopathy, the final visual acuity is not improved by treatment

    2. A 4-month observation period is often recommended before treatment unless decreased visual acuity significantly interferes with the patient's daily functioning (job) or unless multiple prior recurrences have occurred

      a. treatment parameters
        1) wavelength: green
        2) spot size: 100 to 200 microns
        3) duration: 0.1 to 0.2 seconds
        4) intensity: white (Grade I)
        5) pattern: direct treatment to the extrafoveal focal leakage site

G. Miscellaneous

    1. Peripheral retinal neovascularization caused by sickle cell disease, Eales' disease, Behcet's disease, etc., can be treated with peripheral scatter treatment to nonperfused areas

    2. The cryo-ROP study demonstrated a treatment benefit for cryotherapy given to infants with threshold retinopathy of prematurity. More recently, indirect laser (usually diode) has been found to be equally effective in less extensive studies. Threshold disease consists of Stage 3 retinopathy in Zone 1 or 2 with 5 contiguous or 8 cumulative clock hours of NV. A tight scatter pattern of moderate intensity laser burns are placed from the ora to the edge of vascularized retina.

    3. Retinal breaks are frequently treated with laser photocoagulation using moderate intensity 200- to 500-micron spots. Two or three rows of almost confluent photocoagulation is placed around the break and carried to the ora if significant vitreoretinal traction is present. The laser indirect ophthalmoscope has made treatment of peripheral breaks easier, and cryotherapy is used less frequently than in the past.

XI. TREATMENT OF RETINAL BREAKS

A. Cryopexy and Laser Photocoagulation

    1. Definition:
      a. thermal adhesive modalities used to create chorioretinal adhesions and seal retinal breaks

    2. Indications:
      a. acute symptomatic retinal breaks or, rarely, asymptomatic retinal breaks/retinal pathology in eyes at high risk for retinal detachment (RD)

    3. Objective:
      a. to surround retinal breaks with cryoapplications and/or laser photocoagulation in order to create

a permanent chorioretinal scar which prevents fluid vitreous from migrating through the open break (retinal detachment)

4. Method:
   a. general considerations:
      1) transpupillary laser photocoagulation optimal for all breaks if minimal subretinal fluid (SRF) and clear media
      2) cryopexy or transscleral laser useful if breaks 1) very anteriorly located, 2) obscured by media opacities (cortical cataract, vitreous hemorrhage), and 3) surrounded by significant amount of SRF
      3) laser burns more clearly visualized immediately after treatment than cryotherapy; thus, adequacy of treatment easily confirmed at the time of surgery
      4) with either modality, treatment should completely surround breaks and associated SRF or demarcate breaks to the ora serrata
   b. laser photocoagulation:
      1) maximum pupillary dilation
      2) topical anesthesia adequate in most cases; retro/peribulbar anesthetic decreases ocular motility which may be helpful for visualization of lesions
      3) indirect ophthalmoscope laser delivery systems preferable for anterior retinal breaks; if indirect delivery system unavailable, cryopexy (versus transpupillary laser) may be useful for anterior breaks
      4) transpupillary laser photocoagulation easier for breaks closer to the equator; if anticipated, use indirect laser delivery prior to transpupillary laser as contact lens placement may impair corneal clarity
      5) with indirect laser, patient placed in semi-recumbent position; surgeon sits/stands comfortably to minimize extraneous head movement; typical initial settings: 0.1 to 0.2 second duration/0.200 watt power/repeat mode; size of burn relates to dioptric power of condensing lens (bigger with increased power), scleral depression (smaller), and beam focus
      6) 20 or 28 diopter condensing lens; 28 diopter lens provides panoramic view and larger spot size
      7) break visualized (scleral depression used as necessary); to sharply focus aiming beam,

surgeon pulls his/her head back; energy increased in small increments to create gray-white burns; two to three rows to completely surround the tear or demarcate the tear to the ora serrata

8) for transpupillary laser, panfundus/3 mirror fundus contact lens used; typical initial settings: 0.1 to 0.2 second duration/0.150 watt power/100 to 200 micron spot size/argon green or dye wavelengths (yellow for cataract, red for vitreous hemorrhage)/repeat mode

9) two to three rows of gray-white burns applied, completely surrounding retinal break or demarcating to the ora serrata; laser will not "take" in areas of SRF and is placed around the margins of SRF

10) cryopexy or indirect laser used if anterior aspect of the break cannot be adequately treated

c. cryopexy:

1) maximum pupillary dilation

2) subconjunctival anesthetic usually administered, though topical anesthetic adequate if few cryo applications are applied; 0.1 to 0.5 cc lidocaine 2% injected subconjunctively tuberculin (tb) syringe with 27 to 30 gauge needle; inject in quadrant receiving cryo treatment

3) cryoprobe tested by observing ice ball forming and thawing at the tip of the insulated cryoprobe

4) lid speculum placed, topical wetting agents to maintain corneal clarity

5) indirect ophthalmoscopy for visualization; 28 diopter lens provides a panoramic view, helpful in localizing/orienting the cryoprobe

6) tip of the cryoprobe used for scleral depression; slowly moved away from surgeon, from anterior to posterior (posterior to anterior movement difficult due to free rotation of the globe)

7) location of the cryoprobe confirmed by "toeing in" tip; this prevents false localization of the cryoprobe shaft and inadvertent posterior freezes

8) SRF can usually be squeezed through the open retinal break to allow direct retinal treatment

9) pedal depressed as the surgeon observes cryoreaction
10) small holes/breaks can be treated with a single application centered on the break; large breaks should be surrounded with one row of contiguous cryoapplications; treatment delivered directly to the open break causes dispersion of retinal pigment epithelial (RPE) cells, increasing risk of epiretinal proliferation
11) adequate treatment achieved when dull white cryoreaction first appears; intense white applications/ice balls indicate overtreatment
12) if cryoreaction not evident after 5 seconds, freezing should be stopped and position of the cryoprobe reassessed
13) cryoprobe moved to adjacent location after thawing of tip
14) postoperatively, a single application of topical antibiotic drops or ointment instilled if patients received subconjunctival injection
15) mild postop discomfort treated with oral analgesics (e.g., ibuprofen; acetaminophen with codeine) as needed; patients warned that the eye will be hyperemic for a few days

5. Complications:
   a. cryopexy:
      1) cryopexy to eyelids may cause pain, edema, permanent loss of cilia and depigmentation of skin
      2) choroidal effusion/hemorrhage especially with intense or excessive cryoapplication
      3) scleral rupture with forceful treatment over ectatic sclera, or with probe relocation before thawing of iceball
      4) vitreous hemorrhage
      5) posterior RPE fallout usually occurs with intense cryotherapy applied during RD surgery
      6) inadvertent posterior freezes; macular/optic nerve freezes can cause significant visual loss
   b. laser photocoagulation:
      1) choroidal edema/effusion from intense/extensive anterior treatment
      2) rupture of Bruch's membrane from intense (brief duration, small spot size) laser application
      3) inadvertent posterior photocoagulation usually from disorientation/"sliding" off mirror into center of contact lens

6. Prognosis:
   a. treatment of symptomatic retinal break decreases incidence of RD from 40% to less than 10%
   b. prognosis for asymptomatic retinal breaks less certain; treatment of asymptomatic retinal breaks may be advisable for superotemporal tears associated with vitreous traction (elevated flap) in eyes with multiple risk factors for RD
   c. most asymptomatic breaks can be safely observed
   d. treatment benefit for other vitreoretinal lesions (e.g., lattice degeneration) remains unproven
   e. treatment of retinal breaks caused by penetrating trauma or breaks caused by retinitis sclopetaria/retinal necrosis in blunt trauma may be unnecessary as chorioretinal adhesion occurs with inflammatory response
7. Contraindications:
   a. few contraindications to thermal adhesive treatment exist
   b. medically unstable patients should be monitored, especially with cryopexy
   c. cryopexy cannot be applied when significant choroidal edema is present
   d. cryopexy cannot be applied through a scleral buckle
   e. if a significant retinal detachment is present, laser photocoagulation or cryopexy to demarcate the pathology is not sufficient
B. Pneumatic Retinopexy
   1. Definition:
      a. retinal reattachment procedure in which retinal breaks are closed with temporary gas bubble tamponade
   2. Indications:
      a. rhegmatogenous retinal detachment with pathogenic break(s) no greater than 1 clock hour in size and located superiorly between 8 and 4 o'clock; pneumatic retinopexy ideal for patients who are medically unstable and/or unable to tolerate standard retinal reattachment surgery
   3. Objective:
      a. to tamponade pathogenic retinal breaks allowing for resorption of subretinal fluid and retinal reattachment; retinal reattachment maintained by a permanent chorioretinal adhesion produced by cryopexy or laser photocoagulation
   4. Method:

    a. pupil maximally dilated

    b. pure expansile gas (see below—gas) drawn through millipore filter into a 1 cc/3 cc syringe; amount of gas noted and the syringe capped with a 30-gauge needle

    c. retinal break(s) localized with indirect ophthalmoscopy; treated with cryotherapy; scleral depression with cryotherapy softens the globe prior to gas injection; alternatively, breaks treated with laser 24 to 48 hours after gas injection when retina reattached; laser optimal for posterior breaks

    d. anesthesia—surgeon's choice of topical, peri/retrobulbar anesthetic; topical anesthesia allows for light perception checks; peri/retrobulbar provides akinesia and is more comfortable if extensive cryotherapy is needed

    e. aseptic technique; eye prepped with topical iodine solution (e.g., 5% povidone-iodine), sterile lid speculum placed

    f. patient in supine position

    g. under direct visualization with illumination from the indirect ophthalmoscope, needle introduced through the temporal pars plana 3.5 to 4.0 mm posterior to the corneoscleral limbus in phakic patients, 3 mm in pseudophakos; needle directed toward the midvitreous, avoiding areas of bullous detachment; once visualized, the needle is withdrawn slightly toward the eyewall and 0.3 cc of gas briskly injected; as the needle is withdrawn, eye is rotated away from the injection site with a cotton-tip applicator

    h. vision tested for light perception; if no light perception and no perfusion of the central retinal artery after 5 to 10 minutes, anterior chamber paracentesis performed to lower intraocular pressure (IOP); alternatively, pars plana aspiration of vitreous fluid or gas bubble

5. Postoperatively:

    a. topical antibiotic drops for 24 hours

    b. patient instructed to maintain head position so that retinal breaks are uppermost/tamponaded by the bubble for at least 16 hours a day for 7 to 10 days; patients instructed not to sleep in the supine position (avoids gas bubble contact with the crystalline lens/anterior structures)

    c. supplemental laser or cryopexy performed as needed when the retina reattached

6. Complications:

           a. acute central retinal artery occlusion (see above)
           b. endophthalmitis (rare)
           c. macular retinal detachment due to SRF forced posteriorly by gas bubble
           d. subretinal gas
           e. gas entrapment between the anterior hyaloid face and lens (canal of Petit)
           f. new (or missed) retinal breaks in 10 to 15% of cases

      7. Prognosis:
           a. 70 to 80% reattachment with retinopexy procedure alone (higher in phakic eyes); when scleral buckling used for failed pneumatic procedures, final reattachment rates comparable to standard scleral buckling; visual outcome similar in both techniques

      8. Contraindications:
           a. inferior pathogenic retinal breaks
           b. multiple pathogenic retinal breaks extending over several clock hours
           c. significant proliferative vitreoretinopathy (PVR)
           d. inability to position eye postoperatively (children, mental retardation, cervical arthritis)

C. Scleral Buckling
    1. Definition:
        a. retinal reattachment procedure in which retinal breaks are closed and vitreoretinal traction relieved by producing scleral indentation

    2. Indications:
        a. rhegmatogenous RD caused by pathogenic retinal breaks located in peripheral retina (breaks located posterior to the equator may be better suited to vitrectomy techniques due to the difficulty in scleral buckle placement)
        b. traction RDs where vitreoretinal traction can be relieved by scleral indentation

    3. Objective:
        a. to achieve functional closure of pathogenic retinal breaks by decreasing the distance between the retinal break and RPE redirecting intraocular fluid currents and/or plugging the open break with solid vitreous; hole closure allows SRF resorption by RPE pump; retinal reattachment further maintained by permanent chorioretinal adhesion created around retinal break(s) with thermal adhesive modalities (cryotherapy, photocoagulation, diathermy)

    4. Method:
        a. preoperative evaluation:

1) medical evaluation to determine anesthesia risks
2) evaluation of allergies or medical conditions contraindicating commonly used drugs (e.g., antibiotics, acetazolamide, beta blockers)
3) history of glaucoma or outflow obstruction may influence surgical technique (e.g., drainage versus nondrainage)
4) assessment of media clarity for adequate fundus visualization; reason for poor visualization determined (miosis, cataract, vitreous hemorrhage)
5) in pseudophakic/aphakic eyes, presence/absence of posterior capsulotomy noted to determine the risk of vitreous prolapse if anterior chamber paracentesis performed
6) complete fundus examination with binocular indirect ophthalmoscopy and scleral depression performed; specific features include configuration/extent of detachment, macular status (macula-on versus off, macular hole), presence/location of vitreoretinal breaks and associated pathology (e.g., lattice degeneration), ability to close breaks using scleral depression, areas of vitreoretinal adhesion and traction, areas of epiretinal proliferation/PVR
7) patients with macula-on or bullous RDs may benefit by bilateral eye patching and bed rest; decreased eye movement allows partial resorption of SRF
8) head positioning to prevent gravity-dependent spread of SRF into macula may be advisable

b. operative technique:
1) maximum pupillary dilation (e.g., phenylephrine 2.5–10%, tropicamide 1%, and cyclopentolate 1% drops every 15 minutes beginning 1 1/2 hours preoperatively)
2) general or local standby anesthesia depending on patient cooperation, medical status, and the complexity of the surgical procedure
3) for local anesthesia, combination short-acting/long-acting anesthetic (e.g., lidocaine 2%, marcaine 0.75% with Wydase); with retrobulbar or peribulbar anesthetic, adequate volume must be delivered (e.g., > 6 cc) for proper anesthetic effect

4) conjunctiva/adnexa prepped with topical iodine solution (e.g., 5% povidone-iodine)

5) 360 degree conjunctival peritomy; Tenon's capsule dissected off sclera; rectus muscles isolated and tagged with sutures; quadrants examined for scleral ectasia and the position of vortex veins

6) binocular indirect ophthalmoscopy with scleral depression; retinal breaks and other areas to be treated may be marked on the sclera; SRF drainage sites identified

7) cryotherapy applications applied to retinal breaks and areas of vitreoretinal pathology (e.g., lattice degeneration); breaks not causing detachment may be treated by thermal adhesion alone

8) scleral buckle elements selected to provide support from 3 mm posterior to the most posterior aspect of the pathogenic retinal break(s) to 2 mm anterior to the most anterior aspect of the retinal break(s), extending at least 3 mm beyond the lateral aspect of the retinal break(s); scleral buckle should relieve significant vitreoretinal traction

9) nomenclature to describe scleral buckling elements refers to the orientation in which the element is placed:

a) scleral buckle—any material which indents the sclera

b) radial or meridional element—long axis oriented radially; sutures for a radial element placed in a vertical mattress fashion; radial sponges create a focal radial buckling effect ideal for individual tears, reduces radial pleating of the retina and gaping of the retinal break ("fish-mouth" phenomenon)

c) segmental circumferential element—long axis oriented parallel to the ora serrata; sutures placed in a horizontal mattress fashion; useful in supporting multiple tears extending over several clock hours which are located at the same AP distance from the ora serrata; often combined with encircling band

d) encircling element—buckle surrounding the circumference of the globe

e) band—flat piece of material used to create an encircling buckle and to provide permanent support for segmental circumferential elements; often used in aphakic/pseudophakic RDs and in detachments with PVR to relieve vitreous base traction

10) buckling hardware soaked in antibiotic solution (e.g., gentamicin 0.3% ophthalmic solution)

11) nonabsorbable 4-0 or 5-0 scleral sutures (spatulated needles) placed; assistant exposes quadrant by applying traction to the rectus muscle bridle sutures and retracting Tenon's capsule; suture bite width confirmed with caliper; when passing sutures, needle tip position visualized through the scleral lamellae to avoid scleral perforation

12) double arm sutures passed anterior to posterior in vertical mattress fashion for radial elements; single arm sutures placed in a horizontal mattress fashion for segmental circumferential buckling elements or encircling band

13) buckling elements placed and sutures pulled up with temporary ties; adequacy of hole closure assessed; breaks should rest on the crest and anterior slope of the buckling element with broad support of the posterior aspect of retinal break

14) if adequate hole closure not achieved due to buckle malposition, position of breaks reevaluated and additional sutures passed; additional posterior support can be achieved by sliding a piece of buckling material underneath a circumferential segmental element or band; if buckle cannot be pulled up adequately because of severe IOP elevation (CRAO), drainage of SRF or anterior/posterior chamber fluid aspiration may be performed

15) gaping of retinal breaks caused by radial folding of the retina ("fish-mouthing") treated by:

a) injection of intravitreal gas bubble to flatten/tamponade the retina

   i. addition of radial element in the meridian of the fish mouth (spreads redundant retina on buckle)

   ii. drainage of SRF to settle break on the scleral buckle

16) SRF drainage achieves two effects:
   a) reduces the volume of the globe
   b) decreases the height of the detachment; SRF drainage should be considered when
      i. IOP elevation caused by pulling up the scleral buckle compromises central retinal artery perfusion or threatens scleral rupture
      ii. apposition of retinal breaks to the scleral buckle is desirable (e.g., bullous detachments, inferior RDs, tractional elevation in PVR, decreased ability to absorb SRF such as chronic RD)

17) drainage sites chosen away from large choroidal blood vessels/posterior ciliary arteries, in areas with maximum amount of SRF to avoid retinal perforation; nasal sites preferable to avoid submacular blood if subretinal hemorrhage occurs; areas beneath retina fixed by epiretinal membranes ideal as incarceration rarely occurs

18) drainage may be performed within the bed of the scleral buckle or more posteriorly; 3/4 thickness radial sclerotomy developed and a 6.0 suture placed through the lips of the sclerotomy, remaining scleral fibers cut to expose a knuckle of choroid; choroid treated with diathermy cauterization; fine gauge needle tip touched to the choroid barely entering the subretinal space; slow drainage of SRF while maintaining normal IOP by gentle traction on the rectus bridle sutures and by pressure against the sclera with cotton-tip applicators; drainage completed when spontaneous cessation of SRF drainage occurs or when adequate volume has been released; sclerotomy site closed with the preplaced suture; drainage site inspected with indirect ophthalmoscopy for complications

19) intravitreal fluid/air/gas injections performed to replace intraocular volume loss and/or provide tamponade for retinal breaks

20) temporary sutures converted to permanent and suture knots rotated posteriorly; sharp angles or protrusion of the buckling elements trimmed with scissors

21) prior to closure, patency of the central retinal artery (perfusion > 50% of the time) confirmed; patients with compromised outflow may receive systemic acetazolamide/topical aqueous suppressants at the end of the operation

22) irrigation of the retrobulbar space with marcaine (0.5 to 0.75%) prior to conjunctival closure provides excellent postoperative pain control

23) conjunctiva/Tenon's closed over the scleral buckling element with absorbable suture; subconjunctival corticosteroid and antibiotic injections delivered; combination steroid-antibiotic ointment placed followed by patch and shield

c. postoperative care:

1) patients with expanding gas bubbles may be instructed to monitor light perception vision for several hours after the surgery and to seek immediate care if light perception is impaired

2) patients with intraocular gas bubbles instructed to maintain head positioning so that retinal breaks are most superior; instructed not to sleep in the supine position

3) patients with incomplete SRF evacuation instructed to maintain quiet activity/bed rest with SRF pockets directed away from the macula

4) on postoperative day 1, patients should be evaluated specifically for endophthalmitis, elevated IOP, and persistent RD; examination should include vision, IOP, corneal integrity, anterior chamber depth, degree of inflammation (with specific attention to the presence/absence of hypopyon), lens clarity, percent intraocular gas fill, and adequacy of SRF resorption

5) transient IOP elevation is common and usually no intervention is required; fluid aspiration performed as a temporizing measure for compromised central retinal artery blood flow, especially if vision affected; aqueous suppressants often used in eyes with IOP above 30; specific reversible causes for pressure elevation (e.g., hyphema, pupillary block) should be identified and treated

6) if SRF persists, reevaluate buckle position and support of retinal break(s); consider pneumatic retinopexy to treat open retinal breaks within the superior 240 degrees; if gas bubble already present, appropriate positioning may result in resorption of SRF

7) patients should receive topical cycloplegic and combination steroid-antibiotic drops tapered over 4-week period

5. Complications:
   a. intraoperative:
      1) major complications:
         a) choroidal hemorrhage/subretinal hemorrhage can result in permanent severe visual loss; systemic and ocular risk factors for choroidal hemorrhage include systemic vascular disease, increasing age of patient, glaucoma, myopia, and vitrectomy with scleral buckling; subretinal hemorrhage associated with SRF drainage and/or deep scleral suture passes
         b) other major complications (e.g., globe rupture) rarely occur
      2) minor complications:
         a) iatrogenic retinal breaks, retinal incarceration, and loss of vitreous gel associated with deep suture passes or SRF drainage; managed by placement of thermal adhesion and positioning of a buckling element in the affected area
         b) other minor complications include vitreous hemorrhage and extraocular muscle avulsion
   b. postoperative:
      1) elevated IOPs often encountered in the early postoperative period due to several mechanisms including: outflow obstruction secondary to cellular debris, narrow angle from choroidal edema or anterior rotation of the lens-iris diaphragm from intraocular gas bubble tamponade; poor outflow facility related to preexisting glaucoma
      2) mild IOP elevations often transient and do not require treatment; elevations above 30 mmHg often treated with aqueous suppressants (e.g., topical beta blockers/acetazolamide); volume release via aspiration of vit-

reous fluid, vitreous gas or aqueous fluid temporizing measures

3) anterior segment ischemia a rare occurrence associated with encircling buckles and can be related to underlying sickle hemoglobinopathy; patients with sickle cell disease managed perioperatively with hydration, oxygenation, exchange transfusion, and avoiding systemic acidosis

4) choroidal effusion and associated exudative RD occur in 5 to 10% of scleral buckling procedures related to advanced age, thermal adhesive treatment, hypotony, and vortex vein obstruction with broad scleral buckles; in most cases, resolves spontaneously in 2 weeks; systemic steroids may reduce the severity and speed resolution

5) endophthalmitis rare (see below—vitreoretinal surgery)

6) early scleral buckle infections present with chemosis and purulent exudate; systemic antibiotic treatment to temporize while chorioretinal adhesions develop; eventually, infected buckling elements require removal

c. Late complications:

1) late exposure of scleral buckles with erosion through conjunctiva; exposed buckles provide an avenue for infection and usually require removal; incidence of retinal detachment after scleral buckle removal decreases as time from scleral buckling surgery increases

2) migration of scleral buckles

3) intrusion of implanted material with secondary complications of vitreous hemorrhage or recurrent RD (very rare)

4) diplopia with inconcomitant strabismus due to paresis or restriction of extraocular muscles; may spontaneously resolve, especially in younger patients; persistent in approximately 3 to 4% of cases requiring prism correction or strabismus surgery

5) macular pucker formation (epimacular membrane) with decrease of central acuity

6) PVR (extensive epiretinal/subretinal fibrocellular proliferation) develops postoperatively in approximately 5% of primary scleral buckling cases; combined traction-

rhegmatogenous RDs caused by PVR account for the majority of failed operations

6. Prognosis:
   a. anatomically, 85% of eyes with rhegmatogenous RD reattach with one operation and over 90% with reoperation; most common cause of failed scleral buckling operation includes pre- or postoperative PVR and nonclosure of retinal breaks
   b. visually, approximately 50% of patients regain visual acuity of 20/50 or better if the retina successfully reattached, 25%—20/200 or worse; postoperative visual acuity correlates with presence and duration of macular detachment prior to surgery; 75% of patients with macular detachment of less than one week's duration have postop vision of 20/70 or better; with greater than one week of macular detachment, only 50% of patients achieve 20/70 vision or better; visual prognosis in eyes where the macula has not become detached significantly better with approximately 90% of patients maintaining 20/30 acuity or better

7. Contraindications:
   a. contraindications to scleral buckling surgery are few
   b. scleral buckle placement may be hazardous in eyes with severe scleral thinning or undesirable in eyes with posterior retinal breaks (e.g., macular hole detachments); alternative retinal reattachment procedures should be considered in these circumstances
   c. scleral buckling should be combined with vitrectomy for treatment of complex RDs with vitreoretinal traction that cannot be relieved with scleral buckling alone (e.g., PVR)
   d. exudative RDs do not respond to scleral buckling

D. Vitreoretinal Surgery
   1. Definition:
      a. microsurgical technique for dissection and/or removal of intraocular material with minimal tissue traction
   2. Indications:
      a. removal of opacities occluding the optical axis (e.g., cataract, pupillary membrane); release of tissue traction by dissection/removal of intraocular membranes (e.g., vitreous wick, macular pucker, PVR, diabetic traction RD); removal of foreign bodies (e.g., dislocated IOL, traumatic intraocular foreign body); biopsy of intraocular

tissue (e.g., infectious endophthalmitis, large cell lymphoma, viral retinitis)

3. Objectives:
   a. to remove axial opacities, release traction on the retina and other intraocular structures, close retinal breaks, and remove material for diagnosis and treatment; biomechanical properties of vitreoretinal microsurgical instruments optimized to exert minimal traction on intraocular tissues

4. Method:
   a. preoperative:
      1) medical evaluation to assess anesthetic risk
      2) ability of patient to maintain face down position determined when use of long-acting tamponade anticipated
      3) functional tests performed to confirm retinal and optic nerve viability; eyes with no light perception should not be operated on unless due to recent subretinal hemorrhage; electrophysiologic tests especially useful in patients unable to communicate because of age (infants) or CNS dysfunction
      4) standard ophthalmic evaluation performed with special attention to factors influencing surgical approach, including:
         a) presence of corneal opacification requiring use of a temporary keratoprosthesis/ penetrating keratoplasty
         b) miosis requiring mechanical pupillary dilation
         c) iris/angle neovascularization requiring treatment of peripheral RD or ischemic retinal tissue
         d) axial opacities requiring removal to allow for anticipated surgical maneuvers; the need for lensectomy should be anticipated and consent for lensectomy should be obtained on all patients undergoing vitreous surgery in the event that axial opacity (e.g., hyphema, cataract) requires lens removal
         e) instability of the crystalline lens/pseudophakos necessitating need for lens removal/ fixation
         f) position of the peripheral choroid with respect to placement of intraocular instruments; hemorrhagic or serous choroidal detachments requiring external drainage

      g) vitreous anatomy including presence of vitreous detachment and vitreoretinal adherence; complexity and risk of vitreous surgery significantly reduced in eyes with complete posterior vitreous detachment

      h) retinal anatomy with special attention to retinal detachment configuration and position of fixed folds indicating the presence of epiretinal membranes; retinal breaks identified for treatment; bullous anterior retinal and pars plana detachments noted as this impacts on intraocular maneuvers

      i) in eyes with opaque media, combined A/B scan and ultrasonography performed to assess vitreoretinal relationships and presence of peripheral choroidal detachments, retrolental RDs, and intraocular tumors

  b. operative technique:

      1) local standby or general anesthesia as in scleral buckling (see above)

      2) patient's neck extended slightly, coronal plane parallel to ceiling to allow better access to the inferior retina

      3) if scleral buckling performed, open as for buckling surgery; scleral sutures easier to place prior to vitrectomy (closed eye, no cannulas); scleral buckle pulled up after vitreous surgery to avoid interfering with intraocular maneuvers and allowing drainage through peripheral retinal breaks

      4) when no scleral buckle placed, 120 degree conjunctival peritomy temporally, 60 degree superonasal peritomy; hemostasis of episcleral vessels in areas of sclerotomy placement can be considered

      5) sclerotomies for posterior segment vitrectomy placed between the greater arterial circle of the iris and the ora serrata, specific site depending on lens status and position of the ora serrata; in adults, sclerotomies placed 3 to 4 mm posterior to the corneoscleral limbus, more anteriorly in aphakic/pseudophakic eyes (3 mm), more posteriorly in phakic eyes (4 mm); in infants, anterior placement required due to the incomplete development of the pars plana

      6) enriched balanced salt solution (e.g., BSS-Plus) for infusion; 0.3 cc of 1; 1,000 epinephrine added to 500 cc infusion solution to maintain mydriasis; in diabetics, 3 cc of 50% dextrose solution added to prevent development of intraoperative lens opacities; lines cleared of air bubbles

7) infusion cannula placed inferotemporally; occasionally placed in other positions to avoid areas of anterior pathology; 4-0 or 5-0 preplaced horizontal mattress suture engages the infusion cannula flange or cannula system used; infusion cannula placement confirmed with direct visualization before infusion to prevent suprachoroidal or subretinal infusion; if cannula placement cannot be confirmed, an alternative infusion system (e.g., irrigating light probe or irrigating needle) used under direct visualization

8) in making sclerotomies, a 20-gauge microvitreoretinal (MVR) blade directed radially towards center of the eye, avoiding lens and elevated retina/choroid; superotemporal/superonasal sclerotomies positioned just above the horizontal meridian with the superonasal sclerotomy placed to avoid instrument handles hitting the nose; sclerotomy plugs placed to avoid hypotony and tissue incarceration

c. Removal of axial opacities:

1) axial opacities removed if they interfere with vitreoretinal surgical manipulations essential to achieve surgical objectives or patient's visual rehabilitation

2) opacities removed from anterior to posterior

3) edematous corneal epithelium debrided with scalpel blade

4) anterior chamber washout performed with an irrigating needle system for hyphema/inflammatory debris

5) organized pupillary membranes incised and segmented with blade/scissors, then tags excised with vitrectomy cutting instrument

6) cataracts removed either by anterior or posterior segment phacoemulsification; preservation of the lens capsule and intraocular lens implantation considered in uncomplicated cases; lensectomy with capsulectomy often preferred in eyes with active tissue proliferation (e.g., PVR)

       7) core vitreous gel with cellular debris and opacities excised with vitreous cutting instrument
  d. release of retinal traction
       1) vitreoretinal traction induced by vitrectomy instrument a function of flow rate across the aspiration port and cutting rate of the oscillating blade; traction minimized by decreasing the flow rate (low aspiration pressure, reduced port size) and maximizing cutting rate; when removing vitreous from attached retina, cutting port should face the retinal surface to increase cutting efficiency and decrease vitreous traction; when performing vitrectomy near areas of detached (mobile) retina, the port should face 180 degrees away from the retinal surface and retina blocked with the endoilluminator
       2) core vitreous gel removed anterior to posterior, at high cutting (600 cpm), low suction (100 to 150 mm Hg)
       3) surgical plane of the posterior hyaloid face identified; preretinal space entered behind the equator; the posterior hyaloid face circumscribed with the vitreous cutter for 360 degrees to release of anteroposterior traction; vitreous excised anteriorly to the vitreous base area; often, complex membrane dissection is done first to take advantage of clear media, removal of anterior vitreous skirt is done last
       4) tangential traction released by epiretinal membrane dissection (segmentation/delamination), scleral buckling, or retinotomy/retinectomy
       5) circumferential or anterior loop traction in the anterior vitreous base region addressed with vitreous base dissection; using endoillumination and/or coaxial/external illumination, membrane dissection performed with anterior structures exposed by scleral depression
  e. hole closure:
       1) all retinal breaks identified and treated with adhesive modalities
       2) consider cryotherapy prior to buckle placement to treat peripheral retinal breaks; wide field viewing system useful for laser treatment of the peripheral retina

3) breaks identified during vitrectomy marked with diathermy for later treatment

4) retinal reattachment required for laser photocoagulation; achieved by internal fluid-air exchange through a retinotomy/retinal break or by hydrokinetic retinal reattachment with heavier than water perfluorocarbon liquid (see below—perfluorocarbon liquids)

5) optimal placement for retinotomy 1 to 1 1/2 disc diameters superonasal to the optic nerve head away from blood vessels; preexisting posterior retinal breaks (e.g., macular hole) may also be used; drainage through peripheral breaks possible with telescoping silicone extrusion cannula

6) in air-filled pseudophakic or phakic eyes, a high minus (Landers) irrigating contact lens used with the operating microscope focused anteriorly; in aphakic eyes, a flat/no contact lens is utilized

7) after positioning SRF extrusion cannula, infusion line stopcock switched to the air pump; air pressure temporarily increased to approximately 30 to 40 mm Hg to compensate for escape of air through the sclerotomies, thus maintaining the shape of the globe; SRF flows back to the posterior pole and is aspirated through posterior drainage site

8) air prolapse under the retina demonstrates incomplete release of vitreoretinal traction preventing retinal reattachment; indicates need for further membrane dissection and/or relaxing retinotomy/retinectomy

9) after flattening of the retina, the retinotomy site and retinal breaks treated with surrounding rows of laser photocoagulation

10) scleral buckle pulled up and tied permanently; breaks on the scleral buckle treated with laser if not previously treated with cryoapplications

11) in hydrokinetic retinal reattachment, perfluorocarbon liquid injected over the optic nerve head (see below—perfluorocarbon liquids); after reattachment, retinal breaks treated with laser photocoagulation; perfluorocarbon from anterior to posterior removed by fluid-air exchange or fluid-silicone exchange

    12) in fluid-filled eyes, indirect ophthalmoscopy with scleral depression prior to sclerotomy closure performed to identify sclerotomy site tears/dialysis and/or other retinal breaks; small tears in attached retina treated with cryoapplications or laser; dialyses or small detachments may require treatment with gas bubble tamponade and/or scleral buckling; in eyes with poor visualization, prophylactic cryotherapy placed behind sclerotomy sites

  f. closure:

    1) sclerotomy site cleaned of prolapsed vitreous; sclerotomy sites closed with absorbable or nonabsorbable 7-0 or 8-0 sutures using half-thickness scleral bites

    2) long-acting tamponade with gas or silicone oil injected at the time of closure; numerous techniques have been described:

      a) nonexpansile concentration of C3F8 or SF6 gas diluted with filtered air in a 30 cc syringe; after fluid-air exchange, 20 to 30 cc of gas mixture slowly injected into the eye through the infusion cannula venting through an open sclerotomy or a needle placed through the pars plana

      b) 1.0 to 1.2 cc of pure C3F8 gas injected in a soft, air-filled eye to achieve a nonexpansile concentration

      c) partial fluid gas exchange performed and expansile concentration of gas injected

    3) silicone injection performed through the existing infusion cannula system (reinforced at coupling with heavy sutures) or through a large bore cannula placed through a sclerotomy; the eye is tilted to vent remaining air out of the open sclerotomy, thereby achieving maximum silicone fill

    4) after normalizing intraocular pressure, sclerotomy sites closed in air/watertight fashion

    5) conjunctiva and Tenon's closed in standard fashion

  g. special cases:

    1) vitreous sampling/infectious endophthalmitis:

      a) anterior chamber fluid/inflammatory debris and undiluted vitreous specimen obtained prior to infusion and antibiotic injection

b) in cases with chorioretinal lesions, the vitrectomy cutter positioned directly over the lesion prior to sampling of the specimen

c) three-way stopcock connected to the aspiration line of the vitrectomy cutting instrument, 5 to 10 cc syringe placed on the open port

d) after the port of the vitrectomy cutter visualized (using coaxial microscope illumination or endoillumination), assistant gently aspirates with syringe as the cutting mode of the vitrectomy instrument activated, IOP maintained by gentle scleral indentation with a cotton-tip applicator after adequate (0.5 to 1.0 cc) specimen obtained, vitreous infusion turned on and the vitreous cutter removed from the eye; specimen cleared from the dead space of the tubing by aspirating into the syringe

e) the undiluted specimen immediately processed for laboratory studies; contents of vitrectomy cassette later processed for laboratory studies

f) stopcock switched open to the vitrectomy unit if further vitrectomy performed

g) at close of vitrectomy, after sclerostomy closure, slow pars plana injection of 0.1 ml volume intravitreal antimicrobial agent into anterior/midvitreous using tb syringe with 30-gauge needle; eye left slightly soft prior to injection to avoid IOP spike; typical agents include:

   i. vancomycin 1 mg/0.1 ml (gram positive bacteria)

   ii. ceftazidime 2.25 mg/0.1 ml (gram negative bacteria)

   iii. amphotericin 5 to 10 mcg/0.1 ml (fungi)

   iv. ganciclovir 200 to 400 mcg/0.1 ml (CMV/ herpes virus)

h) as an alternative to mechanical vitrectomy, trans-pars plana aspiration of fluid vitreous through 22 to 27 gauge needle followed by intravitreal injection of antimicrobial agents can be performed in the outpatient setting; EVS recommendations for eyes with postoperative bacterial endophthalmitis-vitrectous aspirate performed when vision is hand motions or better, vitrectomy when vision is LP

2) proliferative diabetic retinopathy:
   a) posterior hyaloid face with neovascular/fibrovascular proliferative tissue excised to remove matrix for proliferation; surgical objectives achieved when traction is released from the macula/optic nerve; dissection of membranes from nasal or far peripheral retina may be unnecessary and lead to higher complication rates
   b) in segmentation techniques, a surgical plane established between vitreous membranes and the retina over the macula; membranes around the optic disc and temporal vascular arcades are dissected free from the retina, then segmented; remaining tissue pared back to the retinal surface with the vitreous cutter; bleeding controlled by increasing the infusion (intraocular) pressure and by coagulation of bleeding vessels
   c) in delamination techniques, a horizontal scissors or bimanual approach using lighted multifunctional probe (forceps, pick, tissue manipulator) and scissors, knife used to completely separate membranes from the retinal surface

3) macular/submacular surgery:
   a) in macular surgery, identification and removal of the posterior hyaloid face required; in macular hole surgery, release of tangential traction exerted by the posterior hyaloid and gas tamponade will allow the hole to flatten/close; in submacular surgery (e.g., subretinal neovascular membrane removal) postoperative organization/traction exerted by the posterior hyaloid face may lead to secondary complications
   b) hyaloid face engaged by suction through a silicone tip cannula passed along the retinal surface or by a bent MVR blade;

the hyaloid tents above the retina and the silicone tip deflects towards the retinal surface ("fish strike" sign); hyaloid carefully stripped off the macula and beyond the arcades

4) proliferative vitreoretinopathy:

   a) epiretinal membranes preventing retinal reattachment engaged with pics and stripped tangential to the retinal surface; posterior retina thicker than anterior and therefore retina stripped posteriorly to anteriorly; membranes stripped up to the vitreous base region using a unimanual or bimanual technique

   b) traction on retinal breaks at the vitreous base relieved either by membrane stripping or scleral buckling

   c) vitreous base dissection employed for vitreoretinal traction in the anterior vitreous base region; using coaxial/external illumination, membrane dissection performed with pars plana/ciliary body region exposed by scleral depression

   d) if retina reattachment unsuccessful after removal of epiretinal membranes because of subretinal membranes, subretinal membrane dissection performed; diathermy can be used to lyse membranes when the retinotomy is created, subretinal membranes grasped in the subretinal space and pulled/"spooled" out through the retinotomy. If large retinal breaks or retinotomies present, retina folded over and membranes bimanually dissected.

   e) in cases of intrinsic retinal foreshortening (retinal gliosis) or undissectable membranes, relaxing retinotomy/retinectomy required; relaxing retinotomies made in the periphery circumferential to the ora serrata in areas peripheral to the greatest retinal traction; area large vessels treated with diathermy to achieve coagulation of retinal vessels; scissors or similar cutting instrument used to create the retinotomy; radial and posterior relaxing retinotomy avoided as these tend to gape; small retinotomies (less than 90 degrees) often ineffectual at relaxing retinal traction

   h. postoperative:

     1) during the early postoperative period, acute elevations of IOP should be monitored; maximum expansion rate of long-acting gases occurs during the first 6 to 8 hours after injection; patients instructed to monitor for loss of light perception vision or occurrence of unremitting pain or nausea which may indicate severe IOP elevation

     2) patients with air- or gas-filled eyes instructed as to appropriate positioning to close retinal breaks and instructed not to sleep in supine position, which would predispose angle closure/acute IOP elevation

     3) on postoperative day 1, patients should be evaluated specifically for endophthalmitis, elevated IOP, and persistent RD (see above—scleral buckle)

     4) IOP elevations after vitrectomy are common and usually transient (see above—scleral buckle)

     5) degree of intraocular inflammation assessed; in cases with extensive dissection, especially over the ciliary body region, pronounced inflammation with fibrin response anticipated; infectious endophthalmitis (rare after vitrectomy) suspected when inflammation out of proportion to surgical trauma

     6) inflammation can usually be treated adequately with topical steroid preparations, occasionally, a brief course of systemic steroids for severe inflammation or when topical delivery unreliable; if fibrin reaction persists beyond 10 days, intraocular injection of tissue plasminogen activator (TPA) (5 to 10 mcg in 0.1 cc nonbacteriostatic water) considered; TPA less useful when cellular organization/maturation of fibrin membranes has developed

     7) all patients receive a course of cycloplegic drops to treat discomfort of ciliary spasm and maintain adequate dilation

     8) adequacy of intraocular tamponade assessed; early outpatient fluid-gas exchange (see below—gas) may be indicated when tamponade of inferior retina required and inadequate gas fill present; presence of residual/new SRF may indicate inadequate postoperative head positioning

9) postoperative transpupillary laser indicated for treatment of open breaks; occasionally, need for postoperative laser photocoagulation is recognized at the time of surgery
10) reformation of the anterior chamber angle with viscoelastics may be required for cases of persistent angle closure related to intraocular gas tamponade

5. Complications:
    a. intraoperative:
        1) iatrogenic retinal breaks occur due to vitreoretinal traction (often unavoidable) exerted during vitreoretinal surgery; posterior breaks are commonly encountered in eyes with proliferative diabetic retinopathy during dissection of adherent, plaque-like membranes from atrophic retina; breaks occurring posterior to sclerotomy relate to vitreous base traction as instruments are introduced through pars plana
        2) suprachoroidal/subretinal infusion occurs with malposition of infusion cannula
        3) retinal incarceration in sclerotomy sites occurs with highly elevated mobile retinal detachment; reduced by direct manipulation or fluid-air exchange
        4) fibrin membrane formation may occur during diabetic vitrectomy when excessive hemorrhage develops; difficult to remove and may prevent successful completion of dissection
        5) choroidal/subretinal hemorrhage (see above—scleral buckle)
    b. postoperative:
        1) elevated IOP and inflammation common postoperative complications (see above—scleral buckle)
        2) chronic postoperative hypotony, especially in cases requiring epiciliary dissection or when preoperative hypotony exists
        3) nuclear sclerotic cataract formation, especially in patients greater than 50 years of age; incidence of visually significant nuclear sclerosis increases with time; transient posterior subcapsular lens opacification related to intraocular gas tamponade frequent; traumatic cataracts develop if contact between intraocular instruments and the posterior lens capsule occurs, if the lens cap-

sule ruptured at the time of surgery, lensectomy indicated

4) recurrent/persistent vitreous hemorrhage in
cases of proliferative diabetic retinopathy;
after 10 weeks, outpatient fluid-air exchange
and laser treatment may be considered (see
below); reoperation with vitreous washout
may ultimately be required

5) anterior hyaloidal proliferation after diabetic vitrectomy

6) RD may occur secondary to new retinal
breaks developing from membrane contraction (e.g., sclerotomy site vitreous incarceration); in eyes without significant
traction, fluid-gas exchange with laser or
cryopexy sufficient to treat late rhegmatogenous RDs

7) retinal folds may occur with incomplete
evacuation of SRF and placement of intraocular gas tamponade especially in presence of encircling scleral buckle; SRF
forced posteriorly and fold of redundant
retina compressed by the gas bubble

8) rubeosis iridis/neovascular glaucoma in
eyes with incomplete retinal reattachment
or severe retinal ischemia; aphakia and severe inflammation increase the incidence of
rubeosis

9) postoperative endophthalmitis (rare)

6. Prognosis:
   a. relates to the underlying pathology
   b. in cases of vitrectomy for macular pucker, visual
improvement may occur in 85% of patients
   c. in proliferative diabetic retinopathy, vitrectomy
performed for vitreous hemorrhage alone yields
anatomic success rates of 80%, for traction RDs
approximately 70%, and for eyes with complex
tractional rhegmatogenous detachments, 50 to
60%
   d. anatomic success rate in PVR exceeds 80%

7. Contraindications:
   a. few contraindications to vitreoretinal surgery
   b. except in cases with extensive subretinal hemorrhage of recent onset, performing surgery in
eyes with no evidence for visual function is not
indicated
   c. due to the higher complication rate with vitrectomy (e.g., cataract formation), standard scleral
buckling surgery should be performed for treat-

ment of uncomplicated rhegmatogenous RD; vitrectomy may be indicated in eyes with abnormal scleral anatomy or posterior breaks

E. Intraocular Tamponade—Gas and Silicone Oil
1. Definition—inert substances with high surface tension in aqueous solution; used in retinal reattachment procedures to maintain closure of retinal breaks while chorioretinal adhesions develop
2. Indications:
   a. air:
      1) suitable for short duration tamponade especially when volume replacement required (e.g., to flatten retinal folds on scleral buckle after copious drainage of SRF)
   b. expansile gases:
      1) used when only a small volume (< 0.5 cc) of gas can be injected but large bubble (> 1.0 cc) required for several days' duration (e.g., pneumatic retinopexy)
      2) key features:
         a) slow rate of expansion—avoid IOP spike
         b) large expansivity—small amount of gas forms a large bubble
         c) geometry—a small bubble can unroll/steamroll the retina from center to periphery prior to full expansion (e.g., superior detachment with large tear)
         d) long duration—gas bubble maintains size/tamponade for a long period
   c. nonexpansile gas mixtures/silicone oil:
      1) used in vitreoretinal surgery after retinal reattachment with fluid-air exchange
      2) used when long duration tamponade of retinal breaks required (e.g., PVR)
      3) key features:
         a) minimal/no expansion—IOP controlled; large bubble can be created, final size of bubble can be set at surgery; effectiveness can be determined intraoperatively, i.e., retina reattaches with fluid-air exchange; silicone oil will not expand when atmospheric barometric pressure decreases, thus allowing air travel
         b) geometry—entire vitreous cavity can be filled with bubble, allowing tamponade of inferior retina with face down (gas) or normal (silicone) head position; this property of silicone oil makes it especially useful in patients not able to com-

ply with head positioning requirements (e.g., mentally deficient, arthritis); tamponade of posterior breaks; air-fluid exchange pushes SRF posteriorly allowing for complete internal drainage

  c) long duration—bubble maintains size/tamponade for a long duration (gas) or indefinitely (silicone oil)

  d) vision-optical/visual rehabilitation is possible with silicone oil tamponade; silicone preferable if prompt visual recovery is desirable; must wait for < 40% gas before useful vision is restored

3. Objective:

  a. to atraumatically inject a desired concentration/volume of gas or silicone oil into the vitreous cavity in order to achieve prolonged tamponade of retinal breaks

  b. in selected cases, to remove vitreous debris by exchanging vitreous fluid with gas bubble

4. Method:

  a. preoperative:

    1) determine allergies or medical conditions contraindicating the use of pressure-lowering agents or antibiotics

    2) history of outflow obstruction may influence the use of gas tamponade (expansile versus nonexpansile)

    3) media clarity assessed as gas/silicone injection requires good visualization

    4) integrity of the iris diaphragm; absence of the pupillary sphincter/"floppy" iris increases the risk of angle closure with large gas bubble; need to perform inferior iridectomy in eyes receiving silicone oil should be determined

    5) lens status and presence/absence of posterior capsulotomy specifically noted; determine risk of vitreous, gas, or silicone prolapse into the anterior chamber (especially if paracentesis performed)

  b. operative technique:

    1) general considerations:

      a) choice of tamponade depends on needs with regard to expansiveness, longevity, and patient factors (e.g., ability to maintain head position, air travel, need for immediate visual recovery [silicone])

    2) gas mixtures:

      a) gases (including air) all have the same surface tension (73 mN/m) and therefore the same effectiveness; use of a particular gas relates to the need for gas bubble expansion and longevity:

          i. air
              nonexpansile
              half life—32 hrs
              longevity—6 days

          ii. SF_6 (sulfur hexafluoride)
              expansion (pure gas)—× 2
              nonexpansile concentration—20%
              maximal expansion—24 to 48 hours
              half life—2 1/2 days
              longevity—10 to 14 days

         iii. C_3F_8 (perfluoropropane)
              expansion (pure gas)—× 4
              nonexpansile concentration—15%
              maximal expansion—72 to 96 hours
              half life—5 days
              longevity—60 days

   3) silicone oil:

      a) silicone oil has lower surface tension (53 mN/m) than gas and therefore is a less effective tamponade: a retina that does not flatten with gas tamponade (fluid-gas exchange) will not flatten with silicone oil; a second operation is required to remove silicone oil

   4) gas pneumoretinopexy (see above)

   5) fluid-gas exchange

c. intraoperative: (see above—vitreoretinal surgery)

   1) postvitrectomy (outpatient):

      a) used both to supplement existing gas tamponade and to wash out debris from the vitreous cavity; several techniques have been described; techniques outlined below do not require automated instruments

   2) unimanual technique, transcorneal:

      a) used in aphakic eyes

      b) anesthesia either topical or retrobulbar (retrobulbar particularly useful if laser to be performed immediately after gas exchange)

      c) eye prepped, aseptic technique as in pneumatic retinopexy

d) 10-cc syringe filled with gas mixture, 25- to 27-gauge needle (larger gauge prevents clogging, provides paracentesis tract)

e) patient in prone position, chin resting on hands, head over the end of the stretcher; alternatively, procedure done with patient sitting at slit lamp (gas exchange tends not to be as complete when done in this manner)

f) indirect ophthalmoscope (no condensing lens) for illumination

g) surgeon sits on floor underneath patient if on stretcher

h) under direct visualization, needle introduced through inferotemporal cornea into pupil, directed superiorly just behind the iris plane

i) "push-pull" technique to perform gas exchange; small amount of gas injected until the eye firm, needle then withdrawn out of the enlarging gas bubble into the fluid phase and fluid aspirated until the eye slightly soft; cycle repeated until an adequate/full gas fill achieved; as the exchange completed, patient instructed to put chin down so that remaining fluid runs into anterior chamber and is aspirated

j) when fluid completely evacuated, IOP adjusted to normal range by injecting/aspirating gas

k) eye should be left somewhat firm if laser performed to reduce corneal striae

l) multiple bubbles ("fish eggs") common with this technique; minimized by evacuating all fluid from the needle hub prior to injecting gas and injecting gas directly into the existing gas bubble; bimanual technique better if single bubble desired for immediate postexchange laser

m) central retinal artery patency and LP vision confirmed postop; pressure adjusted by aspirating gas or fluid through closed syringe system; venting the eye to air dilutes the gas mixture

3) unimanual technique, transscleral:
   a) used in phakic/pseudophakic eyes

b) anesthesia/prep as in unimanual technique

c) patient placed in lateral decubitus position, head extended over edge of stretcher; eye to undergo exchange is down or at slit lamp

d) indirect ophthalmoscope or slit lamp for illumination

e) surgeon sits on low stool or floor facing patient

f) 10-cc syringe filled with gas mixture, 25- to 27-gauge needle

g) under direct visualization, needle introduced in the horizontal meridian through temporal pars plana, 3.5 to 4 mm posterior to the limbus; needle directed to the midvitreous away from the lens

h) "push-pull" technique used to perform gas exchange; hand steadied on orbital rim

i) as the exchange completed, patient looks towards the floor so that the temporal pars plana dependent and residual fluid can be evacuated

j) to complete the exchange, a small amount of gas injected to make the eye firm; aspiration performed as the needle slowly removed from the eye, thereby removing residual fluids and normalizing the intraocular pressure

k) central retinal artery patency confirmed; pressure adjusted, closed syringe system

4) bimanual technique:

a) especially useful if a single bubble desired for visualization purposes

b) anesthesia / prep / positionin / ophthalmoscope as in unimanual transcleral technique

c) 20-cc syringe filled with gas mixture connected to IV extension tubing (e.g., K-50); 30-gauge needle placed on the end of the IV tubing and gas injected to clear air from dead space

d) tb syringe with 25- to 27-gauge needle, plunger remover

e) under direct visualization, surgeon introduces needle connected to tubing through the nasal (uppermost) pars plana in the horizontal meridian; needle directed to the midvitreous away from the lens then withdrawn slightly towards eye wall; assistant injects a small amount of gas to firm eye to make passage of second needle easier

f) needle on tb syringe introduced through temporal (lowermost) pars plana in horizontal meridian directed towards midvitreous

g) assistant slowly injects gas through tubing maintaining slight resistance; fluid pushed out of the eye through the lower tb syringe; tb syringe slowly withdrawn, keeping the tip out of the enlarging gas bubble

h) after complete fluid-gas exchange achieved, tb syringe withdrawn, eye pressure adjusted by injection/aspiration through gas tubing, then gas tubing needle withdrawn

i) central retinal artery patency confirmed

d. postoperative:

1) all expanding gases have the maximum rate of expansion in the first 6 to 8 hrs after injection

2) IOP measurement with indentation/applanation tonometry inaccurate in gas-filled eyes with corneal irregularities; pneumotonometer accurate; tonopen accurate below 30 mm Hg

3) patients with expanding gas bubbles monitor light perception vision for several hours; patients instructed to seek immediate care if LP acuity impaired

4) patients instructed to maintain head positioning so that retinal breaks are most superior; in eyes with complete gas fills, face down positioning required to maintain fluid in the anterior chamber

5) patients instructed not to sleep in the supine position in order to maintain the anterior chamber angle and to keep the crystalline lens (if present) from prolonged gas contact

5. Complications:

a. intraoperative:

1) subretinal prolapse of gas may occur during fluid-gas exchange indicating the presence of unrelieved traction; eye refilled with fluid and further membrane dissection/retinotomy should be performed; silicone oil usually injected after retinal reattachment, intraoperative subretinal prolapse rare

2) clarity of cornea, crystalline lens or lens implant may be disturbed after fluid-air exchange due to irregular surface wetting or epithelial desiccation; a drop of viscoelastic spread on the posterior surface of the cornea or lens implant (not crystalline lens) improves visualization; laser may be applied using endolaser with indirect ophthalmoscope if visualization through microscope inadequate

3) entrapment of gas anterior to the anterior hyaloid face (canal of Petit) may occur with pars plana injections; young individuals may require gas bubble aspiration or disruption of the anterior hyaloid to release the gas bubble

4) nitrous oxide is extremely soluble and can cause rapid expansion of gas bubbles with severe IOP elevation; nitrous oxide inhalation anesthesia should be discontinued 15 minutes prior to gas injection

b. postoperative

1) air (or mountain) travel contraindicated in eyes with greater than a 20% gas fill; atmospheric depressurization causes expansion of gas bubbles inducing a dangerous rise in IOP in a gas-filled eye

2) elevated IOP with bubble expansion in eyes with poor outflow facility (e.g., pre-existing glaucoma, hyphema, choroidal edema); angle closure may occur in eyes with a large gas fill due to a pupillary block from gas bubble or forward rotation of the lens-iris diaphragm; pressure elevations often transient (see above—vitreoretinal surgery)

3) keratopathy, including localized opacity, edema; band keratopathy can result from prolonged gas bubble contact with the corneal endothelium

4) transient posterior capsular lens opacities in eyes with gas bubble contact with the posterior lens surface; permanent opacification may occur in eyes with prolonged desiccation of the lens

   a) silicone oil associated with several postoperative complications similar to gas tamponade including keratopathy, cataract formation, hypotony, and glaucoma;

performing inferior iridectomy decreases keratopathy and pupillary block

6. Prognosis:
   a. (see above—gas pneumoretinopexy)
   b. in the treatment of PVR, anatomic (70%) and visual success (40% >= 5/200) of silicone oil and C_3F_8 tamponade are similar (both primary/reoperations considered); both silicone oil and C_3F_8 are superior to SF_6

7. Contraindication:
   a. gases:
      1) huge tears develop when expanding gas used in eyes with extensive tractional membranes on the retina (e.g., PVR with undissected membranes, PDR with TRD)
      2) eyes with severely compromised outflow facility may have severe pressure elevations with expanding gases
      3) patients travelling in planes/mountainous regions in the early postoperative period
      4) patients unable to maintain positioning requirements, especially with regard to avoiding supine positioning during bed rest
      5) complex RDs secondary to viral retinitis (CMV in AIDS) better suited for permanent tamponade with silicone
   b. silicone oil:
      1) no specific contraindications to use of silicone oil; gas preferred (if feasible) as silicone oil requires second operation for removal and has lower tamponade force

F. Perfluorocarbon (PFC) Liquids
   1. Definition:
      a. inert, heavier-than-water, low viscosity liquids used intraoperatively in vitreoretinal surgery to achieve (posterior to anterior) hydrokinetic retinal reattachment and to elevate low density substances (e.g., IOL, crystalline lens) off the posterior retina
   2. Indications:
      a. treatment of extensive (giant) retinal tears or surgical retinotomies prone to posterior rolling/slippage with conventional techniques
      b. sterilization of posterior retina facilitating anterior dissection in eyes with PVR
      c. treatment of dislocated crystalline/artificial lenses especially in the presence of complex RD (rare)

      d. drainage of choroidal hemorrhage (rare)
   3. Objective:
      a. to unroll and fixate peripheral retinal tears by posterior to anterior hydrokinetic reattachment utilizing an enlarging, heavier-than-water PFC bubble ("steamrolling")
      b. to elevate crystalline/artificial lens off the posterior retina allowing surgical maneuvers (e.g., phacofragmentation/IOL fixation) to be performed in an atraumatic fashion
   4. Method:
      a. operative technique:
         1) general considerations:
            a) choice of PFC dictated by FDA as only the perfluoroctane is FDA-approved; PFC liquids have similar specific gravity (1.75 to 2.0), surface tension (16 to 18 dyne/cm) and can be used for the same indications; perfluoroctane (PFO) has high vapor pressure allowing for more complete removal with air-fluid exchange; perfluorphenanthrene (PFA) poorer interface visibility than perfluorodecalin (PFD) and PFO; high viscosity of PFA makes removal more difficult:
               i. PFA
                  refractive index—1.33
                  viscosity—8 centistokes
                  vapor pressure—0.3 torr
               ii. PFO
                  refractive index—1.27
                  viscosity—0.8 centistokes
                  vapor pressure—57 torr
              iii. PFD
                  refractive index—1.31
                  viscosity—2.7 centistokes
                  vapor pressure—13.5 torr
         2) retinal reattachment
            a) standard scleral buckling/vitreoretinal surgical techniques employed; vitreoretinal traction must be completely released to avoid subretinal prolapse of PFC liquid; retinal breaks close as PFC injected
            b) small amount of PFC liquid injected during retinal reattachment to fixate/expose areas for dissection
            c) PFC slowly injected over the optic nerve allowing vitreous infusion to escape

through the sclerotomies around instrument shafts

 d) PFC injected into the enlarging bubble; retina reattaches as SRF forced anteriorly escaping from peripheral breaks/retinotomies; retina monitored for residual traction as interface brought anteriorly; additional membrane dissection/retinotomy performed as required

 e) after retinal reattachment achieved, laser photocoagulation used to treat all breaks/retinotomy sites

 f) PFC-air exchange performed from anterior to posterior to remove all PFC liquid; residual PFO removed by venting the eye with a flute needle allowing PFO evaporation; complete removal of PFA may require multiple washouts

 g) air replaced with long-acting tamponade (gas or silicone oil) and surgery completed

 3) lens removal/repositioning

 a) vitrectomy performed with complete removal of vitreous adherent to the dislocated lens material

 b) PFC slowly injected over the optic nerve elevating crystalline lens material/lens implant off the posterior retina

 c) lens floated up to the equatorial region on the PFC bubble; standard vitreoretinal surgical techniques then employed for lens removal or fixation (phacofragmentation/IOL suture fixation)

 d) after lens removal/fixation, PFC removed by PFC-fluid or PFC-air exchange

 b. postoperative:
 1) special attention paid to identifying/removing retained PFC liquid

 5. Complications:
 a. intraoperative:
 1) retained subretinal PFC is toxic and has been associated with visual loss
 2) subretinal prolapse of PFC liquid through retinal breaks/retinotomy; if subretinal PFC recognized intraoperatively, PFC-fluid exchange performed and the retina redetached to provide access for aspiration of subretinal PFC through existing retinal breaks/retinotomy; alternatively, a posterior retin-

otomy created over the PFC and PFC aspirated

b. postoperative:

1) occasionally, a small amount of preretinal PFC collects over the inferior retina in the postoperative period, probably from material retained in the vitreous base

2) a small amount of retained preretinal PFC usually well tolerated

3) a large amount of retained PFC in the posterior segment or any PFC in the anterior segment should be removed by simple aspiration or transcorneal/transcleral fluid-gas exchange techniques (see above—gas)

6. Prognosis:

a. anatomically, over 90% of eyes with RD due to giant tear reattach with one operation; visually, over 80% of eyes achieve 20/400 or better; visual prognosis best in eyes with macula-on detachments

b. most common cause of failure is PVR

c. prognosis for treatment of dislocated lens similar to that when standard vitreoretinal surgical techniques used

7. Contraindications:

a. no recognized contraindications to the intraoperative use of PFC liquids; standard techniques using pneumatic reattachment preferred, especially if vitrectomy not required

Essentials of Eye Care, edited by Rohit Varma.
Lippincott–Raven Publishers,
Philadelphia © 1997.

16

Optics and Refraction

I. PHYSICAL OPTICS

A. Light is a form of electromagnetic radiation whose behavior can be explained by two theories:

1. the quantum theory: light is considered to be made up of discrete energy particles or photons

2. the wave theory: light behaves as a wave. This interpretation of light best explains the phenomena of diffraction, interference and polarization.

3. Both theories are equally valid and necessary to explain the particle/wave duality of light.

4. The following equation is valid for either waves or particles as light propagates in a vacuum:

Speed of light = wavelength × frequency

5. Light slows down inside transparent materials as the wavelength becomes shorter.

B. Polarization

1. The transverse motion of waves of light occurs in all planes. If the wave motion is made to exist in one plane only, the light is then said to be plane polarized.

2. Light that is scattered by gas molecules in the atmosphere or reflected off a polished surface (e.g., water or snow) becomes partially polarized (usually along the horizontal axis).

C. Interference

1. When two waves of light interact, their electromagnetic fields can add together, resulting in constructive interference, or the fields can neutralize each other, resulting in destructive interference.

D. Coherence

1. This determines the ability of two light beams to interfere with one another.

2. Spatial coherence: defines the ability of two separated portions of a wave to produce interference.

3. Temporal coherence: measures the ability of a beam of light to interfere with another portion of itself.

4. Most lasers approach perfect temporal coherence.

E. Diffraction

1. This is the ability of light to "bend around corners." This phenomenon becomes relevant when light passes through a pinhole or a pupil smaller than 2.5 mm. The original wavefront will continue through the center of the aperture undisturbed, but the wavefront on the edges will bend to create a different pattern (diffraction pattern). If the aperture is round, constructive and destructive interference gives rise to bright and dark rings respectively, and the center of the diffraction pattern thus formed is called an Airy disc. The smaller the aperture, the broader the Airy disc.

2. A pinhole smaller than 1.2 mm placed in front of the eye will create significant diffraction in addition to reducing the amount of light entering the eye.

II. OPHTHALMIC OPTICS

A. Refraction of Light

1. When a light ray travels from a medium with a lower refractive index to a medium with a higher refractive index, it is bent toward the normal, and when it goes from a higher to lower refractive index, it is bent away from the normal.

2. Refraction is governed by Snell's law:

$n \sin (i) = n' \sin (r)$
where i = angle of incidence
r = angle of refraction
n and n' = refractive indices

3. The critical angle is the angle of incidence for which the angle of refraction is 90 degrees (away from the normal) as light travels from a more dense medium to a less dense medium such as a light ray leaving the eye through the cornea. If the angle of incidence is greater than the critical angle, it cannot leave the more dense medium and is said to experience total internal reflection.

B. Prisms

1. Prisms bend rays of light toward the base.

2. However, virtual images (viewed through a prism) are displaced toward the apex of prisms.

3. The power of prisms is measured in prism diopters. A prism diopter is equal to the displacement (in cm) of a light ray measured 1.0 m away from the prism.

    4. The stacked combination of two prisms is different from the sum of the calibrated values, and should not be used as an equivalent way to measure the effect of adding two prism powers over one eye.

    5. Prentice's rule

        a. the prismatic power (PP) of a lens is equal to the distance of a point from the optical axis (in cm) multiplied by the power of the lens (in diopters).

$$PP = h(cm)D$$

where h = distance of a point on the lens from the optical axis
      D = lens power in diopters

    6. The effect of prisms on measured strabismic deviation

        a. plus lenses decrease the measured deviation in all cases of strabismus (ET, XT, or HT). Minus lenses increase any measured strabismic deviation (ET, XT or HT).

        b. the true deviation is changed by approximately $2.5 \times$ (D)%, where D is the power of the glasses (bilaterally) in diopters.

    7. Induced prism generated in prescribing glasses

        a. this phenomenon can cause symptoms when patients read through a part of their glasses that is below the optical centers. This symptom can be treated by:

            1) switching to contact lenses

            2) lowering both optical centers

            3) using a slab-off prism

    8. Prismatic effects created by prescribing bifocal segments

        a. image jump

            1) it occurs when the object which the eye sees in the inferior field suddenly jumps upward when the eye turns down to look at it.

            2) it is caused by the sudden introduction of prismatic power at the top of the bifocal segment.

            3) it is canceled if the optical center of the segment is at the top of the segment.

                a) round-top segment = maximum image jump

                b) flat-top segment = minimal image jump

                c) Franklin (executive) = no image jump segment

        b. image displacement

1) this is the displacement of the image (toward the apex of the prism) by the total amount of prism effective in the bifocal portion.

2) it is more bothersome than image jump.

3) to minimize it, one must use:

    a) round-top bifocal segment — with plus lenses

    b) flat-top bifocal segment — with minus lenses

  9. Prisms and chromatic effects

    a. Blue (short wavelength) light is refracted more than red light (long wavelength). As a result, a chromatic interval of approximately 1.50 to 3.00 D is created and gives rise to chromatic aberration.

    b. This is the basis for the red-green or duochrome test done to refine the sphere of a refraction. The patient should always be approached from the fogged direction (red clearer) to minimize accommodation.

C. Vergence

  1. As light rays travel in space, they can either come together (converge) or spread apart (diverge). Vergence is a measure of this coming together (convergence) or spreading apart (divergence) of the bundle of light rays at a given point in their path.

  2. Collimated light is composed of bundles of light, each having zero vergence.

  3. The unit of vergence is the diopter, which is the reciprocal of the distance (in meters) to the point where the light rays would intersect if extended in either direction.

  4. Lenses change the vergence of light according to the basic lens or vergence formula:

$$U + D = V$$

    U = vergence of light entering the lens
    D = amount of vergence added to the light by the lens
    V = vergence of light leaving the lens

D. Mirrors

  1. A plus mirror adds (+) vergence just like plus lenses add (+) vergence. Therefore, concave mirrors are positive and convex mirrors are negative.

  2. Power of a mirror = $1/f = 2/r$

    where f = focal length of the mirror (in meters)
           r = radius of curvature of the mirror (in meters)

3. The magnification of an object compared to its mirror image is proportional to the respective distances of the image and object from the mirror (as with thin lenses):

mirror magnification = image size/object size
= image distance/object distance

E. Power of a Spherical Refracting Surface in Fluid
1. If a representative portion of the refracting surface and adjacent fluid are enclosed within a rectangle, the surface has plus power if the medium with the higher refractive index is convex and minus power if the medium with the higher refractive index is concave.
2. The refracting power (in diopters) of a spherical surface embedded in a medium is given by:

$$D = (n' - n)/r$$

where $(n' - n)$ = difference in refractive index across the refractive surface
r = radius of surface (in meters)

3. This formula can be used to determine the power of a thin lens (e.g., an IOL) immersed in any fluid as follows:

D (fluid)/D (aqueous) = n (IOL)-n (fluid)/n (IOL)-n (aqueous)

where D (aqueous) = the given power of an IOL
n = refractive index

4. Real vs. virtual objects and images
a. If the object or image is located on the same side as its respective rays, it is called real; if it is on the opposite side, it is called virtual. Virtual objects or images are located by imaginary extensions of their respective rays through the lens.
5. Focal points and focal lengths
a. primary focal point: the point along the optical axis of a lens at which an object must be placed for parallel rays to emerge from the lens.
b. secondary focal point: the point along the optical axis of a lens where parallel incident rays are brought to focus.
c. focal length: the distance from the ideal thin lens to each of its focal points.
6. Changing lens effectivity by altering lens position
a. Moving plus lenses forward (away from the eye) increases effective plus power for distant view-

ing. Moving them toward the eye decreases effective plus power.

   b. Moving minus lenses forward (away from the eye) decreases effective minus power. Moving them toward the eye increases effective minus power.

F. Accommodation

   1. Definition: the ability to increase the convexity of the crystalline lens and thus add plus power to the eye.

   2. Amplitude of accommodation: the total number of diopters which an eye can accommodate.

   3. Far point: the point on the visual axis that is conjugate to the retina when accommodation is completely relaxed.

   4. Near point: the point on the visual axis which is conjugate to the retina when accommodation is fully active.

   5. Range of accommodation: the linear extent of clear vision obtainable through accommodation.

G. Astigmatism

   1. With a spherical lens (where all meridians have the same curvature), the rays coming from a point can be focused as a point. With a regular astigmatic lens, where the principal meridians, at right angles to each other, have different curvatures, rays coming from a point are focused into two focal lines.

      a. interval of Sturm (focal interval): the distance between the two focal lines.

      b. conoid of Sturm: the geometrical figure formed by the rays.

      c. circle of least confusion: the circular cross-section of the conoid of Sturm, and the point where the image is blurred equally in all directions.

   2. Notation of lenses

      a. Cross diagram of an astigmatic lens: the two principal meridians are labeled with the power acting in these meridians.

      b. Rules for transposing between plus cylinder and minus cylinder:

         1) power of new sphere = power of old sphere + power of old cylinder

         2) power of new cylinder = same as old cylinder, but opposite sign

         3) axis of new cylinder = change old cylinder axis by 90 degrees

      c. Spherical equivalent:

power of sphere + (power of cylinder)/2

   d. It places the circle of least confusion on the retina.

  3. Spherical lens aberration is caused by the fact that peripheral rays are refracted more strongly than paraxial rays by typical plus lenses, thus bringing the peripheral rays to focus closer to the lens.

  4. Astigmatism of oblique incidence
    a. Tilting a spherical lens induces a cylinder of the same sign with axis in the axis of tilt.

H. Magnification

  1. Linear (traverse) magnification: is determined by drawing a central ray through the nodal point of the lens and is given by:

$$MAG = I/O = v/u$$

    where u = distance from the object O to the lens
           v = distance from the image I to the lens

  2. Axial magnification: This is magnification along the axis and is always the square of the transverse magnification. It is partially responsible for the distortion in 3-D images as in indirect ophthalmoscopy.

  3. Angular magnification of a lens: is obtained by comparing the angular size of an object when observed through a lens with the angular size of the same object as it is held 25 cm away from the observer's eye. It is given by the following formula:

$$Mag = D/4$$

    where D = lens power in diopters.

  4. Angular magnification of an astronomical telescope
    a. it forms an inverted image and is rarely used in ophthalmic options. It is given by the following formula:

$$Mag = D(eyepiece)/D(objective)$$

    where D = power of the eyepiece or the objective

  5. Angular magnification of a Galilean telescope: A Galilean telescope is made up of a plus objective lens and a minus eyepiece lens (closest to the eye). It forms an upright image, and is frequently used in ophthalmic optics. Its angular magnification is given by the following formula:

$$Mag = D(eyepiece)/D(objective)$$

note: A corrected aphakic eye can be analyzed as a Galilean telescope—the eye's refractive error can be analyzed as a single -12.50 lens in air which is acting 5 mm behind the cornea, and whose primary focal point coincides with the secondary focal point of the corrective spectacle lens. Thus, for a corrective spectacle lens of +10.0 D, the angular magnification is:

Mag = 12.50/10.0 = 1.25X (25% enlarged)

compare this magnification to that obtained with the equivalent corrective contact lens (power +11.75 D)

Mag = 12.50/11.75 = 1.06X (6% enlarged)

6. Knapp's rule: in unilateral high myopia, proper image size is better obtained with a spectacle lens than a contact lens for highly myopic eye. Practically speaking, either may be used.

III. CORRECTION OF AMETROPIAS

A. Emmetropic Eye
1. An object at infinity is focused on the retina.
2. A point on the retina is conjugate with a point at infinity.
3. The far point plane is at infinity.
B. Myopic Eye
1. An object at infinity is focused in front of the retina.
2. A point on the retina is conjugate with a point in front of the eye.
3. The far point plane for a myopic eye is the plane of such a point in front of the eye.
C. The Hyperopic Eye
1. The image of an object at infinity is located "behind" the retina.
2. A point on the retina is also virtual and conjugate with a point "behind" the eye.
3. The far point plane for a hyperopic eye is the plane of such a point "behind" the eye.
D. Correcting Ametropia
1. The far point plane of any eye is conjugate with the retina.
2. Therefore, a correcting spectacle lens must focus parallel rays coming from infinity into the far point plane of the eye. This can be achieved by placing secondary focal point (f) of the correcting lens at the far point plane of the eye.
E. Vertex Distance
1. This is the distance from the back surface of the correcting lens to the cornea.
2. For any correcting lens >5.0 D, changing the vertex distance will significantly change the distance be-

tween the eye's far point plane and the secondary focal point of the correcting lens. This distance should be 0 to create a sharp retinal image.

   3. Vertex distance conversion:
    a. locate the focal point of the present lens
    b. determine the distance of the new lens from the far point
    c. take the reciprocal of this focal length of the new lens to determine the power of the new lens

F. Astigmatism
   1. the refracting corneal surface is toroidal and thus the refracting power of the surface is not the same for all meridians.
   2. Regular astigmatism: the orientation and powers of the principal meridians are constant across the pupil. The principal meridians are those having the greatest and least power.
   3. Irregular astigmatism: the orientation of the principal meridians changes from one point to another across the pupil, or the amount of astigmatism changes from one point to another.
   4. With-the-rule astigmatism: the steepest meridian is vertical; correcting plus cylinder is at axis 90.
   5. Against-the-rule astigmatism: the steepest meridian is horizontal; correcting plus cylinder is at axis 180.
   6. Oblique astigmatism: the principal meridians do not lie at or near 90 and 180 degrees.

G. Intolerance of Astigmatic Spectacle Corrections
   1. Is caused by distortion secondary to unequal magnification of the retinal image in the various meridians (meridional magnification). This distortion is clinically significant only under binocular conditions.
   2. Uncorrected astigmatism does not cause clinically significant meridional magnification.
   3. Clinically significant meridional magnification is introduced by spectacle correction of astigmatism.
   4. Sources of meridional magnification:
    a. "shape factor" of the spectacle lens
     1) only a factor for lenses with the cylinder ground on the front surface of the lens
     2) can be eliminated by prescribing only minus cylinder lenses
    b. power factor magnification
     1) directly proportional to the dioptric power of the correcting cylindrical lens and the vertex distance
    c. axis of orientation of the astigmatic refractive surface

        1) will determine the direction of meridional magnification

        2) oblique aniseikonia is more difficult to tolerate than vertical or horizontal aniseikonia

   5. Blur vs. distortion in astigmatic correction

     a. blur will be determined by the amount of uncorrected or residual astigmatism.

     b. meridional magnification will be determined by the amount of astigmatic correction.

     c. a balance must be achieved between amount of meridional magnification caused by correction of corneal/lenticular astigmatism vs. blur secondary to uncorrected astigmatism. This can be achieved with the following guidelines:

        1) in children, Rx the full astigmatic correction

        2) in adults, try the full astigmatic correction first; try a walking-around trial with trial frames before prescribing

        3) use minus cylinder lenses (almost universally dispensed since 1910) and minimize vertex distance

        4) if necessary, reduce distortion by rotating the cylinder axis toward 180 or 90 degrees (or toward the old axis) and/or by reducing the cylinder power. Balance the resulting blur with the remaining distortion, using careful adjustment of cylinder power and sphere. Residual astigmatism at any position of the cylinder axis may be minimized with the Jackson cross cylinder test for cylinder power. Adjust the sphere using the spherical equivalent concept as a guide, but rely on a final subjective check to obtain best visual acuity.

        5) if distortion is still a problem, consider contact lenses (reduce vertex distance to zero)

H. Guidelines for Prescribing Glasses for Children

   1. Significant myopia

     a. this is refractive error causing vision worse than 20/30 (usually at about −1.50 D OU)

        1) cycloplegic refraction

        2) prescribe the full amount of myopic correction if distance vision is critical

        3) avoid overcorrection, and consider undercorrecting by 0.50 to 0.75D

   2. Significant hyperopia

     a. usually about +5.00 D OU or more

        1) cycloplegic refraction

2) unless there is esodeviation or evidence of reduced vision, it is not necessary to correct iso-
   metropic hyperopia
3) fully correct significant astigmatic errors
4) in cases where esotropia and hyperopia coexist, the initial management includes full correction of cycloplegic refractive error
5) avoid overcorrections
6) in school-age children, a reduction in the
   amount of correction may be necessary to
   avoid blurring of distance vision

3. Anisometropia
   a. full cycloplegic refractive difference between the
      two eyes, regardless of age, presence of strabis-
      mus, or degree of anisometropia

I. Intraocular Lenses
   1. Image magnification from aphakic glasses is 20 to
      35%.
   2. The normal tolerance for spherical aniseikonia is 5
      to 8%.
   3. Clinically, for each diopter of spectacle overcorrec-
      tion at a vertex distance of 12 mm, there is a 2%
      magnification for plus lenses and a 2% minification
      for minus lenses.

J. Calculating the Power of an IOL Preoperatively
   1. In most settings, it is desirable to produce em-
      metropia or slight myopia for three reasons:
      a. because spectacle overcorrection of 21.5 D will
         reduce magnification to essentially zero
      b. hyperopia is more poorly tolerated than an equal
         degree of myopia
      c. this amount of myopia allows the patient some
         degree of function at near unaided by spectacles
   2. When calculating an IOL power, a 1 mm error in ax-
      ial length produces a refractive error of about 2.5 D.
   3. The SRK formula is:

$$P = A + BL + CK$$

P = predicted power of implant
L = axial length in mm
K = average keratometry in diopters
A = constant determined by data
B = constant = -2.5
C = constant = -0.9

4. More sophisticated formulas have provided either
   no improvement or minimal improvement in accuracy in most patients.

5. There is no simple linear relationship between the change in IOL power and the postoperative refractive state.
6. For common values of K, axial length and anterior chamber depth, however, a 1.5 diopter change in the IOL power will give about a 1 diopter change in refractive state at the spectacle plane.

K. Contact Lenses
  1. Types
    a. depending on the surface of the material: soft, rigid or gas-permeable
  2. Characteristics
    a. posterior central curve (PCC)
      1) or "base curve" is the curvature of the center of the posterior surface
      2) its power can be expressed in diopters or in radius of curvature, which are related by the following formula:

$$P = \frac{1000\,(1.3375 - 1.0000)}{R} = \frac{337.5}{R}$$

where R = radius in millimeters
P = power in diopters

      3) it is designed to approximate the curvature of the optic zone of the cornea.
    b. optic zone
      1) central zone of the contact lens containing the refractive power
    c. diameter
      1) is the distance from one of the edges of the lens to the opposite edge
    d. wetting angle
      1) is the angle created by the edge of a bead of water resting on the surface of the lens
      2) the smaller the angle, the more hydrophilic the lens material
    e. toric lenses
      1) have a different radius of curvature in each meridian
      2) used to correct astigmatism
    f. saggital depth or apical height
      1) the distance between a flat surface and the back surface of the central portion of the lens
  3. Lens fitting
    a. to adjust the fitting of a contact lens, two variables can be manipulated: the diameter and the PCC

      b. if the PCC remains constant but the diameter is increased, the lens will fit steeper

      c. if the diameter is kept constant, and the PCC is increased, the lens will fit flatter

    4. Oxygen transmission

      a. is proportional to the permeability of a lens material, where:

$$\text{permeability} = D \times K/\text{lens thickness}$$

      D = diffusion coefficient for oxygen movement in the lens material

      K = solubility coefficient of oxygen in this material

      b. is inversely proportional to the lens thickness

      c. high-performance rigid gas-permeable lenses can provide 90% of oxygenation required by cornea.

    5. Corneal changes associated with prolonged contact lens wearing

      a. spectacle blur

        1) temporary blurring of vision immediately after contact lens removal

        2) it is secondary to a reversible change in corneal curvature and optical power

      b. decreased corneal sensation

        1) adaptive change with chronic contact lens use

      c. microcystic edema

        1) secondary to moderate oxygen deprivation

        2) symptoms include chromatic halos around lights

        3) slit lamp findings include central gray haze (Sattler's veil)

L. Lens-cornea relationships

    1. "Tear lens"

      a. this is the power created by the tears accumulated between the PCC and the anterior corneal curvature.

      b. if the PCC is parallel to the corneal flattest meridian, the tear lens acts as a minus lens, and thus subtracts from the positive power of the steepest corneal meridian.

      c. thus, in fitting a rigid contact lens, the power must be expressed in minus spherocylindrical notation.

    2. Anterior optical zone (AOZ)

      a. this is the central portion of the contact lens.

      b. it provides the new anterior refracting surface of the eye and must be large enough to cover the pupil.

M. Practical guidelines to fitting rigid contact lenses

1. Perform a careful manifest refraction and transpose it to minus cylinder form
2. Measure Ks and choose flatter K
3. Determine the base curve based on the K readings:
   a. if delta K < 1.50 D, fit trial lens 0.50 steeper than flatter K
   b. if delta K > 1.50 D, split the K readings
4. Determine the power from the spherical power of the transposed Rx. The power must be measured in relationship to the flattest K and must therefore be adjusted to compensate any changes in the base curve. That is, if the base curve was chosen to be 0.50 D steeper than the flatter K, the power must be 0.50 D less than the spherical power from the manifest Rx.
5. Choose a trial lens based on the above and evaluate the fit based on:
   a. movement: small amount of vertical movement following a blink is necessary for adequate tear exchange and oxygenation.
   b. fluorescein pattern:
      1) good fit: there should be apical clearance (central cornea → faint green), midperipheral touch (intermediate zone → black), and peripheral clearance (periphery → bright green).
      2) steep fit: heavy touch under the intermediate zone (broad, black intermediate area)
      3) flat fit: central touch (black area) over the corneal apex and a diffuse green pattern in the intermediate and peripheral zones
   c. note: a good fit for an astigmatic cornea will show a black band in the central apical zone over the flattest corneal meridian, a faint green pool over the steeper meridian, and a darker band over the intermediate zone.
6. Overrefract with spheres to determine final power
N. Fitting patients with high refractive errors
   1. Patients with high myopia require CLs with a relatively flat anterior surface, large diameter, and relatively large edge thickness, which ride high and can cause lid irritation. This problem can be reduced by ordering a lenticular bevel which reduces the gripping action of the lids.
   2. High plus lenses are heavy. Their weight can be reduced by using a lenticular cut and designing a peripheral carrier with a minus design or "minus carrier."
   3. Patients with high astigmatism may not be adequately corrected with gas-permeable contact lenses,

requiring toric contact lenses (anterior, posterior or bitoric).

O. Practical guidelines to fitting soft contact lenses
1. Careful manifest refraction
2. Measure Ks
3. Choose the base curve to be flatter than the flattest K reading according to their radii of curvature:
for average Ks (43.00 to 44.00 → BC: 8.4 to 8.6)
for steep Ks (>44.50 → BC: 7.8 to 8.3)
for flat Ks (<42.50 → BC: 8.7 to 9.5)
4. Determine the power by the Rx's spherical equivalent
5. Evaluate the fit by:
a. centration: Look for 1 to 2 mm clearance beyond the limbus
b. movement: 1 to 2 mm movement with a blink
c. steep lenses ride low and show little movement. They can be flattened by increasing the BC or decreasing the diameter.
d. flat lenses ride high and show excessive movement. They can be steepened by decreasing the BC or increasing the diameter.
6. Overrefract with spheres for final power

IV. OPTICAL PRINCIPLES OF SELECTED OPHTHALMIC INSTRUMENTS

A. Indirect Ophthalmoscopy:
1. Works by collecting pencils of light emanating from a large area of the patient's retina and focusing them on the observer's retina by means of a condensing lens
2. An intermediate, inverted image of the patient's fundus is formed near the focal plane of the ophthalmoscopy lens.
3. The observer views this image, with the help of +2.00 or +2.50 lenses in the eyepieces of the ophthalmoscope.
4. Lateral magnification of the aerial image in indirect ophthalmoscopy is expressed as the ratio of the power of the eye (60D) to the power of the condensing lens. Thus, a 20D lens produces 3X lateral magnification, and a 30D lens produces 2X magnification.
5. Axial magnification is the square of lateral magnification. This would ordinarily produce an exaggerated depth effect, but in the design of the indirect ophthalmoscope, the usual PD of 60 mm is reduced

by prisms to 15 mm, and stereopsis is reduced by a factor of 4, compensating for the axial magnification.

6. A 15D lens produces lateral magnification of 4X and an overall depth effect of 4¾ or 4X. Higher power condensing lenses produce relative flattening of images, when the reduced stereopsis of the eyepiece is considered.

7. Most lenses used in indirect ophthalmoscopy are aspheric and have two different curved surfaces. The side with the steep curvature should face the examiner.

8. Moving the eyepieces together increases stereopsis. The effect can be used to increase stereopsis for evaluation of an elevated lesion. The eyepieces can be moved apart to decrease the separation of the viewing paths to enable binocular viewing through a small pupil.

B. The Keratometer

1. This is an instrument for measuring the central anterior corneal curvature by accurately determining the size of a reflected image from the front surface of the cornea (the first Purkinje-Sanson image).

2. The manual keratometer converts the image size into corneal radius using simple vergence relationships of convex mirrors.

$$D(mirror) = 2/r$$

$$r = \text{radius of curvature}$$

3. The resultant standardized keratometric formula is:

$$D \text{ (cornea)} = n(tears) - n(air)/r$$
$$D \text{ (cornea)} = 337.5/r(mm)$$

such that a cornea with a 7.5 mm radius of curvature corresponds to a +45 D refracting surface.

C. The Manual Lensmeter

1. This instrument consists of:

a. an illuminated target consisting of a set of parallel lines located behind a positive lens

b. a source of light behind the target

c. a positive lens (L)

d. a test lens (T) holder located in front of the positive lens

e. an afocal telescope located between the observer's eye and the test lens holder

2. The distance (d) between the illuminated target and the focal plane of the positive lens can be manipu-

lated, thus changing the vergence of the light exiting the lens. That is, when the illuminated target is at the focal point of the positive lens, the vergence of light exiting the lens is zero, but if the target is closer to the lens, the vergence of the light exiting the lens becomes negative. The light exiting the positive lens (L) is then passed through a test lens (T), and the emerging light is viewed by an observer through an afocal telescope. When this light has zero vergence, the target will be seen in sharp focus. The vergence neutralized by the test lens is then proportional to the distance d, and the power of the test lens can be read from a linear scale.

3. To measure cylinder power, the illuminated target is positioned until one set of lines is sharp (P1) and then positioned again until the perpendicular set of lines is sharp (P2). The dioptric difference between P1 and P2 is the cylinder power, and the cylinder axis can be read from the protractor side.

V. OBJECTIVE AND SUBJECTIVE REFRACTION GUIDELINES

A. Objective Refraction (Retinoscopy)
  1. Principles
     a. the blurred image of the retinoscope filament on the patient's retina becomes a light source returning to the examiner's eye. Retinoscopy consists of neutralizing this reflex by placing different lenses in front of the eye. When the reflex is neutralized, the far point of the eye, and therefore its refractive error, can be determined.
     b. at the point of neutralization of the light reflex, the patient's pupil will appear uniformly illuminated with any sweep of the retinoscope.
     c. if the far point is between the examiner and the patient, the movement of the reflex will be in a direction opposite to the sweep of the retinoscope (against motion), and the patient is considered to be a myope. More minus lenses need to be added in front of the patient, in order to bring the far point to the location of the examiner (neutralization).
     d. if the far point is behind the examiner, the movement of the reflex will be in the same direction as the sweep of the retinoscope, and the patient is considered to be a low myope or a hyperope. More plus lenses need to be added to bring the far point to the location of the examiner.

B. Plus Cylinder Technique

    1. For standard retinoscopy, the retinoscope must be in the "plane mirror" setting which is sleeve up in the Copeland retinoscope and sleeve down in the Welch-Allyn retinoscope.

    2. To move the patient's far point to the location of the examiner, place a +1.50 lens working lens in front of the patient.

    3. If manifest RNS, both eyes should be open and the patient should be looking at a fixation light at the end of the room. The fellow eye should be fogged relative to the wall chart at all times to avoid accommodation.

    4. If cycloplegic or aphakic RNS, the patient should be looking directly at the retinoscope and the fellow eye should be occluded.

    5. Observe the retinoscopic reflex in various meridians by sweeping the streak perpendicular to itself.

    6. Add minus sphere until a "with motion" reflex is obtained in all directions.

    7. Add plus sphere until the first meridian is almost fully neutralized.

    8. Rotate the streak 90 degrees and set the cylinder axis parallel to the remaining nonneutralized streak.

    9. Add plus cylinder until the remaining meridian is almost fully neutralized.

    10. Refine the cylinder axis by sweeping at 45 degrees to either side of the axis and changing the cylinder axis toward the narrower, brighter reflex.

    11. Refine the cylinder power by moving closer to the patient to obtain a clear "with motion" reflex and then gradually back off until both meridians neutralize equally. Small changes in the sphere or cylinder power may be necessary to achieve equal neutralization of both meridians.

    12. Once both meridians have been neutralized, dial −1.50 of sphere back into the phoropter to cancel the effect of the working lens and bring the patient's far point to the end of the room.

C. Subjective Refraction (the Cross Cylinder Refraction Technique)

    1. Adjust the sphere to achieve best visual acuity.

    2. Go back two lines larger than the smallest readable line obtained by the previous step prior to introducing the cross cylinder. The cylinder axis must be obtained first, and then the cylinder power.

    3. Cylinder axis: Position the cross cylinder axes 45 degrees to the axis of the correcting cylinder. Determine the preferred flip choice and rotate the cylinder axis toward the corresponding axis of the cross cylinder. Repeat this step until the two flip choices appear equal.

4. Cylinder power: Align the cross cylinder axes parallel and perpendicular to the axis of the correcting cylinder. Determine the preferred flip choice and add or subtract cylinder power according to the preferred position of the cross cylinder. In order to keep the circle of least confusion on the retina, half as much sphere power of opposite sign needs to be added to compensate any changes in the cylinder power.

5. Refine the sphere, cylinder axis, and cylinder power by repeating the steps listed above until no further improvement is obtained.

Note: most of the information in this chapter was abstracted from the notes of David L. Guyton, M.D.

Appendix

Ophthalmic Drug Formulary

The following series of tables is intended to serve as a generalized compilation of the medications most commonly used by ophthalmologists today. This chapter outlines common indications, dosing regimens, and adverse effects, but should not be employed as an exhaustive or authoritative reference regarding dosages, contraindications, side effects, or drug interactions. Pharmacological therapy is continuously evolving with the constant introduction of new medications, changes in formulations, and refinements of indications and usage. Although every attempt has been made to ensure the accurate and up-to-date nature of the information presented here, all indications and dosages should be independently confirmed prior to use. As always, no medication should be administered without complete knowledge of the drug's action, delivery method, and potential adverse interactions or side effects. Comprehensive medication reference materials such as the PDR or drug insert should be consulted for this purpose. It is important to remember that the administration of many of these medications can lead to severe and irreversible complications, including blindness and death. Thus, great care should be exercised at all times, especially with intravenous and intravitreal administration. Indeed, the extensive side effects of many of these medications necessitate that the ophthalmologist work closely with internists and other medical specialists who are intimately familiar with the drug's actions.

In addition, the indications for specific antibiotic, antifungal, and antiviral medications change with time and locality as drug-resistant strains continue to emerge. Physicians prescribing such a medication should do so with an appreciation of the pathogens common to their particular hospital and community. In certain cases, consultation with local infectious disease specialists will be indicated.

Finally, directions for mixing some of the more difficult-to-obtain fortified antibiotics and intravitreal antibiotic injections

644

have been included. Generally, preparation of these compounds should be left to pharmacy professionals well acquainted with appropriate dilutional and sterility technique. However, in some emergency situations it may be useful to have access to this information. Since inappropriate intravitreal antibiotic concentrations can either be ineffective or lead to immediate and permanent visual loss, it is imperative that such medications be prepared with great care and that the doses and dilution be independently confirmed prior to use.

The medication lists in this chapter are arranged alphabetically by generic name within each therapeutic category.

Anesthetic Agents: Local

Generic Name	Example Trade Name	Common Routes & Dosages	Actions	Notes, Contraindications, Adverse Effects
Bupivacaine	Marcaine Sensoricaine	0.25–0.75% up to 50 ml/SC or retrobulbar Maximal Dose 225 mg with, 175 mg without epinephrine	Onset 7–30 min Duration 4–6 hrs (25% longer than tetracaine)	**Adverse effects:** tremor, shivering, nausea, convulsions (rare)
Chloroprocaine	Nesacaine	1–2% solution, Maximal Dose 10–20 mg/kg	Onset very rapid, duration 1 hr	Less toxic than procaine
Hyaluronidase	Wydase	Retrobulbar or subcutaneous	Improves nerve blockade depolymerizes polysaccharides	Decreases duration of local anesthetic effect
Lidocaine	Xylocaine	0.5–2% up to 50 ml/SC or retrobulbar Maximal Dose 3–4 mg/kg	Onset 5–30 min, duration 45 min–2 hr	**Adverse effects:** hypertension, nausea, vomiting, coma, convulsions
Mepivacaine	Carbocaine	1–2% solution, Maximal Dose 7 mg/kg to 1000 mg/24 hr	Onset 5–30 min, duration 2–3 hr	**Adverse effects:** Drowsiness to coma, convulsions

Generic Name	Example Trade Name	Common Dosages	Actions	Notes, Contraindications, Adverse Effects
Procaine hydrochloride	Novocain	0.5%–2% solution SC Maximal Dose 10–15 mg/kg	Onset rapid, duration 30–60 min	Avoid IV injection. Less toxic than procaine. **Adverse effects:** tinnitus, nausea, convulsions (rare)

Anesthetic Agents: Topical

Generic Name	Example Trade Name	Common Dosages	Actions	Notes, Contraindications, Adverse Effects
Cocaine Hydrochloride	—	1–10%	Surface anesthetic, sympathomimetic (blocks re-uptake of norepinephrine). Test for Horner's syndrome (see also Diagnostic Agents)	Epithelial toxicity or erosion, CNS stimulation, respiratory collapse Topical ocular application does not produce measurable urine levels
Proparacaine	Ophthaine	0.5%	Better tolerated than tetracaine	Allergic dermatitis
Tetracaine	Pontocaine	Maximal dose 1.5 mg/kg up to 150mg	Onset 15–45 min, duration 3–6 hr	Corneal epithelial toxic; inhibits mitosis & cell migration. Systemic: drowsiness to coma, convulsions (rare)

Antifungal Agents

Generic Name	Example Trade Name	Common Routes & Dosages	Indications	Notes, Contraindications, Adverse Effects
Amphotericin B	Fungizone	**Intravenous:** 0.25–1.0 mg/kg IV over 6 hr (consult with internist) **Intravitreal:** 5 mg/0.1 ml—add 10cc water to Ampho B vial (50mg/mL), then take 1 mL of this dilution and add to 9 mL water, then take 1 mL of this dilution and add 9 mL more water. **Subconjunctival:** 0.8–1.0 mg **Topical:** 0.1–0.5% solution (dilute with water or 5% dextrose in water)	Blastomyces, candida, coccidioides, histoplasma	**Contraindications:** allergy **Adverse effects:** fever, shaking, chills, hypotension, anorexia, nausea, vomiting, headache, tachypnea (esp. 1–3 hrs after infusion)
Fluconazole	Diflucan	**Loading dose:** 800 mg PO ×1 **Maintenance:** 400 mg/day divided doses (consult with internist)	Candida	**Contraindications:** allergy. **Adverse effects:** anaphylaxis (rare), hepatotoxicity, elevates drug levels (warfarin, phenytoin, cyclosporin, glyburide, tolbutamide, glipizide)

Drug	Trade name	Dosage	Organisms	Contraindications / Adverse effects
Flucytosine	Ancobon	**PO:** 50–150 mg/kg/day in 4 divided doses **Topical:** 1% solution	Candida, cryptococcus	**Contraindications:** allergy **Adverse effects:** cardiac & respiratory arrest, dyspnea, rash, photosensitivity, GI distress, azotemia, anemia, ataxia, vertigo, psychosis
Ketoconazole	Nizoral	**PO:** 200–400 mg q day	Candida, cryptococcus, histoplasma	**Contraindications:** allergy, co-administration with terfenadine or astemizole (arrhythmias) **Adverse effects:** hepatotoxicity, headache, diarrhea, impotence, gynecomastia, oligospermia, anemia, depression
Miconazole nitrate	Monistat	**Intravitreal:** 10–25 μg/0.1cc **Subconjunctival:** 5–10 mg **Topical:** 1% solution	Candida, cryptococcus, aspergillus	**Contraindications:** allergy **Adverse effects:** phlebitis, pruritis, nausea, diarrhea, anorexia, anaphylaxis (rare).
Natamycin	Natacyn	5% suspension	Candida, aspergillus, cephalosporium, fusarium, penicillium	**Contraindications:** allergy

Anti-Inflammatory Agents

Generic Name	Example Trade Name	Common Dosages	Indications	Notes, Contraindications, Adverse Effects
Dexamethasone	Maxidex	0.1% suspension	Intraocular inflammation	**Potency:** 6 times prednisone
Dexamethasone sodium phosphate	AK-Dex, Decadron, Maxidex	0.05% ointment, 0.1% solution, 0.05%, 0.1% solution, 0.05%, 0.1% solution	Decrease in inflammation: Corneal epithelium intact: 19% Corneal epithelium absent: 22%	Water soluble (less penetration with intact corneal epithelium than acetate or alcohol preparations)
Diclofenac	Voltaren	0.1% solution	Postoperative prophylaxis and treatment of intraocular inflammation, cystoid macular edema	Nonsteroidal anti-inflammatory agent
Fluorometholone Acetate	Flarex	0.1% suspension	Mild prolonged anti-inflammatory requirement	Less elevation of IOP than other steroid agents
Fluorometholone	FML S.O.P. Fluor-Op, FML FML Forte	0.1% ointment 0.1% suspension 0.25% suspension	Ocular surface inflammation, mild prolonged anti-inflammatory requirement	Little ocular penetration, fewer adverse effects with prolonged use Less elevation of IOP than other steroid agents

Flurbiprofen	Ocufen	0.03% solution	Inhibition of miosis during intraocular surgery	Nonsteroidal anti-inflammatory agent
Ketorolac	Acular	0.5% solution	Ocular itching (seasonal allergic conjunctivitis)	Nonsteroidal anti-inflammatory agent
Medrysone	HMS	1% suspension	Mild prolonged anti-inflammatory requirement	Less elevation of IOP than other steroid agents
Prednisolone sodium phosphate	AK-Pred Inflamase AK-Pred	0.125% solution 0.125% solution 1% solution	Intraocular inflammation Decrease in inflammation: Corneal epithelium intact: 28%	Water soluble (less penetration with intact corneal epithelium than acetate or alcohol preparations)
	Inflamase Forte	1% solution	Corneal epithelium absent: 47%	
Prednisolone acetate	Pred Mild Econopred AK-Tate	0.12% suspension 0.125% suspension 1% suspension	Intraocular inflammation Decrease in inflammation: Corneal epithelium intact: 51%	Biphasic in solution (good penetration through intact corneal epithelium
	Econopred Plus Pred Forte	1% suspension 1% suspension	Corneal epithelium absent: 53%	

Antiinflammatory Agents (*continued*)

Generic Name	Example Trade Name	Common Dosages	Indications	Notes, Contraindications, Adverse Effects
Rimexolone	Vexol	1% suspension	Post-operative inflammation, anterior uveitis	Equivalent to 1% prednisolone acetate in reducing inflammation but less likely to elevate IOP **Contraindications:** active microbial infection, allergy
Suprofen	Profenal	1% solution	Inhibition of miosis during intraocular surgery	Nonsteroidal anti-inflammatory agent

Antimicrobial Agents: Intravenous, Intravitreal, Subconjunctival, Topical

Generic Name	Example Trade Name	Common Routes & Dosages	Indications	Notes, Contraindications, Adverse Effects
Amikacin sulfate	Amikin	**Intravenous (adult):** 15 mg/kg/day in 2–3 divided doses **Intravitreal:** 0.4 mg/0.1cc— add 1 mL amikacin solution (500 mg/2mL) to 9cc BSS, then take 1 mL of this dilution and add to 5.25 mL BSS **Subconjunctival:** 25 mg **Topical:** 10 mg/mL	Gram-negative bacilli, M. avium	Aminoglycoside **Contraindications:** allergy

Ampicillin sodium	Polycillin	**Intravenous (adult):** 4–12 g/day in 4 divided doses **Intravitreal:** 500 µg **Subconjunctival:** 50–150 mg **Topical:** 50 mg/mL	Gram-positive cocci, Pneumococci, Streptococci, Meningococci, Salmonella, Shigella, Proteus, E. coli, some H. influenza	Semi-synthetic penicillin **Contraindications:** allergy **Adverse effect:** rash more common than other penicillins
Bacitracin zinc	AK-Tracin	**Topical (fortified):** 10,000 U/mL—add 50,000 U bacitracin powder to sterile water to form 5 ml solution. Refrigerate. Expires in 7 days. **Subconjunctival:** 5,000 units/mL **Ointment:** ingredient in many preparations	Gram-positive cocci, Gram-positive bacilli, Gram-negative cocci	**Contraindications:** allergy **Adverse effect:** nephrotoxic if given IV
Carbenicillin disodium	Geopen Geocillin	**Intravenous (adult):** 8–24 g/day in 4–6 divided doses **Intravitreal:** 250–2000 µg **Subconjunctival:** 100 mg **Topical:** 4–6 mg/mL	Gram-negative organisms (enterobacter, serratia), Pseudomonas, Proteus	Semi-synthetic penicillin **Contraindications:** allergy

Antimicrobial Agents: Intravenous, Intravitreal, Subconjunctival, Topical (*continued*)

Generic Name	Example Trade Name	Common Routes & Dosages	Indications	Notes, Contraindications, Adverse Effects
Cefazolin sodium	Ancef	**Intravenous (adult):** 2–4 g/day in 3–4 divided doses **Intravitreal:** 0.4 mg/0.2cc—add 10cc of 0.9% NaCl to Kefzol vial (1g), then take 0.3cc of this dilution and add to 15mL BSS **Subconjunctival:** 100 mg **Topical (fortified):** 50 mg/mL—dilute 500 mg parenteral cefazolin powder in sterile water to form 10 mL solution. Refrigerate. Expires in 7 days.	Gram-positive cocci (except enterococci, MRSA), E. coli, Klebsiella pneumonia, Proteus mirabilis	First-generation cephalosporin **Contraindications:** allergy
Cefotaxime	Claforan	25 mg/kg IV q 8–12 hrs for 7 days	Initial choice for neonatal ophthalmia. Gram-negative bacilli, H. influenza, N. gonorrhoeae	Third-generation cephalosporin **Contraindications:** allergy

Ceftazidine	Fortaz	**Intravenous (adult):** 1 g/day in 2–3 divided doses	Gram-negative bacilli, H. influenza, N	Third-generation cephalosporin better than second-generation cephalosporins for Gram-negative bacilli. Second-generation cephalosporins are better than third-generation cephalosporins for Gram-positive Cocci. **Contraindications:** allergy
	Pentacef	**Intravitreal:** 2.25 mg/0.1cc **Subconjunctival:** 100 mg **Topical:** 50 mg/mL—add 1 gm parenteral ceftazidime powder to 9.2 cc artificial tears. Add 5 cc of dilution to 5 cc artificial tears. Refrigerate, shake well.	gonorrhoeae	
Ceftriaxone	Rocephin	1 gm IM q day for 5 days 125 mg IM x1	Initial choice for gono/meningococcal conjunctivitis Initial choice for neo-natal ophthalmia Gram-negative bacilli, H. influenza, N gonorrhoeae	Third-generation cephalosporin better than second-generation cephalosporins for Gram-negative bacilli. Second-generation cephalosporins are better than third-generation cephalosporins for Gram-positive cocci. **Contraindications:** allergy

Antimicrobial Agents: Intravenous, Intravitreal, Subconjunctival, Topical (*continued*)

Generic Name	Example Trade Name	Common Routes & Dosages	Indications	Notes, Contraindications, Adverse Effects
Ciprofloxacin	Ciloxan	**PO:** 750 mg q 12 hr	Systemic dose can penetrate into vitreous. Staphylococci, H. influenza, Neisseria, enterics, aerobic Gram-negative bacilli	Fluoroquinolone **Contraindications:** allergy
Clindamycin	Cleocin	**Intravenous (adult):** 900–1800 mg/day in 2–3 divided doses **Intravitreal:** 45–200 µg/0.1ml **Subconjunctival:** 15–50 mg **Topical:** 50 mg/ml	Anaerobes Staphylococci in penicillin allergic patients	**Contraindications:** allergy **Adverse effects:** diarrhea, pseudomembranous colitis (PO/IV)
Erythromycin	AK-Mycin, Ilotycin	**Intravitreal:** 500 µg **Ointment:** 0.5% **Subconjunctival:** 100 mg **Topical:** 50 mg/mL	Gram-negative cocci Pneumococci, Group A Streptococci in penicillin allergic patients, Mycoplasma pneumonia, Chlamydia trachomatis, Legionella pneumophilia	**Contraindications:** allergy **Adverse effect:** mild GI distress

Drug	Trade names	Dosage	Spectrum	Class / Contraindications
Gentamicin sulfate	Garamycin, Genoptic, Gentacidin, Gentak	**Intravenous (adult):** 3–5 mg/kg/day in 2–3 divided doses **Intravitreal:** 0.1 mg/0.1 cc—take 0.4 mL from gentamicin vial (40 mg/mL) and add to 15cc BSS. **Ointment:** 3 mg/g **Subconjunctival:** 10–20 mg **Topical:** 0.3% solution **Fortified:** 8–15 mg/mL (14 mg/mL—add 2 ml of parenteral gentamicin (40 mg/mL) to 5 ml of commercially available 0.3% soln)	Gram-negative bacilli Ineffective against anaerobes	Aminoglycoside **Contraindications:** allergy **Adverse effects:** nephrotoxicity, ototoxicity, neuromuscular blockade (myasthenia-like)
Imipenem/ Cilastatin sodium	Primaxin	**Intravenous (adult):** 2 g/day in 3–4 divided doses **Topical:** 5 mg/mL	Broadest antibacterial action. Aerobic Gram-negative bacilli, anaerobes, Staph aureus	β-Lactam **Contraindications:** allergy
Kanamycin sulfate	Kantrex	**Subconjunctival:** 30 mg **Topical:** 30–50 mg/mL	Some Gram-negative bacilli (except Pseudomonas or anaerobes)	Aminoglycoside **Contraindications:** allergy **Adverse effects:** ototoxicity, nephrotoxicity

Antimicrobial Agents: Intravenous, Intravitreal, Subconjunctival, Topical *(continued)*

Generic Name	Example Trade Name	Common Routes & Dosages	Indications	Notes, Contraindications, Adverse Effects
Methicillin sodium	Staphcillin	**Intravenous (adult):** 6–10 g/day in 4 divided doses **Intravitreal:** 1000–2000 μg **Subconjunctival:** 50–100 mg **Topical:** 50 mg/mL	Gram-positive cocci, Gram-positive bacilli, Gram-negative cocci, Group A streptococci, pneumococci	Penicillinase resistant penicillin **Contraindications:** allergy
Neomycin sulfate	ingredient in many preparations	**Subconjunctival:** 125–250 mg **Topical:** 5–8 mg/mL **Ointment:** ingredient in many preparations	Gram-negative cocci	**Contraindications:** allergy **Adverse effect:** severe ototoxicity and nephrotoxicity IV
Norfloxacin	Chibroxin	0.3% solution	Enterobacteriaceae, Enterococcus, Pseudomonas aeruginosa	Fluoroquinolone **Contraindications:** allergy
Penicillin G	—	**Intravenous (adult):** 12–24 million units/day in 4–6 divided doses. 10 million units IV for 5 days 100,000 units/kg/day IV in 4 divided doses for 7 days	Second choice for gono/ meningococcal conjunctivitis or neonatal ophthalmia	**Contraindications:** allergy

Drug	Preparations	Dosage/forms	Spectrum	Contraindications
		Topical: 100,000 units/mL **Fortified:** 333,000 U/ml—dilute 5 million U of parenteral penicillin G in 5 ml artificial tears, then add 5 ml of dilution to 10 ml of artificial tears **Subconjunctival:** 0.5–1 million units	Gram-positive cocci, Gram-positive bacilli, Gram-negative cocci, Group A streptococci, pneumococci	**Contraindications:** allergy
Polymyxin B sulfate	ingredient in many preparations	**Subconjunctival:** 100,000 units **Topical:** 10,000 units/mL **Ointment:** ingredient in many preparations	Gram-negative bacilli	
Sulfacetamide sodium	AK-Sulf Bleph-10 Cetamide Isopto Cetamide Ophthacet Sulamyd sodium Sulf-10	10% solution/ointment, 15%, 30% ointment 10% solution/ointment 10% ointment 15% solution 10% solution 10% solution/ointment 10% solution	E. coli, Staphylococcus aureus, Streptococcus pneumoniae, Streptococcus viridans, H. influenza, Klebsiella, Enterobacter	**Contraindications:** allergy, can be severe, including death (rare)
Sulfisoxazole diolamine	Gantrisin	4% solution/ointment	Bacteriostatic effect on many Gram-negative and Gram-positive microorganisms	**Contraindications:** allergy, infants < 2 months old, pregnancy

Antimicrobial Agents: Intravenous, Intravitreal, Subconjunctival, Topical *(continued)*

Generic Name	Example Trade Name	Common Routes & Dosages	Indications	Notes, Contraindications, Adverse Effects
Tetracycline hydrochloride	Achromycin	1% solution, 4% ointment **PO:** 250 mg	Acne rosacea, meibomitis Gram-negative cocci	**Contraindications:** allergy, children under 8 y/o (discolors teeth) **Adverse effects:** GI upset, pseudotumor cerebri, hepatotoxicity, skin photosensitivity. **Caution:** may alter level of coumadin anticoagulation
Ticarcillin disodium	Ticar	**Intravenous (adult):** 200–300 mg/kg/day in 4–6 divided doses **Subconjunctival:** 100 mg **Topical:** 6 mg/mL	see Carbenicillin	Penicillin **Contraindications:** allergy
Tobramycin sulfate	Tobrex	**Intravenous (adult):** 3–5 mg/kg/day in 2–3 divided doses **Intravitreal:** 100–200 µg **Subconjunctival:** 10–20 mg **Topical:** 0.3% solution, 0.3% ointment. **Fortified:** 14 mg/cc ointment (40 mg/cc) to 5 ml commercial 0.3% tobramycin solution. Refrigerate. Expires in 7 days.	Gram-negative bacilli Pseudomonas aeruginosa	Aminoglycoside **Contraindications:** allergy **Adverse effects:** nephrotoxicity, ototoxicity, neuromuscular blockade (myasthenia-like)

Generic Name	Example Trade Name	Common Routes & Dosages	Indications	Notes, Contraindications, Adverse Effects
Vancomycin	Vancocin	**Intravenous (adult):** 1 g q 12 hrs. **Intravitreal:** 1 mg/0.1cc—add 1 mL of vancomycin solution (500 mg/10 mL) to 4mL of BSS **Subconjunctival:** 25 mg **Topical (fortified):** 50 mg/cc—dilute 500 mg parenteral vancomycin powder in 10 mL sterile water, artificial tears or normal saline (0.9%). Refrigerate. Expires in 4 days.	Gram-positive cocci Methicillin-resistant Staphylococcus aureus and epidermidis	**Contraindications:** allergy **Adverse effects:** nephrotoxicity, ototoxicity

Antiviral Agents

Generic Name	Example Trade Name	Common Routes & Dosages	Indications	Notes, Contraindications, Adverse Effects
Acyclovir sodium	Zovirax	**PO (HSV):** 200 mg 5 times/day for 7–10 days. **PO (HZV):** 600–800 mg 5 times/day **IV:** 10 mg/kg q 8 hr for 7–21 days	Herpes simplex virus Varicella zoster virus	**Adverse effects:** GI upset, headaches, rash IV: irreversible nephropathy, encephalopathy Rare: tremors, hallucinations, seizures, coma
Foscarnet sodium	Foscavir	**Induction:** 60 mg/kg controlled IV infusion over 1 hr q 8 hr for 14–21 days (adjusted for renal function). **Maintenance:** 90–120 mg/kg over 2 hr q day	CMV retinitis	Less tolerated than gancyclovir, possibly less mortality **Adverse effects:** nephrotoxicity, anemia, nausea, seizure, ↑↓ phosphatemia, ↑↓ calcemia, ↓ kalemia, ↓ magnesemia

Antiviral Agents (*continued*)

Generic Name	Example Trade Name	Common Routes & Dosages	Indications	Notes, Contraindications, Adverse Effects
Ganciclovir sodium	Cytovene	**Intravitreal:** 200 µg **Induction:** 5 mg/kg IV q12 hr for 14–21 days **Maintenance:** 5 mg/kg IV q day for 7 days	CMV retinitis	**Adverse effects:** granulocytopenia, thrombocytopenia, fever, rash, phlebitis, confusion
Idoxuridine	Herplex	0.1% topical solution	HSV keratitis	**Adverse effects:** allergy, rare: corneal clouding, punctate epithelial defects
Trifluridine	Viroptic	1% topical solution	HSV keratitis	**Adverse effects:** burning, rare: epithelial keratopathy, hypersensitivity, elevated IOP, stromal edema, keratitis sicca
Vidarabine monohydrate	Vira-A	3% ointment	HSV keratitis	**Adverse effects:** allergy, GI upset, weakness, thrombophlebitis, rare: confusion, renal failure, coma, death

Cycloplegic Agents

Generic Name	Example Trade Name	Common Dosages	Indications & Actions	Notes, Contraindications, Adverse Effects
Atropine sulfate	Atropisol Isopto Atropine	0.5%, 1.0%, 2.0% soln 1% ointment q day, tid	Onset several hrs, Duration 12–14 days. **Additional indications:** malignant glaucoma, cycloplegic retinoscopy, pharmacologic penalization, postop mydriasis	**Adverse effects** (particularly in children): tachycardia, flushing of skin, dryness of skin, thirst, contact dermatitis
Cyclopentolate	Cyclogyl	0.5%, 1.0%, 2.0%	Onset 20–60 min, duration 24 hr	**Adverse Effects:** Confusion, ataxia, dysarthria, personality change
Eucatropine	—	5–10%	Weak cycloplegic, moderate mydriatic. Onset 30 min, Duration 4–6 hr **Additional indications:** Provocative test for narrow-angle glaucoma	see also Diagnostic Agents

Cycloplegic Agents (*continued*)

Generic Name	Example Trade Name	Common Dosages	Indications & Actions	Notes, Contraindications, Adverse Effects
Homatropine	Isopto Homatropine	2%, 5%	Onset 1–2 hr, duration 24–72 hr	Not generally used in infants younger than 1–2 months
Scopolamine	Isopto Hyoscine	0.25%	Onset 20–120 min, duration 5–7 days	**Adverse effects:** CNS stimulation, contact dermatitis (rare)

Diagnostic Agents

Generic Name	Example Trade Name	Routes & Dosages	Common Usage	Notes, Contraindications, Adverse Effects
Cocaine Hydrochloride	—	4–10% topical	Test for Horner's syndrome (4–10%). Sympathomimetic (blocks reuptake of norepinephrine), see also Anesthetic Agents: topical	CNS stimulation, respiratory collapse. Topical ocular application does not produce measurable urine levels.
Edrophonium	Tensilon	10 mg IV	Test for myasthenia gravis: cholinesterase competitive inhibitor. Relieves myasthenic symptoms in 1 min, duration 2 min.	**Adverse effects:** vomiting, diarrhea, urination, cardiac arrest. Reversed by atropine 0.4 mg IV

Generic Name	Example Trade Name	Common Dosages			
Eucatropine	—	5–10% topical		Provocative test for narrow-angle glaucoma **Additional indications:** Weak cycloplegic, moderate mydriatic. Onset 30 min, duration 4–6 hr	see also Cycloplegics
Hydroxy-amphetamine	Paredrine	1% topical		Distinguishing pre- vs. post-ganglionic Horner's syndrome: indirect acting sympathomimetic (onset 30–40 min, duration 2–3 hr), releases norepinephrine from nerve ending	Failure to dilate pupil suggests postganglionic Horner's syndrome. Dilation suggests intact postganglionic neuron (preganglionic Horner's)
Methacholine	Mecholyl	2.5% topical		Diagnosis of Adies' tonic pupil. Similar to acetylcholine, more resistant to cholinesterase	see Other Agents (acetylcholine)

Dry Eye Agents

Generic Name	Example Trade Name	Common Dosages	Preservatives & Composition
Carboxymethyl cellulose	Cellufresh, Celluvisc	0.1%, 1.0%	None
Hydroxypropyl cellulose	Lacrisert	—	None

Dry Eye Agents (*continued*)

Generic Name	Example Trade Name	Common Dosages	Preservatives & Composition
Hydroxypropyl methylcellulose	Isopto Plain, Isopto Tears Tearisol Isopto Alkaline, Ultra Tears	0.5% 0.5% 1.0%	Benzalkonium chloride Benzalkonium chloride, EDTA Benzalkonium chloride
Hydroxyethyl cellulose, povidone	Adsorbotear	—	Thimerosal, EDTA
Hydroxyethyl cellulose	Lytears TearGard	—	Benzalkonium chloride, EDTA Sorbic acid, EDTA
Hydroxyethyl cellulose, polyvinyl alcohol	NeoTears	—	Thimerosal, EDTA
Hydroxypropyl methylcellulose, gelatin A	Lacril	—	Chlorobutanol, polysorbate 80
Hydroxypropyl methylcellulose, dextran 70	Tears Naturale Naturale II Naturale Free	—	Benzalkonium chloride, EDTA Polyquad None

Lubricants	AKWA Tears Ointment	—	White petrolatum, liquid lanolin, mineral oil
	Duolube		White petrolatum, mineral oil
	Duratears Naturale		White petrolatum, liquid lanolin, mineral oil
	HypoTears		White petrolatum, light mineral oil
	Lacri-Lube S.O.P.		Mineral oil (42.5%), white petrolatum (55%), lanolin alcohol, chlorobutanol
	Refresh P.M.		Mineral oil (41.5%), white petrolatum (55%), lanolin alcohol, petrolatum
Methylcellulose	Murocel	1.0%	Methyl-, propylparabens
Polycarbophil	AquaSite	—	EDTA
Polyvinyl alcohol, PEG-400, dextrose	Hypotears	1.0%	Benzalkonium chloride, EDTA
	Hypotears PF	1.0%	EDTA
Polyvinyl alcohol	AKWA Tears, Just Tears	1.4%	Benzalkonium chloride, EDTA
	Liquifilm Tears	1.4%	Chlorobutanol
	Liquifilm Forte	3.0%	Thimerosal, EDTA
Polyvinyl alcohol, povidone	Murine	1.4%	Benzalkonium chloride, EDTA
	Refresh	0.6%	None
	Tears Plus	0.6%	Chlorobutanol

Glaucoma Medications

Generic Name	Example Trade Name	Common Routes & Dosages	Indications & Actions	Notes, Contraindications, Adverse Effects
Acetazolamide	Diamox	**PO:** 250 mg qid-500 mg bid **IV:** 250–500 mg in 5–10 ml sterile water	IOP lowering: **PO:** onset 2 hrs, peak 3–4 hrs, duration 6–10 hrs **IV:** Onset few minutes, peak 30–120 hrs	**Contraindications:** sulfa allergy, metabolic acidosis, adrenal insufficiency. **Relative contraindications:** history of renal stones. **Cautions:** concurrent use of other diuretic or digoxin. **Adverse effects:** paresthesias, lassitude, anorexia, weight loss, GI distress, decreased libido, impotence, dysgeusia, depression, renal stones (calcium oxalate or phosphate), aplastic anemia (rare, idiosyncratic)
Apraclonidine	Iopidine	0.5% q 8 hr 1% q 12 hr prior to and immediately post laser	**Mechanism:** Alpha$_2$ adrenergic agonist Uncertain IOP lowering mechanism Prevents post ALT and ALI pressure spike	Few systemic effects

Betaxolol	Betoptic, Betoptic-S	0.25–0.5%	**Mechanism:** Beta$_1$-selective blockade. Decreases aqueous production 32–47%. Synergistic with epinephrine.	Ocular surface burning (less with Betoptic-S). Cardiac depression, CNS depression. Best choice for reactive airways (eg asthma)
Brimonidine	Alphagan	0.2%	Mechanism: Selective α_2 agonist that reduces the production of aqueous	**Contraindications:** allergy, concurrent use of MAO inhibitors. **Adverse effects:** dry mouth, headache, hypotension, fatigue, drowsiness, ocular allergy, pruritis
Carbachol	Carcholin Miostat	Topical (0.75%, 1.5%, 2.25% and 3%). Intracameral (0.1% solution)	**Mechanism:** direct and indirect acting combination of acetylcholine and physostigmine (inhibits acetylcholinesterase). **Additional indication:** induces intraoperative miosis	Less diurnal fluctuation than pilocarpine. **Adverse effects:** intense miosis, accommodative spasm, conjunctival hyperemia. **Disadvantage:** less corneal penetration than pilocarpine.
Carteolol	Ocupress	1%	**Mechanism:** non-selective β-blocker with intrinsic sympathomimetic activity	**Contraindications:** Asthma, pulmonary disease, heart failure, bradyarrhythmias. **Adverse effects:** similar to timolol. Except does not alter serum lipid profile as much as other β-blockers.
Demecarium bromide	Humorsol	0.125%, 0.25% solution	**Mechanism:** indirect acting (anti-cholinesterase)	see Glaucoma Medications (echothiophate)

Glaucoma Medications *(continued)*

Generic Name	Example Trade Name	Common Routes & Dosages	Indications & Actions	Notes, Contraindications, Adverse Effects
Dipivefrin	Propine	0.1%	**Mechanism:** alpha adrenergic agonist Lowers IOP by increasing uveoscleral outflow Prodrug converted to epinephrine by corneal esterase Better corneal penetration than epinephrine.	May stain soft contact lenses, adenochrome conjunctival deposition from oxidized metabolites, rebound hyperemia, allergic follicular conjunctivitis (20%), cystoid macular edema (aphakes). Minimally additive to beta-blockers.
Dorazolamide	Trusopt	2%	**Mechanism:** topical carbonic anhydrase inhibitor, lowers IOP by decreasing the production of aqueous	**Contraindications:** allergy to sulfonamides **Adverse effects:** ocular discomfort, punctate keratitis, fatigue, and blurred vision
Echothiophate	Phospholine Iodide	0.03%, 0.06%, 0.125%, and 0.25% solution	**Mechanism:** indirect acting irreversible cholinesterase inhibitor **Additional indications:** break posterior synechiae, COAG (0.03–0.25%), strabismus (0.03–0.06%)	Plasma cholinesterase activity may be lowered by 95% **Avoid** depolarizing agents (succinylcholine) during and within 6 weeks of cessation as may cause apnea **Adverse effects:** fibrinous iritis, iris cysts, pseudopemphigoid, eyelid twitching, bronchial constriction

Epinephrine	Epifrin	1:100,000 to 1:200,000 (SC) 1:1000 (intracameral) 1–2% (topical)	**Mechanism:** alpha adrenergic agonist **Actions:** lowers IOP by increasing uveoscleral outflow Prolongs action of local anesthetic by decreasing absorption rate **Additional indications:** hemostasis, mydriasis	**Contraindications:** allergy, narrow angle glaucoma **Adverse effects:** eye pain, browache, headache, conjunctival hyperemia, adenochrome conjunctival deposits, reversible macular edema (in aphakia)
Glycerin	Glyrol, Osmoglyn	1–1.5 g/kg body wt mixed in equal volume flavored water (50% soln) Osmoglyn 4–8 oz., Glyrol 3–4 oz.	Onset of IOP lowering 10 min, peak effect 30 min, duration 4 hr	**Cautions:** glycerin is metabolized to sugar and ketones: resulting hyperglycemia may induce ketoacidosis in diabetic patients
Isoflurophate	Floropryl	0.025% gel	**Mechanism:** indirect acting (anti-cholinesterase)	see Glaucoma Medications (echothiophate)
Isosorbide	Ismotic	**PO:** 1.5 g/kg	Hyperosmotic: onset 30 min, duration 5–6 hours	see Glaucoma Medications (mannitol)
Latanoprost	Xalatan	0.005% refrigerate	**Mechanism:** is a PGF2α analogue that acts on the prostanoid selective FP receptors to increase uveoscleral outflow	**Contraindication:** allergy **Caution:** possibility of permanent increase in brown pigmentation of the iris **Adverse effects:** blurred vision, ocular discomfort

Glaucoma Medications (*continued*)

Generic Name	Example Trade Name	Common Routes & Dosages	Indications & Actions	Notes, Contraindications, Adverse Effects
Levobunolol	Betagan	0.5% every 12–24 hr	**Mechanism:** nonselective beta blocker	Similar to timolol
Mannitol	Osmitrol	**PO:** adults=20% solution in water infants=10% solution in water **IV:** adults=1.5–2 g/kg over 30–45 min infants=1.5 g/kg over 30–45 min	**Mechanism:** increases extracellular water and plasma osmolality moving water out of eye (mostly vitreous) and CSF. Onset of IOP lowering: 30–60 min. Larger the dose, slower eye penetration. Faster the infusion, higher osmotic gradient, more marked IOP lowering. **Indications:** IV osmotic of choice to acutely lower IOP	**Cautions:** cardiovascular overload (increased extravascular volume) leading to congestive heart failure, pulmonary edema **Adverse effects:** headache, backache, mental confusion
Methacholine	Mecholyl	2.5% topical	Similar to acetylcholine, more resistant to cholinesterase Diagnosis of Adie's tonic pupil	See Other Agents (acetylcholine) See also Diagnostic Agents
Methazolamide	Neptazane	**PO:** 25 or 50 mg BID-TID	**Mechanism:** lowers IOP by inhibiting carbonic anhydrase (decreases aqueous production) **Onset:** 2–4 hrs, peak 6–8 hrs, duration 10–18 hrs	**Adverse effects:** see acetazolamide. Renal lithiasis (calcium oxalate or phosphate) less likely than acetazolamide.

Drug	Dose/Formulation	Mechanism/Action	Effects
Metipranolol Optipranolol	0.3% (=0.25% timolol)	**Mechanism:** nonselective beta blocker	Granulomatous uveitis, ocular surface burning, conjunctival leukoplakia, bronchospasm, bradycardia, hypotension
Physostigmine Eserine	0.25% solution/ointment 0.5% topical solution 1–4 mg SC, IV	**Mechanism:** indirect parasympathomimetic (temporarily inactivates cholinesterase)	Increases ciliary contraction. Miosis lasts 12–36 hrs. Kills lice (not eggs). Antidote (IV or SQ) for overdose of anticholinergics: atropine, scopolamine, cyclopentolate
Pilocarpine Pilogel Ocusert 20/40	1–6% (every 6 hrs) Toxic dose: 10 ml of 1% 20–40 μg/hr Polymer "sandwich" once per week	**Mechanism:** direct acting parasympathomimetic **Action:** contracts ciliary muscle, increases aqueous outflow, reduces uveoscleral outflow Pilocarpine 2% will drop IOP 12–40% **Additional indications:** open angle glaucoma, narrow angle glaucoma, symptomatic Adie's pupil	**Adverse effects:** lacrimation, salivation, myopia, brow ache, miosis (less severe with ocusert), iris pigment epithelial cysts, anterior cortical cataract, pupillary block (forward movement of lens-iris diaphragm), inflammation (disrupted blood-aqueous barrier), punctal stenosis, pseudopemphigoid. Rare systemic effects: diarrhea, abdominal cramps, salivation, enuresis. **Contraindications:** may induce retinal detachment in high myopes, worsens ciliary block glaucoma

Glaucoma Medications (*continued*)

Generic Name	Example Trade Name	Common Dosages	Indications	Notes, Contraindications, Adverse Effects
Timolol	Timoptic Timoptic XE	0.25–0.5% every 12 hr 0.25–0.5% every 24 hr	**Mechanism:** nonselective beta blocker Onset of action 30–60 min	**Contraindications:** asthma, pulmonary disease, heart failure, bradyarrhythmias **Adverse effects:** impotence, decrease in HDL cholesterol, increase in triglycerides, lethargy, mood changes, CNS depression, bradycardia, death (33 reported) **Note:** nasolacrimal duct obstruction reduces systemic side effects

Mydriatic Agents

Generic Name	Example Trade Name	Common Dosages	Indications	Notes, Contraindications, Adverse Effects
Hydroxyamphetamine	Paredrine	1%	See also Diagnostic Agents	For distinguishing preganglionic vs. postganglionic Horner's syndrome
Phenylephrine	Neo-synephrine	2.5–10%	Direct-acting alpha agonist stimulates dilator muscle causing mydriasis without cycloplegia. Onset of dilation 15–20 min. Duration of dilation 3–4 hr	Avoid 10% in infants. **Toxicity:** acute hypertension, pulmonary edema, arrhythmia **Contraindications:** MAO inhibitors (sympathetic denervation)
Tropicamide	Mydriacyl	0.5–1%	Onset of dilation 20–30 min. Duration of dilation 4–6 hr	**Adverse effects:** increased IOP, psychosis, cardiorespiratory collapse, headache **Contraindications:** narrow angle glaucoma, allergy

Ocular Decongestants

Generic Name	Example Trade Name	Preservatives & Composition
Naphazoline hydrochloride	AK-Con, Albalon, ClearEyes, Degest 2, Naphcon, Opcon, Vasoclear Vasoclear Regular	Benzalkonium chloride, edetate disodium Phenylmercuric acetate
Phenylephrine hydrochloride	AK-Nefrin, Efricel, Isopto Frin, Prefrin Liquifilm, Tear-Efrin Eye Cool, Velva-Kleen Relief	Benzalkonium chloride, edetate disodium Thimerosal, edetate disodium —
Tetrahydrozoline hydrochloride	Collyrium, Murine Plus, Soothe, Tetracon, Visine	Benzalkonium chloride, edetate disodium
Naphazoline hydrochloride & zinc sulfate	Clear Eyes Allergy Cold Relief	Benzalkonium chloride, edetate disodium
Phenylephrine hydrochloride & zinc sulfate	Prefrin-Z Zincfrin	Thimerosal Benzalkonium chloride
Tetrahydrozoline & zinc sulfate	Visine A.C.	Benzalkonium chloride, edetate disodium

Other Agents

Generic Name	Example Trade Name	Common Routes & Dosages	Indications	Notes, Contraindications, Adverse Effects
Acetylcholine	Miochol	Intracameral	Intraoperative miosis. Duration 10 min	Cannot use topically due to corneal cholinesterase
Aminocaproic acid	Amicar	50 mg/kg PO q 4 hr up to 30 g/day	Hyphema: antifibrinolytic agent to reduce rebleeds	**Contraindications:** pregnancy, intravascular clotting disorder **Adverse effects:** postural hypotension, nausea, vomiting
Chondroitin sulfate Sodium hyaluronate	Viscoat	4% 3% (1:3 mixture)	Viscoelastic: maintain chamber, tissue dissection, prevent mechanical corneal endothelial damage	May cause large post-operative IOP elevation if not adequately removed from the anterior chamber
Hydroxypropyl methylcellulose	Occucoat	2%	Viscoelastic: maintain chamber, tissue dissection, prevent mechanical corneal endothelial damage	May cause large postoperative IOP elevation if not adequately removed from the anterior chamber
Sodium chloride	AK-NaCl, Muro-128 Adsorbonac Ophthalmic	5% solution or ointment 2%, 5% solution	Hyperosmolar agent for corneal edema	May cause burning and irritation

Other Agents (*continued*)

Generic Name	Example Trade Name	Common Routes & Dosages	Indications	Notes, Contraindications, Adverse Effects
Sodium hyaluronate	Healon Amvisc Plus	1.6%	Viscoelastic: maintain chamber, tissue dissection, prevent mechanical corneal endothelial damage	May cause large postoperative IOP elevation if not adequately removed from the anterior chamber

Index

Page numbers in italic denote tables; page numbers in boldface denote appendix.